OPERATIVE SURGERY

Fundamental International Techniques

Cardiothoracic Surgery

OPERATIVE SURGERY

Fundamental International Techniques

Third Edition

Under the General Editorship of

Charles Rob
M.C., M.D., M.Chir., F.R.C.S.

Professor and Chairman of the Department of Surgery,
University of Rochester School of Medicine and Dentistry,
Rochester, New York

and

Rodney Smith (Lord Smith of Marlow)
K.B.E., Hon.D.Sc., M.S., F.R.C.S., Hon.F.R.A.C.S.,
Hon.F.R.C.S.(Ed.), Hon. F.A.C.S., Hon. F.R.C.S.(Can.),
Hon.F.R.C.S.(I.), Hon.F.D.S.

Associate Editor

Hugh Dudley
Ch.M., F.R.C.S., F.R.C.S.(Ed.), F.R.A.C.S.

Professor of Surgery,
St. Mary's Hospital, London

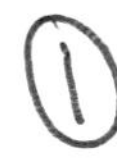

OPERATIVE SURGERY

Fundamental International Techniques

Cardiothoracic Surgery

Edited by

John W. Jackson
M.Ch., F.R.C.S.

Consultant Thoracic Surgeon, Harefield Hospital, Middlesex

BUTTERWORTHS
LONDON - BOSTON
Sydney - Wellington - Durban - Toronto

THE BUTTERWORTH GROUP

ENGLAND

Butterworth & Co (Publishers) Ltd
London: 88 Kingsway, WC2B 6AB

AUSTRALIA

Butterworths Pty Ltd
Sydney: 586 Pacific Highway, Chatswood, NSW 2067
Also at Melbourne, Brisbane, Adelaide and Perth

SOUTH AFRICA

Butterworth & Co (South Africa) (Pty) Ltd
Durban: 152–154 Gale Street

NEW ZEALAND

Butterworths of New Zealand Ltd
Wellington: T & W Young Building,
77–85 Customhouse Quay 1, CPO Box 472

CANADA

Butterworth & Co (Canada) Ltd
Toronto: 2265 Midland Avenue, Scarborough, Ontario M1P 4S1

USA

Butterworths (Publishers) Inc
Boston: 10 Tower Office Park, Woburn, Mass. 01801

First Edition Published in Eight Volumes, 1956–1958
Second Edition Published in Fourteen Volumes, 1968–1971
Third Edition Published in Nineteen Volumes, 1976–1979
This Volume First Published 1978
This Volume Reprinted 1979

ISBN 0 407 00604 4

British Library Cataloguing in Publication Data

Operative surgery. – 3rd ed.
Cardiothoracic surgery
1. Surgery, Operative
I. Jackson, John W II. Rob, Charles
III. Smith, *Sir* Rodney, b.1914 IV. Dudley, Hugh Arnold Freeman
617′.91 RD32 77-30634

ISBN 0 407 00604 4

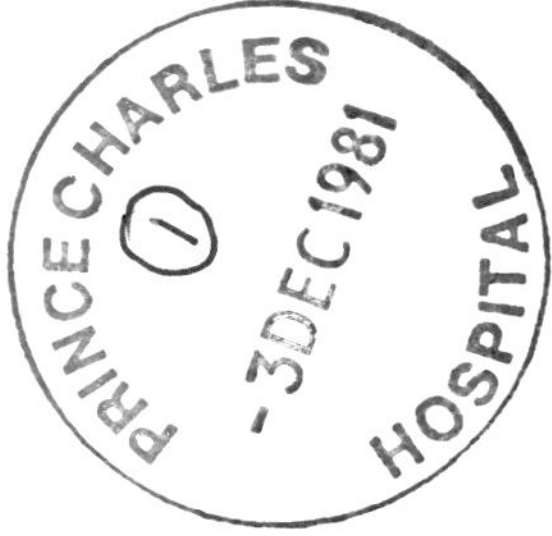

Typeset by Butterworths Litho Preparation Department
Printed in England by The Whitefriars Press Ltd., London and Tonbridge
Bound by The Newdigate Press Ltd., Dorking, Surrey

OPERATIVE SURGERY

Volumes and Editors

ABDOMEN	Hugh Dudley, Ch.M., F.R.C.S., F.R.C.S.(Ed.), F.R.A.C.S. Charles Rob, *M.C.*, M.D., M.Chir., F.R.C.S. Rodney Smith (Lord Smith of Marlow), K.B.E., M.S., F.R.C.S.
ACCIDENT SURGERY	P. S. London, M.B.E., F.R.C.S.
CARDIOTHORACIC SURGERY	John W. Jackson, M.Ch., F.R.C.S.
COLON, RECTUM AND ANUS	Ian P. Todd, M.S., M.D.(Tor.), F.R.C.S.
EAR	John Ballantyne, F.R.C.S., Hon.F.R.C.S.(I.)
EYES	Stephen J. H. Miller, M.D., F.R.C.S.
GENERAL PRINCIPLES, BREAST AND HERNIA	Hugh Dudley, Ch.M., F.R.C.S., F.R.C.S.(Ed.), F.R.A.C.S. Charles Rob, *M.C.*, M.D., M.Chir., F.R.C.S. Rodney Smith (Lord Smith of Marlow), K.B.E., M.S., F.R.C.S.
GYNAECOLOGY AND OBSTETRICS	D. W. T. Roberts, M.Chir., F.R.C.S., F.R.C.O.G.

VOLUMES AND EDITORS

THE HAND	R. Guy Pulvertaft, C.B.E., Hon.M.D., M.Chir., F.R.C.S.
HEAD AND NECK *[in 2 volumes]*	John S. P. Wilson, F.R.C.S.(Eng.), F.R.C.S.(Ed.)
NEUROSURGERY	Lindsay Symon, T.D., F.R.C.S.
NOSE AND THROAT	John Ballantyne, F.R.C.S., Hon.F.R.C.S.(I.)
ORTHOPAEDICS *[in 2 volumes]*	George Bentley, Ch.M., F.R.C.S.
PAEDIATRIC SURGERY	H. H. Nixon, F.R.C.S., Hon.F.A.A.P.
PLASTIC SURGERY	John Watson, F.R.C.S. Robert M. McCormack, M.D.
UROLOGY	D. Innes Williams, M.D., M.Chir., F.R.C.S.
VASCULAR SURGERY	Charles Rob, *M.C.*, M.D., M.Chir., F.R.C.S.

OPERATIVE SURGERY

Contributors to this Volume

EOIN ABERDEEN F.R.C.S., F.A.C.S.	*Director of Cardiovascular Surgery, The Children's Hospital of Newark, New Jersey*
N. R. BARRETT M.Chir., F.R.C.S.	*Consulting Surgeon, St. Thomas's Hospital, London*
J. R. BELCHER M.S., F.R.C.S.	*Surgeon, London Chest Hospital; Thoracic Surgeon, The Middlesex Hospital; Consulting Thoracic Surgeon, North West Thames Regional Health Authority*
RONALD BELSEY M.S., F.R.C.S.	*Consulting Thoracic Surgeon, Frenchay Hospital, Bristol*
H. H. BENTALL F.R.C.S.	*Professor of Cardiac Surgery, Royal Postgraduate Medical School, London; Consultant Thoracic Surgeon, Hammersmith Hospital, London*
R. H. F. BRAIN F.R.C.S.	*Consultant Thoracic Surgeon, Guy's Hospital, London*
A. G. BROM M.D.	*Professor of Thoracic Surgery, University Hospital, Leiden*
L. L. BROMLEY M.Chir., F.R.C.S.	*Consultant Thoracic Surgeon, St. Mary's Hospital, London*
M. MEREDITH BROWN F.R.C.S.	*Thoracic Surgeon, Milford Chest Hospital, Godalming, Surrey*
ALAIN CARPENTIER M.D.	*Professor of Cardiac Surgery, Hôpital Broussais, University of Paris*
D. B. CLARKE F.R.C.S.	*Consultant Cardiothoracic Surgeon, The Queen Elizabeth Hospital, Birmingham*
W. P. CLELAND F.R.C.P., F.R.C.S.	*Surgeon, The Brompton Hospital; Consulting Thoracic Surgeon, King's College Hospital; Senior Lecturer in Thoracic Surgery, Royal Postgraduate Medical School; Civilian Consultant in Thoracic Surgery to the Royal Navy*
J. LEIGH COLLIS M.D., F.R.C.S.	*Professor of Thoracic Surgery and Consultant Surgeon to Queen Elizabeth Hospital, Birmingham; Thoracic Surgeon to the West Midland Health Authority*
MARC DE LEVAL M.D.	*Consultant Cardiothoracic Surgeon, The Hospital for Sick Children, Great Ormond Street, London*
PHILIP B. DEVERALL F.R.C.S.	*Consultant Cardiothoracic Surgeon, Guy's Hospital, London*
CHARLES DREW F.R.C.S.	*Consultant Thoracic Surgeon, Westminster Hospital and St. George's Hospital, London*

F. FONTAN
M.D.
Professor of Cardiac Surgery, University of Bordeaux; Surgeon to the Hôpital du Tondu, Bordeaux

J. W. P. GUMMER
M.S., F.R.C.S.
Consultant Surgeon, Central Middlesex Hospital, London

DAVID I. HAMILTON
F.R.C.S.
Cardiac Surgeon to the Royal Liverpool Children's Hospital

H. R. S. HARLEY
M.S., F.R.C.S.
Consultant Surgeon, University Hospital of Wales and Llandough Hospital

JOHN W. JACKSON
M.Ch., F.R.C.S.
Consultant Thoracic Surgeon, Harefield Hospital, Middlesex

A. W. JOWETT
F.R.C.S.
Consultant Thoracic Surgeon, The Royal Hospital, Wolverhampton

JOHN R. W. KEATES
F.R.C.S.
Formerly, Senior Lecturer, Cardiothoracic Institute, University of London; Consultant Cardiothoracic Surgeon, King's College Hospital, London

G. KEEN
M.S., F.R.C.S.
Thoracic and Cardiac Surgeon, United Bristol Hospitals and Frenchay Hospital, Bristol

S. C. LENNOX
F.R.C.S.
Consultant Surgeon, The Brompton Hospital, London; Senior Lecturer, Cardiothoracic Institute, University of London

CHRISTOPHER LINCOLN
F.R.C.S.
Consultant Paediatric Cardiac Surgeon, The Brompton Hospital, London; Lecturer in Paediatric Surgery, Cardiothoracic Institute, University of London; Thoracic Surgeon, University College Hospital, London

A. LOGAN
F.R.C.S.
Formerly, Reader in Thoracic Surgery, University of Edinburgh

D. G. MELROSE
M.R.C.P., F.R.C.S.
Professor of Surgical Science, Royal Postgraduate Medical School, London

B. B. MILSTEIN
F.R.C.S.
Consultant Cardiothoracic Surgeon, Addenbrooke's Hospital and Papworth Hospital, Cambridge

BRYAN P. MOORE
F.R.C.S.
Consultant Thoracic Surgeon, Brook General Hospital, London

H. C. NOHL-OSER
D.M., F.R.C.S.
Consultant Thoracic Surgeon, Harefield, Hillingdon and West Middlesex Hospitals

M. PANETH
F.R.C.S.
Consultant Cardiothoracic Surgeon, The Brompton Hospital, London

JOHN PARKER
F.R.C.S., M.R.C.P.

Cardiothoracic Surgeon, St. George's Hospital, London and St. Helier Hospital, Carshalton

W. SPENCER PAYNE
M.D.

Head of Section of Surgery, Mayo Clinic and Mayo Foundation; Professor of Surgery, Mayo Medical School, Rochester, Minnesota

F. G. PEARSON
M.D., F.R.C.S.(C.), F.A.C.S.

Professor of Surgery, University of Toronto and Head, Division of Thoracic Surgery, Toronto General Hospital

MARK M. RAVITCH
M.D.

Professor of Surgery, University of Pittsburgh and Surgeon-in-Chief, Montefiore Hospital of Pittsburgh

KEITH D. ROBERTS
Ch.M., F.R.C.S.

Consultant Paediatric Cardiothoracic Surgeon; The Children's Hospital, Birmingham; Senior Clinical Lecturer in Surgery, University of Birmingham

D. N. ROSS
F.R.C.S.

Consultant Surgeon, Guy's Hospital, London; Senior Surgeon, National Heart Hospital, London

J. KEITH ROSS
M.S., F.R.C.S.

Consultant Cardiothoracic Surgeon, Wessex Cardiac and Thoracic Centre, Western Hospital, Southampton

MARY P. SHEPHERD
M.S., F.R.C.S.

Consultant Thoracic Surgeon, Harefield Hospital, Middlesex

R. ABBEY SMITH
Ch.M., F.R.C.S.

Thoracic Surgeon, Walsgrave Hospital, Coventry

JAROSLAV STARK
M.D.

Consultant Cardiothoracic Surgeon, The Hospital for Sick Children, Great Ormond Street, London

ALBERT STARR
M.D., F.A.C.S.

Professor of Surgery and Chief of Thoracic Surgery, University of Oregon Medical School, Portland, Oregon

S. F. STEPHENSON
F.R.C.S.

Thoracic Surgeon, East Birmingham Hospital, Birmingham

M. F. STURRIDGE
M.S., F.R.C.S.

Consultant Thoracic Surgeon, The Middlesex Hospital, London; Consultant Surgeon, London Chest Hospital; Honorary Consultant Thoracic Surgeon, The National Hospital for Nervous Diseases, London

D. G. TAYLOR
F.R.C.S.

Thoracic Surgeon, Sheffield A.H.A.(T.)

VERNON C. THOMPSON
F.R.C.S.

Consulting Thoracic Surgeon to The London Hospital and London Chest Hospital

CONTRIBUTORS TO THIS VOLUME

J. D. WISHEART
M.Ch., F.R.C.S.

Cardiac and Thoracic Surgeon, United Bristol Hospitals and Frenchay Hospital, Bristol

J. E. C. WRIGHT
F.R.C.S.

Consultant Cardiothoracic Surgeon, London Chest Hospital, and Southend-on-Sea Hospital Group

MAGDI H. YACOUB
F.R.C.S.

Consultant Cardiac Surgeon, Harefield Hospital, Middlesex and National Heart Hospital, London

OPERATIVE SURGERY

Contents of this Volume

CONTENTS OF THIS VOLUME

CONTENTS OF THIS VOLUME

Introduction

The third Edition of this volume in the general series Operative Surgery takes its foundations from its predecessors and I am grateful to the previous volume editor, Mr. W. P. Cleland, for his advice and help in re-arranging the text so as to reflect the change in title from Thorax to Cardiothoracic Surgery.

In this re-arrangement, the more complicated and less common operations follow minor and investigatory procedures in a more or less logical manner so that it should be possible to locate any one chapter without continual reference to the index. Where possible each chapter follows the same pattern: an outline of investigations and indications followed by the operation and finally details of post-operative care. All the operations are well-tried, standard procedures calling for a degree of technical competence and considerable surgical experience. Each surgeon has been encouraged to describe his own method, to include pitfalls and complications and to mention or describe alternative procedures where appropriate.

In surgery for congenital heart disease the trend has been more and more away from palliation and multiple-stage operations and towards complete and total correction of the abnormal anatomy and, when this is not possible, a physiological re-arrangement of the haemodynamics. Likewise in adult cardiac surgery the primary aim has been complete repair or correction, with excision and replacement as the alternative when it is considered to provide the better long-term result. Since the last edition vein bypass grafting has replaced the palliative procedures that were then the only available treatment for coronary artery disease and its complications.

In spite of the continued development of new antibiotics, empyema and tuberculosis are still with us, and their careful surgical management remains essential for success and long-term survival. New chapters have been included on post-resection empyema, infected pneumonectomy space and bronchopleural fistula.

In oesophageal surgery the trend has been towards safe reconstruction and replacement, with particular emphasis on the problem of the prevention of oesophageal reflux, and alternative methods in the management of its complications.

I am pleased to have been able to introduce a new group of contributors from Great Britain, France, the Netherlands, the United States and Canada to give the work a new and increased international flavour.

Finally I would like to thank all those who have contributed to earlier editions, because it was on the basis of the quality of their work and reputation that a new edition has been possible.

JOHN W. JACKSON

Treatment of Cardiac Arrest

G. Keen, M.S., F.R.C.S.
Thoracic and Cardiac Surgeon, United Bristol Hospitals and Frenchay Hospital, Bristol

Aetiology

Cardiac arrest has been defined as sudden and usually unexpected failure of the heart to maintain circulation. If this broad definition is accepted, attempts at resuscitating patients dying of chronic disease or of the complications of old age will be avoided. Drowning, electrocution and asphyxia are the commonly encountered causes of cardiac arrest outside hospital, and treatment in these cases may be initiated by laymen. The medical practitioner is more likely to be confronted with cardiac arrest due to anoxia or drug sensitivity, whether in the operating theatre, x-ray department or ward. Myocardial infarction and pulmonary embolism are among the common causes of cardiac arrest occurring in hospital.

Recognition

Absence of major pulses in a collapsed patient is sufficient indication for treatment and no time should be wasted in auscultation or electrocardiographic confirmation. Respiratory arrest and fixed dilated pupils may confirm the diagnosis but should not be awaited, for drugs such as atropine and morphine may influence the pupillary response to anoxia.

Urgency

Circulatory arrest of more than 3 or 4 min duration is likely to be followed by irreversible cerebral damage, and care must be taken to avoid resuscitating the patient to a vegetative existence. However, survival without brain damage has been reported following longer periods of arrest, particularly in children, which deprives an arbitrary period of time of absolute value. Massage of the beating heart is most unlikely to initiate an arrhythmia and the operator should therefore discount the possibility of such an accident arising on account of premature or unnecessary treatment.

External resuscitation

Whereas internal cardiac massage is readily achieved in the operating theatre, this method has considerable disadvantages elsewhere. The introduction of an efficient method of closed massage was therefore timely and this is now well established as the procedure of choice in the first instance in almost all cases of cardiac arrest. Despite theoretical doubts concerning the efficiency of external massage, experimental and clinical observations confirm that under these conditions cardiac output may reach 60 per cent of normal. Clinical experience confirms that an adequate circulation can be maintained for at least an hour, followed by subsequent survival without ill effect. Raising the patient's legs to encourage rapid venous return is a useful preliminary manoeuvre and a hard blow over the sternum with the clenched fist has been known to stimulate the arrested heart into a resumption of normal activity, but too much time should not be wasted, for these manoeuvres are not usually successful alone.

Duration of resuscitative efforts

These must be continued so long as the patient responds. In the presence of a good peripheral circulation and small pupils, persistence cannot be denied. Failure of the peripheral circulation is recognized by stagnant peripheral anoxia with dilated pupils and the condition is usually self-evident. In essentially reversible situations such as asphyxia, electrocution and drug reactions, no effort should be spared and many cases are on record describing unimpaired survival following more than an hour of cardiac massage.

TECHNIQUE

1

Anatomical basis

The heart is limited anteriorly by the sternum, posteriorly by the vertebral bodies and lateral movement is restricted by the pericardium. Anteroposterior pressure forces blood from the heart into the great vessels so long as there is adequate venous return and the valves are competent.

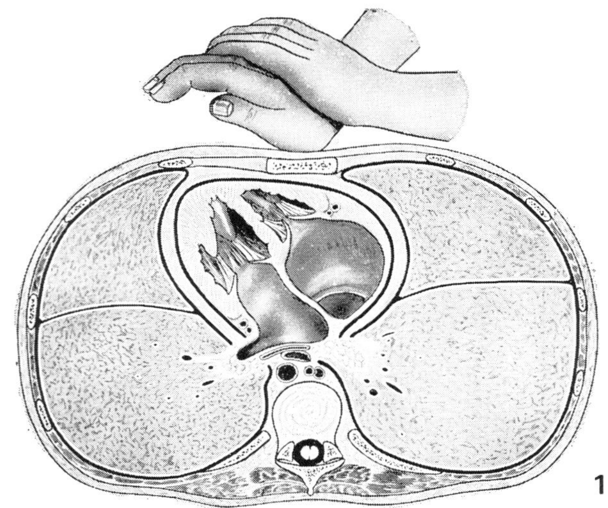

1

2

Position of patient

The patient is placed supine on a firm surface, such as a fracture board or on the floor, to ensure that massage is not rendered inefficient by the oscillations of a sprung bed. The operator stands or kneels beside the patient and massage is applied over the lower third of the sternum. The heel of one hand is placed over this site and the other hand covers it to re-inforce the thrust. In children, external cardiac massage is effective if one hand only is used.

Firm pumping movements at the rate of 70 per minute, each thrust depressing the lower sternum 1–2 inches (less in children) will produce a palpable pulse in the presence of an adequate blood volume. From time to time massage may be discontinued, allowing rapid assessment of the peripheral pulses. In ideal circumstances the patient will have been connected to the electrocardiogram recorder and the rhythm noted. An electrical impulse does not necessarily imply an expulsive heart beat, and the peripheral pulses and blood pressure rather than the monitor must guide the operator as to the adequacy of spontaneous heart action. Effective massage is readily recognizable. The patient's colour will improve and dilated pupils may contract. At the same time respiratory efforts and even consciousness may return. Peripheral pulsation in larger vessels is difficult to assess, for pulsation without flow or mere transmission of body wall movement may convey a false impression. The patient's appearance is probably as good a guide as any.

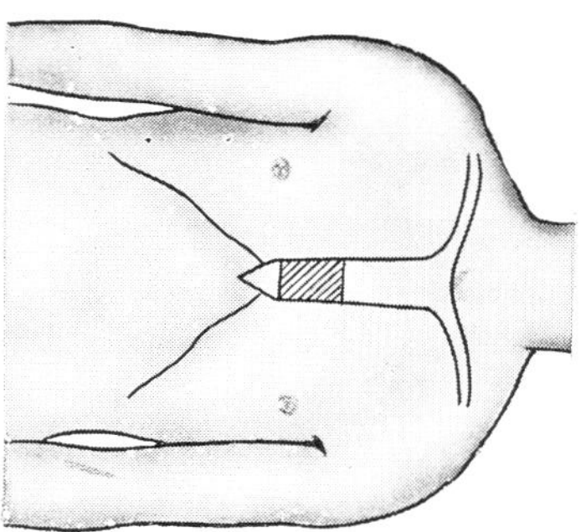

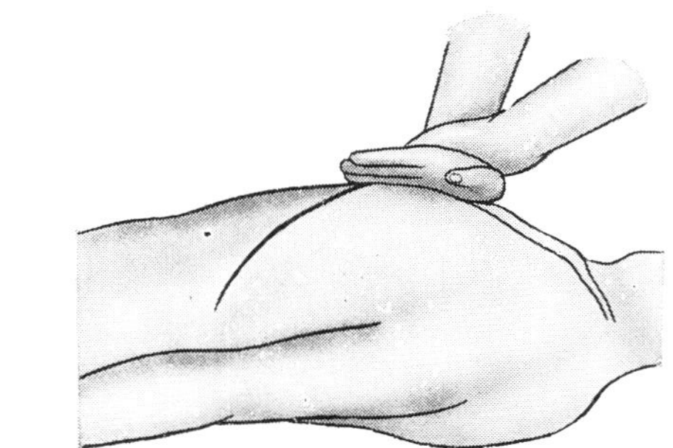

2

Ventilation

3

Mouth-to-mouth

Respiratory failure usually accompanies cardiac arrest and requires artificial ventilation. In an emergency, mouth-to-mouth ventilation is most effective. Care must be taken to extend the patient's neck and occlude the nose, holding the chin down to open the mouth.

3

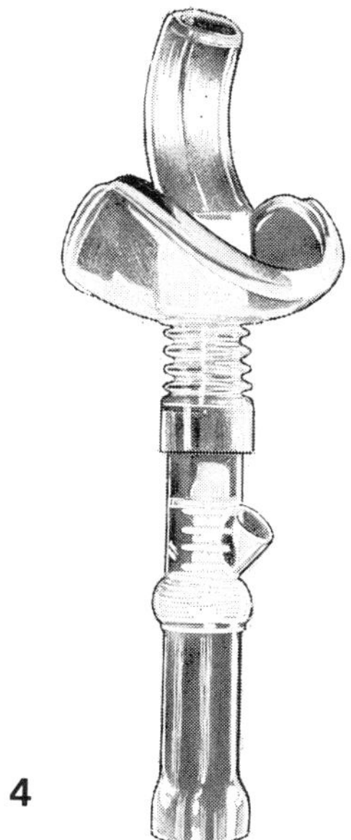

4

Use of Brook airway

A more elegant method of mouth-to-mouth respiration is by means of a double-ended airway, with a one-way valve, such as the Brook airway. Mouth-to-mouth respiration has the disadvantage of ventilation with only 15 per cent oxygen (expired air), but nevertheless appears to be adequate in many cases.

AMBU bag

Several anaesthetic bags which spring back to the distended position (by means of internal support) are available and enable ventilation with room air or oxygen to be achieved most effectively. One of these is the AMBU bag. If facilities are available, ventilation with 100 per cent oxygen via an endotracheal tube is ideal.

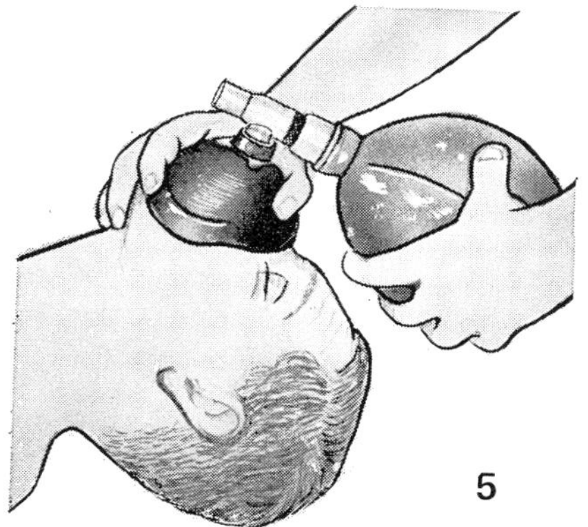

5

6

Ventricular fibrillation

During many episodes of cardiac arrest, the rhythm is true asystole (that is, a flaccid non-contractile heart), and in these patients prolonged massage and the intracardiac use of drugs may often restore tone and heart beat. More frequently, however, ventricular fibrillation is observed and, until defibrillation is achieved, resuscitation is not possible. Should ventricular fibrillation occur, spontaneous reversal to sinus rhythm is unlikely. External defibrillators using a d.c. counter-shock are effective in converting this rhythm and their use will usually avoid thoracotomy. The introduction of the external defibrillator is an important factor in the improved outlook in the treatment of cardiac arrest and it should be regarded as standard hospital equipment. No time should be wasted in attempts to defibrillate using drugs, for although occasionally successful, no known drug will readily convert this serious arrhythmia. Before attempting defibrillation, it is important that a period of efficient massage prepares the myocardium, for an anoxic heart is most difficult to defibrillate. If the heart fails to beat following defibrillation, electrical pacing may be successful.

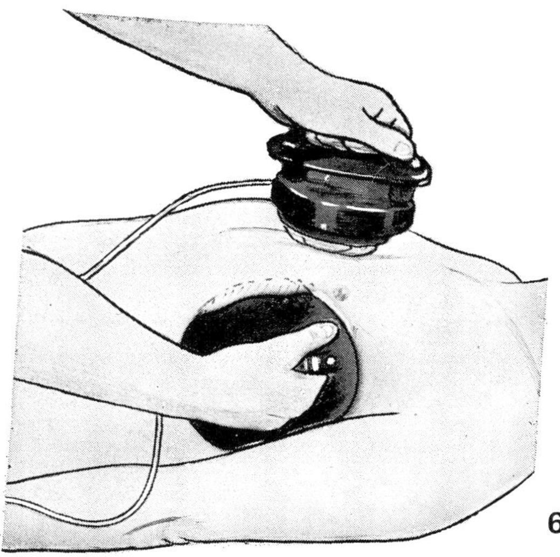

6

Complications of external massage

It is possible, especially in the elderly, for ribs to be broken during external massage, but this is less likely if pressure is confined to the lower end of the sternum. More rarely, rupture of the liver or other viscera has been recorded. However, in the majority of successful cases, there are no untoward traumatic sequelae, perhaps on account of the short period of massage required in these cases. In any event, fear of possible visceral injury should not deter vigorous efforts, as there is clearly no alternative.

Thoracotomy and internal massage

Efficient external massage supported by adequate ventilation and the external defibrillator, has considerably diminished the need for thoracotomy. Apart from the special requirements of cardiac and thoracic surgery, failure of external resuscitation is rarely rendered successful by proceeding to internal massage. However, since individual cases cannot be pre-judged, thoracotomy should be resorted to when external methods fail to achieve adequate cardiac output. Internal cardiac resuscitation may be indicated in pulmonary embolism, cardiac tamponade and massive air embolism, but since in these special situations further procedures may be required, they will not be discussed in this chapter.

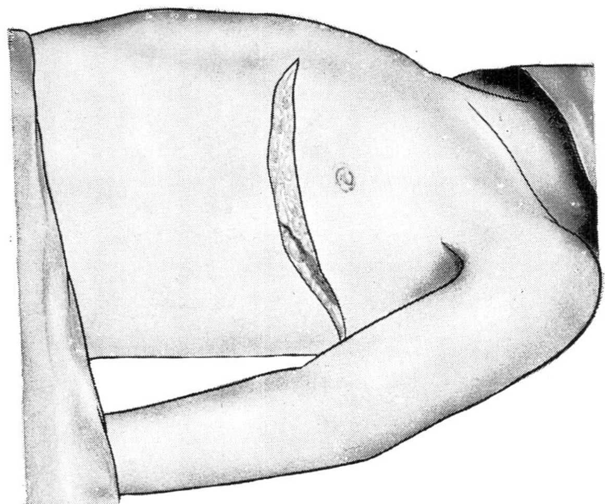

7

7

The incision

The left chest is entered through an incision extending from the mid-line to the mid-axillary line, curving below the breast. The fourth or fifth intercostal space is incised quickly, but care is taken to avoid the lung. The anaesthetist will assist at this stage by avoiding forceful inflation. The internal mammary vessels are best avoided by opening the medial end of the intercostal space by blunt dissection.

8

With the chest held open by an assistant or a retractor (a mouth gag is useful here), the pericardium is widely opened anterior to the phrenic nerve.

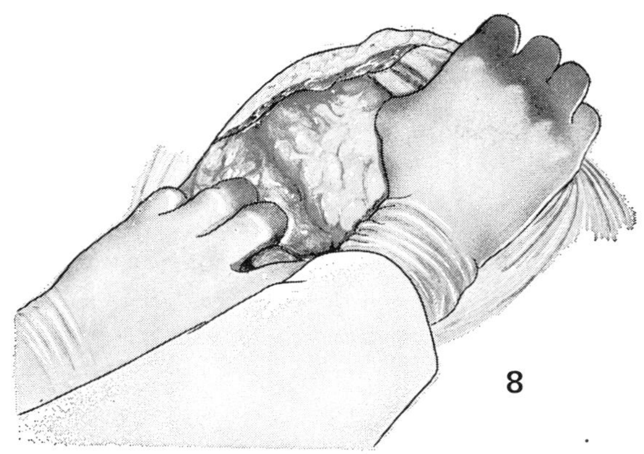
8

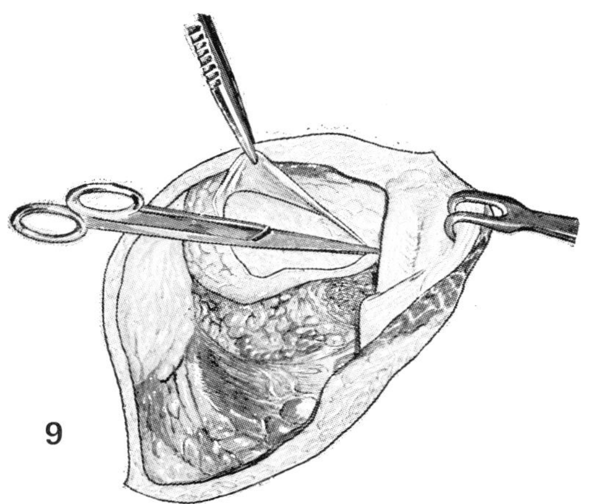
9

9

Massage

Massage should be conducted with both hands, one behind and the other in front of the ventricles, using the flat of the fingers and palm. Massage with one hand using fingers and thumb is both inefficient and tiring, and furthermore the thumb may perforate the heart. A rate of 60 per minute, which allows time for diastolic filling, is ideal.

10

Internal defibrillation

Should ventricular fibrillation supervene, internal defibrillation is undertaken. Two electrode plates are placed one either side of the heart within the pericardium. If there is good myocardial tone a single shock of 15–20 Joules produces organic contractions. If these are not maintained or fibrillation recurs further periods of massage and countershow supported by drugs to improve muscle tone and decrease irritability may be required. Many attempts may be necessary, supported by energetic massage, before successful defibrillation occurs. Procaine amide may facilitate defibrillation and is given intravenously as a dose of 5 mg/kg body weight. However, this drug has a direct depressant effect on the myocardium and should be used with caution, if at all. Following a successful outcome, the chest should be closed in layers and drained.

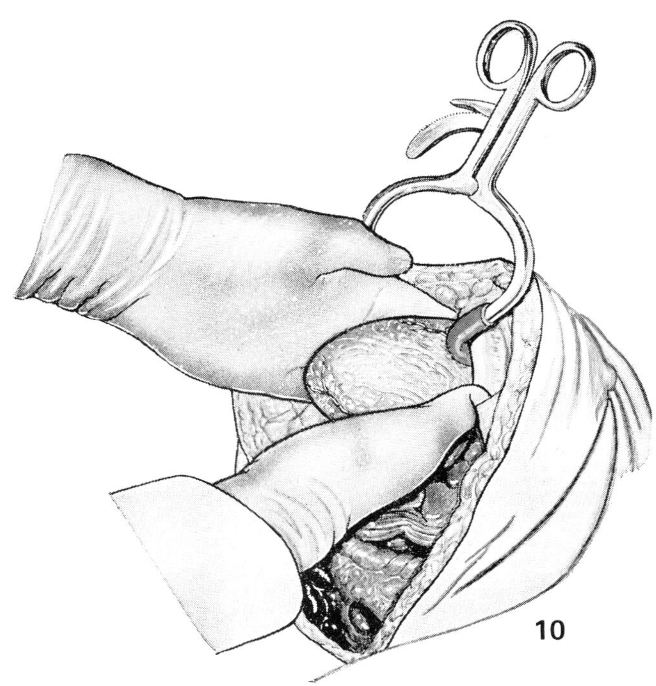
10

Other drugs. The most useful drug is oxygen transported to the myocardium by efficient massage and ventilation. Five to ten ml of 1/10,000 adrenaline given intravenously or into the heart may have a dramatic effect, especially in the restoration of good cardiac tone, but in the presence of anoxia may produce irreversible ventricular fibrillation. A safer drug is calcium chloride or calcium gluconate given by the same route in a dose of 5–10 ml of a 10 per cent solution. Isoprenaline (Isuprel) given intravenously produces a good pressor response, improves heart action and seems to have few toxic effects. Small doses of the order of 5 ml solution of 0·02 mg/ml may produce a good response.

Treatment of metabolic acidosis

Cardiac arrest with resulting tissue anoxia always leads to metabolic acidosis. Its severity is directly related to the duration of circulatory insufficiency and is largely predictable. Early resumption of spontaneous cardiac activity with normal cardiac output is the most effective means of reversal of the acidotic state, by removal of metabolites to the liver, lung and kidneys for disposal. However enthusiastically performed, cardiac massage never provides adequate tissue perfusion to deal completely with these metabolites. There is abundant clinical and experimental evidence that an acidotic state militates against resumption of normal and effective heart beat. Sodium bicarbonate given intravenously will largely correct such an acidosis, thus increasing the chance of success of the resuscitative attempt. An adequate dose of sodium bicarbonate is 1–2 mEq/kg body weight given intravenously over a period of 2–3 min. This should be repeated every 20 min until normal and productive heart action returns. It is important to inject as concentrated a solution as is acceptable to the circulation, as large volumes of dilute intravenous solution may overload an already embarrassed venous circulation. A 7·5 per cent solution of sodium bicarbonate contains 88 mEq/100 ml, and such an initial dose is adequate for a large adult and may be repeated several times without danger of circulatory overload. Myocardial function should improve and there is no evidence to suggest any harmful effects attributable to sodium bicarbonate when employed in this way.

LATER MANAGEMENT

Following resumption of heart action, the patient may recover fully in a very short time but more usually there is some degree of interference with cerebral, respiratory or renal function. Prolonged unconsciousness is compatible with complete recovery, and after the first 48 hr the electro-encephalogram is a useful prognostic guide. However, little reliance can be placed on this investigation in the absence of good apparatus and expert interpretation of the tracings.

Many patients will require artificial ventilation for some days using a reliable volume cycled and humidified respirator. Although nasotracheal intubation is finding favour, especially in children, tracheostomy is sometimes more effective in the management of the profuse and often tenacious and infected secretions of these patients.

Urinary output should be closely watched and daily estimations of serum electrolytes followed. Tubular damage is common after cardiac arrest and resuscitation but is usually transient and not severe, but a rising blood urea and potassium may call for early haemodialysis or peritoneal dialysis. A more comprehensive discussion of the management of respiratory and renal inadequacy is beyond the scope of this chapter but close attention to these complications is frequently required.

Conclusion

External resuscitation is an adequate method of maintaining the circulation and when used in conjunction with artificial ventilation will frequently restore normal heart action. Such maintenance will prevent deterioration while trained personnel and equipment are gathered together. Should external massage fail to produce an adequate cardiac output, resort to thoracotomy and direct cardiac massage should not be delayed. The success of these efforts is determined by the nature of the underlying cause, the speed with which determined resuscitative efforts are begun and the teaching and experience of those at hand. Cardiac resuscitation has passed from the stage of clinical trial to that of regular and recognized therapy. It is our duty to organize the training of hospital medical and nursing staff in the management of this emergency, and the acquisition of adequate and readily available equipment is a necessary part of this organization.

[*The illustrations for this Chapter on Treatment of Cardiac Arrest were drawn by Mr. F. Price.*]

Surgical Access in Cardiac Operations

R. H. F. Brain, F.R.C.S.
Consultant Thoracic Surgeon, Guy's Hospital, London

INTRODUCTION

Simplification, since the last edition, has resulted in the almost universal adoption of the central sternotomy route for open heart operations, and the standard lateral thoracotomy, usually on the left side, for the closed.

Left lateral thoracotomy (see page 255)

This approach is suitable for most closed operations on the heart and those on the aorta, for example the persistent ductus arteriosus, a coarctation, vascular rings, aneurysms of the left arch and descending aorta and for the aortopulmonary anastomotic procedures of the Blalock type.

Anterior thoracotomy (mid-line sternotomy)

For a full exposure of both ventricles, the ascending portions of the great vessels, the thymus, trachea and the anterior mediastinal structures in general, this incision has stood the test of time. The speed with which it can be performed, closed and, when necessary, rapidly re-opened are distinct advantages when compared with lateral thoracotomy. The cosmetic appearance of the incision, which extends from the base of the neck to the upper abdominal wall, appears as a disadvantage.

ANTERIOR THORACOTOMY

1

Position of patient

The patient should be in the full supine position with the left arm slung upwards for intravenous anaesthetic/ medication and often for the administration of blood and other fluids.

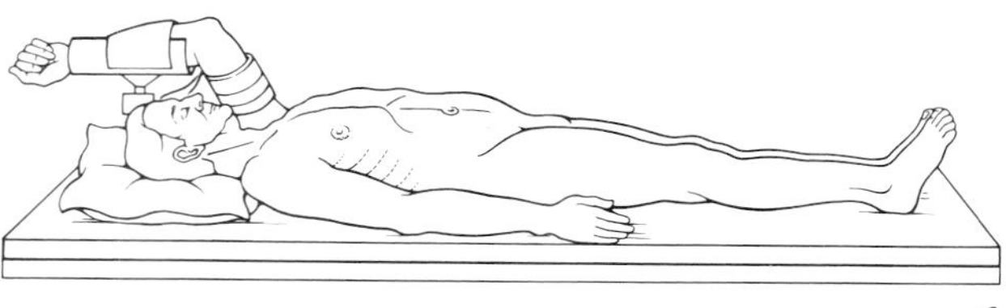

1

2

The incision

This is a simple vertical incision in the mid-line from the suprasternal notch to the tip of the xiphisternum.

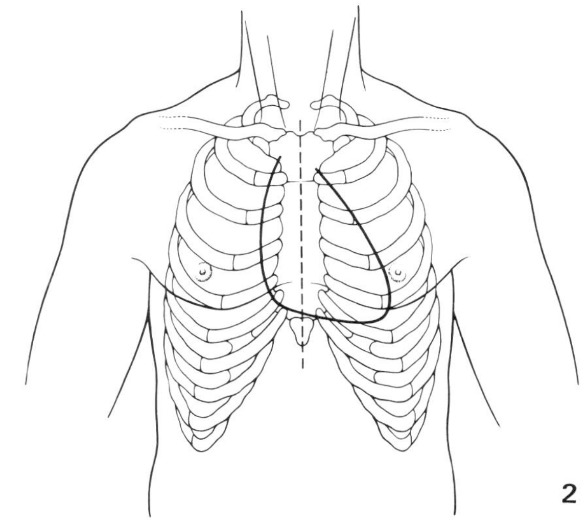

2

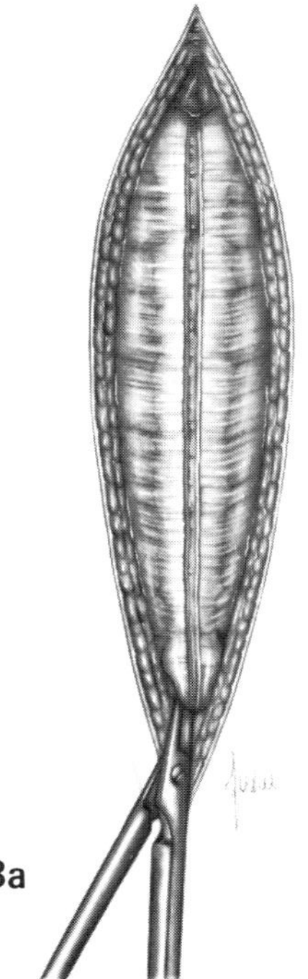

3a

3a

The exposure

The skin is dissected back to approximately the edge of the sternum on either side. Above, the suprasternal notch is clearly defined to its posterior limit. Below, the central tendon of the diaphragm is divided at its attachment to the back of the sternum.

3b, c & d

Division of the sternum

The periosteum over the sternum in line with the skin incision is incised and the bone divided with a pneumatic oscillating saw.

In the absence of this instrument a speedy entrance can be made using the Gigli saw introduced by a long Roberts type forceps that has previously been used to dissect the retrosternal tissues from the back of the sternum using small gauze mops.

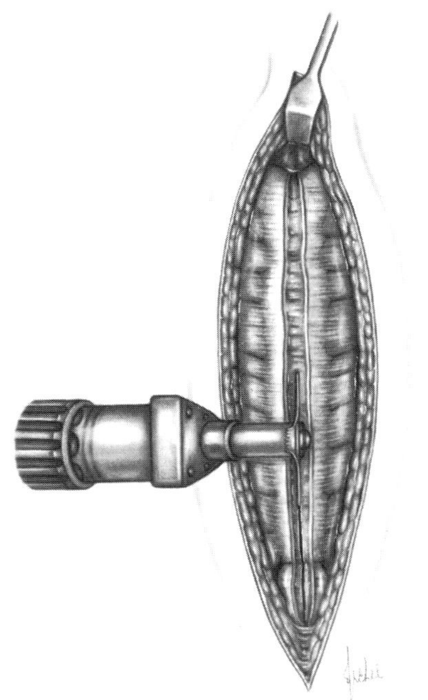

3b

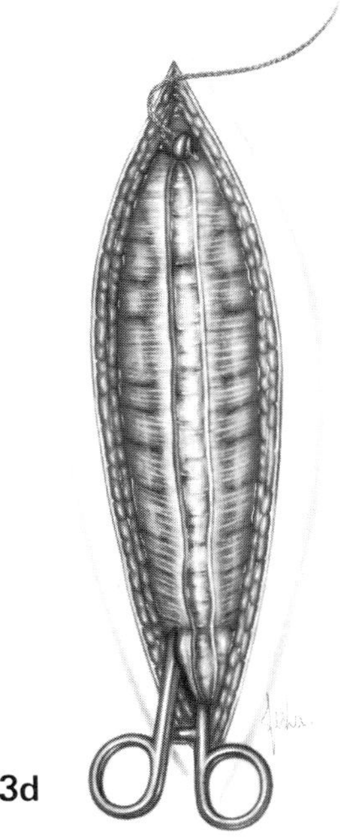

3d

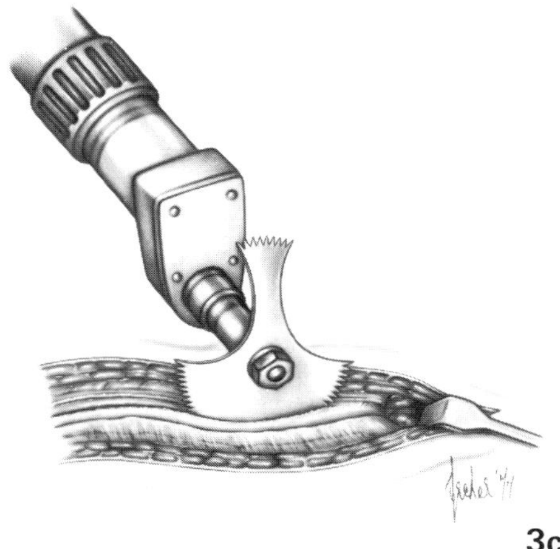

3c

4

Retraction of the sternum and exposure of the pericardium

Achieved by using a mechanical retractor of the Price-Thomas type after such overlying tissues as the edges of the pleural sacs laterally, and the thymus and the left innominate vein above have been dissected clear.

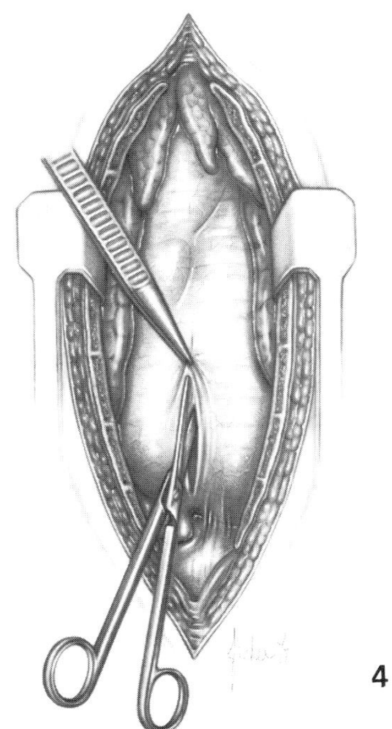

4

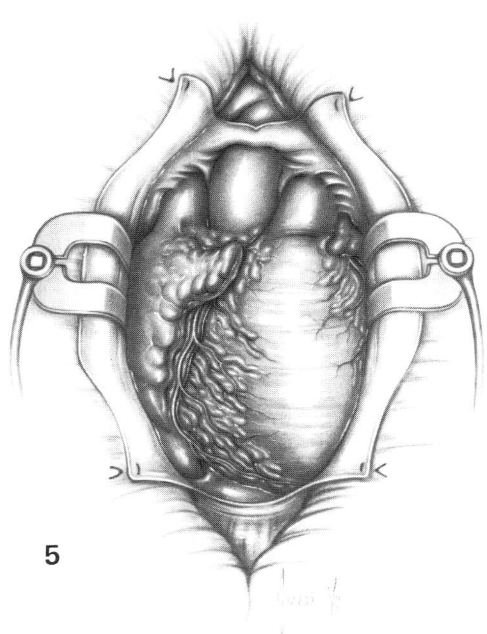

5

5

Exposure of the heart and great vessels

A vertical, or sometimes a cruciate, incision in the pericardium is made, the edges of which are sutured back to the wound.

Closure of the wound

6

The pericardium

Interrupted fine non-absorbable sutures are used over a drainage tube placed on the anterior surface of the heart.

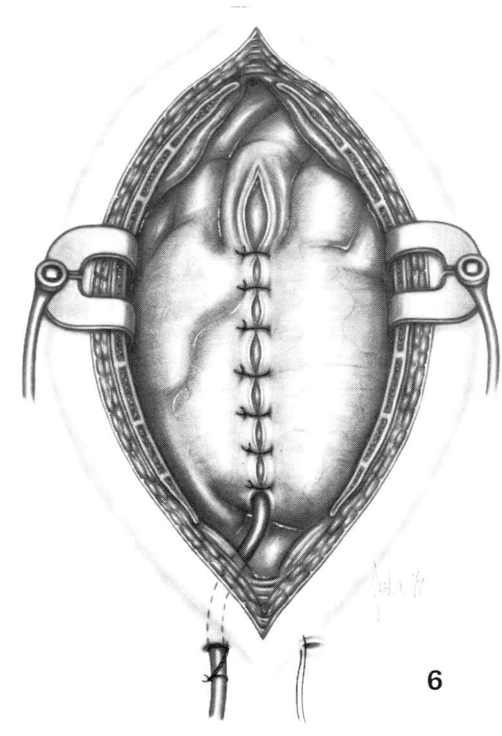

6

7&8

The sternum

The sternum is closed by a series of trans-sternal monofilament, non-absorbable sutures over a second drainage tube placed in front of the pericardium.

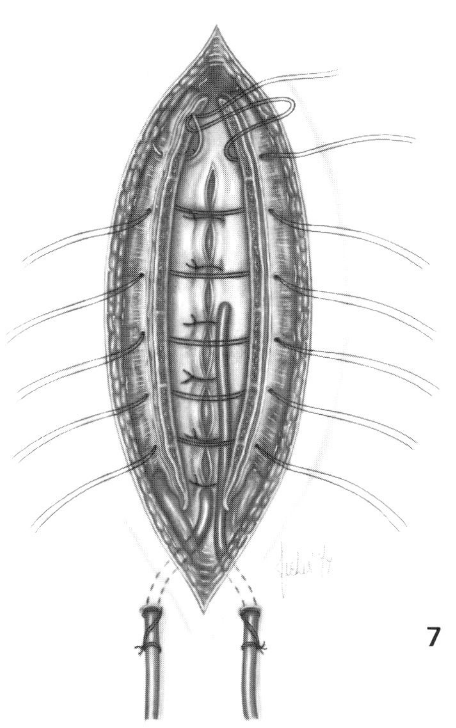

7

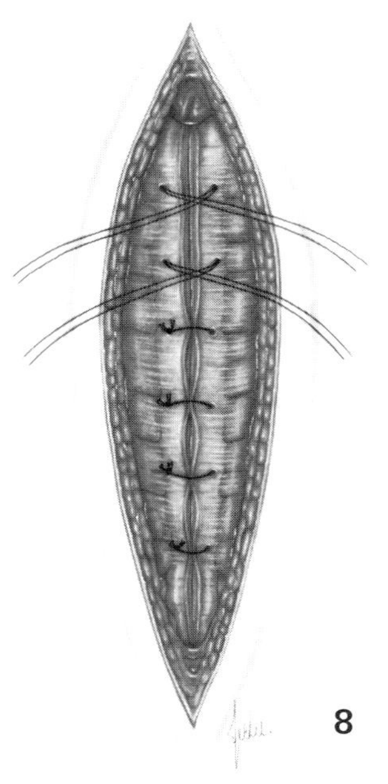

8

POSTOPERATIVE CARE

The need for careful postoperative management of cardiac patients is obvious when it is realized that an adequate cardiac pump depends both on the perfusion of its muscle by blood in full volume, at a proper pressure and containing a full complement of its normal constituents, and at the same time full freedom of movement within the pericardium and the mediastinum. After cardiopulmonary bypass one must expect an increased tendency to haemorrhage and a decrease in lung compliance. The latter may lead to difficulties with ventilation and perfusion – possible sources of serious problems later.

Patient monitoring

Essential to the management of cardiac operations are the continuous measurements of a variety of parameters, varying with individual surgeons, but the following are used frequently:

Venous pressure – a central venous line placed in the superior vena cava.

Arterial blood pressure.

Left atrial pressure – measured on those occasions when a low output and possible failure has been anticipated.

Continuous E.C.G. – fluorescent screen.

Urine secretion – volume, rate and osmolarity.

Peripheral temperature – limbs.

Ventilation/oxygenation/humidification – control.

Arterial blood gas, pH, bicarbonate measurements.

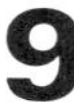

Chest drainage

All tubes are attached to separate underwater seal bottles, including those put into the pleural cavities should these have been opened. Accurate measurement is made of the rate of blood loss. Invariably suction is used.

Radiography

Regular daily, and sometimes more often, chest films are needed if concealed bleeding is suspected or there are problems with ventilation of the lungs.

Pain

Always a postoperative problem, and especially so when lung ventilation is likely to be restricted by depressant drugs affecting deep breathing and coughing. Mechanical ventilation, when used, abolishes these risks and enables a patient to be fully sedated safely. Physiotherapy at frequent regular intervals should be used.

Haemorrhage

This complication, rare from bleeding chest wall vessels, invariably is intrapericardial in origin and when causing tamponade requires thoracotomy, evacuation of the clot and arrest of the haemorrhage by suture.

Wound problems

These are rare but may include dehiscence, infection, osteomyelitis of the sternum and a late fibrous or non-union.

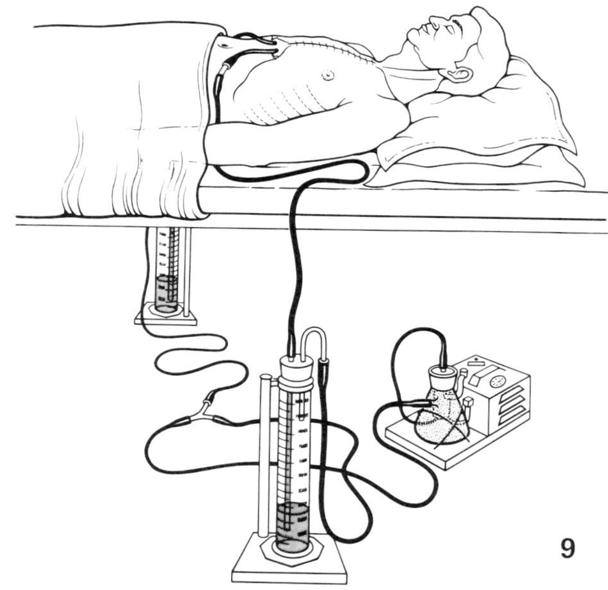

9

Definitive surgical problems

Answers of these should be sought under the various individual operations and the general complications of open heart perfusion techniques.

[*The illustrations for this Chapter on Surgical Access in Cardiac Operations were drawn by Miss P. Archer.*]

Cardiac Pacing

John Parker, F.R.C.S., M.R.C.P.
Cardiothoracic Surgeon, St. George's Hospital, London
and St. Helier Hospital, Carshalton

PRE-OPERATIVE

An artificial cardiac pacemaker may be required in the following situations:

(*1*) chronic complete heart-block;
(*2*) intermittent complete heart-block;
(*3*) sino-atrial disease;
(*4*) complete heart-block associated with acute myocardial infarction or with cardiac surgery.

Although percutaneous wires and electrodes inserted directly into the myocardium were used in emergency situations, they have now been superseded by the use of temporary endocardial pacing catheters which can be inserted percutaneously and advanced into the right ventricle, either blindly or with the aid of x-ray screening. If a pacing wire cannot be inserted for technical or other reasons an infusion of Isoprenaline 4 mg in 500 ml of 5 per cent dextrose run slowly, until the desired increase in heart rate is achieved, can be used.

Emergency pacing is required for recurrent episodes of syncope or near syncope over a short period of time, and is best achieved by the insertion of a temporary endocardial wire. The placement of endocardial wires is usually undertaken by cardiologists and the role of the surgeon is commonly confined to the insertion of the pacemaker units and/or the insertion of electrodes into the epicardial surface of the heart. The stabilization of an endocardial wire in the right ventricle requires some skill to reduce the incidence of displacement to a satisfactory level and is not a procedure that should be too widely shared among too many individuals in any institution.

THE PROCEDURES

Long-term pacing

This involves the implantation of a satisfactory electrode as well as a power source. With new technology different sources of energy are available and Lithium powered units are now widely used. The life span of such units will probably be 5–7 years. Nuclear powered pacing units are also available but their widespread use cannot be justified at the present time.

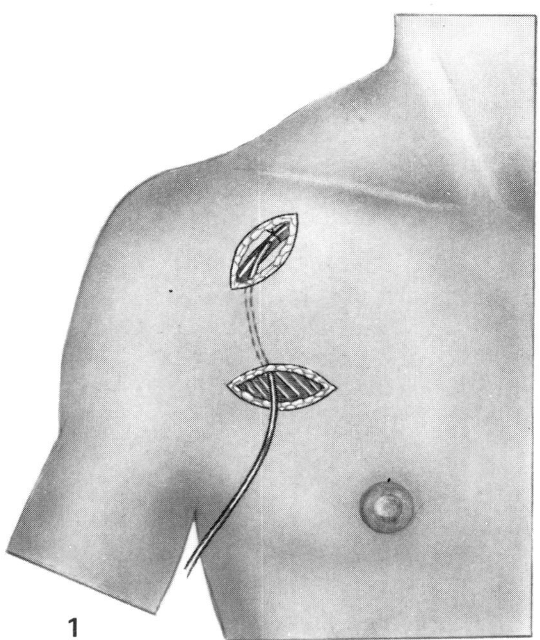

1

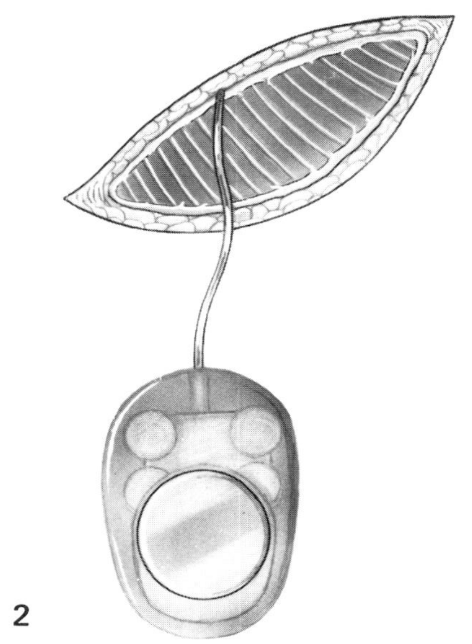

2

Electrode insertion

Pacing established via a wire inserted into the endocardium of the apex of the right ventricle is the first method of choice as an endocardial wire is inserted with a much less extensive operation than for the insertion of an epicardial wire. This is an important consideration as many patients requiring pacing are above the age of 65 years.

ENDOCARDIAL ELECTRODE INSERTION

1

ECG monitoring on a screen, using a limb lead is established. All patients are premedicated and intravenous Diazepam used in small doses is often successful in supplementing the local anaesthesia.

Using local anaesthesia the cephalic vein in the deltopectoral groove is explored and controlled and a flexible unipolar electrode is passed into the subclavian vein and then down the superior vena cava and with screening visualization across the tricuspid valve and into the apex of the right ventricle. Once the electrode has been stabilized and found to have a satisfactory threshold (1 Volt at 2 msec and preferably less than 0·5 Volts), the wire is left with gentle curves and no redundant loops and is then fixed to the vein by a firm ligature. The wire is then brought down to the point selected for the insertion of the pacing unit.

If for any reason the cephalic vein is unsuitable the external jugular vein or if necessary the internal jugular vein can be used. In the latter a simple purse-string suture is used to gain access of the electrode catheter to the vein.

2

Once the wire has been firmly fixed to the vein the free end is brought through to the pocket by tracking it through the subcutaneous fat immediately on top of the fascia to give it as much tissue cover as possible.

If the wire has been inserted in the external jugular or internal jugular vein it is usually best to bring it behind the clavicle unless the patient has an unusual amount of soft tissue over the clavicle.

The site used for insertion of the pacemaker and the technique used is of great importance if pacemaker unit complications are to be avoided. There are three sites that are commonly used:

(*1*) anterior chest wall;
(*2*) axilla;
(*3*) abdominal wall (*see* below).

Anterior chest wall

3

At the present time the anterior chest wall has proved the most successful. The pectoralis fascia is divided to expose the fibres of the pectoralis major. This should be done in females as well even if there is a considerable amount of breast tissue present as doing so will achieve a better cosmetic result and give the unit more protection. It is quite satisfactory to develop the pocket under local anaesthesia.

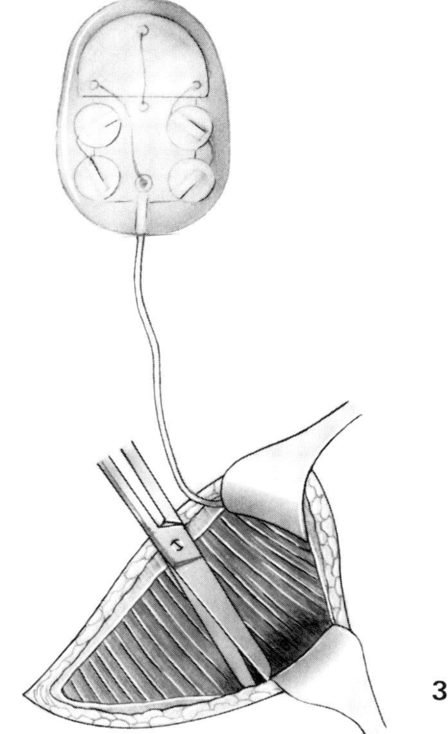

3

4

The pocket is developed by sharp dissection below the line of the skin incision. Haemostasis is achieved and with the pacemaker unit connected to the electrode (carefully following the individual manufacturer's instructions) pacing should commence once the unit is in the pocket. The negative electrode plate is placed facing the fascia and subcutaneous tissue and away from the muscle. Once it is confirmed that pacing is satisfactory and that there is no muscle twitching the wound can be closed. Closure should be in at least three layers – fascia, subcutaneous tissue and skin. Drains should not be used. Subcuticular skin closure with an absorbable suture can be used satisfactorily.

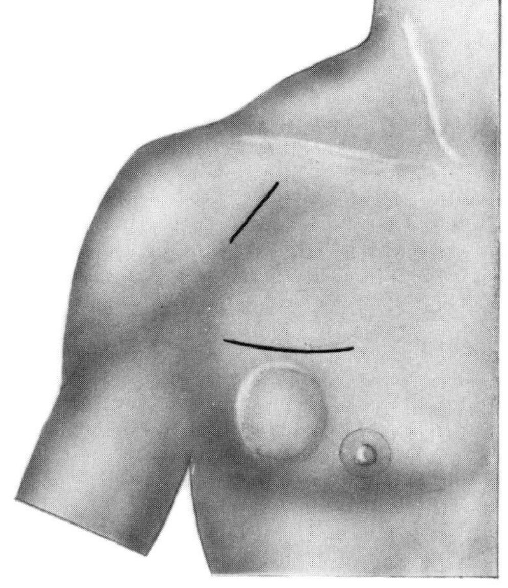

4

Axilla

5 & 6

If the axillary site is selected the skin incision is lower and more lateral on the chest wall just medial to the pectoral fold. The pectoralis major is retracted medially and the pocket developed downwards and laterally.

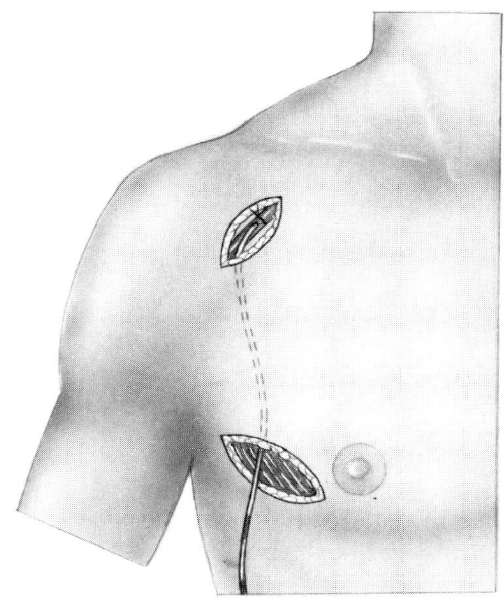

5

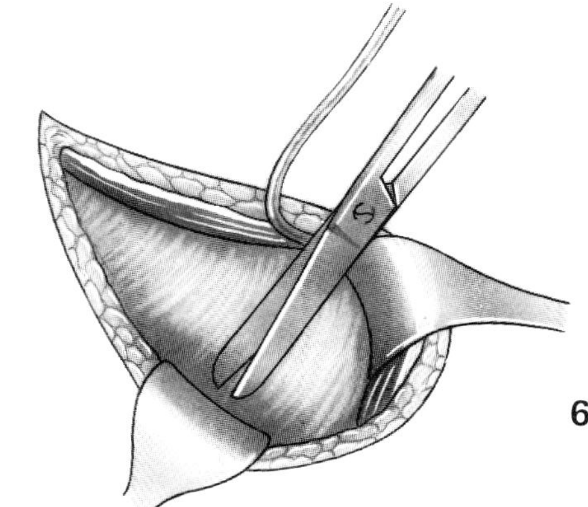

6

7

The pacemaker unit is then inserted and the pectoralis major allowed to cover the anterior and superior part of the unit. Note that the wound closure should be in three layers and that the incision does not overlie the unit directly.

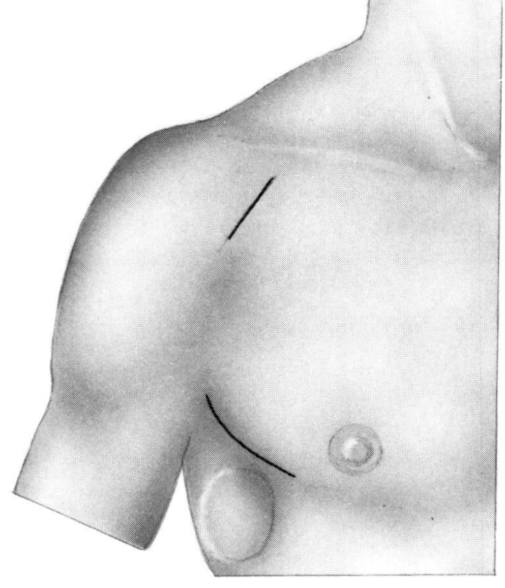

7

EPICARDIAL PACING

The first choice of route for cardiac pacing should be endocardial in most patients. Epicardial pacing is indicated if endocardial pacing has failed because of frequent electrode displacement in the right ventricle or if all available veins have been used to deal with wire and unit complications. Children requiring pacing are best dealt with by an epicardial system. General anaesthesia is required and a temporary endocardial wire should be inserted if one is not already in position before the induction of anaesthesia. The heart may be approached through a left thoracotomy or the subxiphoid route.

Anterior thoracotomy

8

The patient is positioned with the left chest brought a little forward with access to the upper abdominal wall for insertion of the pacemaker unit. In females the incision is submammary.

The chest is opened through the upper border of the fifth costal cartilage and anterior end of the fifth rib. It may be possible to get access to the pericardium without opening the pleura.

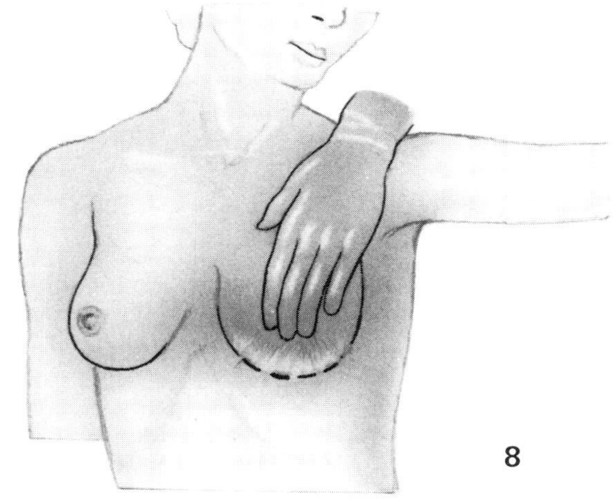

8

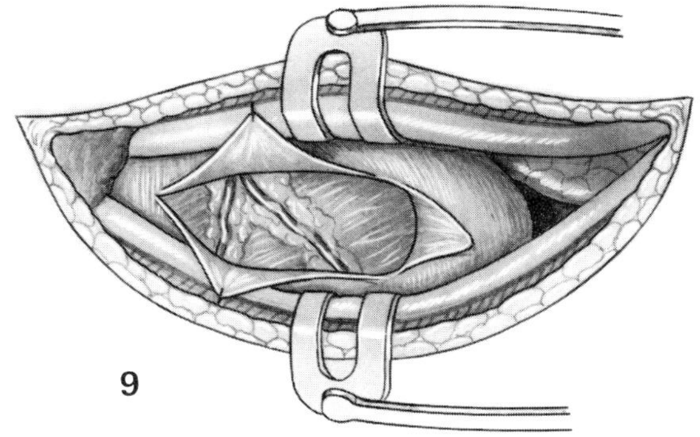

9

9

The pericardium is opened through a cruciate incision to reveal the left ventricle. The most convenient site to insert the electrode is either between the left anterior descending and diagonal coronary arteries or just lateral to the diagonal branch.

10

The standard electrode tip is inserted into the myocardium with a stab incision and is held in place by two sutures placed through the myocardium on either side of the stab and then through the Silastic surround to the electrode. Threshold measurements are then made and should not exceed 1 Volt at 2 msec.

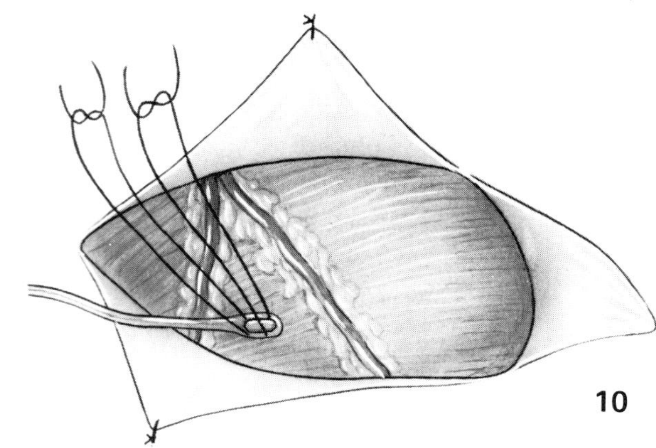

10

11

More recently a screw electrode has been made available and avoids making a stab into the myocardium and any sutures. A three turn electrode is suitable for the left ventricle.

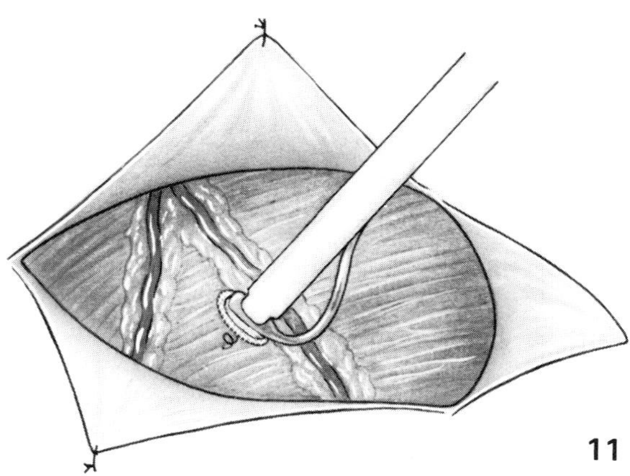

11

12

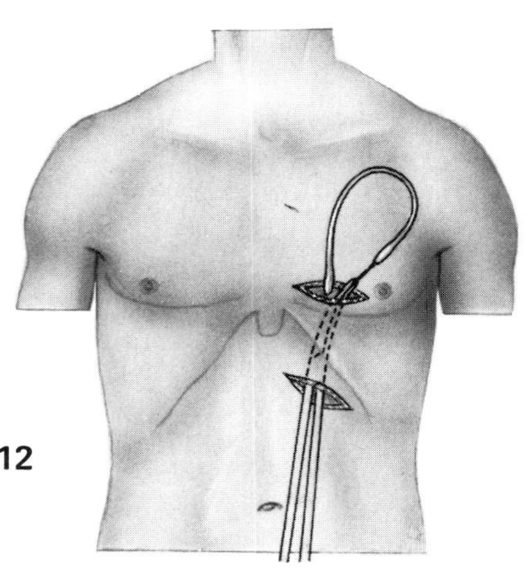

12

Haemostasis is achieved and the pericardium closed. The electrode is then brought down to the abdomen. If there is little tissue over the costal margin the wire is brought down in the chest and passed between the diaphragm and the costal margin. Alternatively it can be brought out into the subcutaneous tissues through a lower intercostal space.

The pocket is then developed below the incision as on the anterior chest wall. If there is almost no subcutaneous tissue the space behind the rectus muscle can be used as described below. Alternatively, the pacemaker unit can be inserted on the anterior chest wall or axilla.

Once satisfactory pacing has been established the chest is closed. A chest drain is only required if there is an air leak or excessive oozing.

The subxiphoid approach

13

This is associated with less discomfort than a thoracotomy and can be used in almost all patients. A very narrow space between the costal margins can make access difficult. A mid-line incision 12 cm long is made.

13

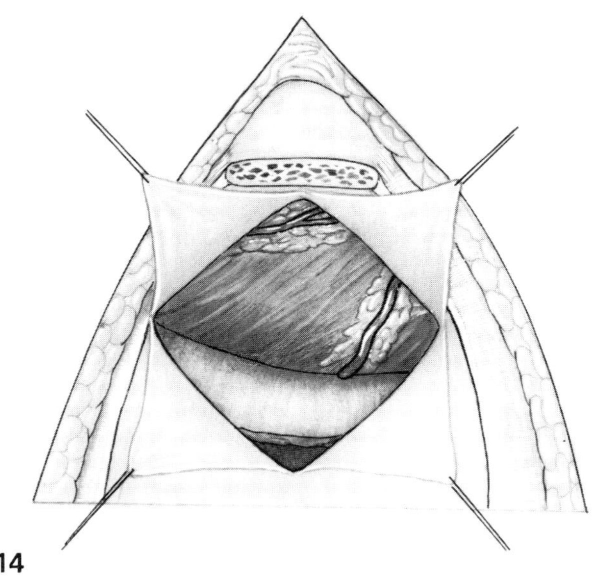

14

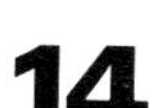

14

The linea alba is divided keeping the peritoneum intact. Unless the xiphoid process is very small and flexible it is resected. The diaphragm is incised to reveal the pericardium which is opened by a cruciate incision. To facilitate access it is helpful to suture the pericardium temporarily to the subcutaneous tissue. The electrode is then inserted usually into the inferior surface of the right ventricle between the posterior descending and marginal branches of the right coronary artery. A two turn screw electrode is now available for this site. If the right ventricle is very thin or if a satisfactory threshold cannot be achieved here it is possible to move onto the left ventricle just to the left of the posterior descending coronary artery.

15

Once a satisfactory electrode position and threshold has been achieved the pocket for the pacemaker is developed. The rectus sheath, usually the left one, is entered through the linea alba. The muscle is retracted laterally and the space behind the muscle is developed. The unit is then inserted into the space with the electrode plate in the unit facing the posterior rectus sheath.

Once satisfactory pacing has been established the rectus sheath and pericardium are closed, the linea alba repaired and the wound closed in layers.

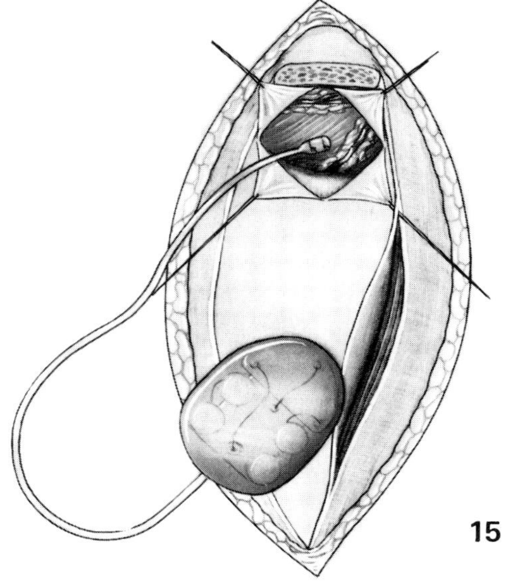

15

Pacemaker unit change

A change of pacemaker unit is usually undertaken on an elective time basis depending on the predicted life of the pacemaker and clinical experience. Alternatively routine tests of pacemaker function may detect premature failure. Different pacemakers have different built in features to warn of failure in the near future. Recurrence of symptoms or a change of pulse rate may indicate a unit failure, electrode failure or an unacceptable threshold rise.

Extraction of the unit and a check on the electrode and its threshold must then be carried out.

16

Routine unit change

This is done under local anaesthesia through the previous incision which should not overlie the unit directly. Carefully avoiding the wire, the capsule that has developed is opened and the unit removed. If the patient's heart will not take over at a rate of 30–40 beats/min then the unit electrode plate must be kept in contact with the patient while the electrode is removed from the unit. Once it is removed pacing is established with the external box and the threshold is measured. A threshold of 1 – 2 Volts at 2 msec is common and acceptable. A threshold of greater than 2·5 Volts is unacceptable and it generally requires a new electrode. If a larger unit is to be inserted or if the capsule cannot be closed then the capsule should be enlarged by incising its deeper side, a three layer closure, capsule, subcutaneous tissue and skin should be carried out.

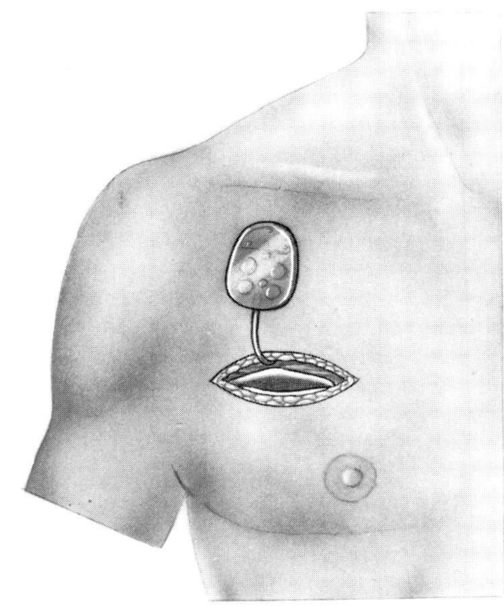

16

Mechanical pacemaker complications

Mechanical problems arising from the wire or the unit may occur. They present as two groups:

(*1*) those in whom the skin is tethered to the unit or wire and often a little inflamed – pre-ulceration;

(*2*) those with frank ulceration or obvious infection with pus present.

Group 1 are easier to deal with and patients should be encouraged to report any discomfort in the area of the pacemaker or wire. Group 2 are best dealt with by removal of the existing system and the insertion of a new system. For a septic pacemaker the unit is removed, the pocket drained and the electrode exteriorized for pacing and the patient treated with antibiotics for a period before a new system is inserted.

For pre-ulceration two procedures are available – reburial of the wire and resiting of the pacing unit.

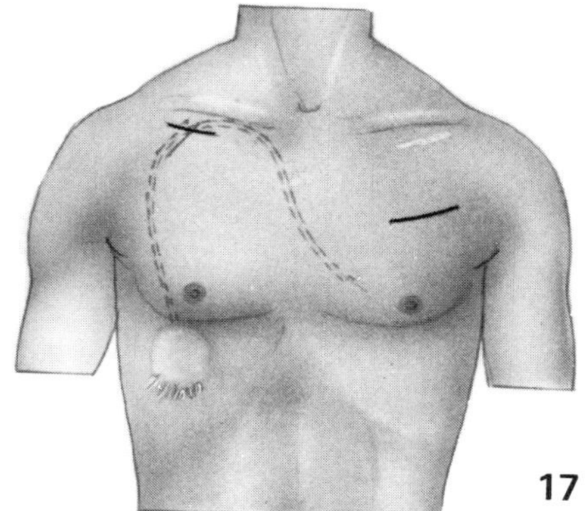

17

Resiting a pacing unit for pre-ulceration

17

This is best done under general anaesthesia. Without disturbing the unit the electrode wire is exposed below the clavicle and divided and pacing continued by an external box as necessary. A new pocket is developed on the other side or in the abdomen but not in the same local area.

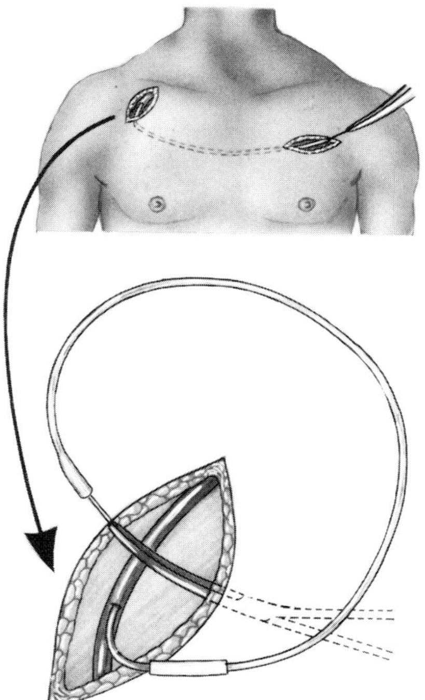

18

18

An electrode extension is then crimped on to the end of the electrode and an insulatory sheath used to cover the join. Using a long forceps the wire is then brought through the subcutaneous tissue planes to the new site and the threshold of the system checked and the new unit then inserted as for a new system. Once these wounds are sealed the pre-ulcerating unit is removed with the attached part of the original electrode wire.

General points

(*1*) Antibiotics are not used routinely for the insertion of new systems or a routine unit change but a 5–7 day course is given if there are any special indications.

(*2*) Anticoagulants should be reduced before doing any procedure on the unit.

(*3*) Diathermy should not be used during pacing procedures.

(*4*) When a new wire has been inserted the patient should be observed for approximately 10 days to ensure that pacing continues satisfactorily as this is the period when wire displacement or threshold rise may occur.

[*The illustrations for this Chapter on Cardiac Pacing were drawn by Mr. F. Price.*]

Methods of Providing Facilities for Open Heart Surgery

D. G. Melrose, M.R.C.P., F.R.C.S.
Professor of Surgical Science, Royal Postgraduate Medical School, London

GENERAL PRINCIPLES

Cardiac surgery demands special surgical conditions. In order adequately to repair intracardiac defects access to the interior of the heart is essential and it can now be obtained. The function of the heart is temporarily suspended to allow such surgery and the well being of the tissues of the body is maintained by substituting for the heart mechanical pumps capable of imitating cardiac function. For particular purposes reduction in body temperature is also used to reduce the metabolic demands of the tissues.

Indications

Of the very wide range of congenital and acquired cardiac defects few remain outside the competence of surgery and as advance in technique continues it is likely that these indications will be extended to all cardiac defects other than those secondary to generalized coronary artery disease in which the integrity of the myocardium cannot be maintained by coronary artery grafting. The special circumstances of transplantation of the heart itself make no additional demands on present perfusion technique.

TECHNIQUES

1

Hypothermia

The general circulation can be halted for only 2–3 min before damage to vital structures ensues. If the patient is cooled to an oesophageal temperature of 28°C this time limit can be extended to approximately 10 min before such changes occur. Hypothermia is the term applied to such partial refrigeration and it is normally induced by exposing the fully anaesthetized patient to an ambient temperature of about 0°C. The illustration shows such an anaesthetized patient shrouded in a special blanket through which iced water is pumped. This technique is now rarely used alone to provide access to the interior of the heart, but is a useful preliminary to connecting a heart-lung machine in infants.

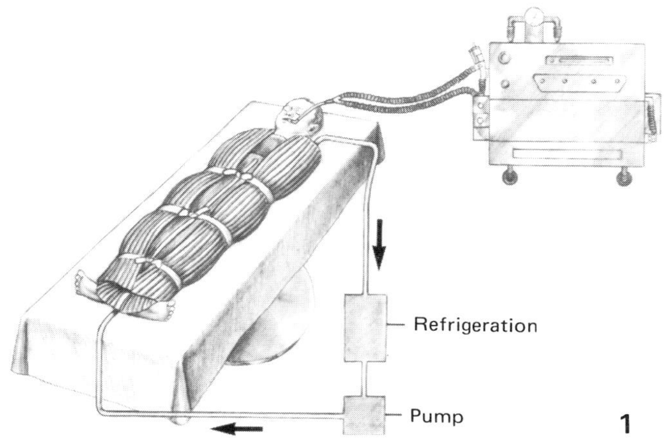

1

2

Heart-lung bypass

Apparatus

The technique now adopted for protecting the tissues of the body whilst the heart is excluded is to supply sufficient artificially oxygenated blood to vital areas to meet their needs. A heart-lung machine is connected to the circulation for this purpose. The diagram indicates a commonly used system and includes the necessary pumps, disposable oxygenator and heat exchanger.

Blood is withdrawn from superior and inferior venae cavae into an oxygenator (A) where respiration is maintained and then it is pumped (B) back into the arterial system through a heat exchanger (C). The coronary arteries may also be perfused by direct cannulation (D) by way of a separate pump as in the illustration or from a branch of the main arterial input.

The heat exchanger may be used to maintain a near normal body temperature or to adjust it to suit special circumstances. In particular, it is convenient to reduce the body temperature of infants to below 20°C when the extracorporeal circulation can be switched off to allow the intracardiac operation to be carried out in a bloodless quiet field. Rewarming is carried out by re-establishing whole body perfusion as soon as the intracardiac procedure is complete.

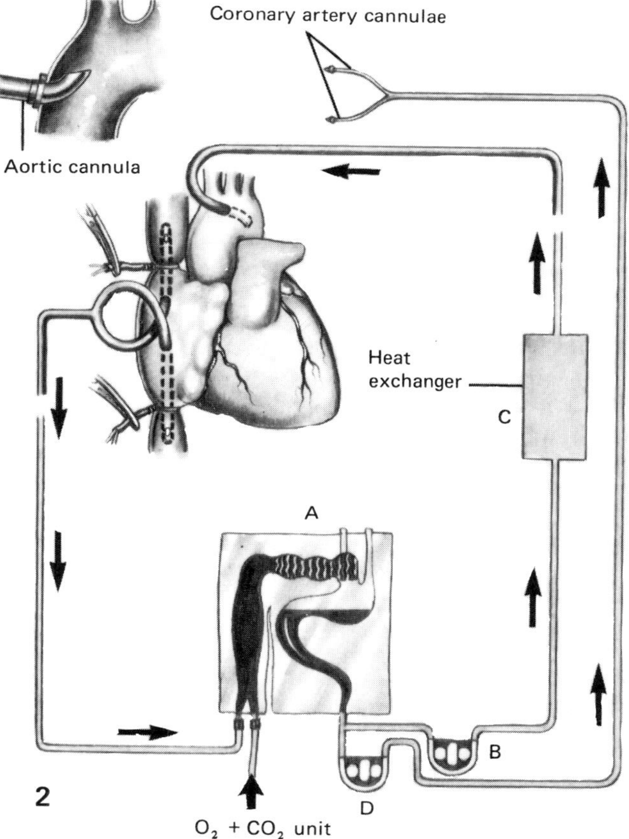

2

3

Intracardiac suction

After the circulation has been diverted into the heart-lung machine the heart can be isolated and its chambers opened. Continuous suction is required to remove blood accumulating within the chambers and it is essential to employ a gentle method. This blood is usually pumped into a defoaming reservoir from whence it is returned to the circulation through a fine filter of 40 micron mesh. Normal high vacuum suction is used only to clear local accumulations and this blood is discarded. Filtration of all blood used to prime the machine is now regarded as essential and many add similar screens to both the venous return and arterial input lines.

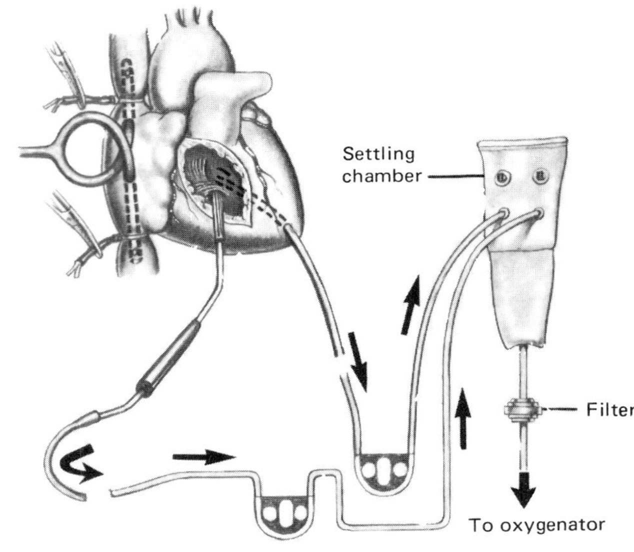

3

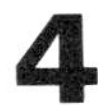

4

Myocardial protection

When it is necessary to isolate the myocardium from arterial blood supplied by the heart-lung machine as occurs in gaining access to the aortic valve, additional steps must be taken to protect the heart muscle. In these circumstances self-retaining catheters can be inserted into the coronary ostia and a blood flow maintained.

While this is the usual method, many attempts have been made to find an alternative to direct coronary perfusion and many have used intermittent ischaemia at near normal temperatures and prolonged ischaemia at low myocardial temperatures to avoid the complexity of coronary cannulation. There is also a return to chemical inhibition of the heart beat by solutions containing potassium or magnesium salts in an effort to reduce metabolic needs. These can be combined with hypothermia as in Bretschneider's technique. A better understanding of myocardial metabolism is still required to determine the best technique or combination of techniques for all circumstances. It is useful to maintain a bloodless field by direct drainage of the left ventricle and this is usually managed by suction on a catheter passed through the apex of the ventricle.

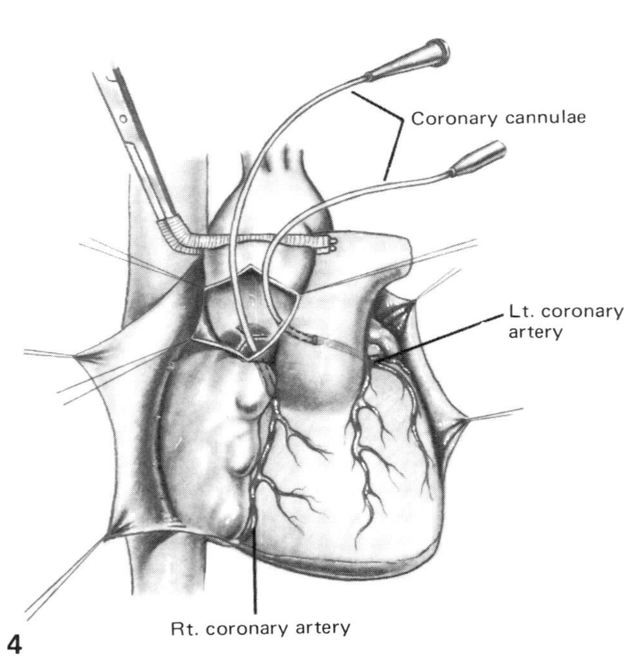

4

5

Supportive perfusion and balloon pumping

The development of oxygenators wherein blood and gas are separated by gas permeable membranes has re-awakened interest in the heart-lung machine as a method of resuscitation. Prolonged perfusion for many days at a time is now possible and it can be expected that supportive perfusion will be added to the armamentarium of the cardiac surgeon. At the same time increasing interest is being shown in balloon pumping as a method of supporting the failing circulation. This device performs as a secondary left ventricle and greatly reduces the work of the heart. The illustration indicates the salient features; an inflatable balloon placed in the aorta whose rhythmical inflation, timed to coincide with natural diastole, imposes a second pressure cycle in the arterial system. Deflation of the balloon has the opposite effect and reduces the pressure against which the heart works in systole. In combination this effect may be life-saving.

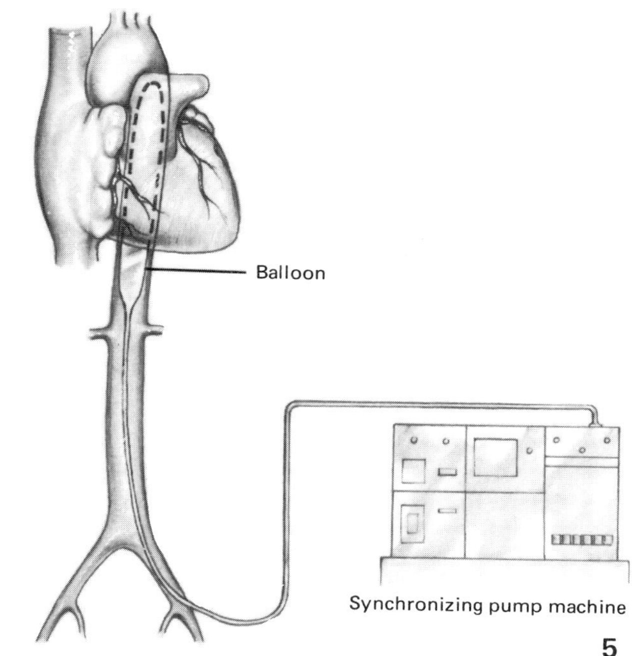

5

6a&b

Left heart bypass

The surgical management of aneurysms of the aorta can best be managed with the help of an extracorporeal shunt between the left atrium and the femoral artery. Blood, oxygenated by the lungs, can be gathered from the left atrium and pumped into the arterial system distal to the aneurysm which can then be isolated between clamps. Alternatively a direct shunt from the left ventricle to the aorta below the lesion can be used if access allows. This has the merit of avoiding any additional equipment other than a special cannula.

These techniques provide an opportunity for deliberate and accurate excision and replacement of the defective area without endangering tissues peripheral to the lesion. Appropriate cannulation of other arteries extends the technique to bridging even aneurysms of the aortic arch.

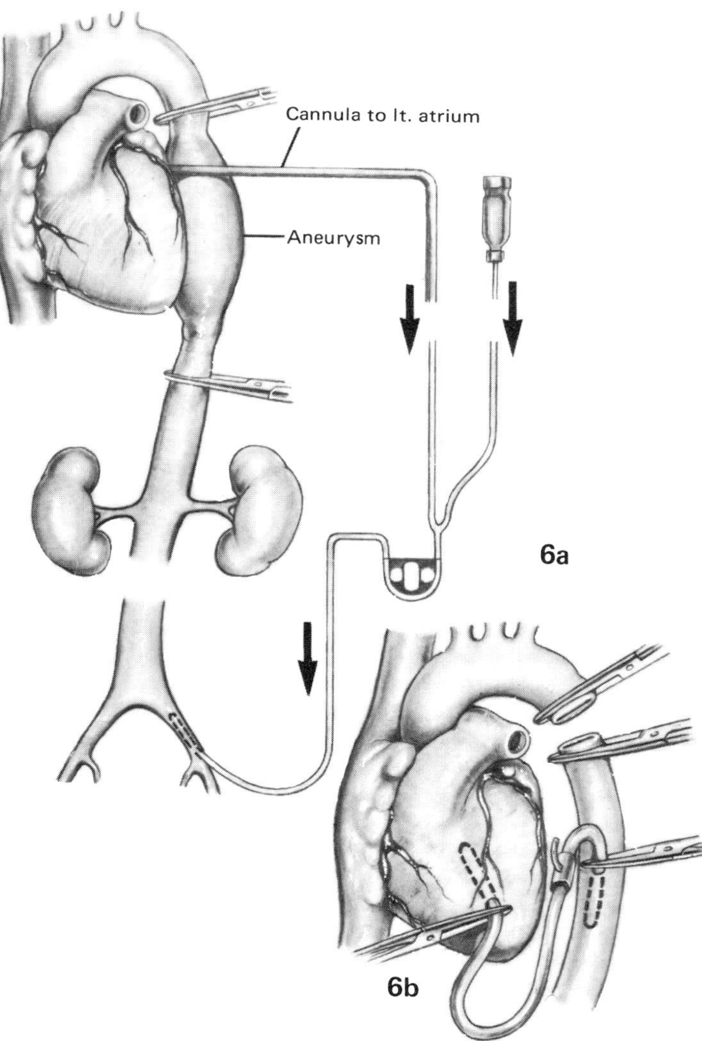

[*The illustrations for this Chapter on Methods of Providing Facilities for Open Heart Surgery were drawn by Mr. G. Lyth.*]

Drainage of the Pericardium and Pericardiectomy

Ronald Belsey, M.S., F.R.C.S.
Consulting Thoracic Surgeon, Frenchay Hospital, Bristol

and

Revised by
Charles Drew, F.R.C.S.
Consultant Thoracic Surgeon, Westminster Hospital
and St. George's Hospital, London

PRE-OPERATIVE

PERICARDIECTOMY

Indications

Fibrous thickening or calcification of the pericardium is not an absolute indication for pericardiectomy as these abnormalities may be found on routine examination of patients showing no evidence of cardiac disability. Only when evidence of cardiac restriction and tamponade is accompanied by subjective and objective disability is pericardiectomy indicated. The rise in the venous pressure, the extent of the ascitic and pleural effusions and the rapidity of their recurrence following aspiration afford some evidence of the severity of the tamponade. Impaired liver function is an indication for surgical treatment as the damage may become irreversible if the tamponade remains unrelieved for too long.

Special pre-operative preparation

If fluid retention is present a course of diuretics is indicated prior to operation. Pleural and ascitic effusions should be aspirated. Oral and dental foci of infection should be eliminated. Vitamins C and K are given. The sooner breathing exercises are started before operation, the quicker will be the postoperative return of full thoracic function. Operation should be delayed until the maximum diuretic effect has been obtained. The final pre-operative aspirations from the serous cavities should be carried out about 4 days before operation.

It is assumed that any previous tuberculous infection of the pericardium will have reached a stage of quiescence, but if a raised sedimentation rate suggests that activity persists, a pre-operative course of antituberculous drugs is given and continued into the postoperative period. The postoperative dosage will be dictated by the operative findings and the histological appearance of the resected pericardium.

DRAINAGE OF THE PERICARDIUM

Indications

Acute suppurative pericarditis may necessitate open drainage of the pericardium but equally good results can usually be obtained by repeated aspiration of the pericardium, injection of the appropriate antibiotic into the pericardium, and systemic chemotherapy. The infection usually complicates a generalized pyaemia or some suppurative intrathoracic infection.

In practice, the diagnosis is frequently missed, the signs of the suppurative pericarditis being overshadowed by those of the primary infection. There should be no hesitation in needling the pericardium if infection is suspected.

Anaesthesia

The operation can be performed under local anaesthesia if the patient is too ill to tolerate a general anaesthetic.

Drainage by aspiration

Two routes are available: (*1*) anterior; the needle is inserted through the anterior end of the fifth intercostal space, 1 inch (2·5 cm) lateral to the left border of the sternum to avoid the internal mammary artery; and (*2*) inferior; the needle is inserted upwards and backwards at an angle of 45° between the xiphoid process and the left costal margin.

The inferior route is to be preferred as aspiration through the anterior approach carries some risk of infecting the left pleural cavity.

Loculation of the pus in the pericardial cavity readily occurs if the infection is not quickly controlled by aspiration and antibiotics. Increasing difficulty in aspiration, accompanied by evidence of continued toxaemia due to the infection, should lead to a revision of the programme. Open drainage should be carried out in order that all loculi may be adequately drained.

THE OPERATIONS

Anaesthesia

In the presence of the more severe degrees of tamponade the patient should be transported to the theatre propped on four or five pillows, and may have to be anaesthetized in this position which can be maintained during operation if the congestion of the head and neck cause embarrassment to the anaesthetist.

Two factors have to be borne in mind by the anaesthetist: (*1*) the presence of liver damage; and (*2*) both pleural cavities may be opened during the operation.

Patients with liver damage tolerate morphine very badly and respiration may become unduly depressed. Alternative premedication is indicated before operation.

OPEN DRAINAGE OF THE PERICARDIUM

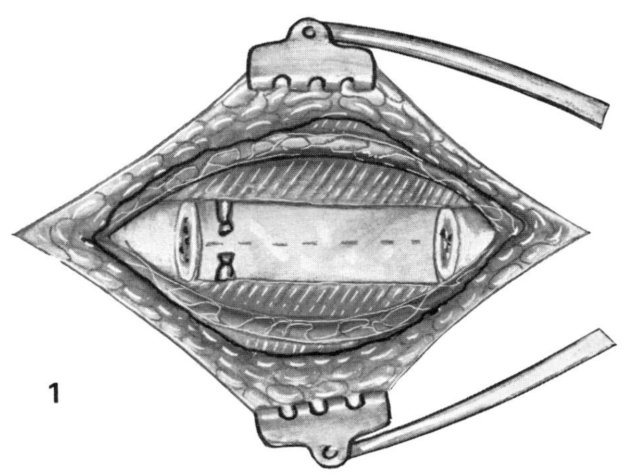

1

1

A short transverse incision is made over the fifth costal cartilage. The whole of this cartilage is resected subperichondrially. The internal mammary vessels are ligated and divided. The pericardium is then opened through the bed of the cartilage taking care to avoid opening the left pleural cavity.

The finger is then inserted into the pericardial cavity to ensure that no loculated collections of pus remain undrained. Drainage is maintained by several strips of soft rubber drain, securely anchored with safety pins, but owing to the complicated nature of the pericardial cavity loculation is prone to occur, especially posterior to the heart.

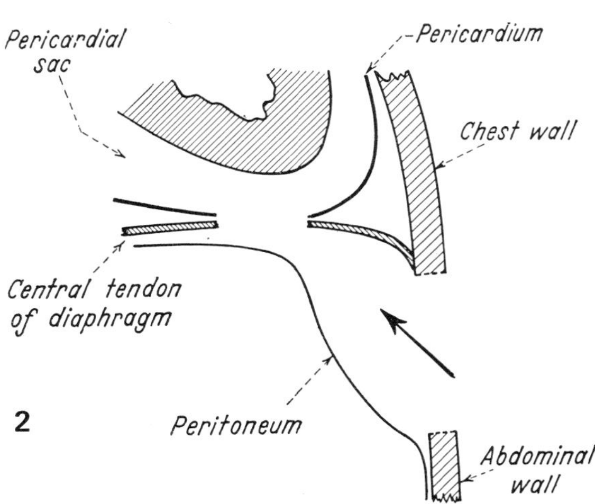

2

2

Inferior route

A vertical incision is made in the angle between the xiphisternum and the left costal margin. The rectus sheath is incised vertically and the incision deepened in the extraperitoneal plane, through the gap between the xiphoid and costal portions of the diaphragm. The pericardial cavity is then opened and drained on its inferior aspect at the most dependent point.

A schematic representation of the inferior approach to the pericardial sac for purposes of open drainage is shown.

PERICARDIECTOMY

Aim of the operation

The aim of the operation is the removal of the restricting layer of fibrous tissue that surrounds the ventricles. The phenomenon of tamponade and its sequelae are largely a manifestation of ventricular restriction. Constriction of the orifices of the great veins, or the auriculoventricular groove, plays little or no part in the functional disability that results. It is therefore not necessary to increase the risk of the operation by extending the pericardial resection to these areas.

It is of the greatest importance that the left ventricle be released before the right ventricle; re-

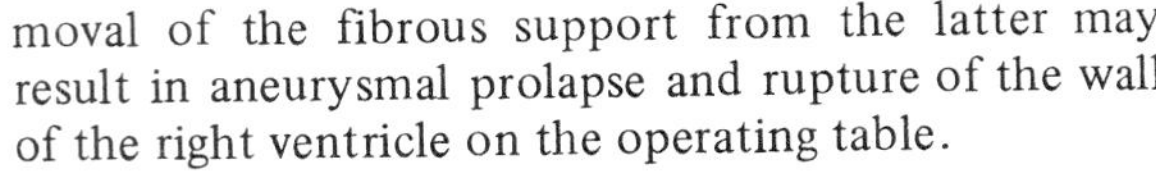

moval of the fibrous support from the latter may result in aneurysmal prolapse and rupture of the wall of the right ventricle on the operating table.

Blood transfusion

A saline drip should be started before operation and blood should be available in case a ventricle is perforated, but routine transfusion during operation is contra-indicated by the circulatory congestion already present.

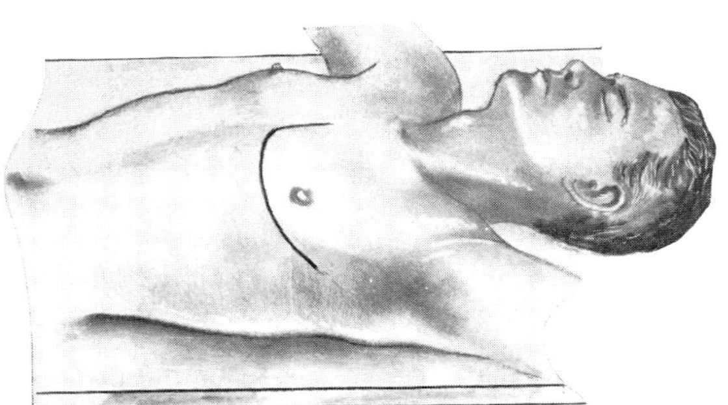

3

3

The incision

The patient is placed on the operating table in the dorsal supine position. A curved anterolateral incision is made over the fourth left interspace, carried laterally upwards towards the axilla and curved up medially over the sternum to the level of the third costal cartilage. In the female patient the incision follows the submammary sulcus. The pectoral muscle is dissected from the ribs, cartilages, and sternum, and reflected upwards with the breast.

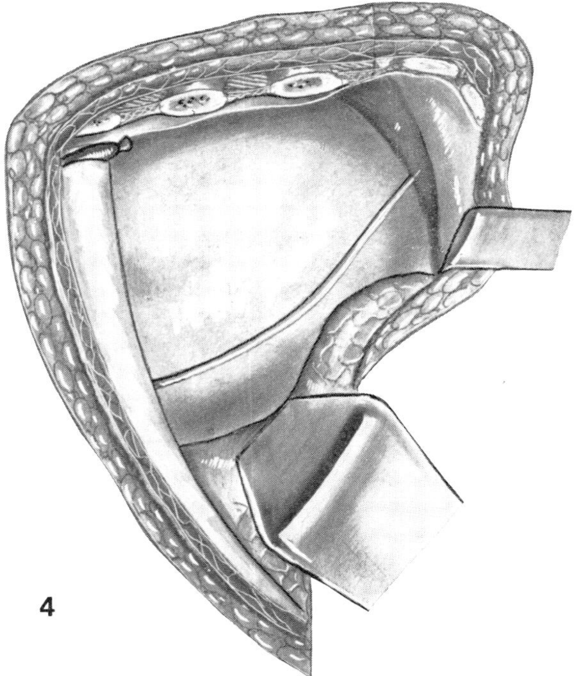

4

4

Exposure

The periosteum is stripped from the upper border of the fifth rib and the left pleural cavity entered through the bed of this rib. If this exposure is inadequate half-inch segments are now resected subperichondrially from the third, fourth and fifth costal cartilages close to the sternum. The internal mammary artery is ligated and divided. The anterior ends of the third, fourth and fifth intercostal bundles are divided. Mechanical retraction should give an adequate exposure, but further costal cartilages can be divided if necessary.

There is no point in attempting to perform the operation in the extrapleural plane. The pleura is usually torn during the operation and in the event of any postoperative haemorrhage the blood is more easily aspirated from the pleural cavity than it is from the mediastinum.

5

Additional exposure

The mediastinal pleura is unusually adherent to the parietal pericardium. The phrenic nerve is dissected free, carefully preserved and displaced backwards towards the hilum of the lung.

The restriction of ventricular activity is immediately obvious. A cruciform incision is made with great care into the thickened parietal pericardium over the left ventricle and deepened until the edges of the incision spring apart. Using the corners of the flaps for retraction, a plane of separation is sought beneath them by gentle finger dissection or with a small swab on a holder. The interventricular branches of the left coronary artery are constantly sought, to obviate their damage and as a guide to ventricular topography.

Whether the plane of cleavage corresponds to the original pericardial cavity or runs between the visceral pericardium and the myocardium is not easy to determine. There may still appear to be a thin layer of fibrous tissue overlying the myocardium, but this appears to play little part in restricting the ventricles and any attempt to remove it incurs the risk of damage to the coronary vessels or perforation of the myocardium.

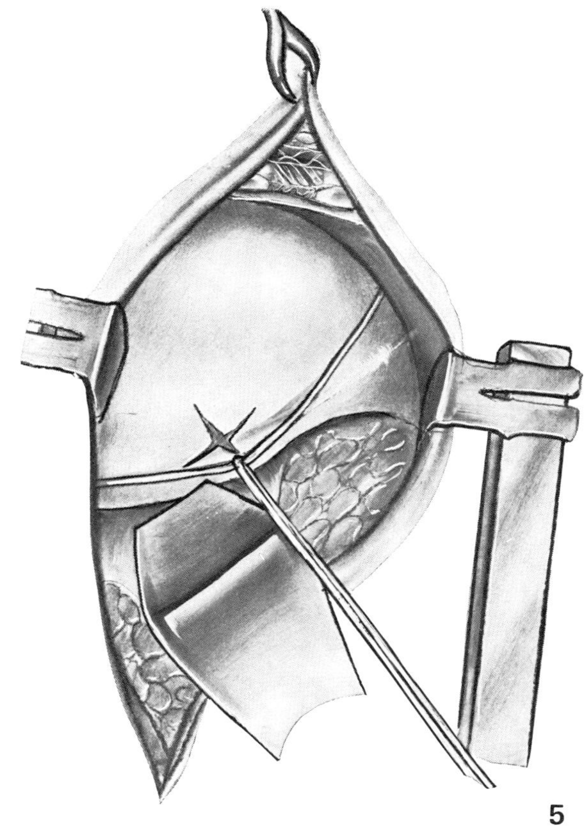

5

6

Left ventricle

The pericardial incisions are extended and the plane of separation developed over the left ventricle. As the ventricle is released from its fetters so the amplitude of cardiac movement increases dramatically. The anaesthetist may detect an immediate improvement in the patient's circulation.

The raised flaps of thickened pericardium should not be excised until the dissection is complete. The myocardium is atrophic as a result of disuse and may be perforated by the dissecting finger or instrument. The perforation can be closed by suturing a flap of thickened pericardium down to the myocardium, provided the flaps have been retained against this eventuality.

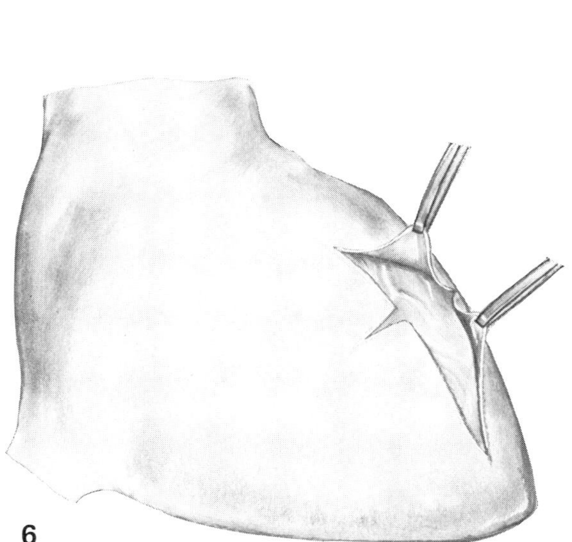

6

7

Right ventricle

After the left ventricle has been uncovered the pericardial resection is extended over the right ventricle. Ideally the whole of the ventricular pericardium should be resected but this is seldom possible.

The pericardial resection must be pursued with extreme caution to avoid damage to the coronary vessels. The restricting membrane is usually the outermost layer and to carry the dissection too deep in an effort to resect visceral pericardium may end in disaster.

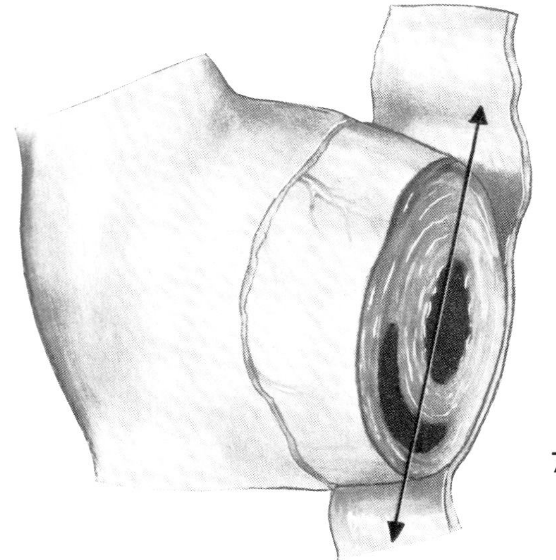

7

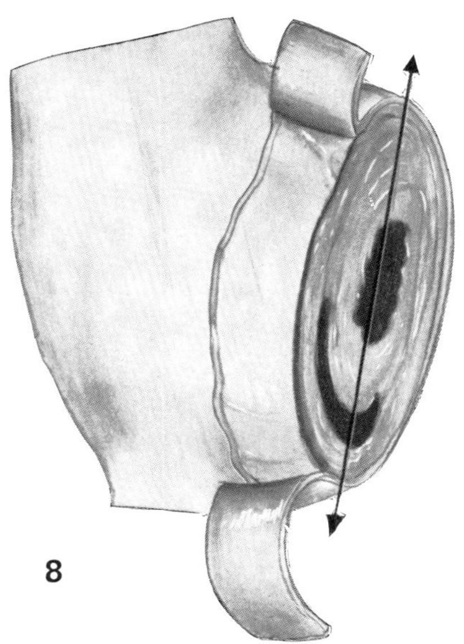

8

8

Further resection

A satisfactory functional result can be obtained by carrying the resection beyond the 'meridian' of the ventricles in all directions, so that any contraction of the remaining portion of pericardium tends further to uncover the ventricles. It is unnecessary to extend the resection beyond the atrioventricular groove, or to include the orifices of the great veins.

The calcified pericardium is removed in the same manner. The calcification may extend into the myocardium. The dissection should be discontinued in this area in view of the risk of perforating the ventricle, and the islands of calcified pericardium thus abandoned will probably not jeopardize the success of the operation.

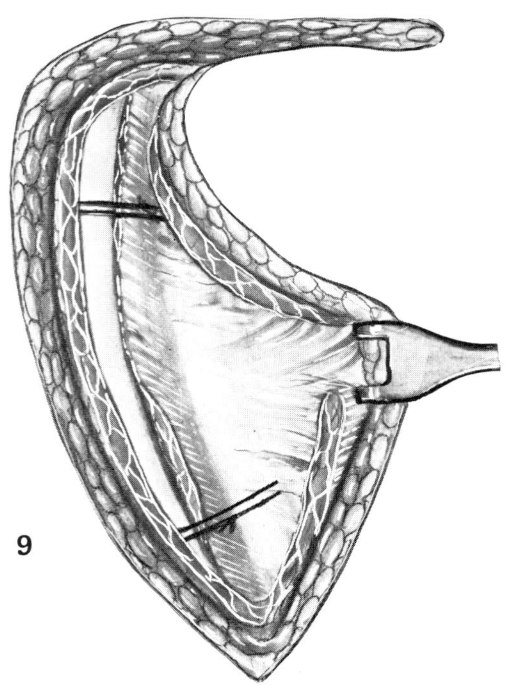

9

9

Closure

An intercostal catheter is inserted into the left pleural cavity for later attachment to an underwater seal. The fourth and fifth ribs are approximated by pericostal sutures and the intercostal layer repaired. The divided costal cartilages will not require any fixation. The pectoral muscle is sutured back into position by interrupted or continuous sutures and the skin incision closed.

POSTOPERATIVE CARE

The intercostal catheter can be removed as soon as the lungs are fully expanded, usually within 24 hr of operation. The myocardium is in a state of disuse atrophy as a result of the prolonged restriction of its activity and acute cardiac dilatation may occur after operation. Oxygen therapy may be indicated, and good nursing can spare the patient any undue exertion likely to aggravate the cardiac dilatation. Digitalis is indicated if excessive tachycardia or auricular fibrillation supervene. Breathing exercises should be resumed as soon as the patient regains consciousness. Postoperative administration of morphine is avoided if possible, and replaced by other analgesics.

Aspiration of the serous cavities may have to be repeated once or twice after the operation, but once the myocardium has regained its tone the effusions rapidly disappear. Assuming that histological examination of the resected pericardium reveals no evidence of active tuberculous infection, the rehabilitation of the patient can proceed rapidly.

References

Churchill, E. D. (1936). *Ann. Surg.* **104**, 516
Hewer, G. J. and Stewart, H. J. (1939). *Surgery Gynec. Obstet.* **68**, 979
Sellors, T. Holmes (1946). 'Constrictive pericarditis.' *Br. J. Surg.* **33**, 215
Stewart, H. J. and Bailey, R. L. (1941). *Am. Heart J.* **22**, 169

[*The illustrations for this Chapter on Drainage of the Pericardium and Pericardiectomy were drawn by Mr. G. Lyth.*]

Pulmonary Embolectomy

M. Paneth, F.R.C.S.
Consultant Cardiothoracic Surgeon, The Brompton Hospital, London

GENERAL CONSIDERATIONS

There are two lines of treatment available for the management of the critically ill patient with acute massive pulmonary embolism. These are: (*1*) pulmonary embolectomy; (*2*) thrombolytic therapy.

Which of these is appropriate will depend on the clinical state of the patient, the effectiveness of resuscitation and the response to pharmacological support.

After the usual resuscitative measures an accurate assessment of the patient's clinical status is obtained by measurement of the following parameters:

(*1*) the central venous pressure;

(*2*) the arterial pressure obtained by radial artery cannulation;

(*3*) hourly urine flow;

(*4*) peripheral skin temperature.

Patients may broadly be divided into two groups:

'Non-shock' group. In this group the urine flow does not fall below 20 ml/hr, the central venous pressure is not rising, the blood pressure is maintained at 80 mmHg or above without the use of increasing doses of peripheral vasopressors and the peripheral skin temperature rises.

For these patients thrombolytic therapy with streptokinase is justified and will produce excellent results if administered for 72 hr. Improvement in the patient's clinical state will be noticeable during the first 12 hr. Failure to respond to this treatment is an indication for urgent embolectomy.

'Shock' group. These patients are not expected to survive 12 hr, their urine flow falls below 20 ml/hr, the blood pressure has to be maintained by the administration of increasing amounts of vasopressors and the skin temperature fails to rise. Emergency pulmonary embolectomy should be performed.

Conventional anticoagulation, i.e. Heparin, followed by Warfarin, has no place in the primary treatment of massive acute pulmonary embolism. Pulmonary embolectomy is also indicated if there are other contra-indications to thrombolytic therapy, and these are:

(*1*) an operation within the preceding 72 hr;

(*2*) severe systemic hypertension or previous cerebrovascular accident;

(*3*) coagulation defect;

(*4*) recent history of gastro-intestinal ulceration or haemorrhage.

PULMONARY EMBOLECTOMY

Optimum operating conditions are obtained by the use of total cardiopulmonary bypass; the immediate availability of sterile, disposable oxygenators of various types has made any other technique obsolete and only necessary when an 'open heart team' is not available on a standby basis.

Contrary to the reports from some other centres our experience with patients from a distance of up to 60 miles suggests that, after successful initial resuscitation and inspite of progressive deterioration, they can still be transported to a suitable centre equipped for modern pulmonary embolectomy.

General anaesthesia should be delayed until the surgical team is scrubbed-up, the bypass equipment is fully primed, the patient is connected in the operating room to the electrocardiograph and with the arterial and central venous pressures continuously displayed. Intermittent estimations of the blood pressure by cuff techniques are unsuitable in these severely vasoconstricted patients. Intravenous thiopentone and succinylcholine anaesthesia at a minimal dosage is used to permit intubation. The inevitable fall in blood pressure, which accompanies this, is anticipated and counteracted by adding a small dose of metaraminol (Aramine) to the thiopentone syringe. Further small doses of this vasopressor or even adrenaline may be required to maintain a recordable blood pressure up to the moment of instituting cardiopulmonary bypass.

The incision and exposure

A vertical median sternotomy with longitudinal incision of the pericardium affords immediate access to the ascending aorta and right atrium.

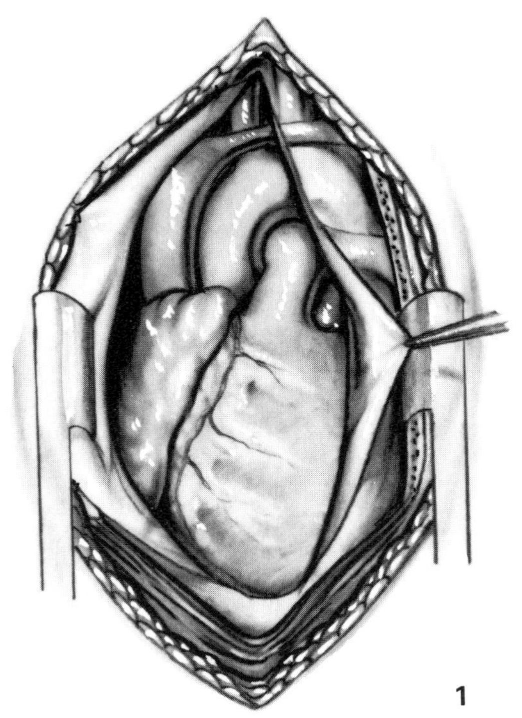

1

2

Placing of cannulae

Heparin in a dose of 2 mg/kg body weight is administered as soon as adequate haemostasis has been achieved and due allowance must be made for the grossly retarded circulation time. If time allows a purse-string suture is placed at the aortic cannulation site, but if the blood pressure is critically depressed, immediate cannulation of the aorta for arterial return and single right atrial cannulation, via its appendage, for venous drainage is performed and these two cannulae are rapidly connected to the arterial and venous limbs of the 'sash' of the bypass circuit in the usual way.

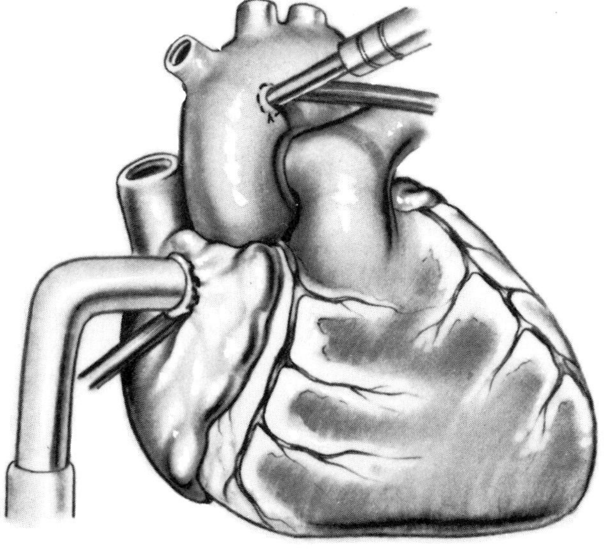

2

Bypass is commenced and continued with the heart beating for a suitable period to allow correction of the severe acid base imbalance and re-adjustment of the high arteriovenous oxygen difference. The institution of cardiopulmonary bypass in itself is beneficial for the following reasons:

(*1*) the right ventricle is relieved of its 'overload';

(*2*) the 'systemic output' and blood pressure (perfusion pressure) are improved;

(*3*) arterial oxygen tension is raised improving cerebral, coronary and renal oxygen supply;

(*4*) general tissue oxygen tension is improved by the reduction in the high arteriovenous oxygen difference.

3

Incision of pulmonary trunk

After a suitable interval of total body perfusion the heart is electrically fibrillated and the pulmonary trunk is opened by a longitudinal incision extending from just distal to the pulmonary valve almost to its bifurcation.

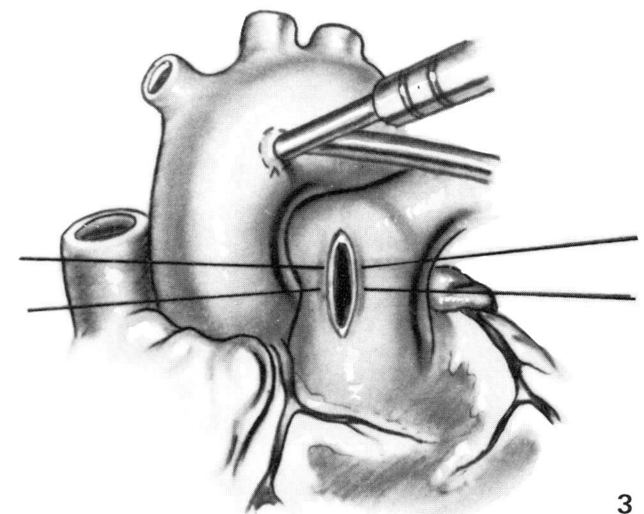

3

4

Embolectomy of pulmonary arteries

By careful use of the cardiotomy sucker the pulmonary trunk is emptied and emboli invariably present in the main pulmonary arteries are slowly and gently extracted with a Desjardin forceps until each pulmonary arterial tree has been inspected to its basal divisions. The strong sucker is next passed down each pulmonary artery in turn to remove impacted embolic fragments and finally the anaesthetist inflates both lungs (Valsalva manoeuvre) to demonstrate reflux of red blood from the pulmonary capillaries into each pulmonary artery in turn thereby demonstrating that the pulmonary arterial tree has been completely cleared on both sides.

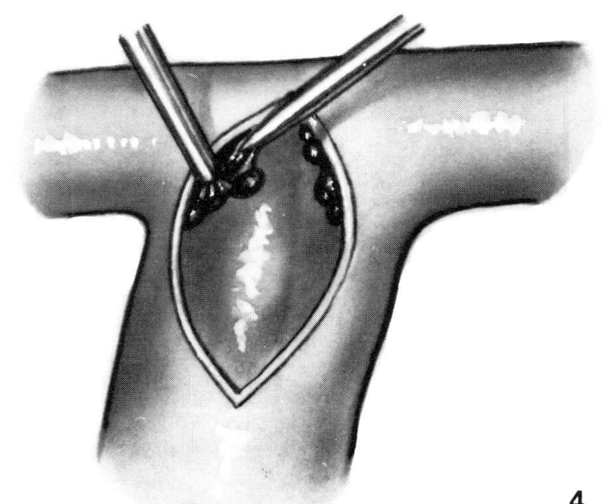

4

5

Closure and drainage

Following repair of the incision in the pulmonary trunk in two layers by continuous monofilament suture, the heart is defibrillated. A period of supportive perfusion may be necessary in cases of severe right ventricular failure and at this stage Isoproterenol (Isoprenaline) may be required by continuous intravenous infusion. After 'weaning off', decannulation and the administration of Protamine in suitable dosage, the pericardium is loosely closed and the sternum approximated over two drainage tubes.

Artificial ventilation may be necessary for a few hours on return to the intensive care unit.

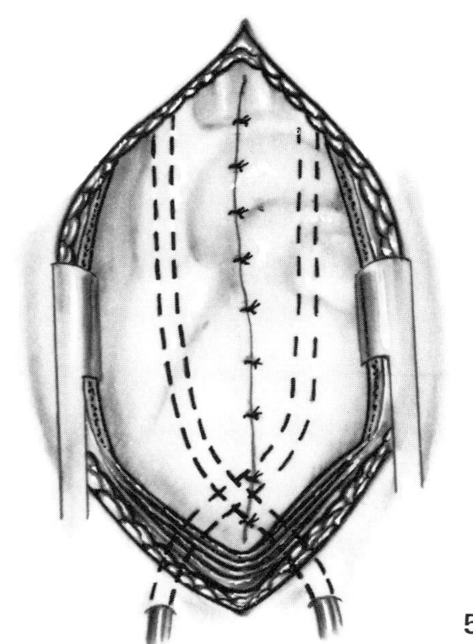

5

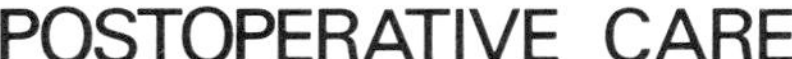

POSTOPERATIVE CARE

Inferior caval ligation has been advocated by some while others have claimed that it significantly lowers the recurrent embolic rate. The author has never interrupted or narrowed the inferior vena cava nor interfered with the systemic venous system in any way. It is advisable that all patients after successful operation or thrombolytic therapy are maintained on oral anticoagulants for a minimum period of 3 months, unless there are overt signs of venous obstruction when anticoagulants should be continued until these have completely resolved or for a minimum period of 6 months, whichever is the longer.

PULMONARY EMBOLECTOMY WITHOUT BYPASS

If a perfusion team is not available then it may be necessary to perform the operation by the technique of inflow occlusion. A vertical median sternotomy is used and after inserting stay sutures in the pulmonary trunk, the inferior vena cava and superior vena cava in that order are occluded with Crafoord clamps. When the cardiac output has fallen, the pulmonary trunk is opened by a longitudinal incision and each pulmonary artery is cleared of emboli with the sucker. The circulation should be restored by clamping the incision of the pulmonary trunk temporarily and then releasing the superior vena cava completely followed by a gradual release of the inferior vena cava so as not to overfill the heart. The whole manoeuvre should not last more than 3 min, but may be repeated after suitable intervals of restoration of the circulation, until satisfactory clearance of each pulmonary artery has been obtained and an adequate circulation has been restored. The operation is completed by suturing the incision in the pulmonary trunk over the clamp and closing the incision routinely.

Summary

Patients with suspected acute massive pulmonary embolism should be resuscitated by external cardiac massage and transferred to the intensive care unit. The diagnosis may then be confirmed by pulmonary arteriography and their treatment will depend on the clinical state.

'Non-shock group'

Blood pressure 80 mmHg or above, urine production 20 ml/hr or more, increasing doses of vasopressors not required. Treatment: *Thrombolytic therapy with streptokinase.*

'Shock group'

Blood pressure 80 mmHg or below, requiring increasing doses of vasopressors, urine production below 20 ml/hr, failure of rise of peripheral skin temperature. Treatment: *Emergency pulmonary embolectomy, preferably with cardiopulmonary bypass.*

The emergency pulmonary embolectomy rate has fallen since this treatment protocol based on clinical trials has been established.

References

Cooley, D. A., Beall, A. C. and Alexander, J. K. (1961). *J. Am. med. Ass.* **177**, 283
Crane, C., Hartsuck, J., Birtch, A., Couch, N. P., Zollinger, R., Matloff, R., Dalen, J. and Dexter, L. (1969). *Surgery Gynec. Obstet.* **128**, 27
Hall, R., Sutton, G. C. and Kerr, I. H. (1975). *Circulation* **52** (suppl. 2), 131
Little, J. M. and Lowenthal, J. (1968). *Surgery Gynec. Obstet.* **127**, 777
Miller, G. A. H., Sutton, G. C., Kerr, I. H., Gibson, R. V. and Honey, M. (1971). *Br. med. J.* **2**, 681
Sasahara, A. A. and Barsamian, E. M. (1973). *Ann. thorac. Surg.* **16**, 317
Sharp, E. H. (1962). *Ann. Surg.* **156**, 1

[*The illustrations for this Chapter on Pulmonary Embolectomy were drawn by Mr. G. Lyth.*]

Patent Ductus Arteriosus

J. D. Wisheart, M.Ch., F.R.C.S.
Cardiac and Thoracic Surgeon, United Bristol Hospitals
and Frenchay Hospital, Bristol

INTRODUCTION

Isolated patent ductus arteriosus is the second most common congenital cardiac anomaly, accounting for 12 per cent of the total. Spontaneous closure is usual in the first few days of life but is rare after the third month. The ductus runs between the pulmonary artery, arising to the left of its bifurcation, and the aorta just distal to the origin of the left subclavian artery. It is thin-walled and may be conical, with the wider part at the aortic end. Its most important anatomical relations are the vagus nerve and its recurrent laryngeal branch, the left main bronchus and the 'lappet' of pericardium which overlies the pulmonary end of the duct.

Blood flow along the ductus is determined by the relative resistances, and hence pressures, in the pulmonary and systemic vascular beds. Patients may present for surgery at any time in the natural history of the lesion. As the neonatal pulmonary vascular resistance falls, the left-to-right shunt increases and left ventricular failure may develop. Later, as pulmonary vascular resistance slowly increases, shunt flow moderates, the threat of left ventricular failure recedes and the patient is usually free of symptoms. Eventually in about 5–7 per cent of cases, pulmonary vascular resistance will rise sufficiently to cause reversal of the shunt and the development of the Eisenmenger complex. In those who survive without shunt reversal, aneurysmal dilatation or calcification of the duct may occur. At any time the small threat (probably about 1 per cent) of bacterial endocarditis is present. A patent ductus arteriosus in association with other congenital abnormalities should be closed at the time of the definitive operation and prior to going on bypass. Finally, the presence of a patent ductus arteriosus in a premature neonate with the respiratory distress syndrome may contribute to pulmonary dysfunction and thus threaten life.

Special investigations are not required for the classical clinical picture of patent ductus arteriosus in childhood. Catheterization is required (*1*) to elucidate any unusual findings and any associated abnormality, (*2*) to determine the level of pulmonary vascular resistance, (*3*) in infants and adults. Surgery should be carried out between the second and fifth years, or at the time of diagnosis if complications are present. Surgery is contra-indicated in the presence of severe pulmonary hypertension with shunt reversal. When associated with other cardiac anomalies, the ductus should usually be closed at the time of total correction and not surgically treated in isolation.

The object of surgery is to interrupt the communication between the pulmonary and systemic circuits, either by division or ligation of the duct. Panagopoulos *et al.* (1971) have shown that ligation is a safe and satisfactory technique in most cases, while division is reserved for the short, wide or high pressure duct. The operative mortality in the uncomplicated ductus is less than 0·5 per cent but is higher in infancy, when associated with other abnormalities, and in the presence of pulmonary hypertension.

In the uncomplicated case pre-operative bacteriological screening and blood count should be carried out and two units of blood should be cross-matched; prophylactic antibiotics should be commenced prior to surgery. An arterial cannula should be inserted in infants; they may also require postoperative mechanical ventilation. When left ventricular failure is present it should be treated with digoxin and diuretics; subacute bacterial endocarditis should be treated with the appropriate antibiotics for at least 6 weeks and some authorities advise a further delay of up to 3 months prior to surgery.

THE OPERATION

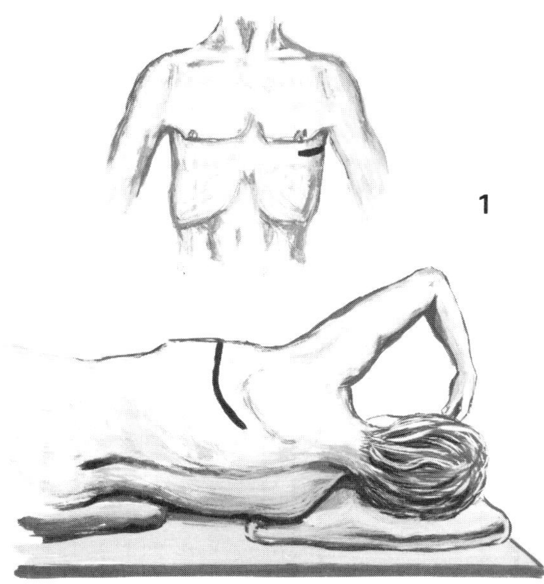

1

1

The incision

Left posterolateral thoracotomy is carried out through the third or fourth intercostal space.

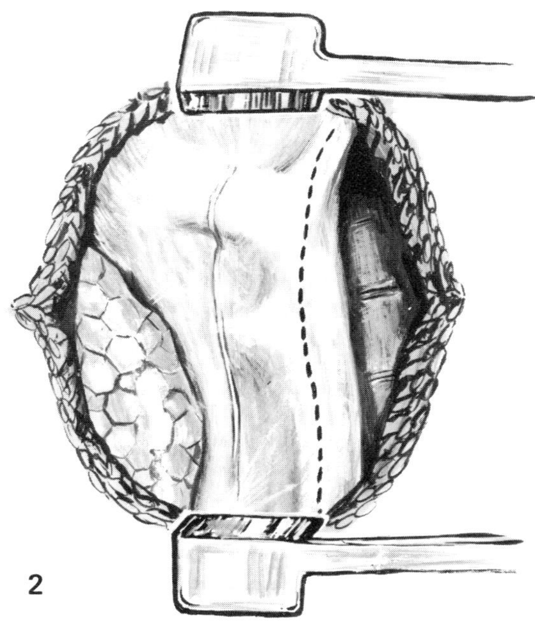

2

2

Surgical anatomy

When the left lung is retracted forward and downward the aortic arch, the left subclavian artery, the pulmonary artery and the vagus and phrenic nerves may be seen. A thrill is palpable, but it is not usual to see the ductus clearly at this stage. The aortic sheath is opened by a vertical incision extending from the left subclavian artery to below the ductus.

3

Dissection of the aortic sheath

After the aortic sheath is reflected forward, using sharp and blunt dissection to maintain the correct plane, it is retracted by stay sutures which also serve to keep the left lung out of the immediate operative field. The posterior part of the aortic sheath is dissected next and tapes passed around the aorta, above and below the ductus, avoiding the intercostal arteries.

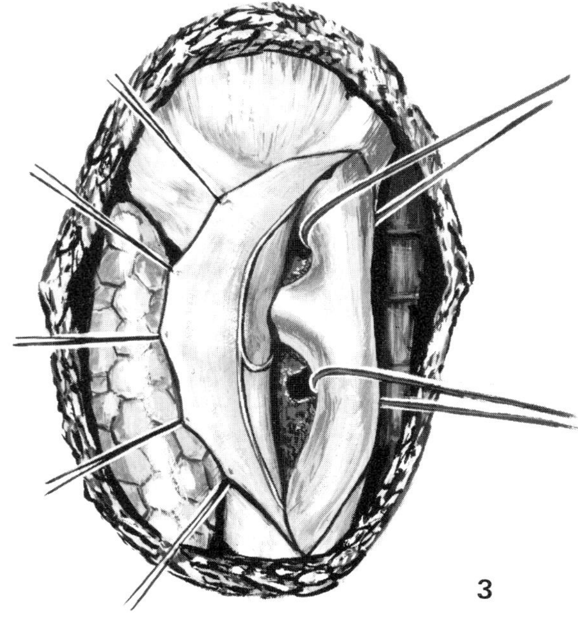

3

4

Identification of the ductus

The aortic end of the ductus may now be seen, and the anatomy of the arch of the aorta is confirmed by identification of the left common carotid artery proximal to the left subclavian artery. Further reflection of the aortic sheath anteriorly permits dissection of the anterior, superior and inferior aspects of the ductus, still in the same tissue plane. The vagus and recurrent laryngeal nerves are reflected safely with the pleura and sheath.

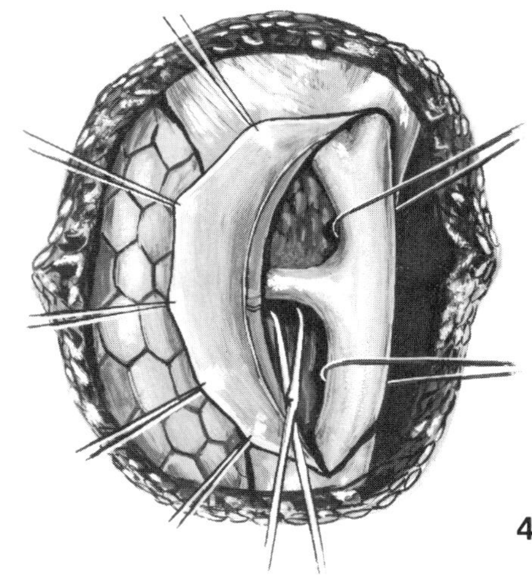

4

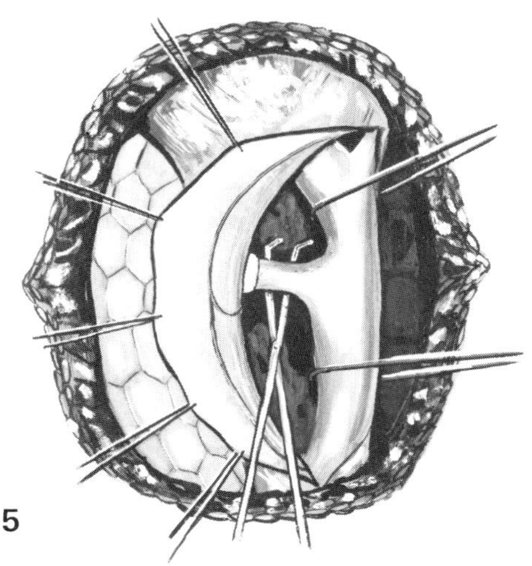

5

5

Dissection of the ductus

Development of the same plane usually permits a right-angled dissecting instrument to be passed around the back of the ductus. If it is difficult to free the back of the ductus, the aorta may be lifted forwards using the tapes, and the dissection completed under direct vision. Gentle lateral retraction of the aorta facilitates dissection of the pulmonary end of the ductus; in particular it may be freed from the pouch of overlying pericardium.

6

Ligation of the ductus

The effects of occluding the ductus should now be observed by 'test-clamping' with a vascular clamp. It is usually sufficient to observe arterial pressure and heart rate. Should the arterial pressure fall, the heart rate rise and, in the presence of known pulmonary vascular disease, the pulmonary artery pressure should be measured before and after clamping. Failure of the pulmonary artery pressure to fall indicates that the operation should not be carried further.

Two ligatures of 1/0 linen or plaited silk are now passed around the ductus, and the aortic end ligated first. Temporary reduction in aortic pressure makes this safe, and is most easily achieved by cross-clamping the aorta above the ductus for the 20 sec needed to apply the first two throws to the knot, which is then completed with the aorta released. The second ligature is applied to the pulmonary end of the ductus, which has now been decompressed. It is important that the two ligatures should be separated.

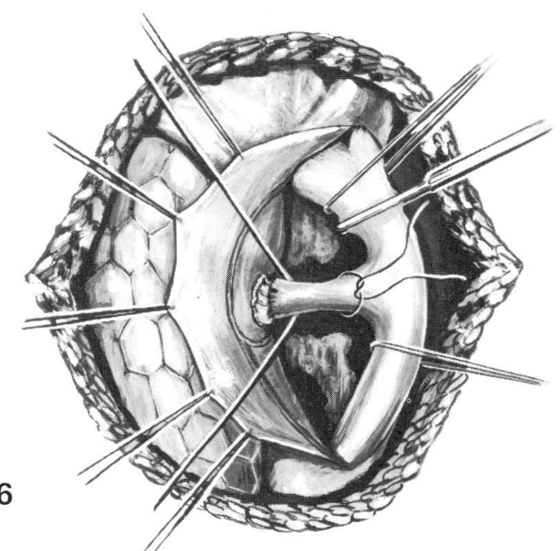

6

7

Closure

When haemostasis is secured, the pleura should be reconstituted over the aorta, a basal intercostal drain inserted, the lung carefully re-inflated and the chest closed.

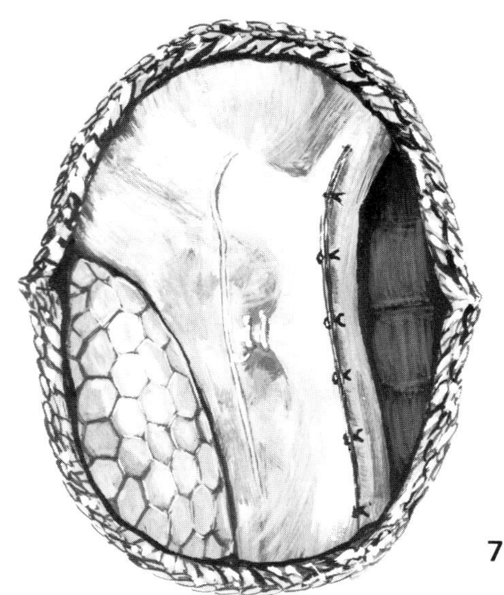

7

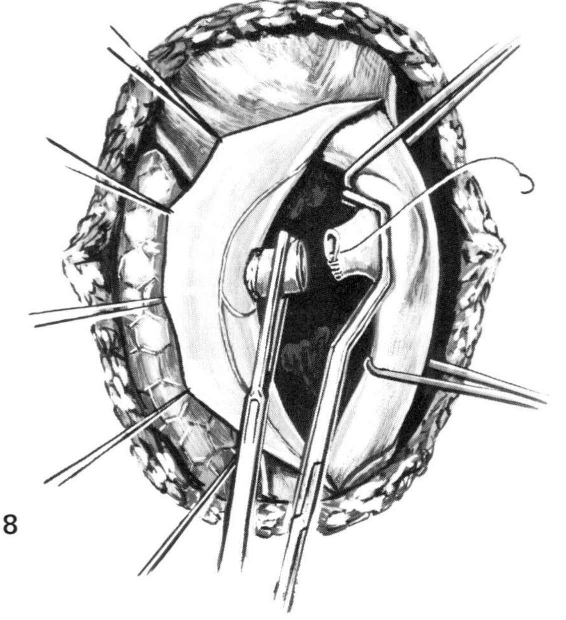

8

8

Division of the ductus

When the ductus is to be divided, two clamps should be applied to the aortic and pulmonary ends. Traditionally a pair of Potts clamps has been used, but if a side-biting clamp is applied to the aorta at the origin of the ductus more secure control is achieved and more room provided for suturing. A Potts clamp is applied at the pulmonary end of the ductus, which is now divided, and its two ends secured with running sutures of 3/0, 4/0 or 5/0 Mersilene or Prolene mounted on an atraumatic needle.

9

Closure of a ductus associated with intracardiac abnormalities

In these circumstances the ductus should be closed at the time of correction of the intracardiac anomaly (McGoon, 1964); control of the ductus should be achieved prior to instituting cardiopulmonary bypass in order to avoid loss of perfusion to the lungs. The most widely used method is that described by Kirklin and Silver (1958), in which the bifurcation of the pulmonary artery is brought into view by digital retraction of the main trunk. The pericardial reflection at the bifurcation is opened, permitting the ductus to be identified and dissected. Ligatures are passed around it, and after cardiopulmonary bypass is established the ductus is closed by multiple ligation. Alternative techniques describe suture closure of the ductus from within the pulmonary artery after cardiopulmonary bypass is established; in these circumstances control of ductal flow may be achieved either by digital pressure followed by hypothermic circulatory arrest, or by placing a Fogarty catheter within the ductus.

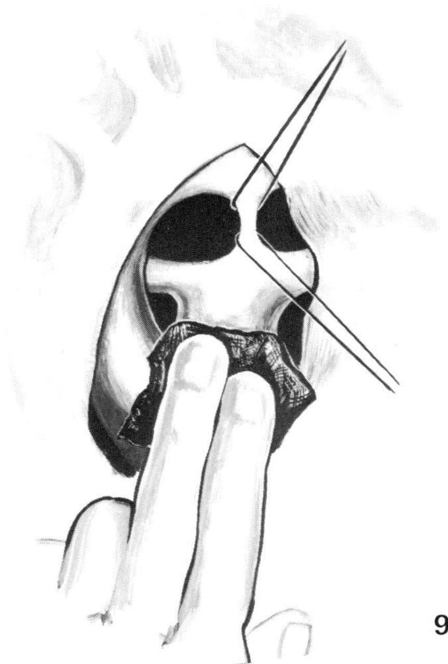

9

10

10

Closure of a calcified or aneurysmal ductus

None of the above techniques is appropriate when closing a complicated ductus in an older patient, as any direct approach is very hazardous. Pifarre, Rice and Nemickas (1973) described a technique in which the aortic end of the ductus is exposed by opening the descending aorta between clamps, and the orifice closed by a patch applied under direct vision. The distal circulation is supported by left atriofemoral or aorto-aortic bypass; heparinization may be avoided if a Gott shunt is used (*see* Chapter on 'Methods of Providing Facilities for Open Heart Surgery', pages 22–25). Flow through the ductus from the pulmonary end may be controlled when the aorta is opened by applying a side-clamp to the pulmonary artery at the origin of the ductus. Alternatively, full cardiopulmonary bypass may be used with both proximal and distal arterial cannulation as described by Morrow and Clark in 1966. With this technique the distal circulation is supported and flow through the ductus is satisfactorily reduced.

POSTOPERATIVE CARE

Most children have an uneventful postoperative course. Antibiotics should be maintained for 5–7 days, the intercostal drain may usually be removed on the day after surgery and the patient mobilized as soon as possible. Hoarseness due to recurrent laryngeal nerve damage is uncommon and usually temporary. Chylothorax is described following surgery for a patent ductus.

In infants full haemodynamic monitoring, with regular arterial gas analysis and ventilatory support may be needed. In those who have had a complicated ductus closed from within the aorta, full postoperative cardiac surgical intensive care is required.

References

Kirklin, J. W. and Silver, A. W. (1958). 'Technique of exposing the ductus arteriosus prior to establishing extracorporeal circulation.' *Mayo Clin. Proc.* **33**, 423

McGoon, D. C. (1964). 'Closure of patent ductus during open heart surgery.' *J. thorac. cardiovasc. Surg.* **48**, 456

Morrow, A. G. and Clark, W. D. (1966), 'Closure of clacified patent ductus arteriosus: A new operative method utilising cardiopulmonary by-pass.' *J. thorac. cardiovasc. Surg.* **51**, 534

Panagopoulos, P. G., Tatooles, C. J., Aberdeen, E., Waterston, D. J. and Bonham-Carter, R. E. (1971). 'Patent ductus arteriosus in infants and children. A review of 936 operations (1946–69).' *Thorax* **26**, 137

Pifarre, R., Rice, P. L. and Nemickas, R. (1973). 'Surgical treatment of calcified patent ductus arteriosus.' *J. thorac. cardiovasc. Surg.* **65**, 635

[*The illustrations for this Chapter on Patent Ductus Arteriosus were drawn by Mr. C. Tyrell.*]

Coarctation of the Aorta

A. Logan, F.R.C.S.
Formerly, Reader in Thoracic Surgery, University of Edinburgh

and

Revised by
Charles Drew, F.R.C.S.
Consultant Thoracic Surgeon, Westminster Hospital
and St. George's Hospital, London

PRE-OPERATIVE

Indications

Coarctation of the aorta is rare except in close relation to the attachment of the ligamentum arteriosum or ductus arteriosus. Most cases are asymptomatic and a firm prognosis in the individual case cannot usually be made. The indications for surgical removal of the aortic obstruction are based on the frequency of death before the age of 40 from some complication of arterial hypertension, such as intracranial haemorrhage, heart failure or aortic rupture. Resection of the coarcted segment of the aorta with end-to-end anastomosis, providing a lumen of approximately normal size, is the operation of choice (Crafoord and Nylin, 1945; Gross, 1945). Patients between the ages of 5 and 40 years found to have coarctation of the aorta severe enough to cause hypertension in the upper limbs and delay or weakness of the femoral pulse should have the coarctation resected. The operation is best performed about the age of 8 years when the aorta has the elasticity of childhood and yet has a large lumen. Above the age of 40 and below the age of 5, operation may be necessary for the relief of symptoms, or because of increasing left ventricular hypertrophy, or because an aneurysm has developed above or below the coarctation. The operation is performed in infancy when heart failure caused by the coarctation does not fully respond to medical treatment.

Contra-indications

There is nothing to be gained from resection of the coarctation when there is an associated anomaly with a worse prognosis unless this too can be corrected, as in the case of associated congenital stenosis of the aortic valve.

Special equipment

Clamps, such as those designed by Potts, are required for aortic occlusion.

A Dacron (Terylene) prosthesis of aortic size must be available to allow reconstruction of the aorta if the gap after removal of the coarctation should be too great to allow approximation of the aortic ends; a rare occurrence except when an aneurysm is resected along with the coarctation.

Blood is prepared for transfusion.

Anaesthesia

General anaesthesia with tracheal intubation and controlled respiration is ideal. Manipulation of the aorta and its branches is made easier, especially in adults, if hypotension is induced by a ganglion-blocking drug such as a hexamethonium or thiophanium derivative (Arfonad).

Position of patient

The right lateral position for standard left throacotomy is used.

THE OPERATION

1

Thoracotomy

A long left lateral thoracotomy is made (*see* Chapter on 'Surgical Access in Pulmonary Operations', page 255). Although the parietal arteries, particularly those in the substance of the latissimus dorsi muscle, are abnormally large, there is little blood loss if the muscles are divided a short segment at a time, while firm digital pressure is applied on each side of the incision until the vessels are secured. They are ligated, not sealed with diathermy. The upper border of the fourth or fifth rib is stripped of its periosteum from the tip of the transverse process to the costochondral junction and the pleural space is opened through the bed of the rib.

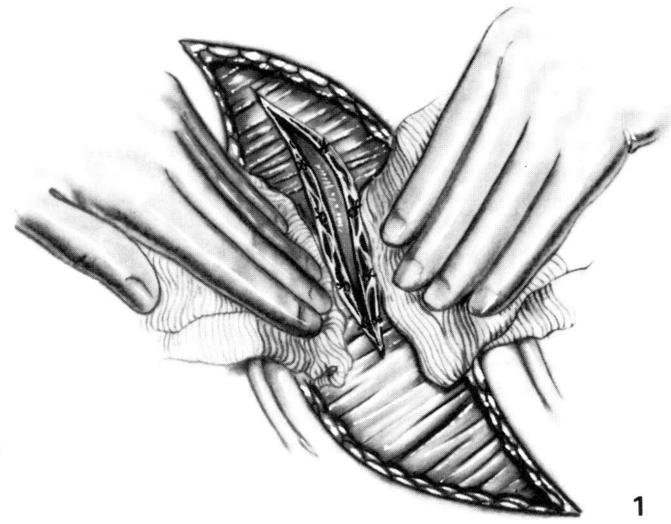

1

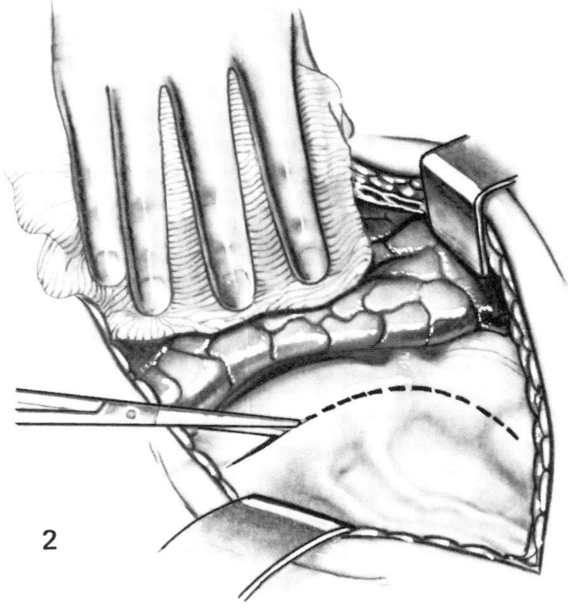

2

2

Exposure of aorta

The wound is opened to its full extent. The lung is displaced downwards and forwards to expose the left subclavian artery, the coarctation and the post-stenotic dilatation of the descending aorta. The left superior intercostal vein is divided as it passes across the aortic arch near the origin of the left subclavian artery. The mediastinal pleura and aortic sheath are incised to expose the coarctation and the proximal part of the descending aorta, and the incision is continued upwards on the left subclavian artery.

3

Mobilization of aorta

The aortic sheath is reflected and fixed by sutures to the wound towels. In addition to giving a constant exposure this helps in the retraction of the lung and displaces the vagus nerve and its recurrent branch from the area of operation. The lower part of the left subclavian artery and the aortic arch from the left common carotid origin to the coarctation are mobilized. The lower border of the whole aortic arch is brought into view. It is rare to need to tie any vessel during this dissection. The ligamentum arteriosum is ligated and divided or the ductus arteriosus is divided between clamps and each end is closed with a fine suture. It is then safe to mobilize the aorta distal to the coarctation. This sometimes requires the division of one or more intercostal arteries. The arterial sheath is opened and fine silk ligatures are placed before the division of the artery.

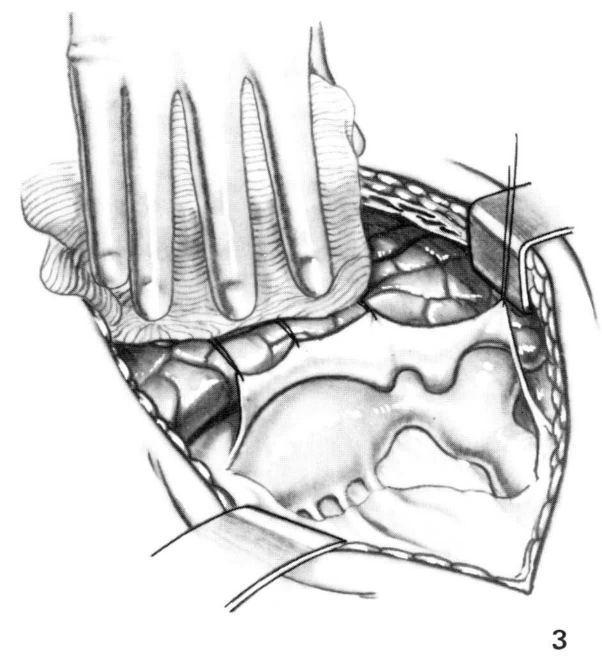

3

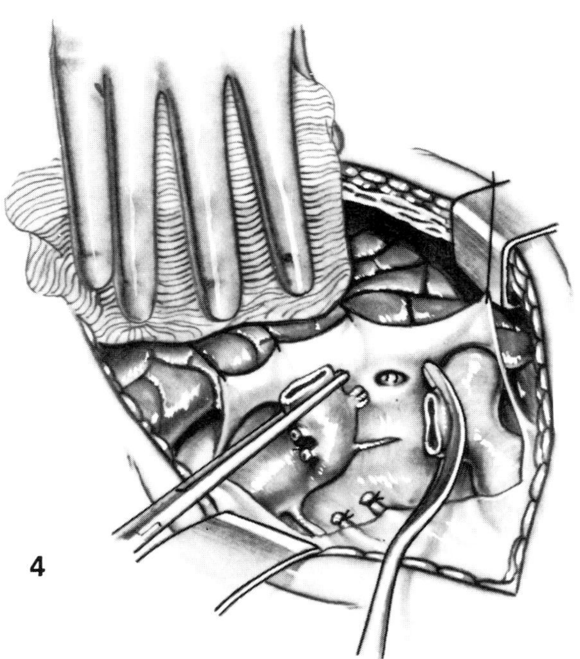

4

4

Control of right intercostal arteries

Recognition and ligation of the right intercostal arteries are aided by light traction on tapes placed round the aorta close to the coarctation. If difficulty is encountered in ligation of the right intercostal arteries or if bleeding occurs the aorta, already mobilized, may be divided between clamps close above and below the coarctation. This allows the distal segment to be turned down, giving a good exposure of its deep surface and the vessels to be dissected.

5

Occlusion of aorta and excision of coarctation

The extent of coarcted aorta which must be removed in order to leave a channel equal to that of the aorta at the origin of the left subclavian artery is estimated. Clamps are applied 1 cm from the proposed lines of section, their handles lying in the posterior end of the parietal incision. When the segment of aorta between the subclavian artery and the coarctation is short, it is necessary to include both the subclavian artery and the aortic arch in the proximal clamp or to occlude them separately. The aorta is divided at the upper and lower limits of the coarctation. The upper line of section may be oblique, higher on the left than on the right, to adapt the size of the upper lumen to that of the lower and to give a smooth line to the left wall of the aorta.

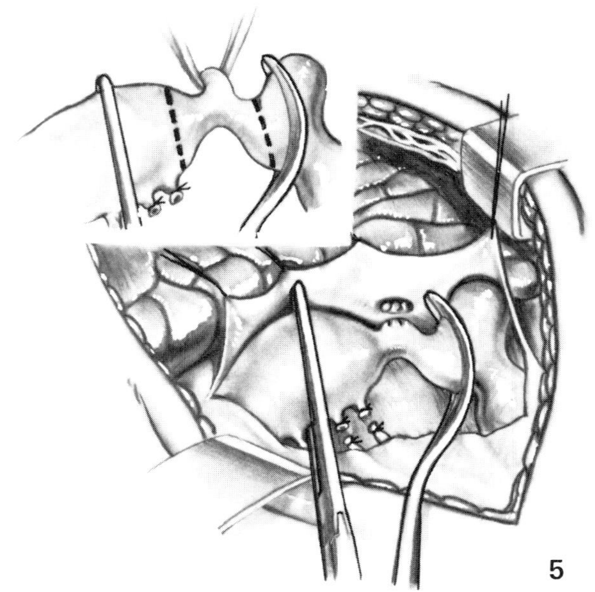

5

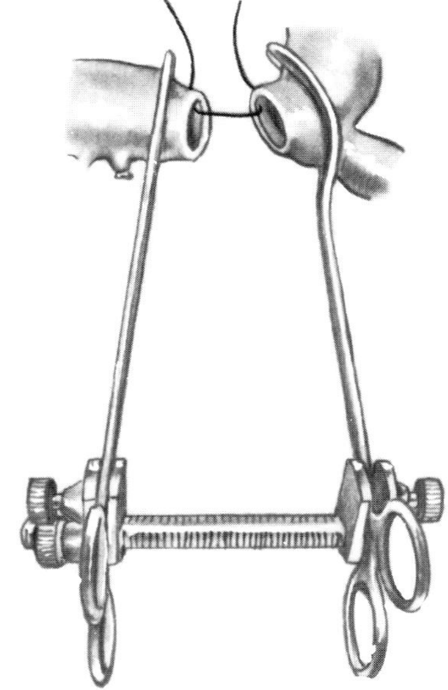

6

6

Control of aortic clamps

For reconstruction of the aorta, constant approximation of the clamps must be maintained so that the introduction of sutures is easy and the suture line takes no strain while it is incomplete. The approximation can usually be done manually by the first assistant. Sometimes, however, the tension on the aorta is such as to make it difficult to keep the open ends of the aorta in a steady relationship. This difficulty can be overcome by the use of the vice designed by Brom which holds and approximates the clamps. The handles of the clamps are divergent when they are first fixed in the vice but narrowing the gap between them by the thumbscrew, with consequent traction on the aorta, renders the clamps parallel.

7

The anastomosis

For the anastomosis, atraumatic sutures of 4/0 Mersilk are used but fine Prolene sutures are probably more suitable in children. A continuous over-and-over or mattress posterior suture is introduced first, beginning at the side furthest from the operator where defects in the suture line are most liable to occur; care must be taken to leave no gap. The posterior aortic wall is exposed by rotation of the clamps so that their handles lie anteriorly. If this cannot readily be done, the suture, after the first fixed loop, can equally well be introduced from the lumen of the aorta. In an adult, a similar suture closes the anterior wall, but in a child the anterior sutures should be interrupted in the hope of favouring increase in size of the lumen at the suture line.

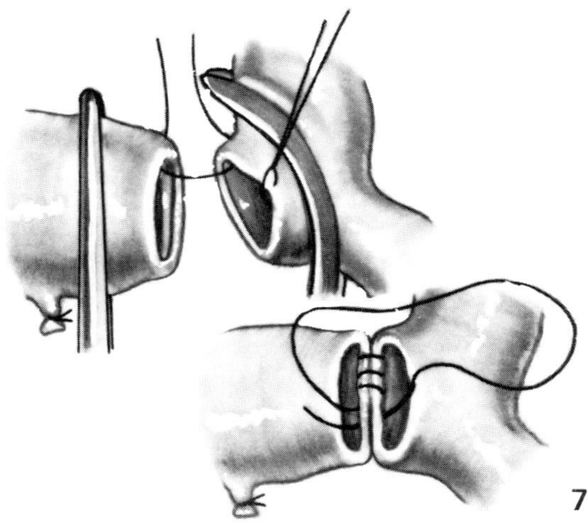

7

8

Removal of clamps

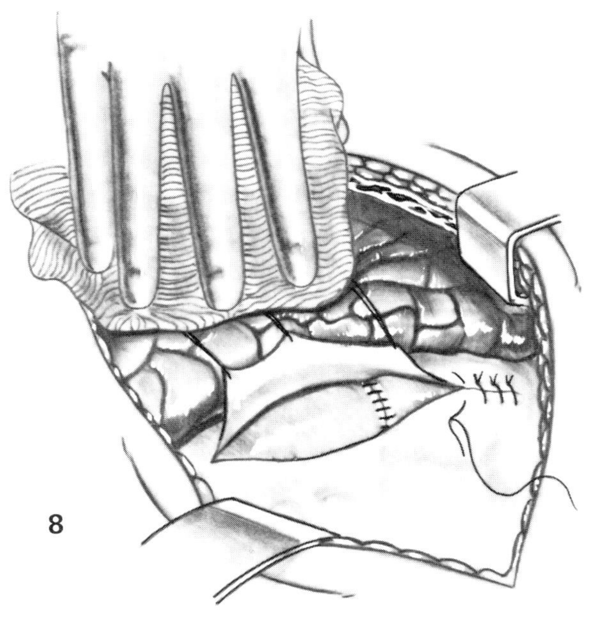

8

When the anastomosis is complete and approximation of the clamps is no longer necessary, the distal clamp is loosened. If there is free bleeding from a gap in the suture line the distal clamp is re-applied and an additional suture is introduced. If there is little bleeding or bleeding only from needle holes, both clamps are removed and digital pressure is applied to the anastomosis until bleeding has ceased. Removal of the clamps may be followed by an immediate and excessive fall in blood pressure. Transfusion of blood and partial occlusion of the aorta will restore the pressure.

Induced hypotension is ended. The mediastinal pleura and aortic sheath are repaired with interrupted fine catgut sutures. A low intercostal drain is introduced and attached to a water-seal. Particular care is taken in the final inspection of the wound to ensure haemostasis. On recovery from anaesthesia the systemic blood pressure may rise even above its pre-operative level and cause bleeding from the very large parietal vessels.

The chest wall is closed in layers.

9a-d

Long coarctations

Rarely the excised segment is so long that reconstruction by end-to-end anastomosis of the aorta is impossible. In an adult a prosthetic tube of Terylene is used to bridge the gap.

Alternatively, the coarcted segment may be slit open in its whole length and a gusset of Terylene fabric introduced. This has the merit of retaining all the potentially growing aortic tissue (Vosschulte, 1961).

When coarctation of the aorta occurs at a rare site, such as the distal end of the thoracic aorta or upper end of the abdominal aorta, the length of the narrow segment usually prohibits end-to-end anastomosis and a prosthetic tube or gusset is required.

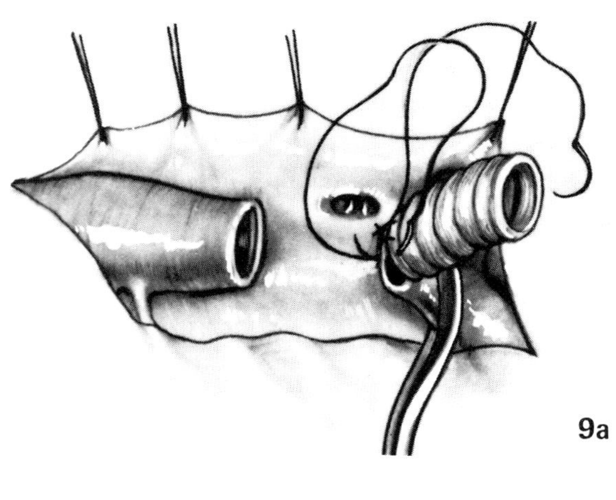

9a

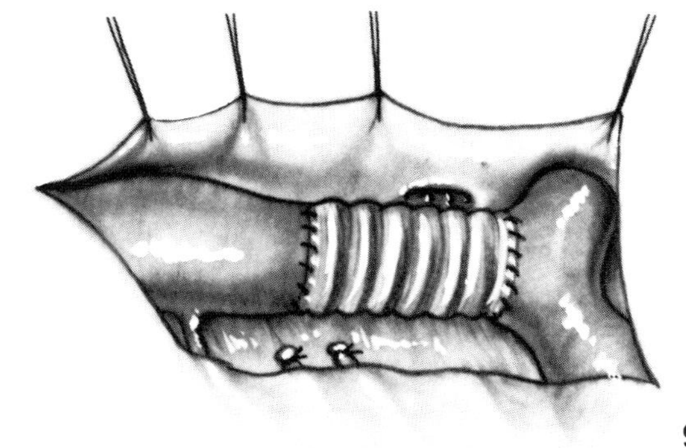

9b

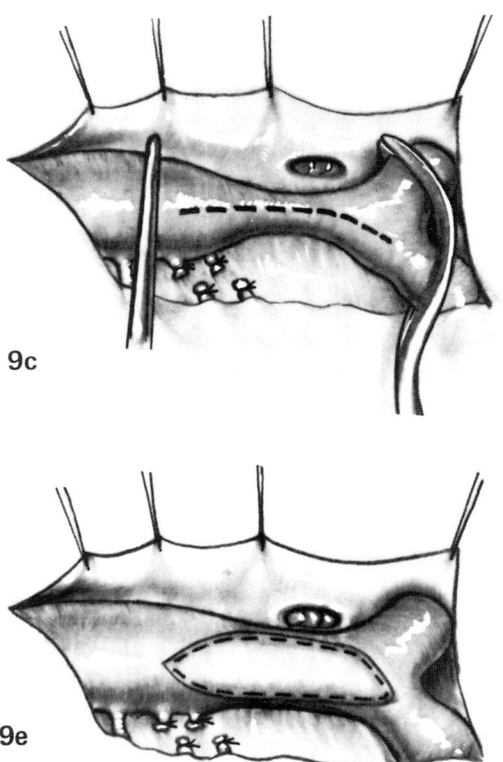

9c

9e

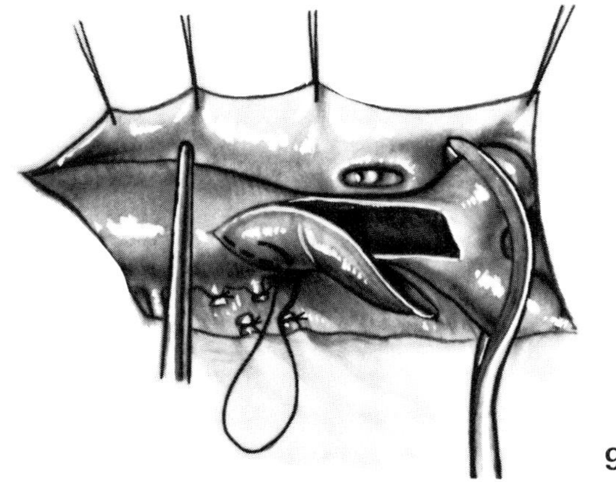

9d

POSTOPERATIVE CARE

The drainage tube is removed after 24 hr. In a few cases, after removal of the tube, blood-stained effusion accumulates in the left pleural space and should be aspirated. There is a theoretical danger from puncture of a large vessel during thoracentesis.

The patient is allowed out of bed in 7 days. The patient should avoid strenuous effort for 3 months. Postoperative complications are infrequent.

Persistent hypertension

Reduction of the arterial pressure in the upper part of the body to a normal level, which is an important object of operation, may be delayed for 2 or 3 weeks. Rarely, the pressure, although lowered, may never fall to a normal level. The older the patient the more likely is this failure of adjustment of the pressure. Provided that an anastomosis of good size has been made, immediately after the operation the pulses in the lower limbs become palpable and the femoral arterial pressure becomes greater than the brachial.

Aneurysm

A false aneurysm may occur at a point of leakage from the suture line (Gross, 1950). It calls for re-exposure of the aorta, control of its lumen with clamps as for resection, and repair of the defect in its wall.

Haematoma in chest wall

Bleeding may occur in the chest wall, especially from vessels in the substance of the latissimus dorsi. Evacuation of a haematoma may be required (Crafoord, Eirup and Gladnikoff, 1947).

Infection

The special danger of infection is involvement of the aorta. As soon as infection is suspected antibiotic therapy should be begun and adjusted to the causal organism when it has been isolated. Suppuration in the chest wall or loculated in the pleural space may require drainage. The abnormal size of the parietal vessels must be taken into consideration. If it becomes apparent that the infection is uncontrolled and the organism can be cultured from the blood stream and an increasing radiographic shadow indicates disruption of the aortic suture line with formation of a false aneurysm, the complication is likely to be fatal. If, nevertheless, it is decided to attempt reconstruction of the aorta with a prosthesis, the aneurysm can probably best be exposed using a bypass from the left atrium to the femoral artery.

Abdominal pain

In a few patients, 2–5 days after operation, severe generalized abdominal pain occurs. It usually subsides in 48–72 hr without specific treatment. Gangrene of the small bowel, however, has been recorded, along with acute arteriolar necrosis in the abdominal viscera, possibly the result of sudden exposure of these vessels to a high pressure (Benson and Sealy, 1956).

The same authors have recorded postoperative hypertension, the rise in the diastolic pressure being especially marked, and relate the abdominal symptoms to this. They propose the use of sympathicolytic drugs in the management of both hypertension and the abdominal pain.

Other complications

Injury of the para-aortic structures is unlikely since they are excluded from the operative field by the aortic sheath, but laryngeal paralysis from interruption of the left vagus nerve or its recurrent branch may occur. Similarly, chylothorax may follow damage to the thoracic duct. Traumatic chylothorax usually responds to repeated pleural aspiration.

Late re-operation

If, several years after the primary operation, a defect becomes apparent in the repair of a coarctation, for example an aneurysm at or near the suture line or inadequacy of the lumen after resection in infancy, a second operation is required. Especially if a prosthesis has been used, the aorta at the site of operation is likely to be embedded in dense fibrous tissue. Since it must be assumed that the collateral circulation has largely disappeared, prolonged occlusion of the aorta is no longer safe without maintenance of the renal and spinal circulation by another route. In these circumstances, before occlusion of the aorta, a bypass is established from the left atrium or left ventricle to the femoral artery or descending aorta (*see* Chapter on 'Methods of Providing Facilities for Open Heart Surgery', page 25) to permit unhurried reconstruction.

References

Benson, W. R. and Sealy, W. C. (1956). 'Arterial necrosis following resection of coarctation of the aorta.' *Lab. Invest.* **5**, 359

Crafoord, C. and Nylin, G. (1945). 'Congenital coarctation of the aorta and its surgical treatment.' *J. thorac. Surg.* **14**, 347

Crafoord, C., Eirup, B. and Gladnikoff, H. (1947). 'Coarctation of the aorta.' *Thorax*, **2**, 121

Gross, R. E. (1945). 'Surgical correction for coarctation of the aorta.' *Surgery* **18**, 673

Gross, R. E. (1950). 'Coarctation of the aorta–surgical treatment of one hundred cases.' *Circulation*, **1**, 41

Vosschulte, K. (1961). 'Surgical correction of coarctation of the aorta by an "isthmusplastic" operation.' *Thorax*, **16**, 338

[*The illustrations for this Chapter on Coarctation of the Aorta were drawn by Mr. G. Lyth.*]

Congenital Abnormalities of the Aortic Arch

David I. Hamilton, F.R.C.S.
Cardiac Surgeon to the Royal Liverpool Children's Hospital

Developmental considerations

During fetal development six pairs of aortic arch vessels connect the ventral and dorsal aortae which will become the ascending and descending portions of the thoracic aorta. The six pairs of arch vessels are never all present simultaneously. The first, second and fifth pairs regress. The third pair become the carotid arteries. The fourth right arch vessel is absorbed leaving the left to form the normal aortic arch. The sixth pair are involved in the formation of the pulmonary arteries and the ductus arteriosus. Developmental abnormalities are the result of unusual persistence or absorption of these vessels. Only those encountered more frequently in clinical practice are described here.

Right aortic arch

This is a mirror image of the left aortic arch and is seldom associated with an entirely normal heart. It is frequently present in Fallot's tetralogy, persistent truncus arteriosus and tricuspid atresia. Usually there are no symptoms. The condition is noted on the chest radiograph, barium swallow or on angiography.

Right aortic arch passing behind the oesophagus

This anomaly may form a ring completed by the ligamentum arteriosum which is tight enough to cause tracheal and oesophageal compression. The aortic arch may descend on either the right or the left side.

Anomalous right subclavian artery from a left descending aorta

This is a relatively common finding on routine radiological and postmortem examination. The right subclavian artery arises from the descending thoracic aorta distal to the left subclavian artery and passes upwards and behind the oesophagus to the right upper limb. There may be no symptoms and signs but compression of the oesophagus is quite common. This is demonstrated as a posterior indentation during the barium swallow.

Bayford used the term 'dysphagia lusoria' in describing this condition (1789). The mirror-image situation is present when a right aortic arch gives origin to an aberrant left subclavian artery.

Anomalous innominate artery

The origin of this vessel is situated further to the left of the transverse aortic arch than is usual and, therefore, the artery must spiral across the trachea to reach the right side of the neck. If the vessel is short, tracheal obstruction is likely.

Anomalous left carotid artery

A similar situation occurs when this artery arises unusually far to the right from a left aortic arch. Both of these conditions cause stridor and dyspnoea rather than dysphagia.

Pulmonary arteries arising from the ascending aorta

Anomalous left pulmonary artery

Bilateral persistent ductus arteriosus

These conditions are rarely encountered in clinical practice. The left pulmonary artery may arise from the main pulmonary artery and swing behind the trachea, but in front of the oesophagus, to reach the lung hilum. Stridor and dyspnoea are the most usual symptoms.

Double aortic arch

This condition was described by Hommel (1737) and was treated successfully surgically by Gross (1945).

Persistence of both fourth arch vessels produces a vascular ring which encircles the trachea and the oesophagus. The right arch artery passes behind the oesophagus and is usually the dominant vessel. The smaller left arch component passes in front of and to the left of the above structures. When the aorta descends on the right side there may be dominance of the right or left arch components.

Symptomatology

Symptoms result from tracheal and/or oesophageal compression and depend upon the degree of tension exerted by the 'vascular ring' or aberrant vessel.

In some cases there are no symptoms. Presentation is common in infancy but can be delayed until the second year of life or later. The usual symptoms are stridor, wheezing, cough or recurrent chest infections causing an increase in respiratory rate. Intercostal recession and cervical extension are present in severe cases. Moist sounds may be heard on auscultation of the chest. Dysphagia can occur early or may be delayed until solid food is taken.

Investigation

Chest radiograph

An abnormal vascular shadow is seen in the presence of a right aortic arch. The trachea may be displaced or compressed.

Barium swallow

The swallow is observed during fluoroscopy with the patient in the postero-anterior, lateral and oblique positions to assess the degree of indentation of the oesophagus and trachea.

Aortography

Studies of the aortic arch or aberrant vessel are obtained either by retrograde aortic or by left ventricular injection. Pulmonary artery injection may also be required.

Endoscopy

Bronchoscopy and oesophagoscopy are performed under general anaesthesia. The site and nature of any narrowing is noted. Palpation of the upper limb and femoral pulses is performed during manipulation of the oesophagoscope. Obliteration of any pulse, for example, in the right upper limb may be produced by pressure on the aberrant artery with the endoscope.

Considerations in diagnosis and management

(*a*) Is a vascular anomaly present?
(*b*) Is it causing symptoms?
(*c*) Has the anomaly been demonstrated clearly so that surgical correction can be planned?
(*d*) Seventy-five per cent of patients having a double aortic arch will have a dominant right arch with the aorta descending on the left side.

Up to 80 per cent of the patients who have a dominant left arch will still have their descending aorta on the left side. This means that approximately 95 per cent of patients having a double aortic arch can be treated surgically through a left thoracotomy.

Pre-operative management

Respiratory infection should be treated and controlled by physiotherapy, antibiotic therapy and humidity. Surgery may be indicated as an emergency measure.

Anaesthesia

An endotracheal tube is used and may have to be passed through any tracheal obstruction which is usually 2–3 cm above the carina. Nitrous oxide, oxygen and muscle relaxants are usually employed.

THE OPERATION

1

Position of patient

In the majority of patients satisfactory access is obtained through a left posterolateral thoracotomy with the patient on his right side. The third or fourth intercostal space is opened.

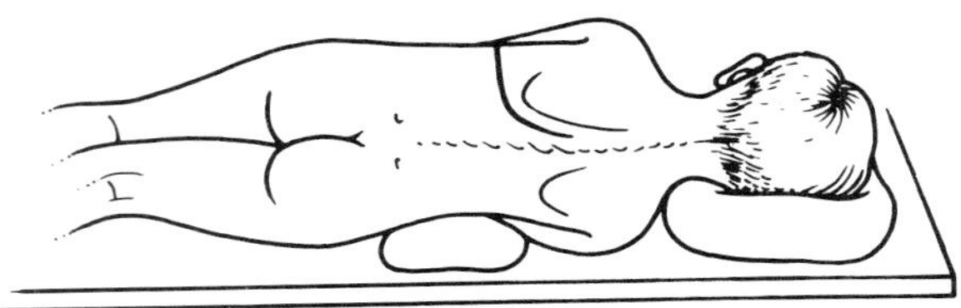

1

Incision

A standard posterolateral thoracotomy is made from below the nipple, curving posteriorly below the angle of the scapula and passing upwards mid-way between the vertebral border of the scapula and the vertebral spines. The latissimus dorsi muscle is divided in the same line. The fascia within the triangle of auscultation is opened following the posterior border of the serratus anterior muscle anteriorly and posteriorly below the rhomboid muscles until the underlying fibres of the erector spinae muscle are exposed. The attachment of the serratus anterior muscle is separated from the fifth rib so that its periosteum can be reflected from its superior border. The pleura is opened and a rib-spreader is inserted. The upper lobe of the lung is retracted inferiorly and anteriorly by the surgical assistant.

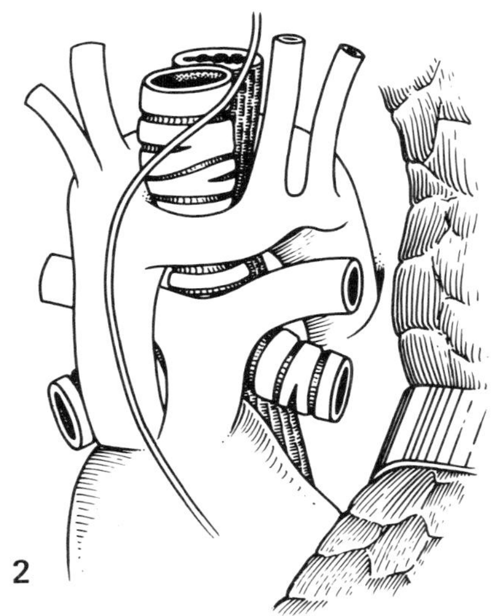

2

2

Exposure of the aortic arch

The mediastinal pleura is opened posteriorly to the vagus nerve from above the lung hilum towards the apex of the chest. The pleura is reflected off the underlying vessels which are then dissected out carefully. It may be helpful to pass a stomach tube into the oesophagus to assist in identifying this structure.

A careful inspection of the anatomical disposition of the normal and anomalous vessels is made. The ligamentum arteriosum or persistent ductus arteriosus is examined and, if necessary, divided.

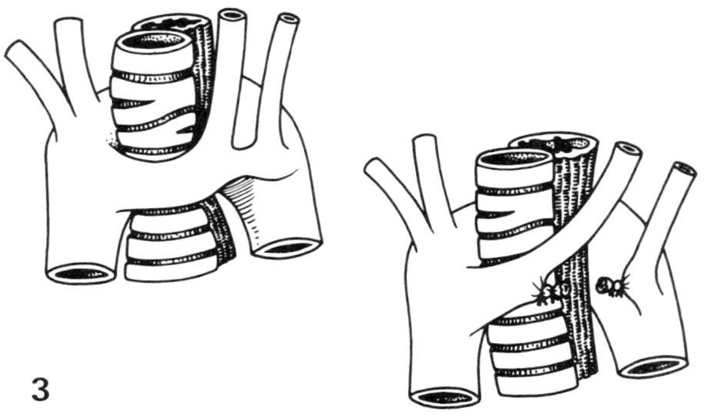

3

3

Division of a vascular ring (double aortic arch)

The correct site for division is selected after trial clamping of the anomalous vessel. An assessment is made of the pulsation in all the vessels arising from the anomalous artery and in the descending aorta itself. Only when it is clear that blood flow in them will not be impeded is the division completed. The divided vessel ends are either ligated or are sutured. It is usual for the separated ends of the anomalous artery to spring apart quite widely after division, thus reflecting the degree of tension previously present.

4

Division of an aberrant subclavian artery

This vessel usually arises distal to the left subclavian artery.

It passes behind the oesophagus and crosses the mid-line towards the right axilla.

If this vessel is compressed, the right upper limb pulse will disappear. Although it is usually safe to divide this vessel, it may also be possible to anastomose it to a major vessel nearer its correct site of origin.

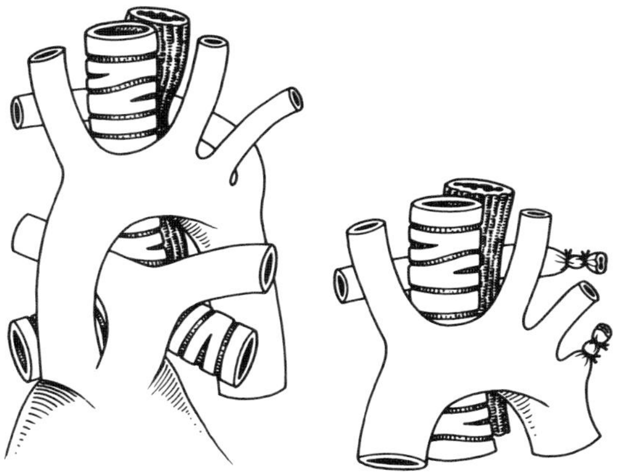

4

Closure

The edges of the mediastinal pleura are sutured together and the chest is closed in layers with drainage of the pleural space by means of an underwater seal system.

POSTOPERATIVE CARE

Dysphagia is usually relieved immediately. Although stridor is frequently improved from the day of operation, it can be disappointingly slow to regress. This is due to severe deformity of the trachea at the site of compression and this may take several weeks or even months to disappear. Treatment with humidity and oxygen may be necessary whilst improvement is awaited.

Tracheostomy is seldom required for the removal of secretion from the bronchial tree.

RESULTS

The long-term results following the relief of pressure on the trachea and oesophagus are almost uniformly good. Patience is sometimes required whilst the trachea is recovering from the effects of compression but, even in such cases, the long-term result can be entirely satisfactory.

[*The illustrations for this Chapter on Congenital Abnormalities of the Aortic Arch were drawn by Mrs. D. H. Blundell.*]

Atrial Septal Defects

Donald N. Ross, F.R.C.S.
Consultant Surgeon, Guy's Hospital, London
Senior Surgeon, National Heart Hospital, London

and

John R. W. Keates, F.R.C.S.
Formerly, Senior Lecturer, Cardiothoracic Institute, University of London;
Consultant Cardiothoracic Surgeon, King's College Hospital, London

PRE - OPERATIVE

Indications

The presence of an atrial septal defect with a significant left-to-right shunt at cardiac catheterization is an indication for surgical closure. Ideally the operation should be carried out before puberty but there is no contra-indication to operation in the older age groups.

Contra-indications

The presence of an increased pulmonary vascular resistance increases the risk of closure. Where this is responsible for a balanced or reversed shunt, closure is contra-indicated.

Classification

(*1*) Persistent foramen ovale.
(*2*) Secundum defects.
(*3*) Sinus venous defects.
(*4*) Primum defects.

The secundum defect is the one most commonly encountered surgically, while the persistent foramen ovale is a normal finding in 10–20 per cent of the population. The latter only becomes surgically important in relation to other lesions such as pulmonary valve stenosis, when it may be responsible for a right-to-left shunt and cyanosis. Primum defects are of importance because of the associated abnormalities of the atrioventricular valves and the possibility of a concomitant ventricular septal defect.

THE OPERATIONS

These are all performed with the aid of cardiopulmonary bypass.

SECUNDUM DEFECTS

1

Incision—external appearances of the heart

Usually a vertical sternotomy gives the best exposure. Occasionally a right anterolateral thoracotomy through the fourth rib-bed is used. It gives an adequate exposure and a less prominent scar.

The right atrium, right ventricle and pulmonary artery are enlarged while the aorta is small, reflecting the heavy left-to-right shunt. A search is made for anomalies of pulmonary venous drainage.

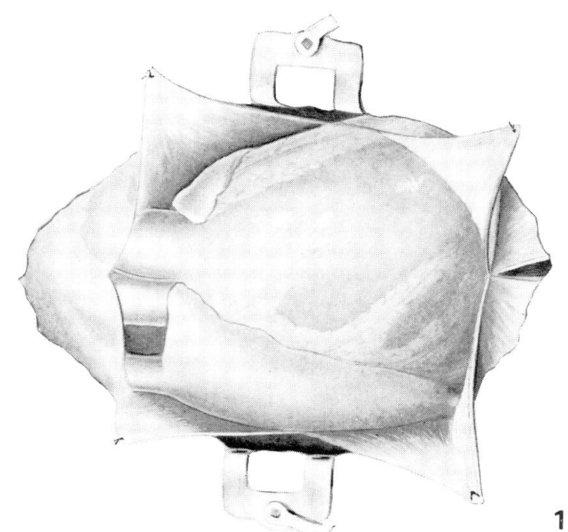

1

2

Digital exploration of the interior of the right atrium

The right index finger is inserted through the right atrial appendage and the size and position of the atrial defect is assessed. The ostium secundum defect has a sharp crescentic anterior border. The mitral valve is palpated to exclude associated mitral valve disease and a search is made for anomalous pulmonary venous drainage.

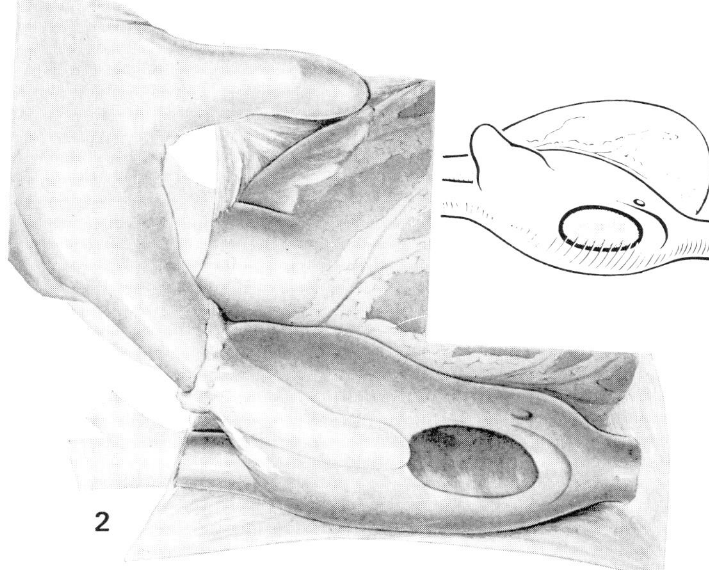

2

3

Preparation for exposure of defect

Two vena caval cannulae are introduced via the right atrial appendage. Slings are placed around the venae cavae. The arterial cannula is inserted through a purse-string suture in the ascending aorta.

On achieving full bypass the heart is electrically fibrillated, the left ventricle vented and the ascending aorta clamped.

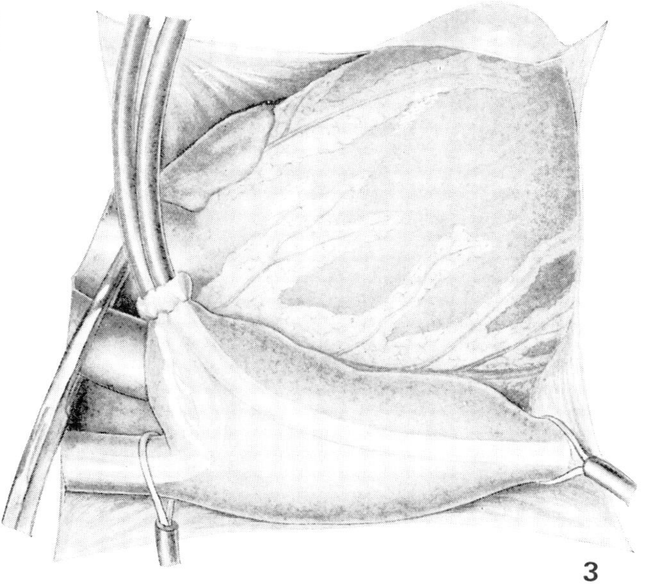

3

4

Atrial incision

The atrial incision should be made with care to avoid the area of the sino-atrial node around the insertion of the superior vena cava. This incision should not be unnecessarily large so as to avoid postoperative arrhythmias.

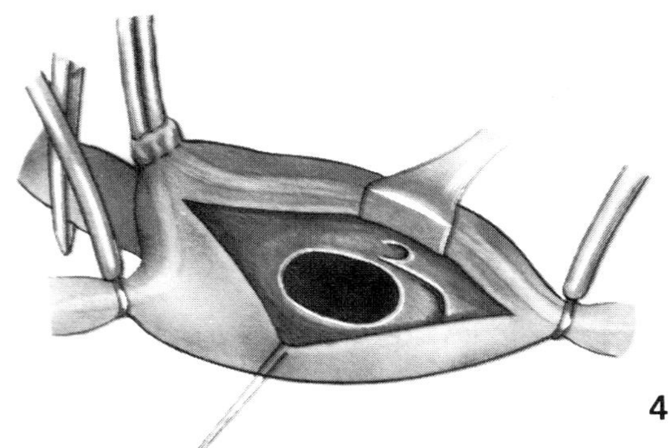

4

5

Closure of defect

On opening the atrium the defect is defined and the mitral valve inspected. A stitch is placed across the lower margin of the defect, thus defining it, avoiding the Eustachian valve. The suture starts at the inferior margin and is carried up as a continuous whip stitch incorporating the thick muscular margins of the defect. The thin fenestrated tissue sometimes seen in the vicinity of the defect is not suitable to take sutures. Finally, one or two additional interrupted sutures are advisable.

The large defects seen in older patients when there is a deficiency of tissue may be closed with a pericardial patch.

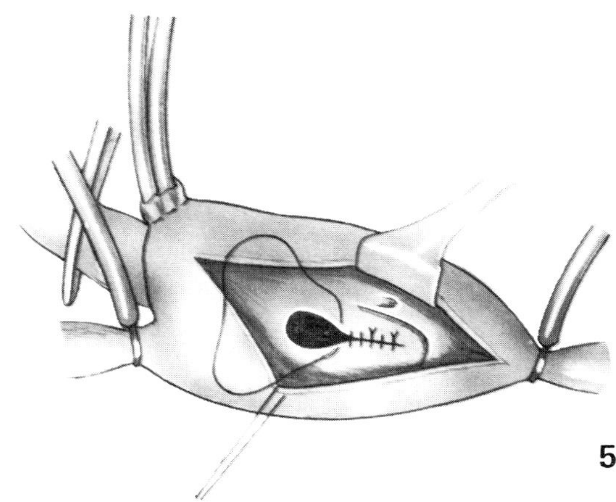

5

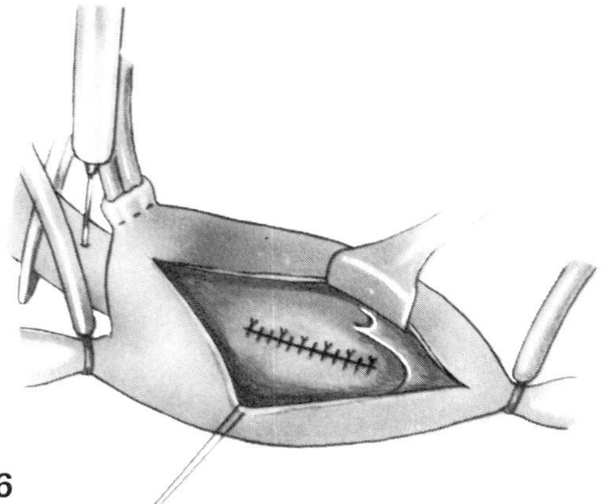

6

6

Elimination of air

Air trapped in the left heart is a hazard in atrial septal defects. It is released (*1*) from the ascending aorta with a wide-bore needle before removal of the aortic cross-clamp (*2*) from the left atrium by aspiration with a wide-bore needle through the septum and left atrial appendage and (*3*) the left ventricle by flushing blood through the left ventricular vent-hole whilst massaging the heart. Hand-ventilation of the lungs by the anaesthetist is helpful during this procedure as the flow of blood flushes out any air trapped in the pulmonary veins. The vena caval snares can now be released and the bypass is discontinued.

SINUS VENOUS DEFECTS

7

Diagnosis

In this condition there are always anomalous pulmonary veins entering the terminal superior vena cava. A finger in the right atrium will confirm these and identify the defect which is normally small and lies within the entrance of the superior vena cava. It has a sharp crescentic *inferior* margin. A number of sinus venous defects have an associated left superior vena cava.

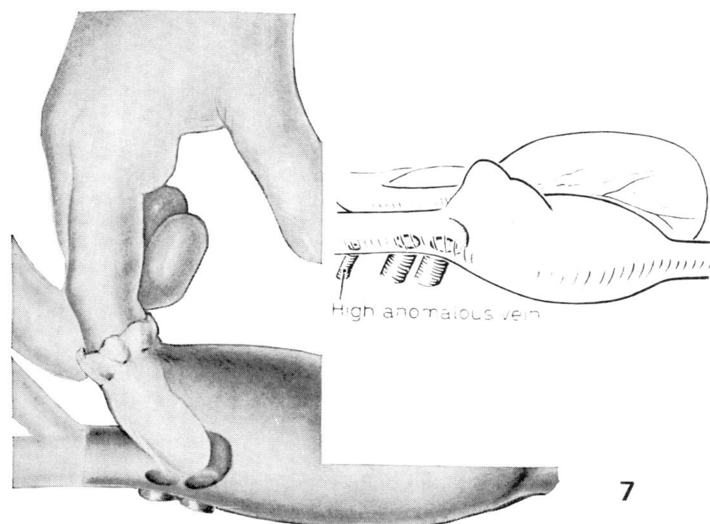

7

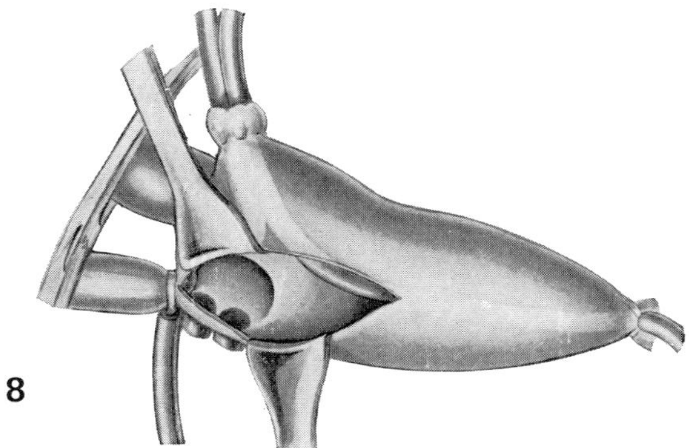
8

8

Exposure

The preliminary preparation of the patient is as for a secundum defect, but the incision in the right atrium will be higher and more posterior.

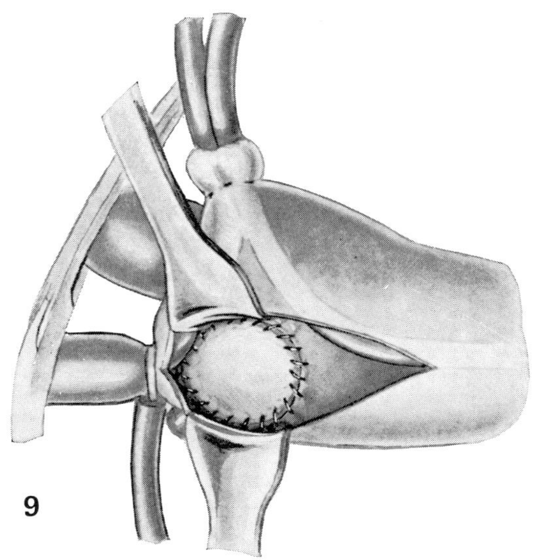
9

9

Closure

The superior vena caval catheter is then retracted and the defect closed with a patch which also covers the anomalous veins deflecting the pulmonary blood flow into the left atrium. The patch may be of pericardium or prosthetic material. Attempts to mobilize the veins and attempt a direct suture of the defect are often associated with thrombosis of the pulmonary veins. When a single small pulmonary vein enters high on the superior vena cava it is better ignored as the corresponding shunt will be haemodynamically unimportant.

PRIMUM DEFECTS

The correction of these defects can pose many problems, particularly the identification and correction of the abnormal anatomy and the avoidance of heart-block.

10

Diagnosis

A finger in the right atrium confirms the presence of the defect which is low-lying and immediately above the atrioventricular valves. It has a sharp crescentric *superior* border. Feeling through the defect a mitral regurgitant jet may be palpable but this can be variable in intensity and intermittent.

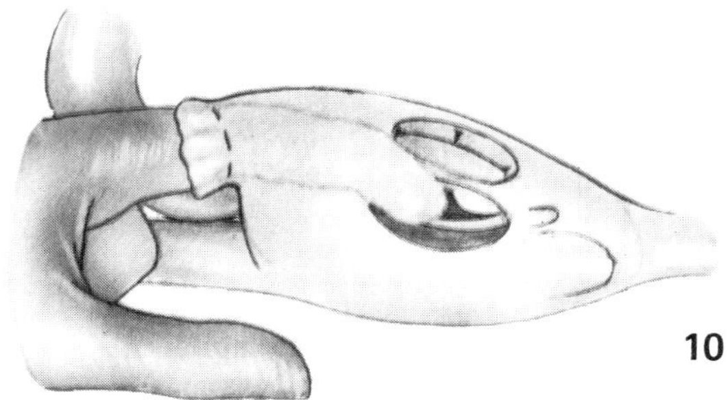

10

11

Exposure

Initial preparation of the heart is similar to that in a secundum defect. A large oblique incision in the right atrium extending from the inferior vena cava to the atrial appendage gives a good exposure. A deep curved retractor through the tricuspid valve now lifts the atrioventricular rings and atrial and ventricular septa into view and allows one to identify the mitral cleft and its spatial relationships. Careful examination and probing of the ventricular septum excludes a high ventricular septal defect.

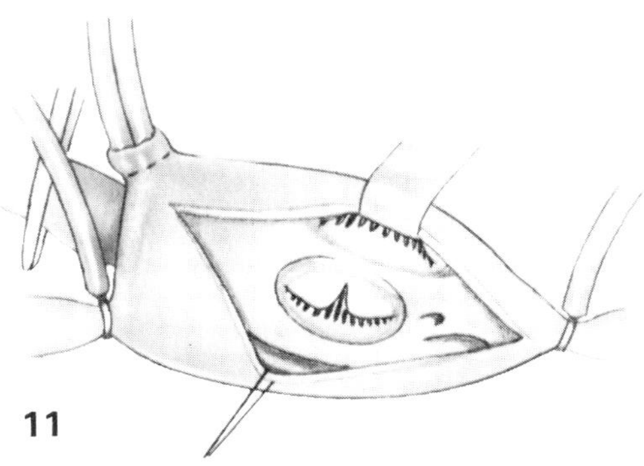

11

12

Closure and repair

The mitral cleft is identified as it runs from the mitral orifice to the middle of the ventricular septum. It normally has thickened and slightly rolled margins. These are brought together with multiple interrupted sutures.

A patch of pericardium or thin prosthetic material is then used to close the atrial septal defect. This can be fixed in place with a continuous suture and with an arrested heart. However, in the danger area between the coronary sinus and the mid-point of the ventricular septum, it is safer to have the heart beating so that damage to the conducting tissue will be detected early. Also, sutures should be placed in the tricuspid leaflet close to the septum but not penetrating it as a further precautionary measure.

Even if conduction disturbances have not been a feature of the closure it is usual to fix pacemaker leads in position in the right ventricle at the end of the operation to deal with possible postoperative heart-block.

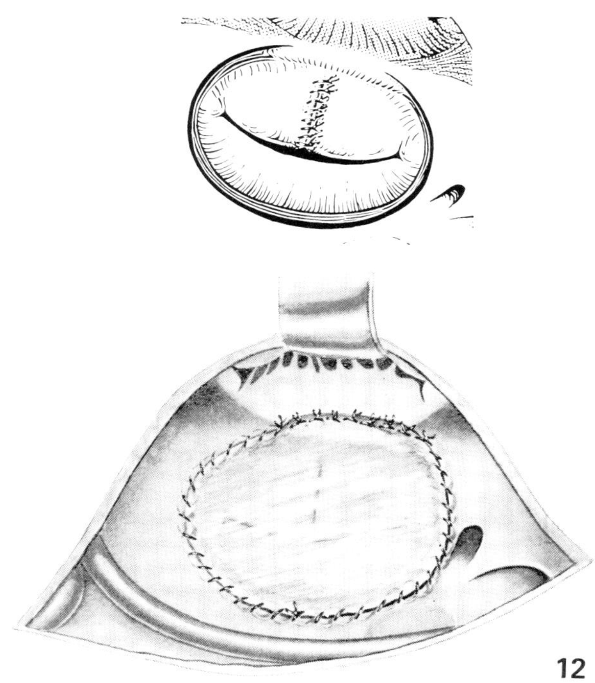

12

POSTOPERATIVE CARE

Cases of atrial septal defect usually run an uncomplicated postoperative course but should have routine intensive care nursing as for any other heart procedure.

Secundum defects rarely cause problems but atrial arrhythmias may occur. The most common arrhythmia is atrial flutter but in older age groups atrial fibrillation may be present pre- or postoperatively. These arrhythmias may require control with digitalis and if they do not revert spontaneously electrical defibrillation should be considered.

Sinus venous defects may develop pulmonary complications as a result of distortion of the pulmonary veins with super-added pulmonary venous thrombosis. This is rare when a patch is used for closure of a defect and this is an added reason for using a patch instead of attempting direct suture.

Primum defects have as their special complication the likelihood of atrioventricular dissociation because of the proximity of the conducting tissue to the atrial repair. For this reason special care is required and in the danger area stitches are placed in the root of the tricuspid valve.

Persistent mitral regurgitation is also a possibility but accurate repair of the cleft should mean that this will be haemodynamically unimportant.

[*The illustrations for this Chapter on Atrial Septal Defects were drawn by Mr. F. Price and Mrs. C. Dawbarn.*]

Pulmonary Valve Stenosis

W. P. Cleland, F.R.C.P., F.R.C.S.
Surgeon, The Brompton Hospital; Consulting Thoracic Surgeon, King's College Hospital;
Senior Lecturer in Thoracic Surgery, Royal Postgraduate Medical School;
Civilian Consultant in Thoracic Surgery to the Royal Navy

PRE - OPERATIVE

Aim of operation

The aim is to relieve stenosis of the pulmonary valve accurately under direct vision.

Indications

The operation is indicated in patients who have appreciable obstruction to the forward flow of blood from the right ventricle to the lungs. The valve stenosis may occur with intact septa or with a ventricular or atrial septal defect.

Evidence of significant obstruction is provided by the signs of right ventricular hypertrophy, radiologically and electrically, and the demonstration of a gradient across the valve at cardiac catheterization.

The patients are not cyanosed unless shunt reversal has taken place through a septal defect.

The ideal time for open valvotomy is between the ages of 5 and 12 years, but the operation may be necessary at an earlier age in severe cases. Minor degrees of valve obstruction carry little risk for the patient and do not demand operation. Moderate and severe obstruction requires surgical relief.

Severity can best be assessed as follows:

(*1*) Mild–Normal sized heart; normal lung vascularity. Grade I right ventricular hypertrophy on ECG and a right ventricular pressure less than 50 mmHg.

(*2*) Moderate–Moderate right ventricular enlargement and oligaemic lungs. Grade II right ventricular hypertrophy on ECG and a right ventricular pressure between 50 and 100 mmHg.

(*3*) Severe–Considerable right ventricular hypertrophy, radiologically and electrically. Oligaemic lungs and a right ventricular pressure of over 100 mmHg.

Contra-indication

The only patients who do not require operation are those with mild obstruction. Absence of symptoms, however, is no criterion.

Pre-operative investigations

Apart from routine chest radiography and electrocardiography, all patients should ideally have right heart catheterization and angiography to determine the severity of the lesion and to demonstrate associated anomalies.

Anaesthesia

The patient is premedicated with an endotracheal intubation performed with thiopentone induction.

Anaesthesia is maintained by nitrous oxide and oxygen.

Although the operation can be performed with inflow occlusion or with the aid of surface cooling, the vast majority of operations are done with conventional heart-lung bypass. This provides conditions for careful inspection of the valve and deliberate and accurate mobilization of the leaflets and division of commissures.

THE OPERATION

The best incision is a mid-line sternal splitting one; a left anterior or left anterolateral can be employed if desired but it does not provide any specific advantages.

Cardiopulmonary bypass is instituted in the usual way (*see* page 23) with cannulation of the cavae separately. The latter is necessary as the right atrium should be explored to identify and deal with any patency of the atrial septum.

With full flow bypass established the caval snares should be tightened and a low-pressure suction tube inserted into the right atrium to remove coronary sinus blood.

1

The incision

The illustration shows the view obtained of the heart from the mid-line approach; the incision into the base of the pulmonary artery is indicated with a dotted line. Before opening the artery stay sutures are placed on either side of the proposed incision. The artery is opened sufficiently to obtain a good view of the valve. If the view of the valve is obscured by right ventricular blood, the heart should be electrically fibrillated.

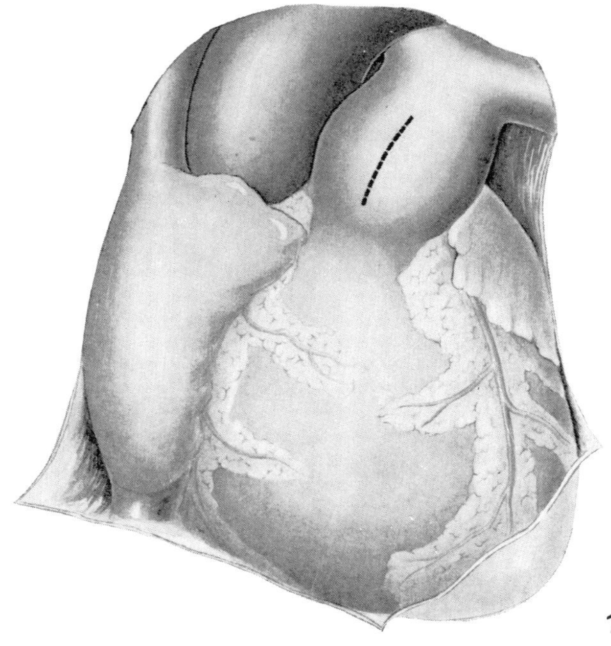

1

2

Fusion of cusps

The incision in the pulmonary artery is held open with further stay sutures and small retractors. Fusion of the cusps to each other and of the commissures to the artery wall is well demonstrated. The illustration shows the classical valve stenosis but in practice the anatomy of the valve shows considerable variation and is often severely disorganized.

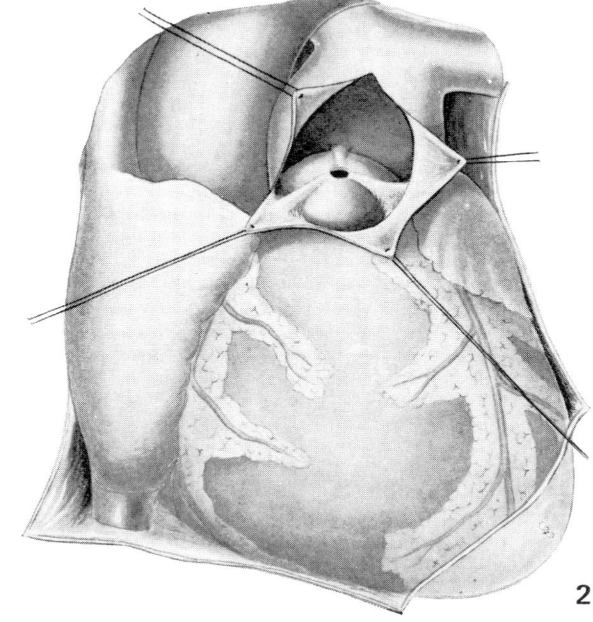

2

3

Separation of valve dome from artery wall

The valve dome is separated from the artery wall with scissors down to the base of the cusps.

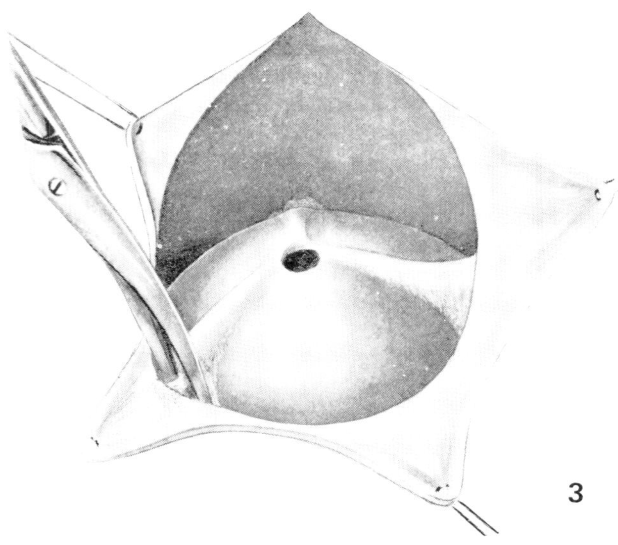

3

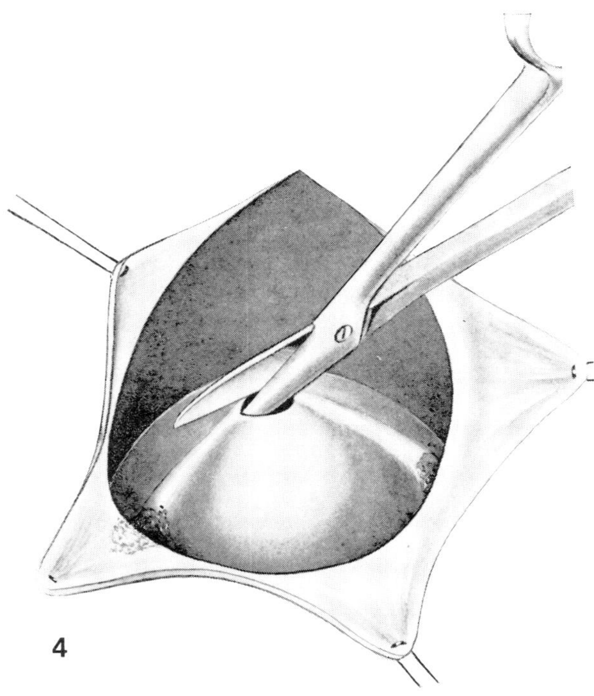

4

4

Division of fused cusps

The fused cusps are now divided with scissors or with a knife as far as the cusp base. The valve can now be gently dilated to ensure maximal relief of obstruction.

Next inspect the atrial septum and close any defects.

5

Valvotomy completed

This illustration reveals the fully divided commissures. The valve should admit the little finger in a child or index finger in an adult. The arteriotomy is closed and bypass discontinued. Pressures in the right ventricle and pulmonary artery are taken to record the gradient. If the right ventricular pressure is above 100 mmHg further action is probably needed – either resection of obstructing infundibular muscle or enlargement of a small valve ring (*see* Chapter on 'Complete Intracardiac Repair of Fallot's Tetralogy', page 104).

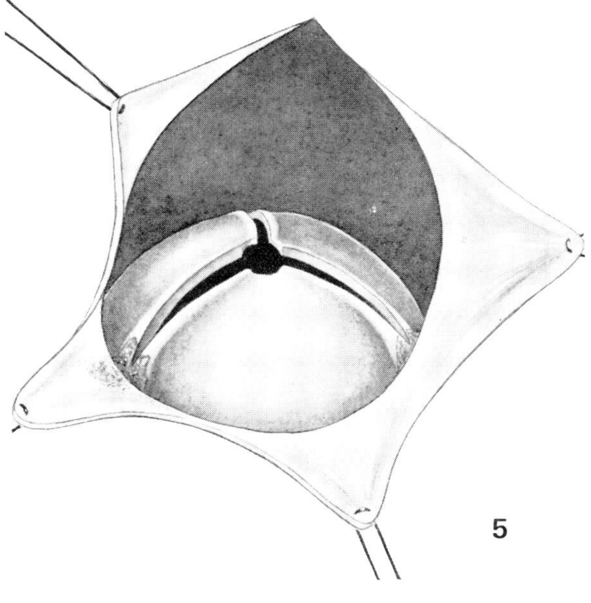

5

POSTOPERATIVE CARE

The operation requires little beyond the routine care for any bypass procedure, due attention being paid to blood loss and fluid replacement.

The patient may have evidence of right ventricular failure with a high venous pressure for several days or weeks and should be given digitalis.

Results

The operation is amongst the safest of the open heart procedures. Operative mortality lies between 1 and 2 per cent. The results are excellent in the majority with normal right ventricular pressures found at subsequent catheterization. Moderate residual right ventricular hypertension demonstrated on the table after a good valvotomy will resolve in most instances, although in a few it may persist.

Reference

Edwards, F. R. (1960). 'Pulmonary valvotomy and infundibulectomy.' *Br. Heart J.* **22**, 472

[*The illustrations for this Chapter on Pulmonary Valve Stenosis were drawn by Mrs. C. Dawbarn.*]

Ventricular Septal Defects

W. P. Cleland, F.R.C.P., F.R.C.S.
Surgeon, The Brompton Hospital; Consulting Thoracic Surgeon, King's College Hospital;
Senior Lecturer in Thoracic Surgery, Royal Postgraduate Medical School;
Civilian Consultant in Thoracic Surgery to the Royal Navy

PRE-OPERATIVE

Aim of operation

The closure of defects of the ventricular septum.

Aetiology

The majority of defects are the result of developmental anomalies. A few are caused by direct or indirect trauma and cardiac infarction.

Anatomy

Defects occur most commonly in the inflow portion of the right ventricle between the crista and the tricuspid valve (infracristal). A smaller group are located between the crista and the pulmonary valve (supracristal). Others arise in the muscular part of the septum. Multiple defects are found in 10–15 per cent of patients.

Infracristal defects (see Illustration 1)

These vary considerably in size from a few millimetres to 3–4 cm in diameter. The larger defects occupy the area between the crista and the tricuspid valve. The edges of the defect are as follows: (*a*) superiorly the aortic valve ring with the parietal band of the crista overlying it; (*b*) posteriorly the tricuspid valve ring; (*c*) inferiorly the upper rim of the muscular septum with the papillary muscle of the conus attached; and (*d*) anteriorly the crista. The atrioventricular bundle of His runs in close relationship to the posterior and inferior quadrants of the defect as it passes from the atrioventricular node beneath the tricuspid valve ring to the vicinity of the conus where it divides into right and left branches. It is vulnerable to trauma along this part of its course.

Supracristal defects (see Illustration 2)

These occupy the area between the crista and the pulmonary valve ring. The margins of the defect are made up successively by the pulmonary valve ring, aortic valve ring, crista and anterior portion of the muscular septum. The aortic valve is often poorly supported and valve anomalies are not infrequent.

Bulboventricular defects

These represent a combination of infracristal and supracristal defects. The deficiency is large and elongated and extends between the pulmonary valve and the tricuspid valve. The body of the crista is absent but its two limbs are present.

Muscular defects

These may be anywhere in the muscular septum but usually near the apex. They are often partly concealed by thickened trabeculae and are then difficult to expose.

Left ventricular–right atrial defects (Gerbode)

These are caused by a deficiency of that part of the membranous ventricular septum which presents on the right atrial wall. Shunting takes place into the right atrium.

Haemodynamics

Defects of the ventricular septum result in a shunt of blood from the left to the right side of the heart.

The magnitude of the shunt is governed by the size of the defect, the presence or not of pulmonary valvular or infundibular stenosis and the resistance of the pulmonary circulation (pulmonary vascular resistance). A large hole with no pulmonary stenosis and normal pulmonary vessels produces a considerable shunt and a pulmonary blood flow of 2–4 times the normal. Conversely a small hole, severe pulmonary valve stenosis or considerable pulmonary vascular disease may result in a very small shunt from left to right or even a reversal of the shunt (Fallot's tetralogy; Eisenmenger complex).

Clinical features

Infants may present with heart failure which carries a considerable mortality. Feeding difficulties and failure to thrive are likely during the first year. Thereafter, symptoms are less pronounced but repeated respiratory infections and slow progress are usual. After adolescence there is a progressive risk of severe pulmonary vascular disease and shunt reversal (Eisenmenger complex).

An occasional defect may close spontaneously perhaps by secondary adherence of the tricuspid valve to the defect.

Investigations

All patients require full cardiological investigations with catheterization and angiocardiography, not only to determine the severity of the condition but also to demonstrate anatomical variations.

Indications for operation

(*1*) *In infants:* Usually present in failure. If the latter uncontrolled with digitalis and diuretics, then closure advised.

(*2*) Patients with small shunts (less than 2:1 ratio) and right ventricular pressure below 50 mmHg are not at risk and do not require operation for haemodynamic reasons.

(*3*) Patients with shunts of over 2:1 and right ventricular pressures above 50 mmHg are in urgent need of closure in order to avoid the development of pulmonary vascular disease.

(*4*) Progressive pulmonary vascular disease raises the pulmonary resistance above the systemic and results in reversal of shunt and cyanosis (Eisenmenger complex). These patients will not benefit from operation.

Approach

The majority of defects are best approached through the ventricular wall. Some, especially those situated near the tricuspid valve, can be exposed very adequately from the right atrium by retracting the tricuspid valve. Accurate closure is thus possible but it is important not to damage any part of the tricuspid mechanism.

THE OPERATION

The operation is carried out with the aid of cardiopulmonary bypass or profound hypothermia (*see* page 23). The ventricle is best approached through a mid-line sternal splitting incision.

Before setting up bypass, pressures should be taken from the various cardiac chambers and the right atrium explored with a finger. With bypass established, caval occlusion is carried out and a 'vent' inserted into the apex of the left ventricle. The ventricle is opened with an incision so placed as to avoid major branches of the coronary artery. Either a transverse or longitudinal incision in the outflow tract of the ventricle is used.

At this stage the aorta is cross-clamped and the ventricles fibrillated to improve operating conditions.

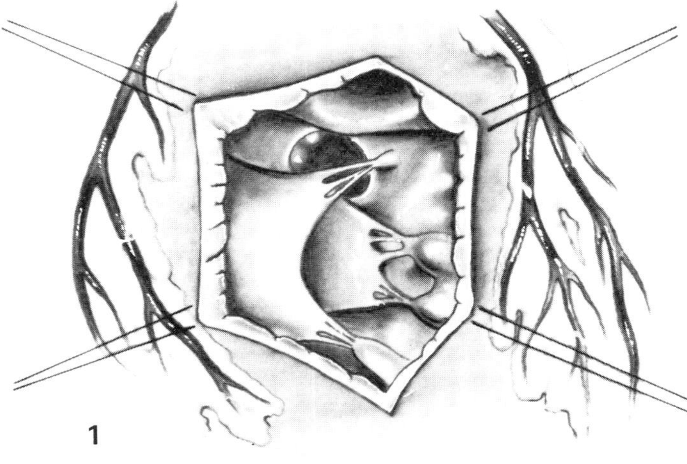

1

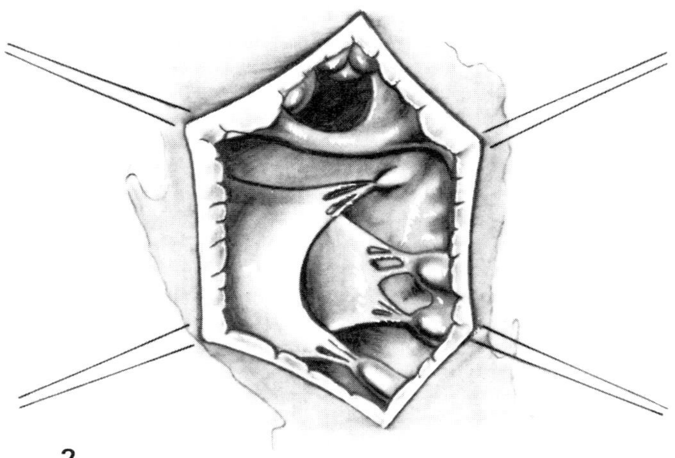

2

1&2

Inspection of ventricle

The ventriculotomy can be held open by suitably placed stay stitches to avoid mechanical retraction. A careful inspection of the ventricle is carried out.

The size of defect, its site and the quality of its margins are noted. The atrium should be inspected through the tricuspid valve for an atrial defect or patent foramen ovale (which should be closed if present). The outflow tract of the right ventricle and pulmonary valve are inspected for obstruction. The intracardiac part of the operation is facilitated by temporary aortic clamping. If the body is cooled to 30°C the aorta can be clamped safely for periods of 20–30 min. Before releasing the aortic clamp all air should be carefully expelled from the ascending aorta lest it be driven into the coronary vessels.

If the defect is large, it should be closed with a patch of Teflon felt, woven Dacron or pericardium.

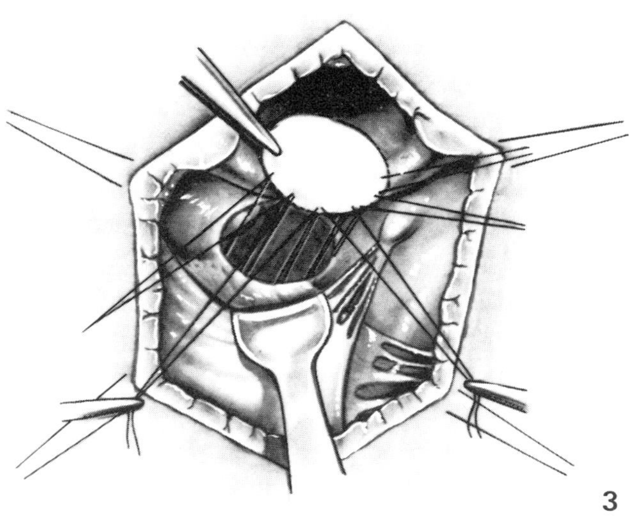

3

3&4

Placing of mattress sutures

Mattress sutures are first placed in the margins of the defect.

Posteriorly, in order to avoid the bundle, these are placed either into the tricuspid annulus (*Illustration 3*) or the base of the septal leaflet of the tricuspid valve (*Illustration 4*). Inferiorly they must be placed either into the precise rim of the defect or about 0·5–1·0 cm from the rim in order to avoid the bundle. Anteriorly, larger bites of the crista can be taken, whilst superiorly the stitches should be inserted either into the aortic valve ring itself or into the crista limb which lies superficial to it.

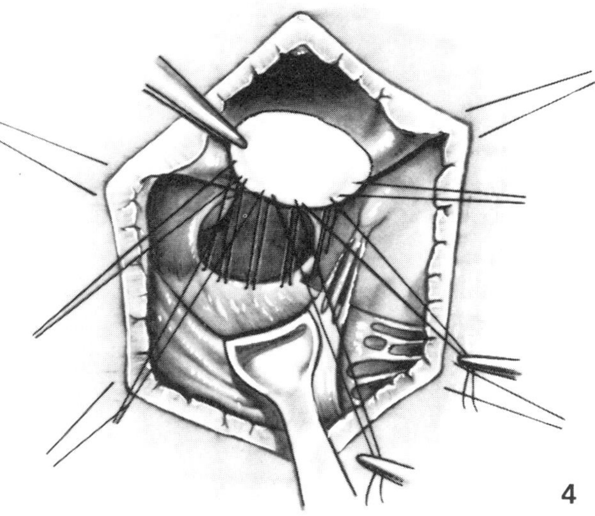

4

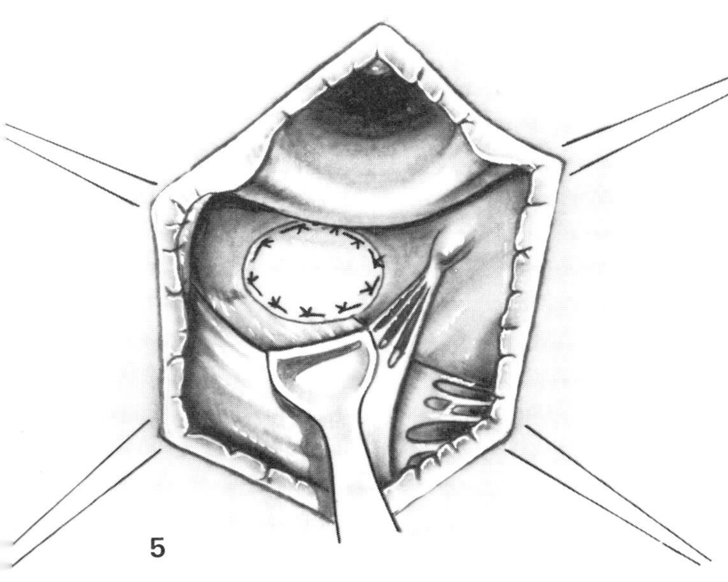

5

5

Tying of patch

When all stitches are passed the patch is lowered down and the sutures tied. The completeness of closure is then tested and additional stitches placed if necessary.

All air must be expelled from the left ventricle before defibrillation. The closure should again be verified with the heart beating and before the right ventricular incision is closed.

6

Closure of small defects

Small defects and those with fibrous margins can be safely closed with direct sutures. Mattress sutures are passed through the margins of the defect and tied. A second layer is then passed and tied over a strip of Teflon felt to prevent the pin hole leaks between the first layer of sutures.

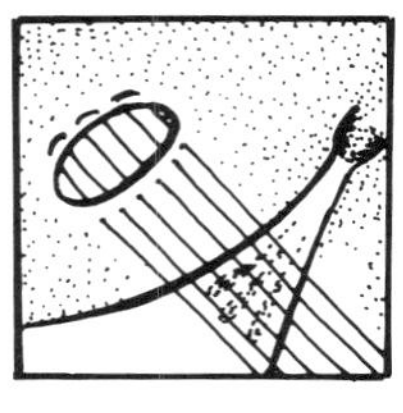
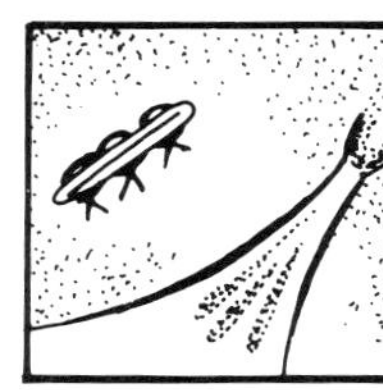
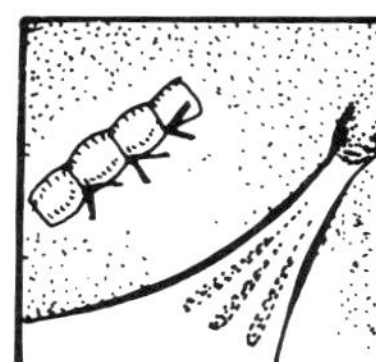

6

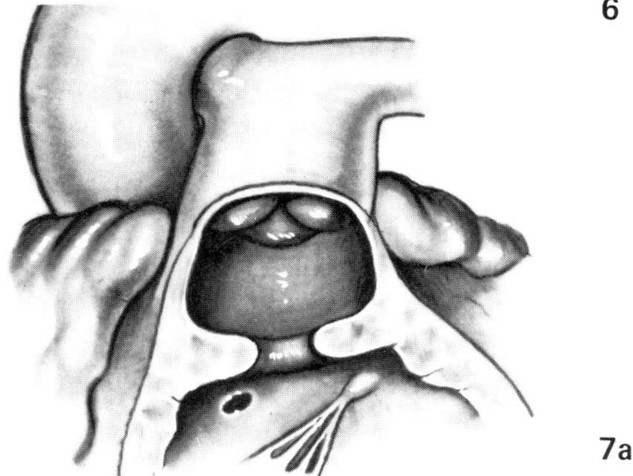

7a

7a & b

Excision of infundibular muscle

If there is any obstruction by infundibular muscle this should be adequately excised.

Similarly, any stenosis of the pulmonary valve should be relieved.

7b

POSTOPERATIVE CARE

Should the bundle be damaged and heart block produced, a pacemaker unit must be connected to the ventricle with embedded wire electrodes.

Replacement of blood lost through drainage tubes must be meticulously carried out.

The central venous pressure is monitored and additional blood is slowly given to maintain a pressure of 8–10 cm above the sternal angle.

Fluid is given intravenously as $^{1}/_{5}$ N saline and dextrose at a rate of 1 litre/m^2 body surface in 24 hr. Approximately half of this amount is given during the day of operation and the first postoperative night.

[*The illustrations for this Chapter on Ventricular Septal Defects were drawn by Mrs. C. Dawbarn.*]

Pulmonary Artery Constriction

Eoin Aberdeen, F.R.C.S., F.A.C.S.
Director of Cardiovascular Surgery,
The Children's Hospital of Newark, New Jersey

PRE - OPERATIVE

Absence of the ventricular septum, a very large ventricular septal defect or multiple ventricular septal defects result in an excessive pulmonary blood flow which may cause two main complications.

(*1*) Persistent heart failure, with pulmonary oedema in the early months of life, which is resistant to medical therapy.

(*2*) Pulmonary vascular obstructive disease which usually does not develop until after the first or second year of life.

Closure of a single ventricular septal defect if most of the ventricular septum is still present is preferred in infants of any age, but closure of very large or multiple defects in the first months of life still carries a higher risk than repair at a later age. Since a large ventricular septal defect is relatively innocuous in infancy when combined with pulmonary outflow tract obstruction, as in Fallot's anomaly, it is logical to imitate this combination of defects by narrowing the pulmonary artery in infants who have persistent heart failure as a result of an excessive left to right ventricular shunt. Pulmonary artery constriction (banding) was first proposed by Muller and Dammann in 1952, and has been widely used to palliate heart failure resulting from large ventricular septal defects in the early months of life, and to prevent the development of pulmonary vascular disease in infants. Ventricular septal defects, in association with transposition of the great arteries large enough to raise the pulmonary artery pressure to systemic levels, must either be closed at the time of operative correction of the transposition, or have pulmonary artery banding well before the end of the first year of life or, inevitably, severe pulmonary vascular obstructive disease will develop.

Special contra-indications

Constriction of the pulmonary artery should not be attempted when the pulmonary vascular resistance exceeds or equals the systemic vascular resistance.

The pulmonary artery should only be constricted if a very large ventricular septal defect or defects are present. If an isolated single ventricular septal defect of medium size is present, it is unusual to find the infant presenting in severe heart failure in the first weeks of life. Such lesions can be closed at open heart operations with a risk of less than 5 per cent, so primary closure is always preferred.

Special equipment

Pressure recording equipment and adequate technical assistance should be available in the operating room. But even with accurate pressure recording, pulmonary artery banding is an imprecise operation. Technical problems prevent the accurate measurement of flow in the pulmonary artery during the pulmonary artery constriction, and even if measured accurately with the chest open the flow could change significantly when the chest is closed.

Pre-operative investigations

As in other forms of congenital heart disease requiring operation, adequate pre-operative investigation is essential to determine the lesion or lesions present, to calculate relative flows and resistances, and also to exclude the presence of other additional heart defects. This requires angiocardiography with injection of dye into each ventricle and the x-ray beam projection inclined to show the ventricular septum in silhouette so that the position, size and number of defects can be precisely assessed.

Anaesthesia

Halothane or endotracheal nitrous oxide with oxygen and muscle relaxants is preferred.

Position of patient

The child is placed in the left oblique or left lateral position with the right side down.

THE OPERATION

1

The incision

The left lateral thoracotomy is made through the third interspace with a submammary skin incision. The interspace is opened from the edge of the sternum anteriorly to near the vertebral column posteriorly. The third interspace opening makes pressure recording in the pulmonary artery much simpler than does an opening in the fourth interspace. If the child is female, the incision can be placed lower than shown in this illustration so that it will lie in the submammary fold. The posterior part of the incision can be kept almost horizontal in an infant, and the upper edge of the incision is retracted to expose the third interspace. The conventional method of making the incision curve posterosuperiorly about the scapula is to be avoided because it makes a scar which is obvious and ugly.

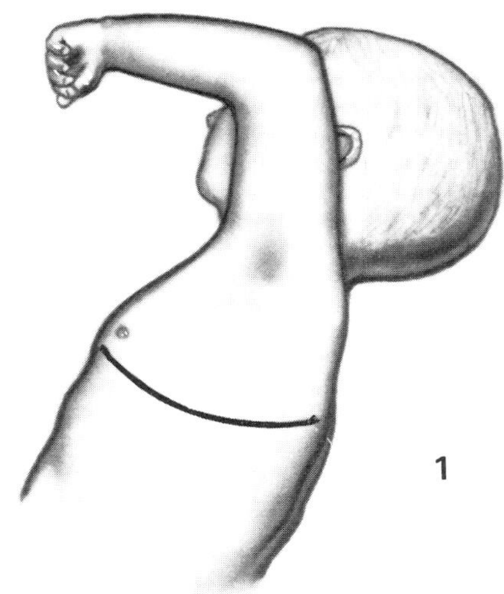

1

2 & 3

Examining the ligamentum or ductus

Dissection can be made around the ligamentum or ductus, adding only a few minutes to the operative procedure. If two ligatures of thick plaited silk (No. 6, 1·2 mm diameter) are tied around the structure, no question of patency remains, and it is suggested that routine ligation is wise in this operation, since duct ligation is so reliable if done in this manner (Panagopoulos *et al*., 1971).

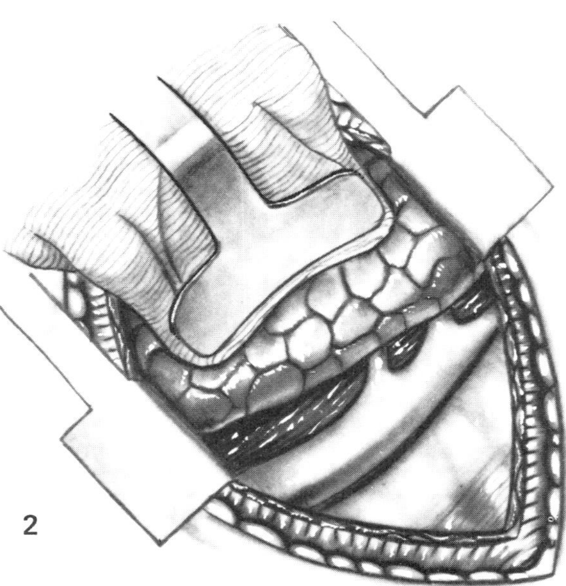

2

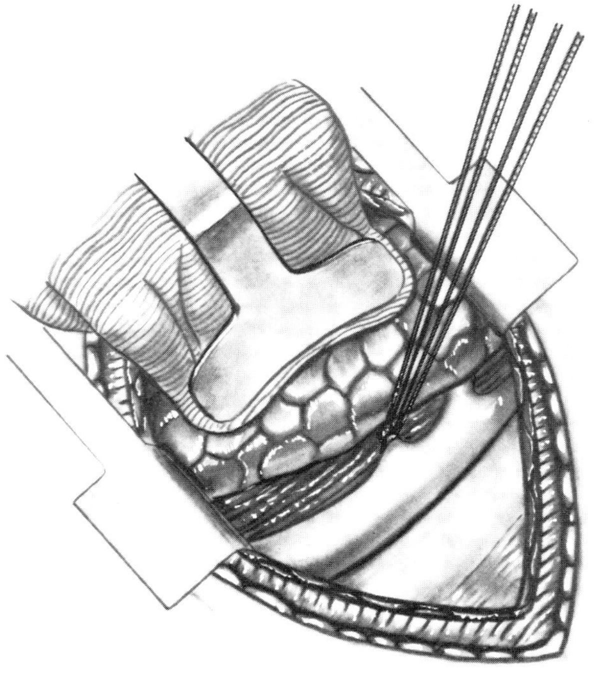

3

4

Opening the pericardium

The lung is retracted posteriorly and the lower portion of the left lobe of the thymus is mobilized upward. An incision is then made in the pericardium parallel to the phrenic nerve and 1–2 cm anterior to it. This incision is extended for 4 cm or more in length but should not be extended down over the apex of the ventricle as this allows the heart to dislocate too readily.

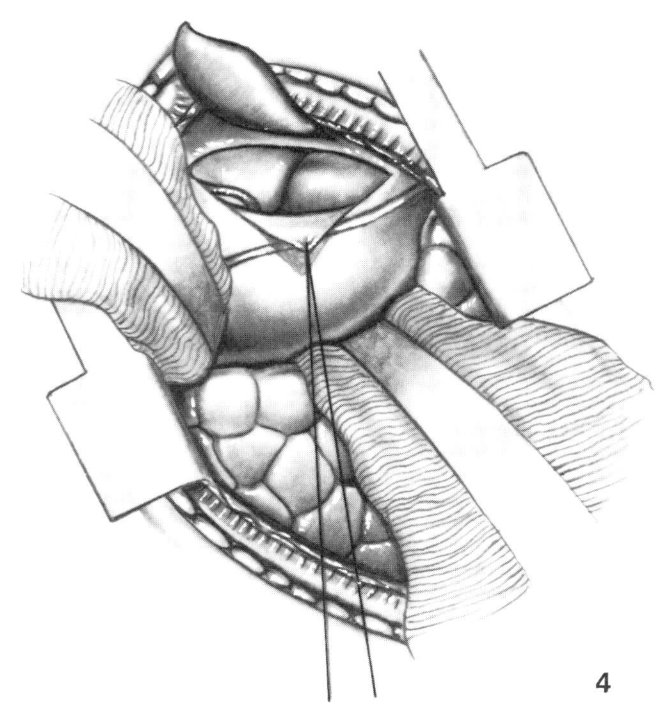

4

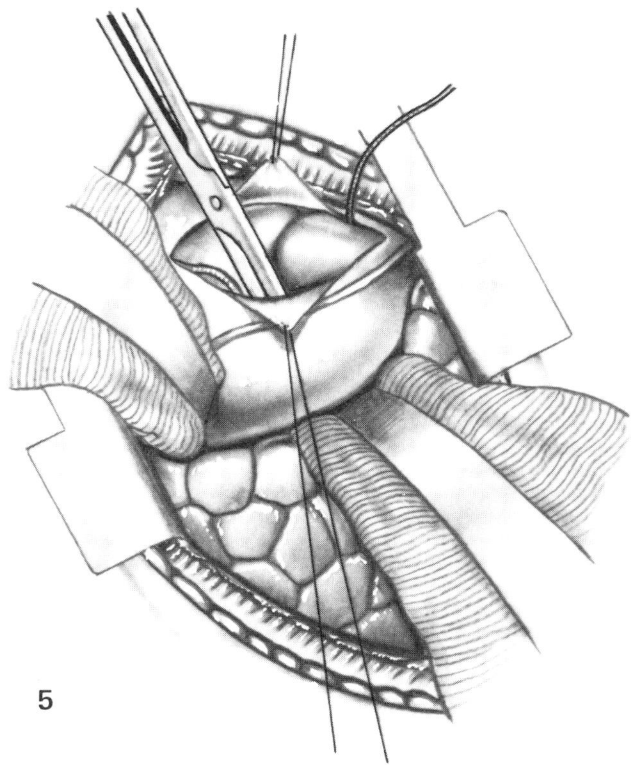

5

5

Dissection of pulmonary artery

Dissection is made around the pulmonary artery using a blunt dissecting instrument. The Denis Browne dissector has an olivary shaped tip which makes it very suitable for dissecting around arteries. Care should be taken to keep proximal to the right pulmonary artery. A vein lying parallel to and between the pulmonary artery and the aorta is often surprisingly large and should be avoided by commencing the dissection in this region under vision. When the pulmonary artery is very large and the aorta is very small, be sure that the dissection is, in fact, anterior to the aorta. In all cases check that the vessel being constricted is not the vessel which gives origin to the coronary arteries.

6

Placing the constricting ligature

The ligature is now placed around the pulmonary artery, again checking to ensure that it does not include the aorta. Many types of ligature have been used, including umbilical tape and Teflon tape. One satisfactory method is to use thick (No. 8 1·8 mm diameter) plaited silk; this has the advantage that it can be tied in a simple square knot (triple tied) which makes a desired circumference simpler to achieve precisely than some other methods. The silk ligature is deliberately chosen because it excites a fibrous reaction and is less likely to rupture the pulmonary artery, but it cannot be completely removed at the subsequent corrective operation. Then the pulmonary artery can be enlarged with a gusset of pericardium, or a plastic closure of the pulmonary artery incision. Pulmonary artery rupture has occurred using other materials such as a Teflon ligature (Rohmer, Brom and Nauta, 1967). The hope in using a non-irritant material is that it can be removed later and permit the pulmonary arteries simply to expand. However, extensive animal experimentation has shown that any material which constricts the pulmonary artery tightly will produce scar tissue in the portion of artery wall which is compressed by the band. Clinical experience has shown that Teflon bands often produce fibrosis in humans.

When the great arteries are transposed the pulmonary artery can usually be constricted from either a left or a right thoracotomy, although a left thoracotomy is usually best in complete transposition of the great arteries. A pre-operative angiocardiogram is wise since the relative positions of the great arteries is not constant, and the pulmonary artery may be to the right of the aorta (so called d.TGA). Dissection around the posterior pulmonary artery is not necessary. Dissection need be made only posterior to the aorta and when one end of the ligature is drawn through this space the other end is passed through the transverse sinus posterior to the two great vessels and the pulmonary artery is completely encircled.

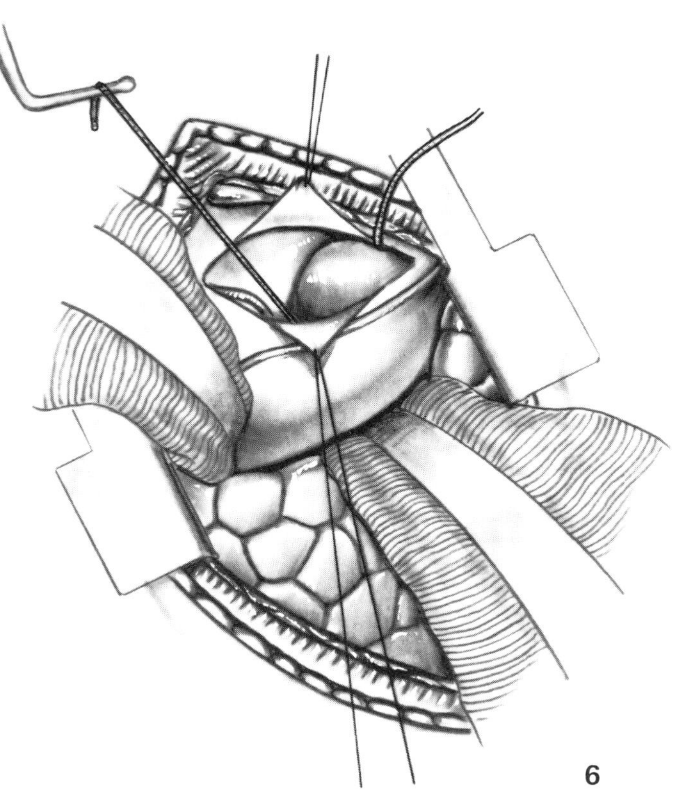

6

7

Tightening the ligature

Pressures are now taken simultaneously in a systemic artery cannula (e.g. the radial) or in the anterior ventricle, and in the pulmonary artery distal to the ligature. This pulmonary artery monitor needle should not be close to the band. The ligature is tightened until its internal diameter is about 6–7 mm. Usually the ventricular pressure will rise 10–20 mmHg and the distal pulmonary artery pressure will fall to 25–30 mmHg. If pulmonary vascular disease is severe, the pulmonary artery pressure may fall little or not at all, even though the pulmonary artery has been tightly constricted. The actual diameter of the narrowed portion of the artery is more important than the relative degree of narrowing of the artery. If the artery is very dilated, an allowance must be made for the infolding of the arterial wall, which will reduce flow in the artery more than would be expected by calculation from the outside diameter. The desirable degree of constriction is more than that required simply to produce a coarse thrill, and if a pulsatile blush is present in the lung this should be abolished. Any measurement which does not include flow in the pulmonary arteries is obviously less than satisfactory. At present the flow meter heads available give inaccurate readings if the wall is not firmly applied to the recording head, and these are not satisfactory in this operation. Monitoring the peripheral artery saturation will indicate when the shunt has been reversed to give a right-to-left flow. Production of a right-to-left shunt indicates that the constriction is too tight. There is at present no ideal method of calculating the change of pulmonary artery flow and the exact diameter to which the artery should be narrowed, when the chest is opened at operation and the lung retracted.

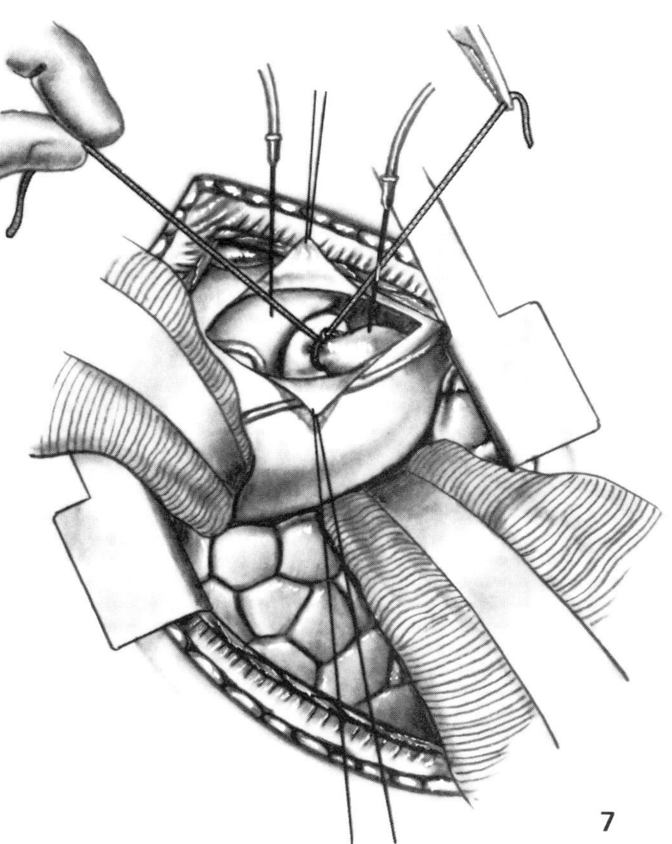

7

8

Securing the ligature

When the ligature has been secured with a second tie of a square knot, it is firmly secured with a third tie. The ligature has in some cases, slipped peripherally to the pulmonary artery bifurcation. The ligature can be secured by suturing it to the adventitia of the pulmonary artery but when this has been done with interrupted sutures it has resulted in pulmonary artery rupture. If the ligature is to be fixed to the pulmonary artery it should be done with a continuous suture over at least half the circumference of the ligature.

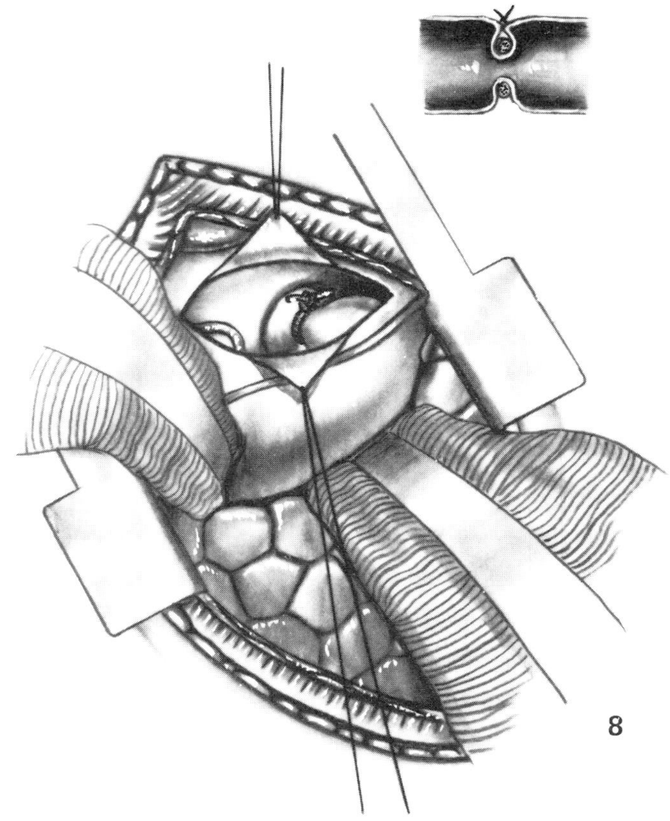

8

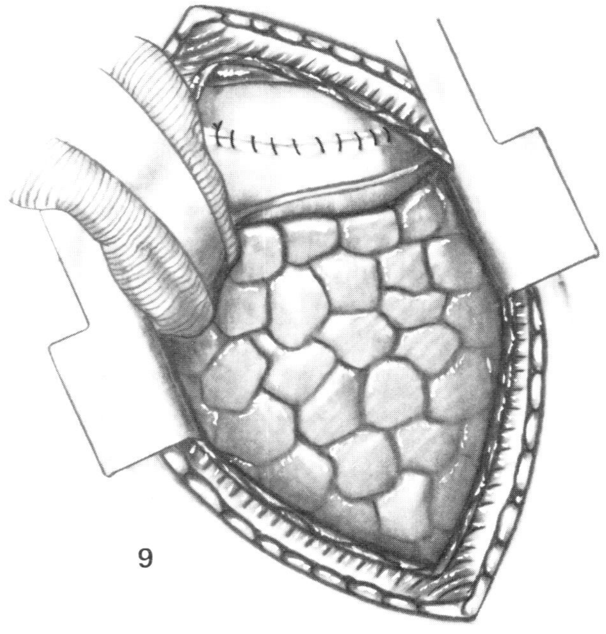

9

9

Closing the pericardium

When the needle puncture sites are completely dry, the pericardium is closed with continuous 5/0 or 6/0 suture, leaving a small opening superiorly for drainage.

Wound closure

The chest wound is closed with pericostal catgut (No. 1) with continuous 3/0 chromic catgut to the muscle layers and continuous 4/0 chromic catgut subcutaneously. The skin is closed with a continuous subcuticular suture. The pleural cavity is drained routinely.

SPECIAL POSTOPERATIVE CARE AND COMPLICATIONS

Lung compliance is often poor and this is usually one of the indications for the operation. All inhaled gases should be fully saturated with water vapour and careful nursing attention given to aspirating the nasopharynx and to chest physiotherapy. If pulmonary insufficiency is severe, an artificial airway, usually a nasotracheal tube, is used to help with aspiration of the tracheobronchial tree and with artificial ventilation. Frequent assessment of arterial blood gas and pH levels is most valuable when the infant is severely ill, and is best done by an indwelling arterial cannula.

Results and prognosis

This palliative operation for ventricular septal defect has resulted in mortality rates of between 5 and 12 per cent when no other cardiac defect is present. For more complex lesions the mortality rate has been higher and therefore less acceptable. The results have been quite unacceptable in the banding for truncus arteriosus. Banding continues to be of value when a ventricular septal defect in a young infant with transposed great arteries has resulted in severe heart failure, and is also of help in double outlet right ventricle and in some cases of endocardial cushion defect and with a large ventricular septal defect when heart failure in early infancy is a problem (Somerville *et al.*, 1967). At the subsequent corrective open heart procedure, the intrapericardial adhesions which are a result of the banding operation are an inconvenience but rarely a major problem. Restoring the pulmonary artery outflow is usually not difficult and adds about 15–20 min to the perfusion time, which does increase the risk of correction, but usually only by a small degree. Although pulmonary artery banding is usually an operation which cannot be judged precisely and adds another mechanical lesion, it still continues to have a limited place in the treatment of complex forms of congenital heart disease. Obviously primary correction of a lesion at the time when it first becomes a problem is the most desirable course of treatment, both for the patient and their anxious family, but in some lesions the results of pulmonary artery banding and subsequent later correction still offer a higher survival rate than radical correction performed when the patient is first seen in early infancy. Better methods of cardiac and pulmonary support and preservation will no doubt make this unnecessary in the future, but a careful appraisal of surgical results indicates that this state has not been reached.

References

Hallman, G. L., Cooley, D. A. and Bloodwell, R. D. (1966). 'Two-stage surgical treatment of ventricular septal defect. Results of pulmonary artery banding in infants and subsequent open-heart repair.' *J. thorac. cardiovasc. Surg.* **52**, 476

Muller, W. H. and Dammann, J. F. (1952). 'The treatment of certain malformations of the heart by creation of pulmonic stenosis to reduce pulmonary hypertension and excessive pulmonary blood flow.' *Surgery Gynec. Obstet.* **95**, 213

Panagopoulos, R., Tatooles, C. J., Aberdeen, E., Waterston, D. J. and Bonham-Carter, R. E. (1971). 'Patent ductus arteriosus in infants and children.' *Thorax* **26**, 137

Rohmer, J., Brom, A. G. and Nauta, J. (1967). 'Bands inside the pulmonary artery. A complication of the Dammann-Muller procedure.' *Ann. thorac. Surg.* **3**, 449

Somerville, J., Agnew, T., Stark, J., Waterston, D. J., Aberdeen, E., Bonham-Carter, R. E. and Waich, S. (1967). 'Banding of the pulmonary artery from common atrioventricular canal.' *Br. Heart J.* **29**, 816

[*The illustrations for this Chapter on Pulmonary Artery Constriction were drawn by Mr. G. Lyth.*]

Total Anomalous Pulmonary Venous Drainage

Jaroslav Stark, M. D.
Consultant Cardiothoracic Surgeon, The Hospital for Sick Children, Great Ormond Street, London

PRE-OPERATIVE

Introduction

Total anomalous pulmonary venous drainage occurs in only about 1·5 per cent of children born with congenital heart disease. Most patients become symptomatic within the first months of life. Without treatment, 80 per cent of the symptomatic infants die before they reach their first birthday (Bonham-Carter, Capriles and Noe, 1969).

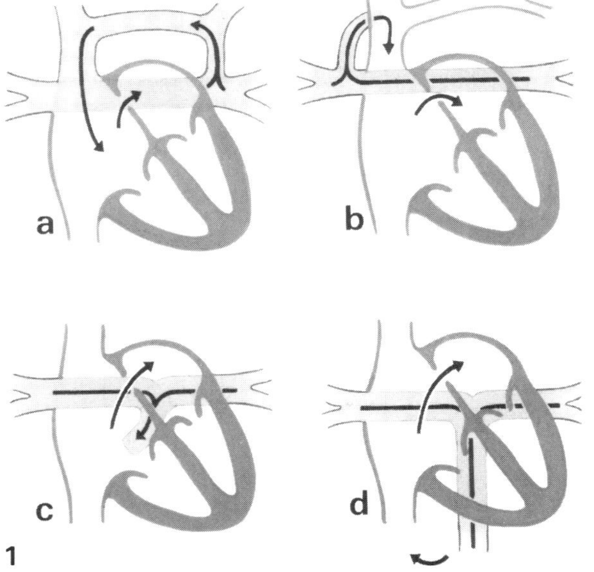

1

Diagnosis

Infants with total anomalous pulmonary venous drainage usually present with heart failure and/or cyanosis. Pulmonary oedema is common. An electrocardiogram shows right axis deviation, right atrial and right ventricular hypertrophy. A heart that is not enlarged, together with pulmonary oedema and hepatomegaly is almost diagnostic of obstructive total anomalous pulmonary venous drainage. Complete diagnosis is established by cardiac catheterization and angiocardiography. Additional lesions should be excluded and the exact type of drainage from all parts of the lungs established.

1

Various types of total anomalous pulmonary venous drainage are recognized: supracardiac (*a*, *b*); intracardiac (*c*); and infracardiac (*d*).

Indications

All infants with total anomalous pulmonary venous drainage and pulmonary hypertension should be operated on immediately. In the absence of pulmonary hypertension and/or pulmonary venous obstruction, surgery can be delayed, but patients in the latter category usually do not have symptoms in infancy. If they do, an early operation is preferred.

Anaesthesia

Patients are often severely ill on admission. They may require insertion of arterial and central venous lines for pressure and blood gas monitoring. If they hypoventilate, or if they are suffering from gross pulmonary oedema, they should be intubated and ventilated. A catecholamine drip is often helpful to treat severe heart failure. Premedication and anaesthesia do not differ from that in other open heart procedures in sick infants. Monitoring devices are often inserted before or during diagnostic cardiac catheterization. For sick infants with total anomalous pulmonary venous drainage, the author prefers to use the technique of circulatory arrest under deep hypothermia (Hikasa, Shirotani and Satomura, 1968).

THE OPERATION

Surface cooling

Once the arterial monitoring cannula is inserted, the patient is placed on a water mattress and surrounded by ice packs. Extremities, the area of the skin incision and the lumbar region (kidneys) are not cooled. It is felt that surface cooling is safer for very young and sick infants with congenital heart defects. If cardiac arrest or ventricular fibrillation occurs in the initial stages of operation, the lower temperature provides protection of the vital organs before cardiopulmonary bypass is established.

The incision

A mid-line sternotomy is performed when the nasopharyngeal temperature reaches 26° – 28°C. These infants are often dystrophic and a further drop of 2°C in nasopharyngeal temperature can be expected. The pericardium is opened in the mid-line, the aorta, superior vena cava and inferior vena cava are then dissected.

Persistent ductus arteriosus

It is very important to check for patency of ductus arteriosus. It may not be demonstrated on the preoperative angiocardiogram because the pressures in the aorta and the pulmonary artery are often equal. Furthermore intra-operative diagnosis may be difficult because, under circulatory arrest, excessive pulmonary venous return, as a warning sign of a patent ductus arteriosus, will not be present. Apart from the haemodynamic consequences, the patent ductus arteriosus can cause air embolization when circulatory arrest is introduced and pressure in the aorta drops to zero. (For the technique of ligation of the ductus from the mid-line sternotomy, *see* Chapter on 'Patent Ductus Arteriosus', pages 37–42.)

Cannulation and perfusion

The ascending aorta is cannulated with a right-angled metal cannula and a plastic cannula is placed into the right atrial appendage. The patient is connected to the heart-lung machine and further cooled to a nasopharyngeal temperature of 19° – 20°C. The oxygenator is primed with fresh blood and Ringer lactate, so that when the perfusate and patient's blood are mixed, a haematocrit of about 30 per cent is achieved. During the cooling phase, CO_2 is added to keep the arterial P_{CO_2} between 40 – 50 mmHg (corrected for temperature). When the desired temperature is reached, perfusion is stopped, the patient's blood is drained into the oxygenator, the aorta is cross-clamped, the superior vena cava and inferior vena cava are snared and the venous cannula is removed from the right atrium.

In older children, the operation is performed using standard cardiopulmonary bypass with moderate hypothermia. Both venae cavae are cannulated with right-angled cannulae with semirigid tips (Rygg), the left ventricle is vented and the aorta cross-clamped. Care should be taken to open the common pulmonary vein as soon as the ascending vein is ligated to avoid complete obstruction of pulmonary venous drainage with distension and subsequent damage to the lungs.

The surgical technique depends on the anatomical type of total anomalous pulmonary venous drainage.

INTRACARDIAC TYPE

2

The right atrium is opened and anatomy visualized. The most common site of intracardiac drainage is the coronary sinus, although separate entry of the pulmonary veins to the right atrium is possible.

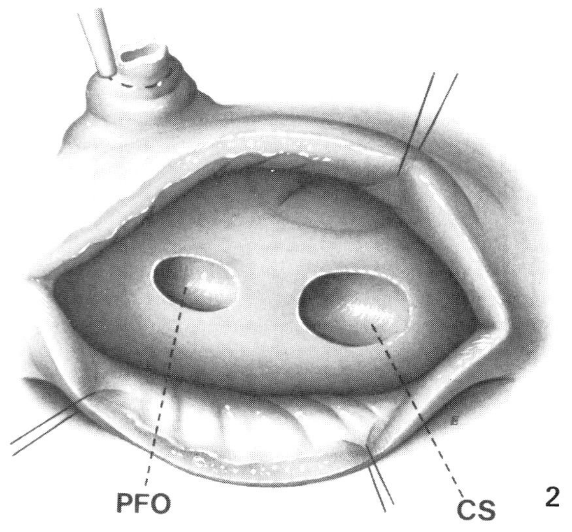

2

3a

3a

The septum between the coronary sinus and patent foramen ovale is excised. This creates a large communication between the coronary sinus and the left atrium.

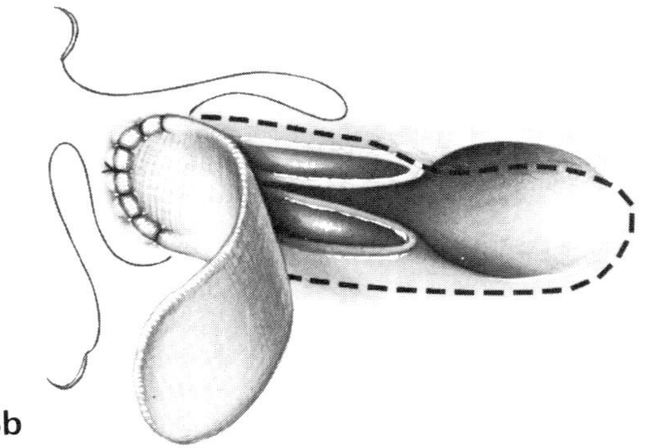

3b

3b

A patch of pericardium or thin Dacron is then stitched in to divert all pulmonary venous blood together with the coronary sinus blood to the left atrium. A small right to left shunt resulting from the coronary sinus blood admixture is not significant and is usually not detected on oxymetry at postoperative cardiac catheterization. Note that anteriorly the suture line runs through the floor of the coronary sinus away from its anterior rim. This is to avoid any damage to the tail of the atrioventricular node.

SUPRACARDIAC TYPE

The vein connecting the pulmonary vein to the innominate vein is dissected outside the pericardium. Care is taken not to damage the phrenic nerve and to pass the ligature above the entry of the left upper pulmonary vein. This may be rather high. When the circulation is stopped the vein is doubly ligated. Premature ligation of this vein would completely obstruct pulmonary venous drainage and damage the lungs.

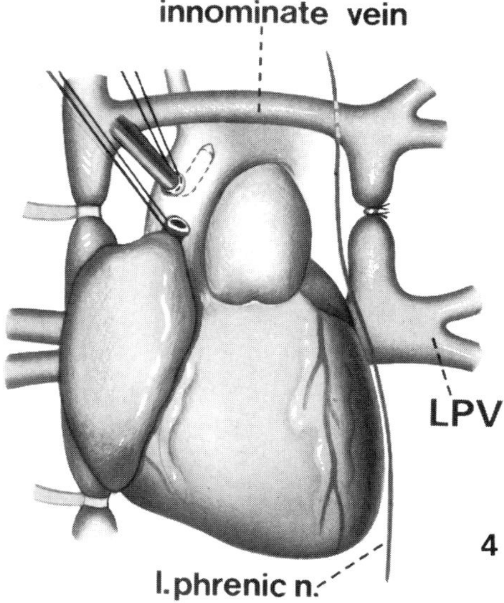

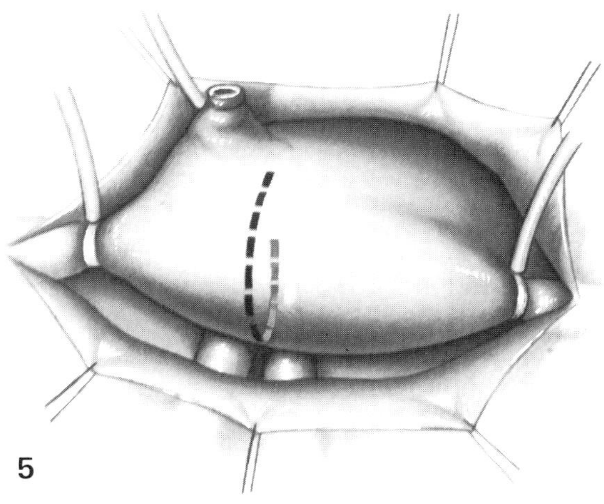

5

The right atrium is opened transversely, i.e. from the atrioventricular groove across the crista terminalis over the septum.

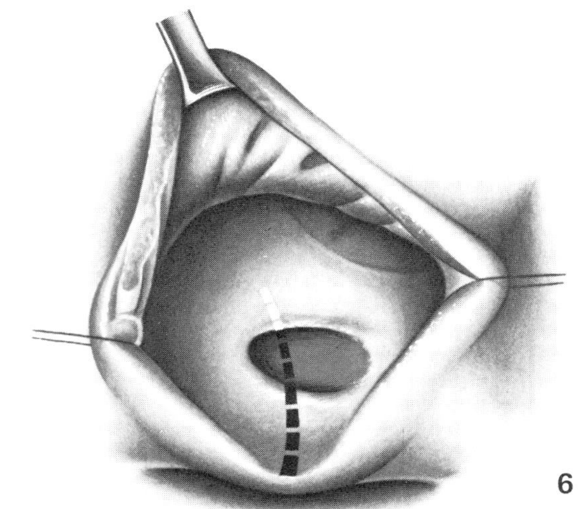

6

6&7

The incision then continues through the patent foramen ovale to the posterior wall of the left atrium down to the base of the left atrial appendage.

The horizontal confluence of the pulmonary veins lies just beneath and is incised. A ligature is placed on the tip of the left atrial appendage which is retracted to the left.

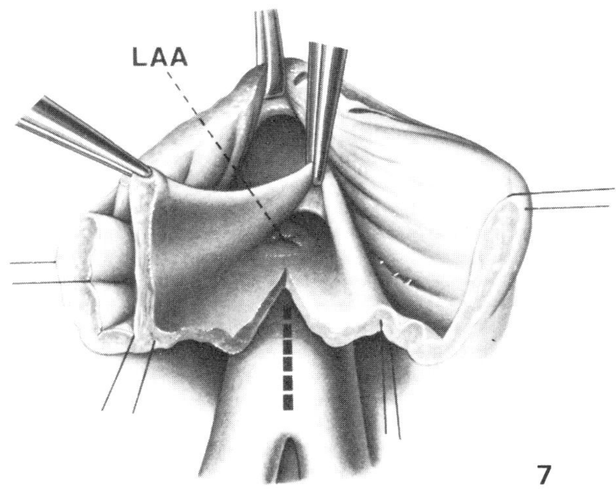

7

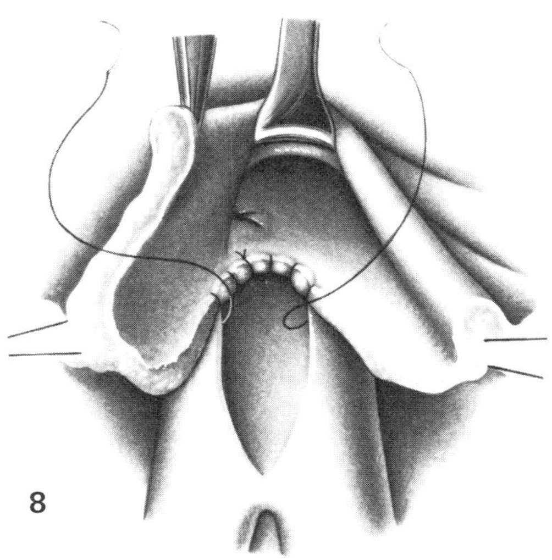

8

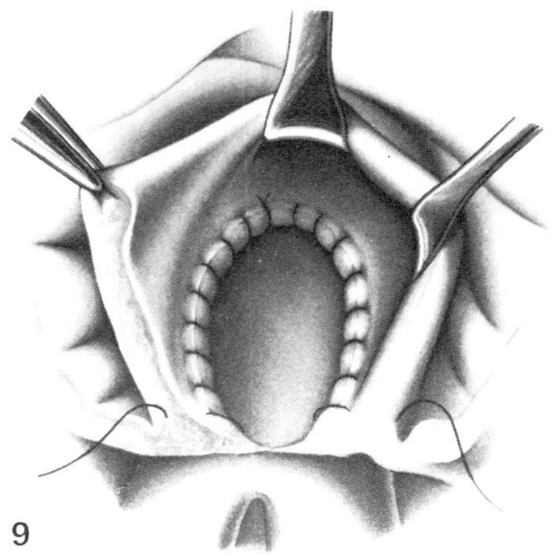

9

8&9

The posterior wall of the left atrium and the common pulmonary veins are joined by a suture of 5/0 or 6/0 Prolene. As long an anastomosis as possible is created. Care must be taken when both sides of the posterior left atrial wall and the septum are joined to the right side of the common pulmonary vein. Avoiding a constriction of this vein is of great importance.

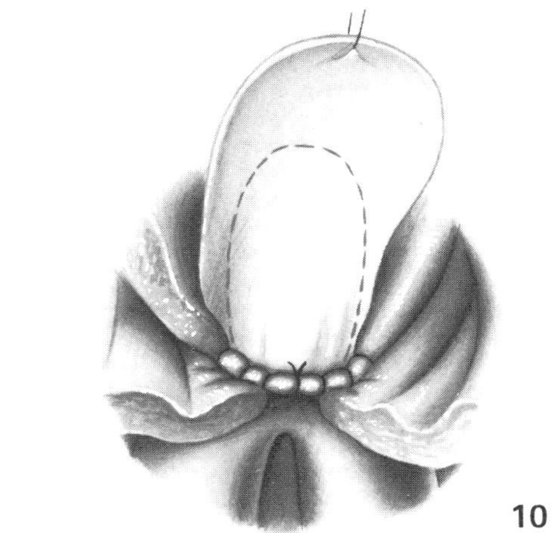

10

10 & 11

The atrial septal defect can be closed directly. When the size of the left atrium is small, the atrial septal defect can be closed with a pericardial patch, thus enlarging the small left atrial cavity at the expense of the right atrial cavity which is always large in this condition.

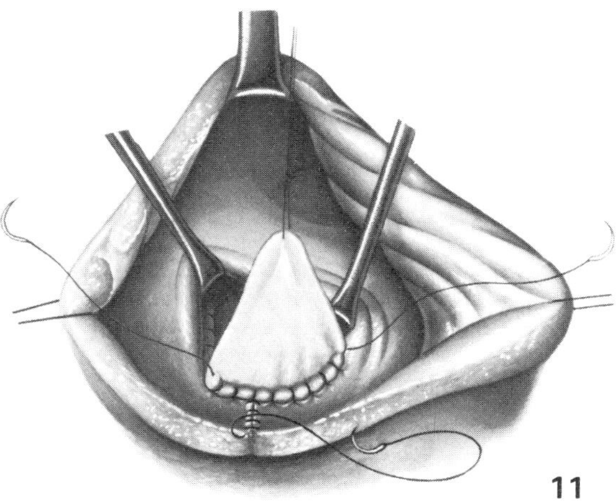

11

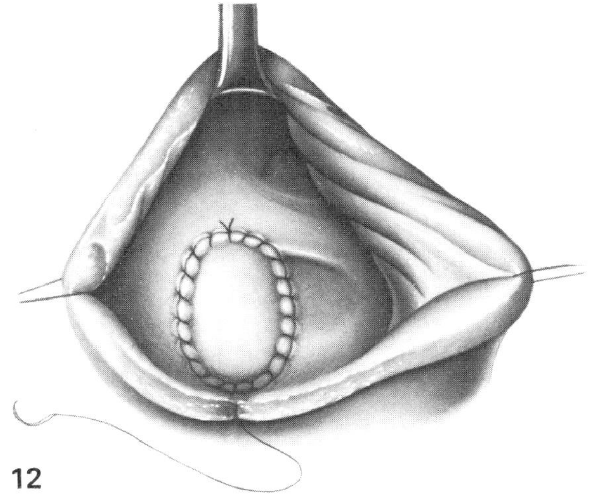

12

12

Completed closure of the septum is illustrated.

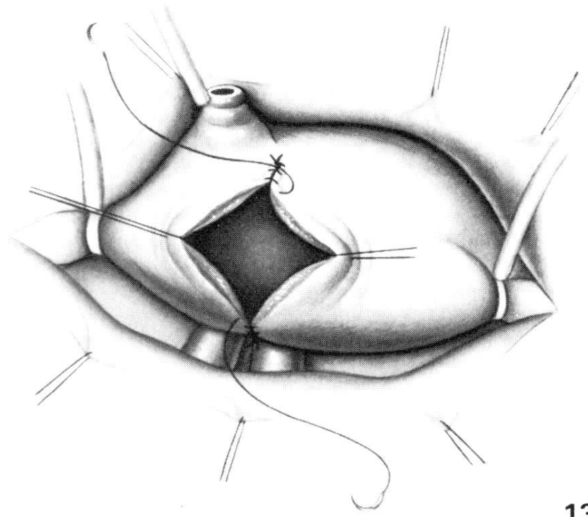

13

13 & 14

The atriotomy is closed with a running Prolene stitch.

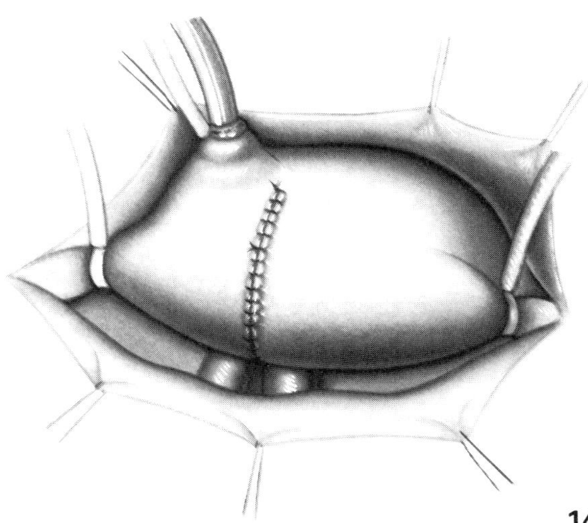

14

INFRACARDIAC TYPE

15

For the repair of this type, a retrocardiac approach is preferred, again using the technique of deep hypothermia and circulatory arrest. This allows better exposure of the common vein which is usually orientated vertically.

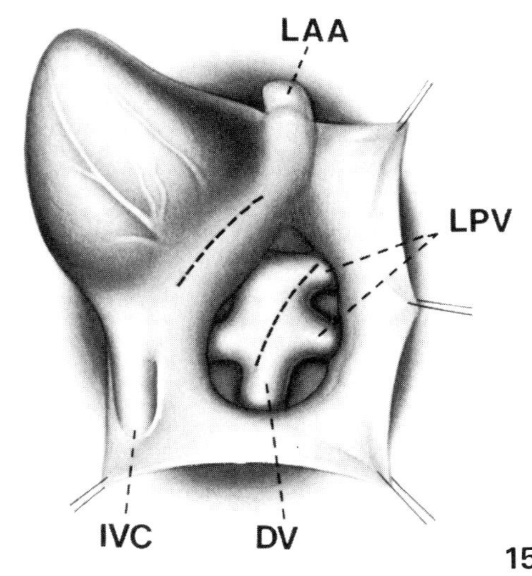

15

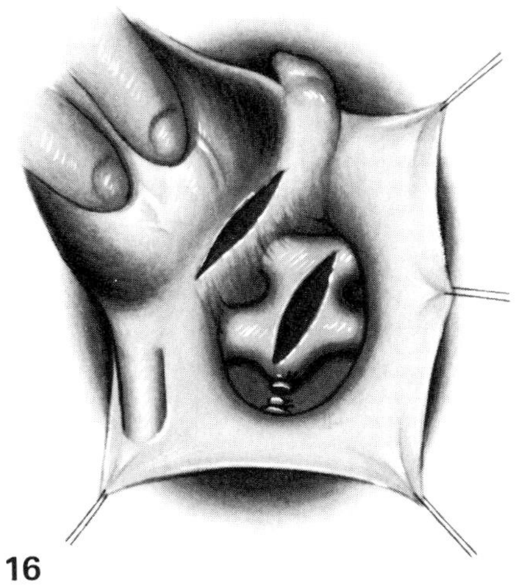

16

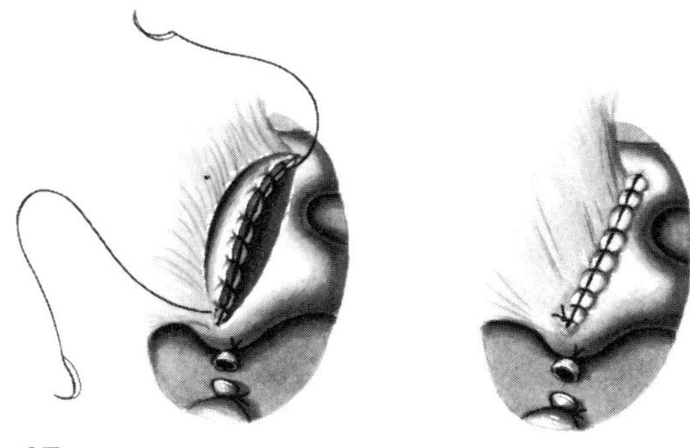

17

16 & 17

The first step is ligation of the connecting anomalous vein. In patients in whom there is a long distance between the confluence of the pulmonary veins and the left atrium, the descending vein (DV) can be doubly ligated and divided allowing the site of the anastomosis to come into closer apposition to the left atrium. Oblique parallel incisions are then made in the confluence of the pulmonary veins and in the posterior wall of the left atrium. The incision can start from the origin of the left upper pulmonary vein and extend into the upper portion of the dilated ascending vein allowing for a larger anastomosis to be created. The atrial septal defect or patent foramen ovale is closed through a separate right atriotomy.

MIXED TYPE TOTAL ANOMALOUS PULMONARY VENOUS DRAINAGE

Almost any combination of the standard types of drainage can exist in one patient. If one lobe drains differently from the rest of the lungs, it can be left uncorrected without great physiological consequences. Commonly the left upper lobe drains to the innominate vein while the remaining drainage is intracardiac.

Rewarming and terminating the perfusion

When the repair is completed, the heart is filled with saline. The venous cannula is replaced into the right atrium and the patient slowly transfused from the oxygenator. When the superior vena caval pressure reaches 12 – 15 mmHg, the caval snares are loosened and air is aspirated from the venous line. The left ventricle and ascending aorta are aspirated of air, the bypass is then restarted and aortic clamps released.

In some infants, the pulmonary veins are very small and in these we do not leave the left atrial line for fear of narrowing the pulmonary vein with a purse-string suture. In these patients, the right atrial line is inserted after the termination of bypass. During rewarming, the left atrial pressure is kept at 8 – 10 mmHg, allowing the heart to eject. It is believed that the pulsatile flow achieved at this stage is beneficial. When the temperature reaches 36°C, bypass is discontinued and the venous cannula removed. Occasionally, it is necessary to remove the aortic cannula quickly as the aorta is usually small and the cannula may cause partial obstruction. Because of the tendency of patients with total anomalous pulmonary venous drainage to pulmonary oedema, the central venous pressure or left atrial pressure is kept lower than in other lesions. Usually 8 – 10 mmHg is enough for an adequate cardiac output. Pacemaker wires are inserted and the chest is closed leaving mediastinal and pericardial drains.

POSTOPERATIVE CARE AND COMPLICATIONS

We prefer to intubate and ventilate all infants with total anomalous pulmonary venous drainage for the first 12 – 24 hr after operation. Constant positive airway pressure with spontaneous breathing is often used to wean them off the ventilator. Fluid restriction is important. Other supportive measures, such as catecholamines, Digoxin, diuretics etc., are used in the usual indications.

Complications

Pulmonary oedema is common, even if a large anastomosis has been constructed. Segmental or lobar atelectasis is treated with intensive physiotherapy; occasionally deep suction is required.

Results and prognosis

The operative mortality depends on the anatomical type of total anomalous pulmonary venous drainage. In the intracardiac type, the risk is below 10 per cent, supracardiac type 35 per cent, while infracardiac type drainage still carries about a 50 per cent risk (Gersony *et al.*, 1971; Wukasch *et al.*, 1975; Clarke *et al.*, 1977; Barratt-Boyes, 1973). Late deaths due to the development of pulmonary vascular disease or late stenosis of the anastomosis have been described. The majority of survivors are leading normal lives.

References

Barratt-Boyes, B. G. (1973). *Advances in Cardiovascular Surgery,* page 127, Edited by J. W. Kirklin. New York: Grune & Stratton

Bonham-Carter, R. E., Capriles, M. and Noe, Y. (1969). 'Total anomalous pulmonary venous drainage: A clinical and anatomical study of 75 children.' *Br. Heart J.* **31**, 45

Clarke, D. R., Stark, J., de Leval, M., Pincott, J. R. and Taylor, J. F. N. (1977). 'Total anomalous pulmonary venous drainage in infancy.' *Br. Heart J.* **39**, 436

Gersony, W. M., Bowman, F. O., Steeg, C. N., Hayes, C. J., Jesse, M. J. and Malm, J. R. (1971). 'Management of total anomalous pulmonary venous drainage in early infancy.' *Circulation* **43**, 44 (Suppl. I)

Hikasa, Y., Shirotani, H. and Satomura, K. (1968). 'Open heart surgery in infants with an aid of hypothermic anaesthesia (II).' *Archs Jap. Chir.* **37**, 399

Hikasa, Y. *et al.* (1967). 'Open heart surgery in infants with an aid of hypothermic anaesthesia.' *Archs Jap. Chir.* **36**, 495

Wukasch, D. C., Deutsch, M., Reul, G. J., Hallman, G. L. and Cooley, D. A. (1975). 'Total anomalous pulmonary venous return. Review of 125 patients treated surgically.' *Ann. thorac. Surg.* **19**, 623

[*The illustrations for this Chapter on Total Anomalous Pulmonary Venous Drainage were drawn by Mr. M. J. Courtney.*]

Blalock - Taussig Operation

Philip B. Deverall, F.R.C.S.
Consultant Cardiothoracic Surgeon, Guy's Hospital, London

PRE - OPERATIVE

Indications

The Blalock-Taussig operation, i.e. anastomosis of the subclavian artery to the pulmonary artery, is indicated as a palliative procedure for increasing pulmonary blood flow in various forms of cyanotic congenital heart disease. The procedure can be performed at all ages, but requires microvascular suturing techniques in infancy. Occasionally, in infants, the subclavian artery is too short or too small to permit a satisfactory shunt; then a direct aorta-to-pulmonary artery anastomosis is constructed. However, in most instances a satisfactory Blalock can be created and is the author's choice of shunt. The size of the subclavian artery is such that too large a shunt is only rarely created, unlike direct shunts between the aorta and pulmonary artery. Similarly the development of pulmonary vascular disease after a Blalock shunt is very rare.

A further advantage of the Blalock shunt is that local damage or distortion of the pulmonary artery is rare. Closure of the shunt at the time of a subsequent repair of the basic cardiac defect is relatively safe and uncomplicated, and the presence of a Blalock shunt does not increase the risk of complete correction in, for example, tetralogy of Fallot.

Assessment

Cardiac catheterization and angiography is performed to make a precise diagnosis. The Blalock shunt is ideally performed on the side of the innominate artery, i.e. on the right when the aortic arch is left-sided and vice versa. Although the position of the arch can usually be assessed by study of a plain chest x-ray, angiography is valuable in precisely defining the anatomy of the aortic branches and pulmonary arteries.

Pre-operative preparation

Standard pre-operative preparation is used. Patients with severe cyanosis or cyanotic spells should be operated upon on an urgent basis. Polycythaemic patients should have a careful haematological assessment. Gross abnormalities of bleeding and/or clotting times are best treated by staged haemodilution.

THE OPERATION

1

The chest is opened through a third-space thoracotomy; the child having been positioned in a lateral position.

After incising the skin, the subcutaneous tissues and the lower parts of the trapezius and latissimus dorsi muscles with diathermy, the scapula is retracted upwards and forwards and the intercostal muscle between the third and fourth ribs is divided with diathermy. After inserting a suitable rib spreader the intercostal incision can be extended slightly anteriorly and posteriorly.

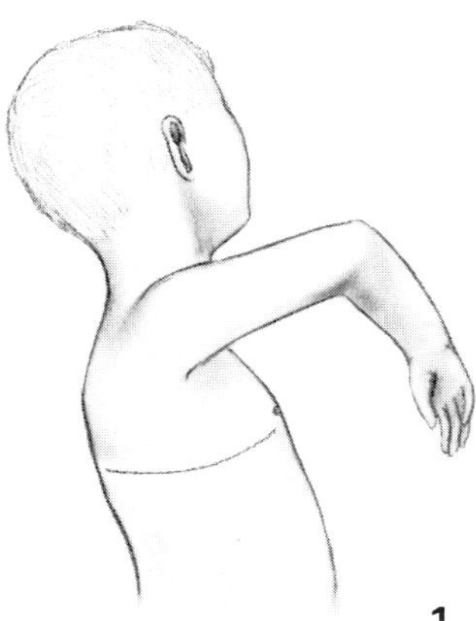

1

2

Exposure of mediastinum and mobilization of pulmonary artery

The lung is retracted posteriorly exposing the structures on the root of the lung. Before any dissection is commenced, a check is made that the mediastinum is moving satisfactorily with ventilation, i.e. the opposite lung is ventilating well. The main right or left pulmonary artery is then mobilized by a combination of sharp and blunt dissection. Small collateral vessels are cauterized. 2/0 Silk ligatures are looped around the main distal branches of the pulmonary artery and medially the pulmonary artery is mobilized behind the superior vena cava (on the right side) or to the pericardial reflection (on the left side). It is important that this dissection is completed fully as this gives extra mobility.

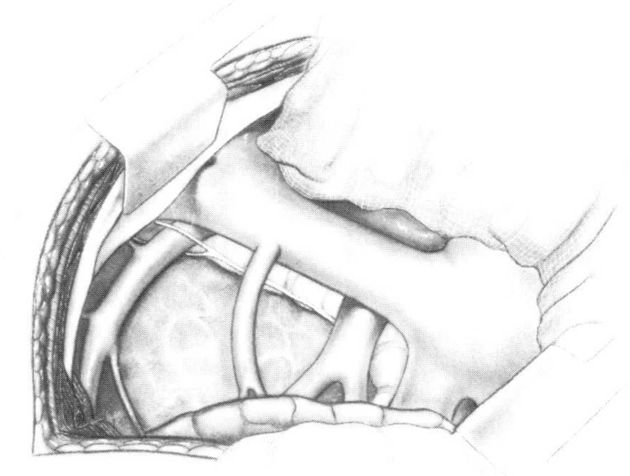

2

3

Mobilization of subclavian artery

The mediastinal pleura is then incised from the pulmonary artery up to and along the subclavian artery as far as the neck of the first rib. The azygos vein and any small veins crossing the subclavian artery at the apex of the chest are mobilized, ligated and divided. The vagus nerve is identified together with the site of the recurrent laryngeal branch. Small sympathetic nerve fibres loop around the subclavian artery and usually have to be divided. A heavy plaited silk ligature is then placed around the subclavian artery and by gentle retraction the branches of the artery are exposed. These are the vertebral, internal mammary, thyrocervical and costocervical branches. They are ligated with 2/0 or 3/0 silk and then divided.

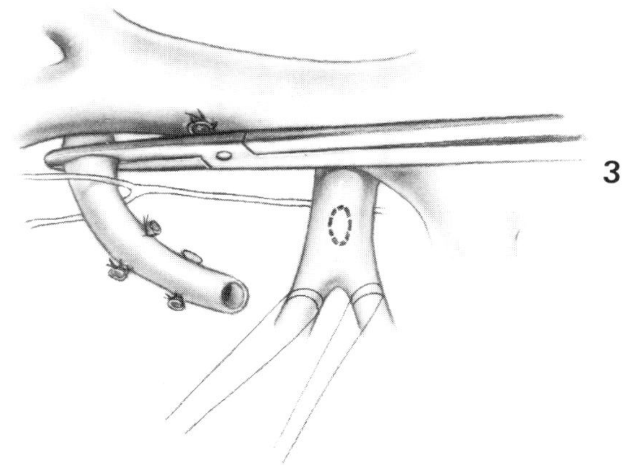

3

Division of subclavian artery

Following complete mobilization of the subclavian artery, it is then ligated and transfixed close to the neck of the first rib. The subclavian artery is then controlled with an atraumatic vascular clamp medial to the vagus nerve and the artery divided distally. Its lumen is irrigated with heparinized saline and the artery is drawn under the vagus/recurrent nerve loop. The adventitia over the innominate and carotid artery is incised and these arteries gently mobilized. This facilitates mobilization of the subclavian artery.

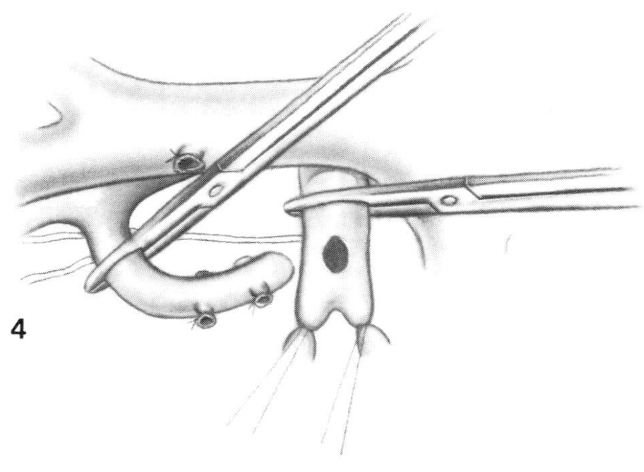

4

4

Preparation for anastomosis

The proximal end of the pulmonary artery is clamped with an atraumatic vascular clamp and the distal loop ligatures tightened. A small incision is made in the anterosuperior portion of the artery about midway between the clamp and the distal branches with sharp scissors and this incision gently dilated with blunt forceps.

The divided end of the subclavian artery is prepared by removing the adventitia. As wide an anastomosis as possible is made by incising any surplus subclavian artery, which will have narrowed as it approaches the first rib.

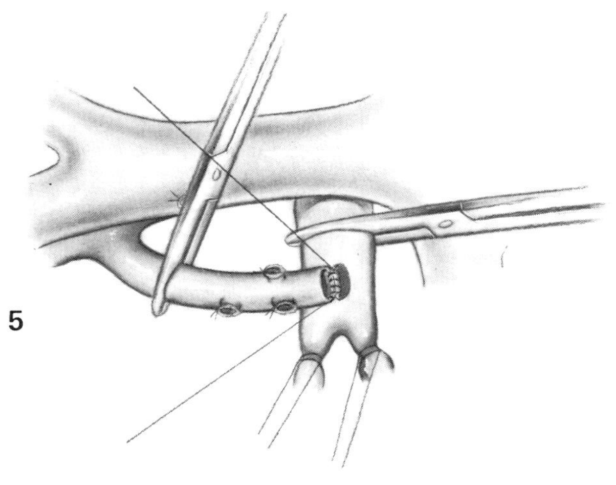

5

5

Anastomosis

The anastomosis is made using 6/0 silk or Prolene sutures. We use interrupted sutures in all infants and whenever the anastomotic diameter is less than 4 mm. Simple sutures with the knots on the outside of the lumen are used starting with the mid-point of the posterior layer. With larger anastomoses a continuous 6/0 Prolene suture is used starting at the medial angle and continuing as a simple over-and-over suture and placing the single knot on the outside. Anastomotic patency is checked with a fine probe before placing the final anterior sutures. It is particularly important to avoid dragging any adventitia into the lumen of the anastomosis.

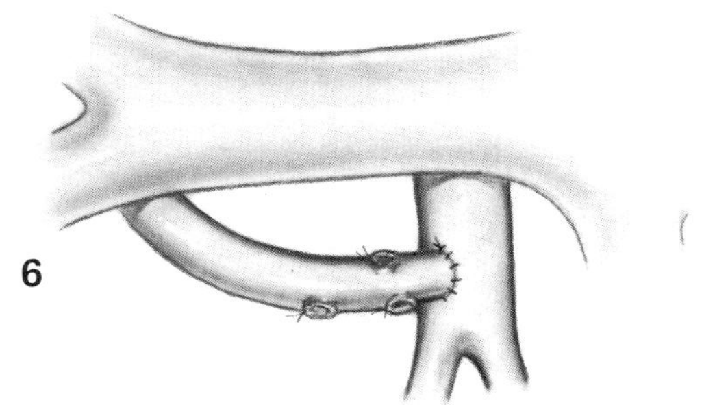

6

6

The distal loops of the pulmonary artery are then loosened followed by the pulmonary artery clamp. Minor bleeding is packed; only major bleeding is secured by a further suture. Finally, the subclavian artery is unclamped.

Assessment of shunt

On release of the clamp a continuous soft thrill should be present over the anastomosis or pulmonary artery. If this is present immediately the anastomosis is satisfactory. If no thrill is palpated, a check should be made to see that the patient's blood pressure is adequate; if not this is treated. If there is still no palpable thrill the anastomosis should be re-explored and if necessary, revised. It is our experience that the anastomosis is unsatisfactory if no thrill at all is present. By performing the shunt on the side of the innominate artery, the problem of kinking of the origin of the subclavian artery is avoided.

POSTOPERATIVE CARE AND COMPLICATIONS

Most patients will not require any blood replacement during the operation. A degree of haemodilution can be obtained in polycythaemic patients by using a non-haemic plasma expander. We prefer to maintain assisted ventilation postoperatively until a stable cardiovascular state exists. The patient is then extubated and placed in a humidified oxygen-enriched environment. An intercostal tube is always left in position and is removed usually on the day following operation.

Excessive bleeding should usually be treated by re-exploration. Occasionally a serous effusion develops which may require drainage or intermittent aspiration. A chylothorax is rare.

Horner's syndrome is common and is caused by division of the sympathetic nerves around the subclavian artery. Very rarely, transient abnormalities of cerebrovascular function occur following the Blalock shunt and are thought to be due to a subclavian steal phenomenon. If a satisfactory shunt has been constructed it is unusual for clotting and obstruction of the shunt to occur in the early postoperative period. However, if a shunt murmur ceases to be audible and is associated with a deterioration in the patient's clinical condition, re-exploration is probably needed. Clotting is usually due to a clumsy anastomosis and particularly to adventitia, which has been drawn into the anastomotic lumen.

Late complications are uncommon, though occasionally there is evidence of mild ischaemia of the arm on the side of the shunt. Closure of the Blalock-Taussig shunt at the time of a subsequent corrective operation is described in the Chapter on 'Complete Intracardiac Repair of Fallot's Tetralogy', page 101.

[*The illustrations for this Chapter on Blalock-Taussig Operation were drawn by Mr. G. Lyth.*]

The Waterston Operation. Ascending Aorta-Right Pulmonary Artery Anastomosis

Eoin Aberdeen, F.R.C.S., F.A.C.S.
Director of Cardiovascular Surgery,
The Children's Hospital of Newark, New Jersey

PRE-OPERATIVE

When Drs. Blalock and Taussig introduced the subclavian-pulmonary artery shunt in 1945, they began the surgical treatment of cyanotic congenital heart disease.

Some forms of pulmonary valve atresia and severe Fallot's anomaly in early infancy, transposition of the great arteries with ventricular septal defect and pulmonary stenosis, and tricuspid atresia are the three most common types of congenital heart disease which may require palliative treatment by a systemic-pulmonary artery shunt. The Blalock anastomosis is still the palliative operation of choice for these conditions, but when the anatomy does not allow this anastomosis to be made satisfactorily, a direct anastomosis between the aorta and pulmonary artery is required. A Potts-Smith anastomosis which joins the descending aorta to the left pulmonary artery is effective, but it has proved difficult to close at a later radically corrective operation. An anastomosis of the ascending aorta to the right pulmonary artery is much more easily corrected later. This operation was first performed by Waterston in 1960 (Waterston, 1962) and has become a widely used palliative operation of special value in infants (Fuller, 1965; Edwards, Mohtashemi and Holdefer, 1966; Cooley and Hallman, 1966).

Indications

If an infant or child is constantly and severely cyanosed or is having severe cyanotic attacks, or is unable to thrive, surgical relief is necessary. If a systemic-pulmonary artery shunt is required, a Blalock-Taussig anastomosis is preferred. If the anatomy is not suited to a classic Blalock-Taussig shunt, then a Waterston shunt is a desirable alternative, especially in the very young infant. The Waterston shunt is an easier operation to perform than the Blalock shunt.

Radical correction of Fallot's anomaly is being performed in the first few years of life with increasingly good results, and when radical correction can be achieved with a mortality rate less than 10 per cent it is to be preferred at any age, but the current risks of Blalock-Taussig shunt or a Waterston shunt in experienced hands has been less than 2 per cent in older children for many years and is now approaching this low rate even in early infancy.

Special equipment

Partial occlusion clamps designed for infants are strongly advised for this operation. Cooley's modification of the Satinsky clamp is ideal.

Pre-operative investigations

Any infant who is severely ill with congenital heart disease should be fully investigated before operative treatment is performed. Assessment of the lung vascularity by plain postero-anterior x-ray is inadequate. Angiocardiography will help to establish the diagnosis and left ventricular injection or aortography will also outline the great arteries and their branches, and so enable an accurate decision to be made about the most suitable type of systemic-pulmonary arterial anastomosis.

Anaesthesia

Endotracheal halothane or nitrous oxide and oxygen with muscle relaxants are preferred.

Position of patient

The child is placed on the table with the right side uppermost, the shoulders being closer to the operator's side of the table than the lower part of the body. This causes the rib space to lie at right angles to the edge of the table.

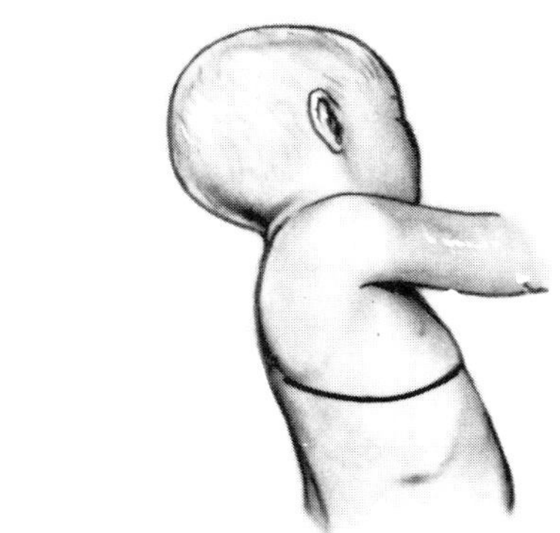

THE OPERATION

1

The incision

The fourth interspace is opened widely after a submammary skin incision has been extended posteriorly almost to the vertebral column. The skin incision need not be extended posterosuperiorly around the scapula as in adults, because the more horizontal scar is less unsightly.

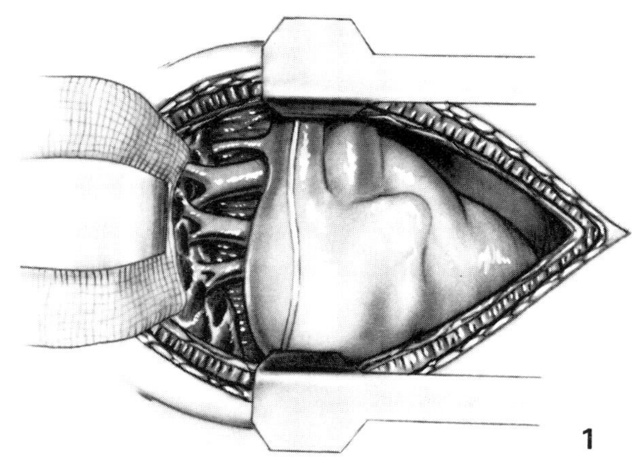

1

2

Dissection of pulmonary artery and aorta

The mediastinal pleura is incised, the azygos vein is divided and the mediastinal pleura overlying the superior vena cava is gently drawn forward and to the patient's left by two stay sutures. (The azygos vein is not necessarily divided in cases with transposed great arteries.)

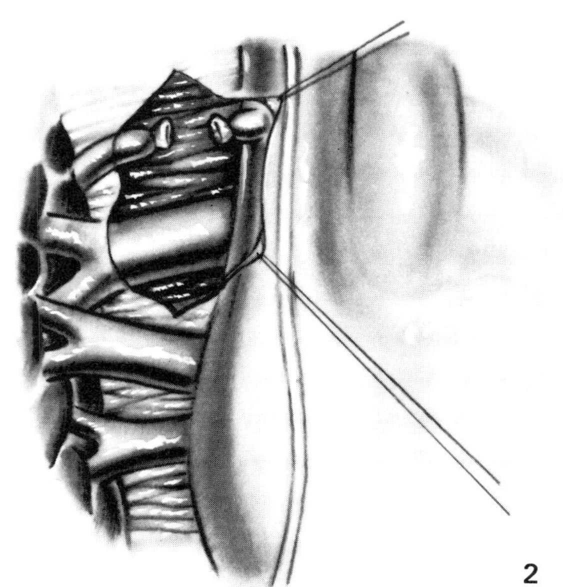

2

3

Mobilization of pulmonary artery

Dissection is commenced over the lung hilum and the pulmonary artery identified and mobilized. Peripherally, dissection is carried out to the lung root where the primary branches are identified and dissected separately and held by two snares of silk or silicone rubber. Medially, the right pulmonary artery is dissected posteriorly to the superior vena cava, as far centrally as the main pulmonary artery.

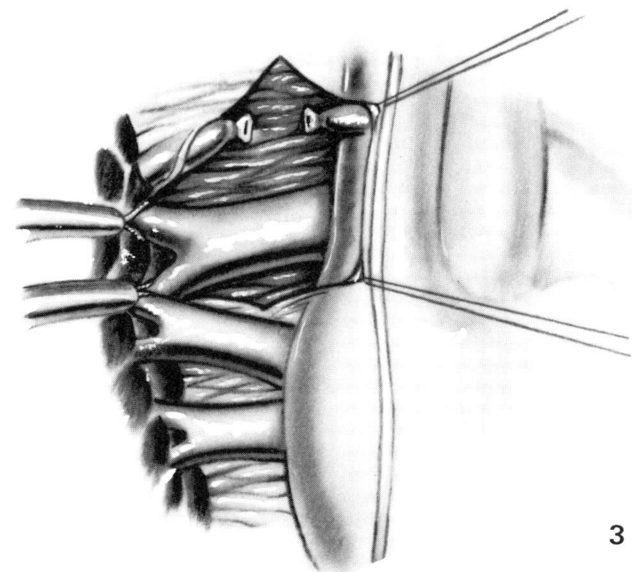

3

4

4

Exposure of aortic wall

The aorta can be identified behind and medial to the superior vena cava, the more dextroposed the aorta, the easier it is to identify. The pericardium is divided in the long axis of the aorta to expose the aortic wall.

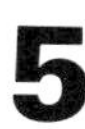

5

Placement of partial occlusion clamp

The peripheral artery branches are drawn laterally by two thick (No. 3) plaited silk or silicone rubber ligatures, which have been passed around them and held by rubber snares (catheter size 8 Ch, length 5 cm long). A partial occlusion clamp is then passed with one jaw posterior to the right pulmonary artery and the other jaw anterior to the artery, and so placed that when closed it will occlude a small portion of the aortic wall. The left coronary artery may be seen arising from the aorta posteriorly, and should not be obstructed by the partial occlusion clamp.

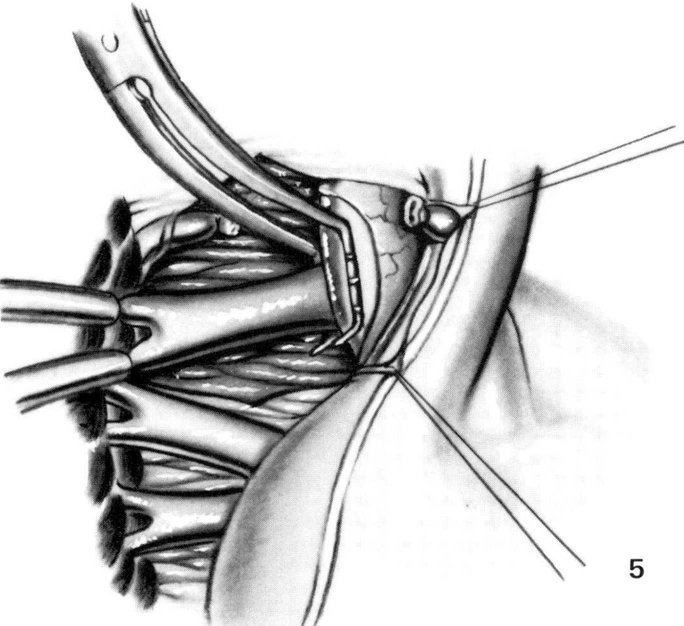

5

6

Closure of partial occlusion clamp and rotation of the aorta

The amount of aorta drawn into the clamp can be controlled by using tissue forceps to grasp the aortic wall at this point. The aorta should be grasped directly posteriorly and rotated to the right anteriorly. This allows the incision in the aorta to be made in the posterior aortic wall. When the anastomosis is completed and the occlusion clamp removed the anastomosis thus lies directly posterior to the aorta and so does not kink the right pulmonary artery. (Two sutures may be placed in the posterior aorta and used to rotate the aorta so the posterior portion is pulled into the clamp and is correctly placed for the anastomosis.) Enough aorta is drawn into the clamp to leave a cuff of 2 or 3 mm after the aortic wall has been incised. If too much aortic wall is drawn into the clamp, it may narrow the aortic lumen and reduce the cardiac output. Once this clamp has been firmly closed the snares are tightened around the primary branches of the pulmonary artery.

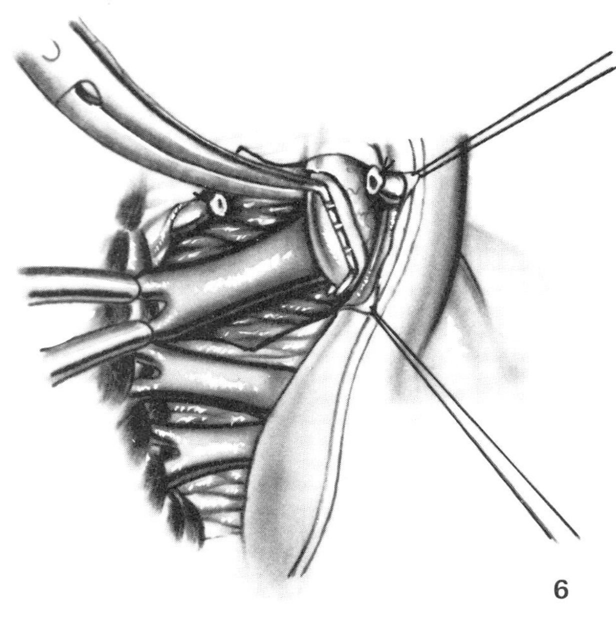

6

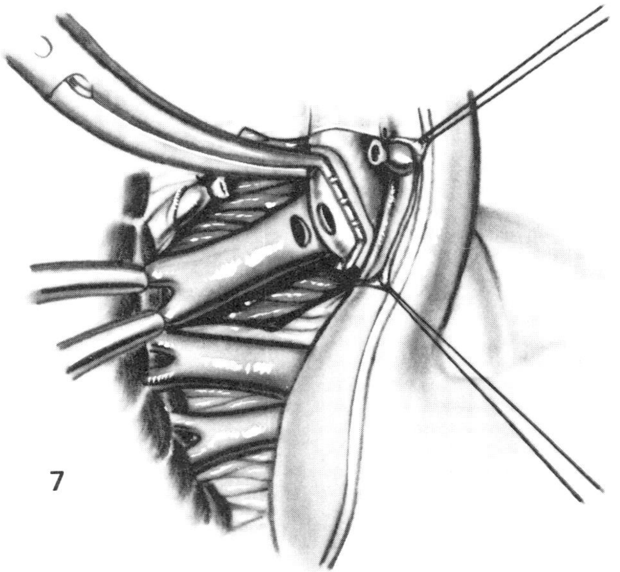

7

7

Incision of aorta and pulmonary artery

The ascending aorta is incised with a scimitar scalpel blade. The precise length of this incision is *critical* (a specially designed caliper has been produced to make accurate measurement easier (Donahoo and Aberdeen, 1976)). In a newborn infant an incision no longer than 3 mm should be made in the aorta. In an infant 1 year old, an incision of 4 mm long should be made and in older children, the incision should be 5 mm long. The length of the incision should be measured precisely and not judged by the eye.

The pulmonary artery is then opened transversely to provide an opening of the same size as the aortic incision. The loose adventitia around the adjoining parts of the pulmonary artery and the aorta should be removed before suturing is commenced.

8 & 9

The anastomosis

The anastomosis is made using continuous 6/0 monofilament arterial suture. The posterior layer is placed first in a continuous suture. The same suture is then continued around anteriorly, the suture being finally tied to the point where it commenced.

The anastomosis is made with a continuous suture because growth of the anastomosis should be limited. A band of heavy silk or Teflon of measured length placed around the anastomosis has been suggested as a more certain method of limiting later growth (Trusler, 1973).

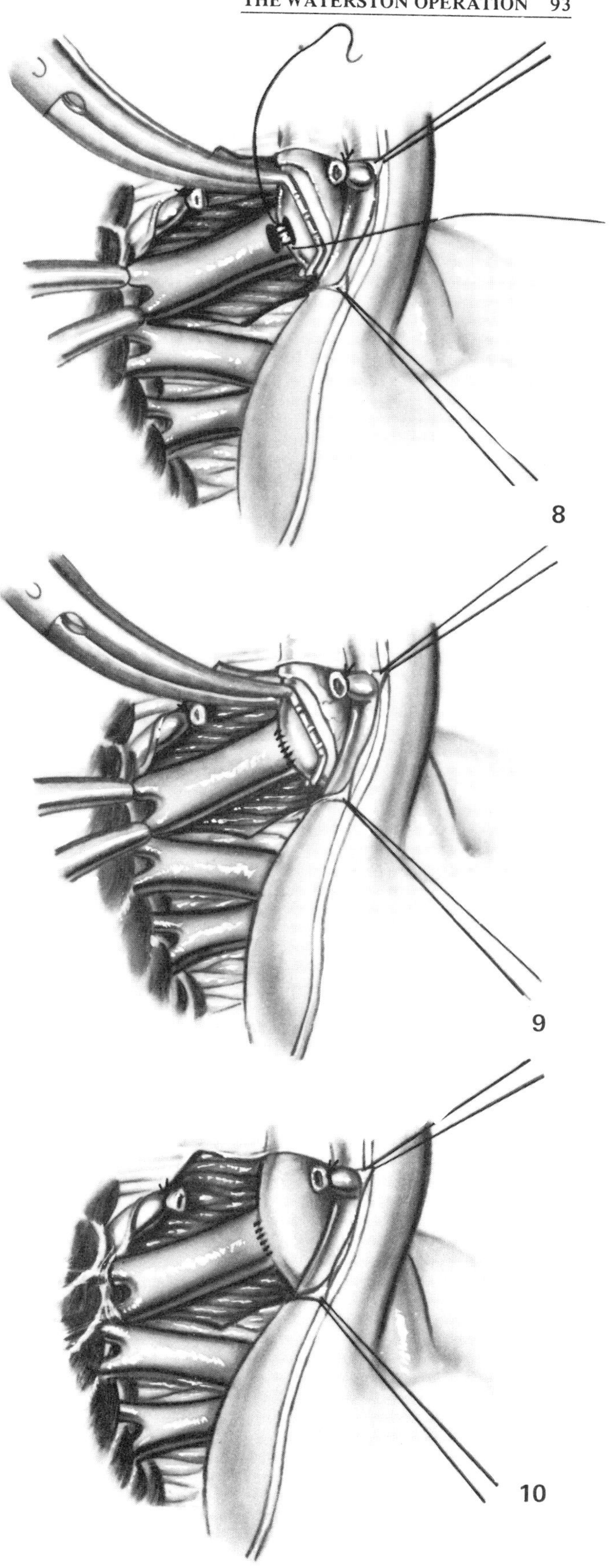

10

Removal of clamp

The snares around the primary branches of the pulmonary artery are first released and then the partial occlusion clamp is released. If leaking of the suture line is severe, an extra suture should be placed at this time. If bleeding is not severe, the partial occlusion clamp is completely removed and the anastomosis packed with gauze and haemostasis awaited. Palpation of a thrill in the right pulmonary artery indicates that the shunt is patent and the increased pressure in the pulmonary artery is usually obvious. The anaesthetist may note an improvement in the child's colour at this time also. If the pulmonary artery feels tense the pulmonary artery pressure should be taken by needle, and if this is higher than 40 mm, or more than half of the systemic pressure, it probably indicates that the shunt is too large. The shunt can easily be narrowed by placing a mattress suture through the corner of the anastomosis. A small difference in the diameter of the anastomosis can make a very large difference to the size of the shunt, because there is practically no length to the shunt.

POSTOPERATIVE CARE AND COMPLICATIONS

Two complications should be watched for in the early postoperative period. An excessive shunt may lead to congestive heart failure which should be treated with medical therapy. If severe and persistent it may require re-operation and narrowing of the shunt, but this is most unusual if the shunt was carefully measured at operation. Rarely the shunt may thrombose postoperatively, in which case the chest should be re-explored promptly and the clot removed from the anastomosis and pulmonary artery using a Fogarty embolectomy catheter. The anastomosis should then be resutured and allowed to function again.

Over a longer period a large shunt can result in the development of pulmonary vascular disease. This complication is more likely to develop following a Waterston or Potts shunt than it is with a Blalock-Taussig anastomosis, because the length of the subclavian artery better controls flow through the shunt.

Respiratory complications are unusual in the postoperative period but occasionally a nasotracheal tube and artificial ventilatory support may be required in the very young infant.

Results and prognosis

As with most other arterial systemic-pulmonary shunts, the operative risk is low (less than 2 per cent mortality rate) in the older infants and children. In very small infants the Waterston operation is easier than the Blalock-Taussig anastomosis, although this latter operation can be performed safely in infants from the day of birth. For those with limited experience of these operations the Waterston shunt is to be preferred, but great care should be taken to make the incision in the aorta the correct length.

In the long term, the prognosis is that of the underlying lesion for which palliative surgery is required. In Fallot's anomaly the long-term results are excellent after total correction if the shunt was correctly made. Even in tricuspid atresia the improvement is surprisingly well maintained after many years.

References

Blalock, A. and Taussig, H. B. (1945). 'The surgical treatment of malformations of the heart in which there is pulmonary stenosis or pulmonary atresia.' *J. Am. med. Ass.* **128**, 189

Cooley, D. A. and Hallman, G. L. (1966). 'Intrapericardial aorto-right pulmonary arterial anastomosis.' *Surgery Gynec. Obstet.* **122**, 1084

Donahoo, J. S. and Aberdeen, E. (1976). 'A new instrument for measurements in cardiovascular surgery.' *Ann. thorac. Surg.* **22**, 494

Edwards, W. S., Mohtashemi, M. and Holdefer, W. F. (1966). 'Ascending aorta to right pulmonary artery shunt for infants with tetralogy of Fallot.' *Surgery* **59**, 316

Fuller, D. (1965). 'Aorta-right pulmonary artery anastomosis.' *S. Afr. J. Surg.* **3**, 117

Trusler, G. A. and Kanzaki, Y. (1973). 'Controlling the growth of aorto-pulmonary anastomoses in piglets.' *Archs Surg.* **106**, 72

Waterston, D. J. (1962). 'The treatment of Fallot's tetralogy in infants under the age of one year.' *Rozhl. Chir.* **41**, 181

[*The illustrations for this Chapter on The Waterston Operation. Ascending Aorta-Right Pulmonary Artery Anastomosis were drawn by Mr. G. Lyth.*]

Closed Infundibular Resection The Brock Procedure

D. G. Taylor, F.R.C.S.
Thoracic Surgeon, Sheffield A.H.A.(T.)

PRE - OPERATIVE

Indications

Fallot's tetralogy is a significant cause of failure to thrive. In the more severe cases central cyanosis may be intense and associated with syncopal attacks and death. The relevant pathology is a large volume right ventricle with right ventricular outflow obstruction consisting of variable combinations of pulmonary infundibular stenosis, pulmonary valve stenosis and pulmonary artery hypoplasia. An important associated feature is a large ventricular septal defect with right to left shunting related to the severity of the right outflow obstruction. The severe category characteristically shows considerable disproportion between the aorta and pulmonary artery.

A surgical approach to this problem can be initially palliative with a view to later total correction (staged procedures) or, alternatively, one-stage total correction. A method of palliation is that originally described by Brock and Campbell (1950). This aims at a partial relief of the right outflow obstruction with increased pulmonary blood flow and is a valuable procedure in the surgical treatment of Fallot's tetralogy in infancy (Taylor, Grainger and Verel, 1963). A notable long-term advantage of this procedure is the development of the hypoplastic right outflow following the increased function resulting from partial relief of obstruction. Intense cyanotic and syncopal attacks with failure to thrive are a general indication for surgical relief of Fallot's tetralogy in infancy. The specific indication for the Brock-type procedure is poor development of the right ventricle outflow tract. Angiographic assessment showing an aortic diameter three times (or more) that of the pulmonary artery is a strong indication for a staged operation as a prelude to total correction.

Precautions

This group with intense cyanosis have haemoglobin concentrations in excess of 15 g per cent, and blood transfusion should be restricted to those few cases in which occasionally a relatively large haemorrhage occurs. An adequate intravenous infusion should always be maintained for immediate blood transfusion if required. In general, intravenous fluid administration should be minimal.

THE OPERATION

Special instruments

1

Expanding dilator

The expanding dilator is simply a scaled-down version of the mitral valve dilator originally designed by Mr. O. S. Tubbs.

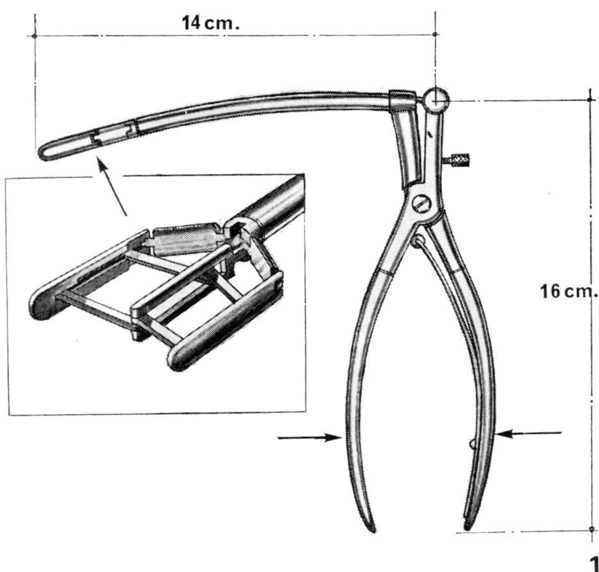

1

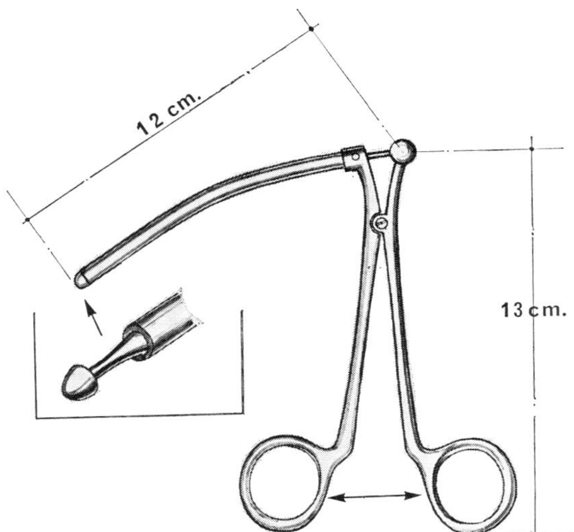

2

Infundibular punch

This type of infundibular punch is used for closed resection of infundibular muscle.

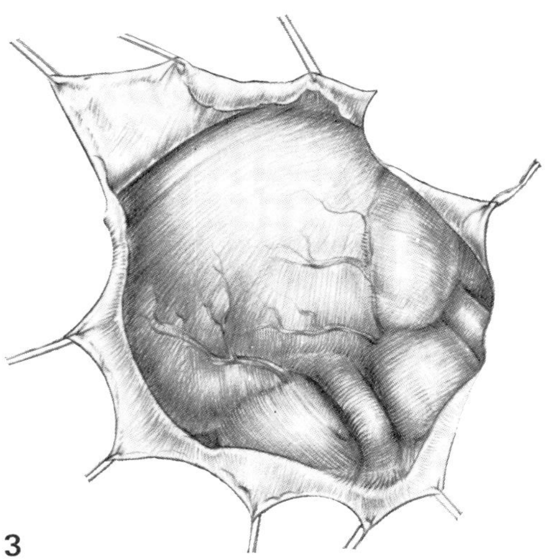

3

3

Exposure

The large right ventricle and pulmonary artery are readily exposed by a left anterior inframammary incision extended through the fourth space. Alternatively, a mid-line sternal splitting incision can be used.

The exposed pericardium is incised with flap formation in such a fashion as to expose the right ventricular outflow and the pulmonary artery. The thymus, which is usually prominent, requires mobilization and is excluded from the operative field by a stay suture. The diameters of the pulmonary artery and aorta are then measured and a withdrawal trace from the pulmonary artery to the right ventricle is then taken. This indicates the degree and levels of obstruction.

4

Dilatation and resection of infundibular muscle

A purse-string suture is inserted high in the right ventricular outflow immediately below the infundibular obstruction. The purse-string control is placed in such a way that it does not inconvenience subsequent instrumentation. The line of direction and level of the obstruction in the right ventricular outflow tract is then determined by the careful passage of a malleable probe. Failure to do this may result in a perforation posteriorly at the junction of the pulmonary artery and right ventricle creating a hazardous situation. When the line of the right outflow tract has been defined the ventriculotomy is dilated sufficiently to take the appropriate valvotome which is then passed through the stenotic valve. Progressive dilatation is carried out with graduated dilators, with intermittent use of the valvotomes and expanding dilator as required. Finally, resection of infundibular muscle is performed by a punch similarly inserted through the area of ventricle enclosed by the purse string. It is important that a large type of dilator should be passed proximally into the right ventricular cavity to exclude significant organic obstruction. The aim is to produce a long, easily palpable, systolic thrill in the pulmonary artery, and this should be associated with a measurable increase in diameter of at least several millimetres. Sufficient monitoring is provided by an electrocardiograph and pulse counter and pressure recording equipment is required for the determination of intracardiac and pulmonary artery pressure.

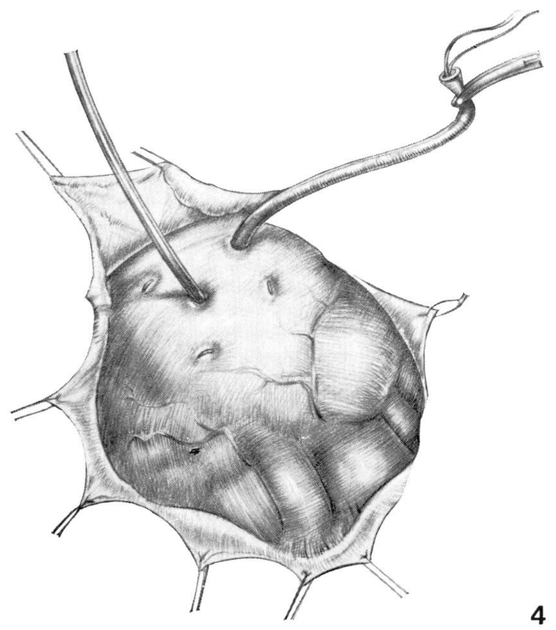

4

5

Closure of ventriculotomy

The ventriculotomy is closed by interrupted sutures and the purse-string suture is removed. A further withdrawal trace is taken across the right ventricular outflow tract. The pulmonary artery and aortic diameters are again measured and, characteristically, there is a measurable increase in the diameter of the pulmonary artery.

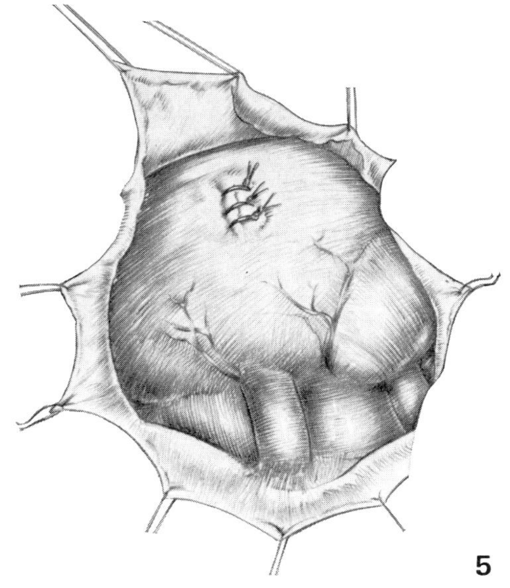

5

POSTOPERATIVE CARE

Postoperative management is along conventional lines. The patient is nursed in an oxygen tent in an adequately humidified atmosphere. Intermittent suction is maintained on the chest drain, and any blood loss is carefully measured and replaced. Haemorrhage is normally slight, but if replacement on any scale is required, it should be controlled by hourly—or more frequent—haematocrit estimations. A small gastric tube is normally passed in the theatre, and as soon as consciousness is recovered 2-hourly glucose saline feeds are commenced, making sure that no gastric residue remains before each feed. This regimen is maintained for 12 hr, and is followed by a gradual return to full-strength feeds with normal feeding commencing after 24 hr.

Following infundibular resection cyanosis often temporarily increases on the third to the fifth day, and this is particularly notable in the smaller infants. This is apparently due to local reaction following instrumentation, and generally responds to rest and inhalation of a humidified enriched oxygen mixture. Drug therapy is of little value at this stage, although recent experience with propranolol suggests that it may be of some assistance in relieving a spasmodic element. There is generally a marked reduction in cyanosis from the eighth to the ninth day onwards, with improved capacity to take feeds and early weight gain.

References

Brock, R. C. and Campbell, M. (1950). 'Infundibular resection or dilatation for infundibular stenosis.' *Br. Heart J.* **12**, 403

Taylor, D. G., Grainger, R. G. and Verel, D. (1963). 'Closed pulmonary valvotomy for the relief of Fallot's tetralogy in infancy.' *J. thorac. cardiovasc. Surg.* **46**, 77

[*The illustrations for this Chapter on Closed Infundibular Resection. The Brock Procedure were drawn by Mr. A. S. Foster.*]

Complete Intracardiac Repair of Fallot's Tetralogy

Christopher Lincoln, F.R.C.S.
Consultant Paediatric Cardiac Surgeon, The Brompton Hospital, London;
Lecturer in Paediatric Surgery, Cardiothoracic Institute, University of London;
Thoracic Surgeon, University College Hospital, London

PRE-OPERATIVE

Indications

Complete intracardiac repair is the operation of choice for patients with Fallot's tetralogy. In the specialist units equipped and staffed to treat patients with complex congenital heart disease, operation is performed in infancy and/or before the age of 3 years. Occasionally a palliative operation may be carried out, either a subclavian artery-pulmonary artery anastomosis (Blalock-Taussig) or an ascending aortic-pulmonary artery anastomosis (Waterston), after which total correction can be performed at 3–4 years of age, even though good palliation still exists. Experience with complete correction at all ages suggests that an operative mortality of between 5 and 15 per cent can be achieved.

Pre-operative study

Patients require specialist investigation by cardiac catheterization and angiography. This should demonstrate:

(*1*) concordant atrioventricular relationships;
(*2*) right ventricular infundibular stenosis, pulmonary valve stenosis, and/or pulmonary artery hypoplasia;
(*3*) a single high ventricular septal defect or multiple ventricular septal defects;
(*4*) the aorta over-rides the right ventricle but is placed above both right and left ventricles;
(*5*) there is no patent ductus arteriosus;
(*6*) a functioning systemic–pulmonary artery shunt (when previously palliated).

Extracorporeal circulation

Intracardiac surgery is facilitated by means of extracorporeal circulation. In this, blood from the venous circulation is returned to the pump oxygenator and the arterialized blood is returned to the ascending aorta, thereby excluding the heart from the circulation. Moderate hypothermia to 28°C can be used. When moderate hypothermia is used intermittent cross-clamping of the aorta for a maximum of 10 min provides a quiet, dry operative field.

In small patients (6 kg and under) previous surface cooling to 28°C, followed by a limited period of cardiopulmonary bypass when the heart and body is further cooled to 15°C, at which temperature the circulation is stopped. This is an alternative method of obtaining ideal intracardiac operating conditions. Circulatory arrest for an arbitrary period of 60 min has evolved, in which complete intracardiac repair can be carried out. Following this, cardiopulmonary bypass is re-instituted and the patient is rewarmed.

Perfusion to the patient is maintained at 2–2·4 litres/min/m^2 of body surface area.

CARDIAC MORPHOLOGY

The aortic valve is dextroposed in relation to the origin of the tricuspid and mitral valves. The mitral valve is in fibrous continuity with the aortic valve.

The pulmonary valve is abnormally posterior, inferior and leftwards in its position. The valve commissures may or may not be fused, and the pulmonary valve annulus is usually hypoplastic.

The infundibular septum is rotated and anteriorly deviated forming a prominent supraventricular muscle mass. The septal and parietal insertions of the infundibular septum form two prominent muscle bundles on either side of the ventricular septal defect. The medial papillary muscle is a key structure identifying the right lateral and inferior border of the ventricular septal defect.

The atrioventricular (A-V) bundle of His and Kent lies in the inferior posterior wall of the ventricular septal defect on the left side beneath the crest of the ventricular septum. The left bundle branch (L.B.B.) runs an endocardial course on the left side of the septum. The right bundle branch (R.B.B.) passes through the inferior aspect of the defect and proceeds on the trabecula septomarginalis (*see Illustration 7*).

SURGICAL ANATOMY

Hypertrophied septal and parietal insertions of the infundibular septum encroach upon the outflow tract of the right ventricle, and in addition the infundibular septum projects anterosuperiorly, thus raising the floor of the cavity of the right ventricular infundibulum, causing further obstruction to the outflow of blood. Therefore, varying degrees of hypertrophy of these muscle bars will cause differences in the severity of the condition. Pulmonary valve stenosis may or may not be added to the above morphological abnormalities.

Damage to the left bundle branch of the conducting tissue can be avoided by placing sutures to the right side of the interventricular septum 2–4 mm back from the crest of the interventricular septum and the rim of the ventricular septal defect. These sutures, however, invariably cause right bundle branch block, since it is difficult to avoid damage to this structure (*see Illustration 7*).

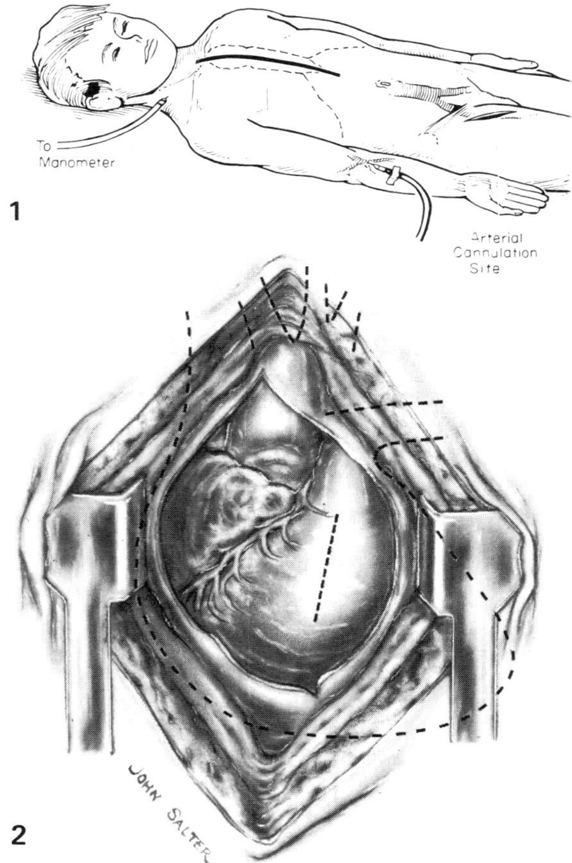

1

2

THE OPERATION

1

Position of the patient

The patient is placed in the supine position with arms at the sides. Plastic cannulae are inserted percutaneously into the internal jugular vein for intravenous administration of fluids and medication, and a plastic cannula is inserted percutaneously into the radial artery for monitoring systemic arterial pressure. A urinary catheter is placed in the bladder for accurate measurement of urinary flow during and after the operation.

2

The incision

A median sternotomy incision offers good exposure for intracardiac repair as well as for closure of previously constructed shunts. After the sternum has been divided with a saw, meticulous haemostasis must be achieved. The thymus, if large, can be partially excised. Care is taken to avoid entering the pleural spaces. The pericardium is incised longitudinally to expose the heart.

3

CLOSURE OF PREVIOUSLY CONSTRUCTED SHUNTS

Right Blalock-Taussig anastomosis and left aortic arch

If a previous anastomotic operation has been performed, this must be closed prior to the intracardiac repair. A right subclavian artery–pulmonary artery anastomosis is the preferred palliative operation in patients with the aortic arch on the left, and such an anastomosis can be closed with relative ease. Prior to heparinization and the institution of extracorporeal circulation, the subclavian artery just proximal to the anastomosis is exposed by retracting the superior vena cava laterally. Two ligatures are placed about the subclavian artery and tied immediately after extracorporeal circulation is instituted.

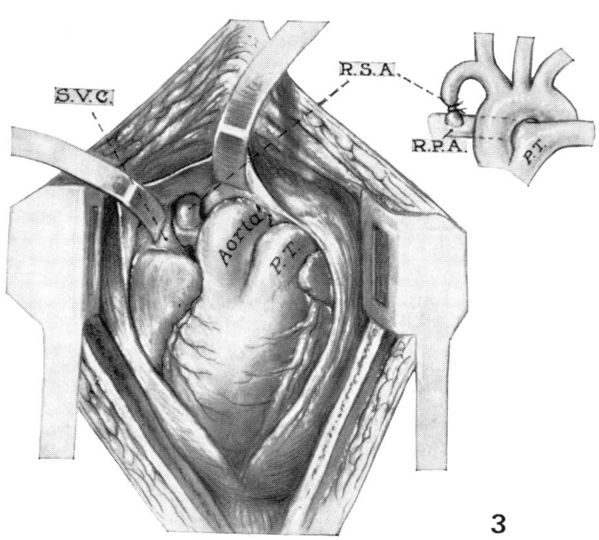

3

4

Left Blalock-Taussig anastomosis and left aortic arch

Ligation of the left subclavian artery is more difficult when a left subclavian artery-pulmonary artery anastomosis has been performed in a patient with a left aortic arch. The region of the anastomosis is exposed by careful extrapleural dissection, care being taken to avoid injury to the phrenic nerve.

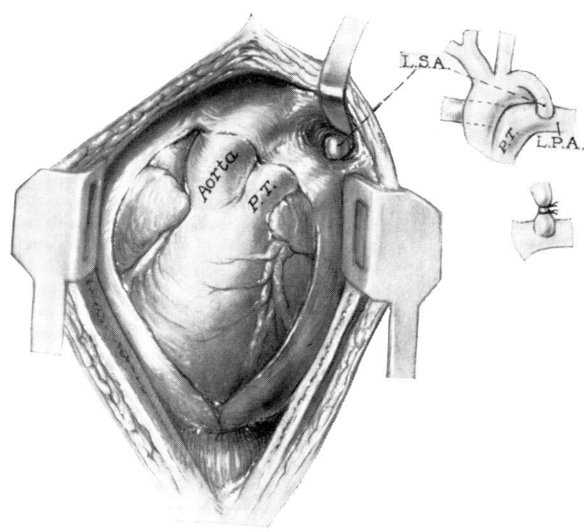

5

Left Blalock-Taussig anastomosis and right aortic arch

A left subclavian artery-pulmonary artery anastomosis is preferred in patients with the aortic arch on the right. To close such a shunt, the subclavian artery is approached by a dissection distally along the innominate artery to the origin of the subclavian artery. The vessel is ligated at its origin immediately after extracorporeal circulation is instituted.

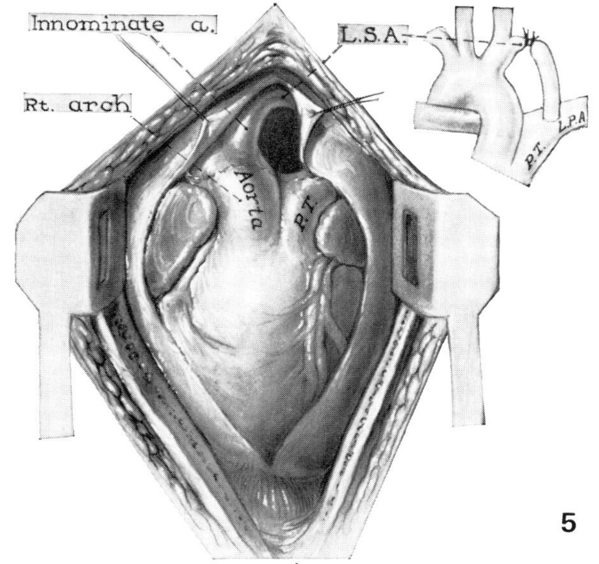

5

6

The Waterston anastomosis

An ascending aorta to right pulmonary artery anastomosis can be constructed for palliation, particularly in infants with very small pulmonary arteries (Waterston's anastomosis). Closure of this anastomosis at complete correction is carried out by clamping the aorta proximal to the aortic perfusion cannula immediately on establishing cardiopulmonary bypass. An oblique incision is made in the first part of the ascending aorta, and the stoma of the anastomosis can be closed by direct suture. The aortotomy is then closed, the aortic clamp is released, and the heart perfused and cooled to the desired temperature. Occasionally the construction of this anastomosis causes distortion of the right pulmonary artery. Growth may also cause distortion of this vessel. In this event, it is necessary to detach the right pulmonary artery from the posterior aspect of the ascending aorta, and the pulmonary artery is then reconstructed by an angioplastic repair. The defect in the posterior aspect of the ascending aorta is closed by direct suture.

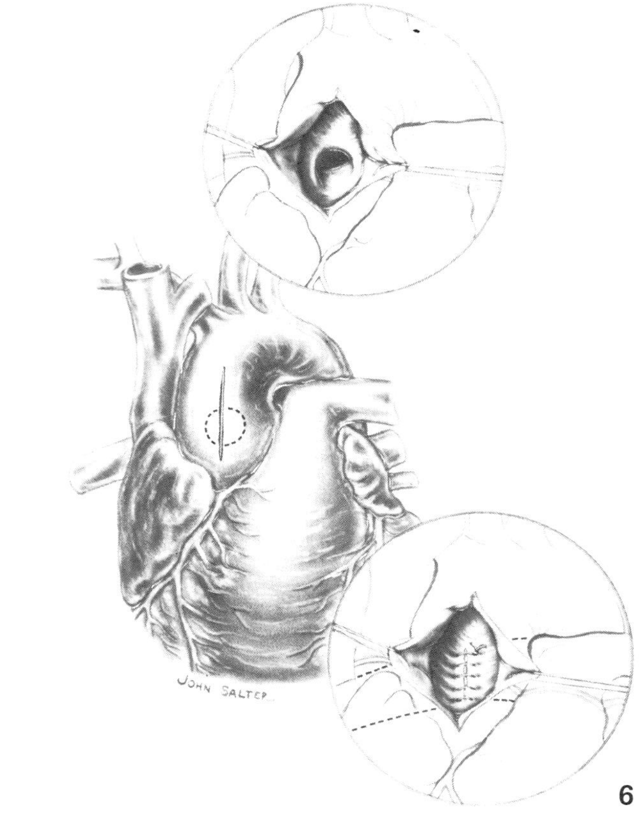

6

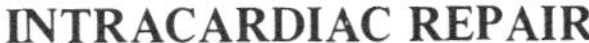

INTRACARDIAC REPAIR

Criteria for successful intracardiac correction

Successful intracardiac repair of tetralogy of Fallot must fulfil the following criteria:

(*1*) the ventricular septal defect or defects must be securely closed;

(*2*) right ventricular outflow tract obstruction must be relieved at ventricular, pulmonary valve, and pulmonary artery level;

(*3*) the myocardium must be preserved from prolonged ischaemia or from damage to coronary arteries.

7

The intracardiac repair is performed through a vertical right ventriculotomy, avoiding branches of the coronary arteries. The region of infundibular stenosis is treated by excision of the hypertrophied parietal and septal insertions of the infundibular septum, and mobilization of the free wall of the right ventricle. Failure to relieve satisfactorily right ventricular outflow tract obstruction will occur in between 40 and 60 per cent of patients, when outflow tract reconstruction will be required to enlarge this channel.

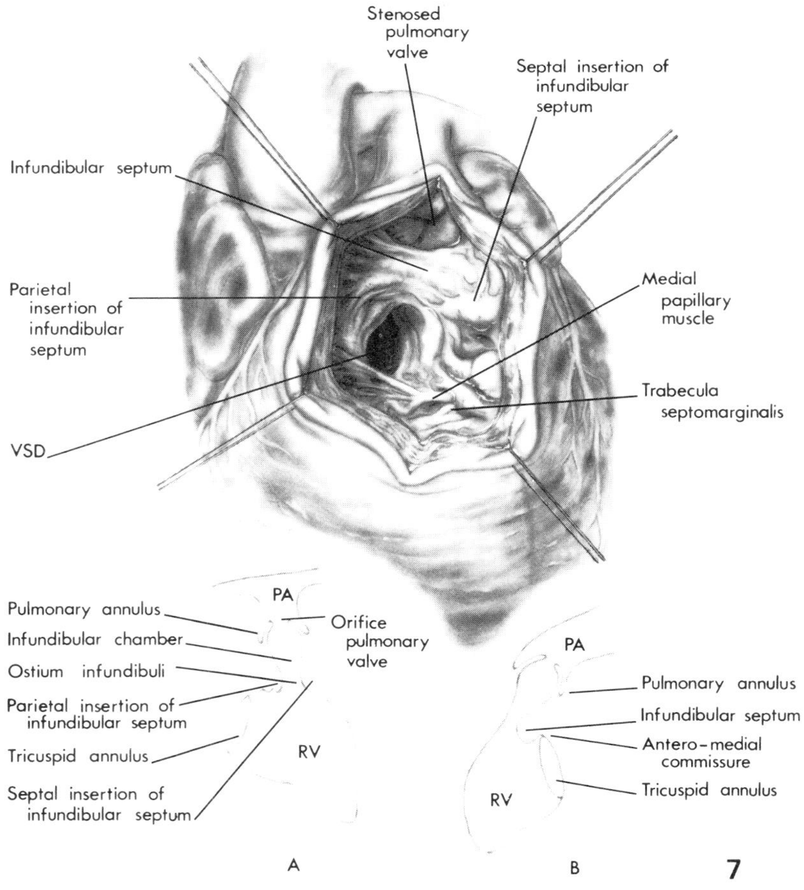

7

Closure of the ventricular septal defect

The ventricular septal defect is closed with a Teflon patch sutured in place with interrupted or continuous 4/0 monofilament sutures. This is facilitated by a dry field in a non-beating heart, and by knowledge of the pathways of the conducting bundle.

8&9a,b&c

Placing the sutures

The initial suture is placed at the base of the medial papillary muscle. Gentle traction on this suture delivers the base of the septal leaflet of the tricuspid valve, where further sutures are placed. Continuing traction on the sutures as placed paripassu delivers the periphery of the ventricular septal defect, thus facilitating placement of the sutures throughout its circumference. In the region of the muscular septum, the sutures are placed well back from the margin of the defect till the region of the septal leaflet of the tricuspid valve is reached (the medial papillary muscle is detached for illustrative purposes). A metal probe is used to detect any small defects between sutures, and if present, they are closed with additional sutures. Sutures are placed around the superior edge of the defect, avoiding distortion of the aortic valve cusps.

The ventriculotomy incision is closed with continuous 4/0 sutures. The left atrium which has been vented either through the patent foramen, if present, or an incision made in the fossa ovalis, is then closed.

Care is taken to remove air from the left atrium, left ventricle, and right ventricle. The heart is then allowed to beat, and eject blood from the ventricles into the great arteries. Extracorporeal circulation is then gradually discontinued, continuously monitoring the left atrial pressure as an index to the amount of perfusate that can be administered to the patient from the pump oxygenator, and also as an index of left ventricular function. On discontinuing cardiopulmonary bypass the heart is allowed to support the circulation for approximately 5 min, when peak pressures in the left and right ventricles are measured. If the right ventricular peak pressure is 75 per cent, or less than the left ventricular pressure, relief of the right ventricular tract obstruction is considered to be adequate. Decannulation of the heart is then performed, and the site of the cannulation is repaired. Meticulous haemostasis is then achieved. Drainage catheters are placed in the mediastinum and the pericardial space. A left atrial pressure-line is inserted in the left atrium prior to closing the chest. The sternum is approximated with sutures, and the skin wound is closed.

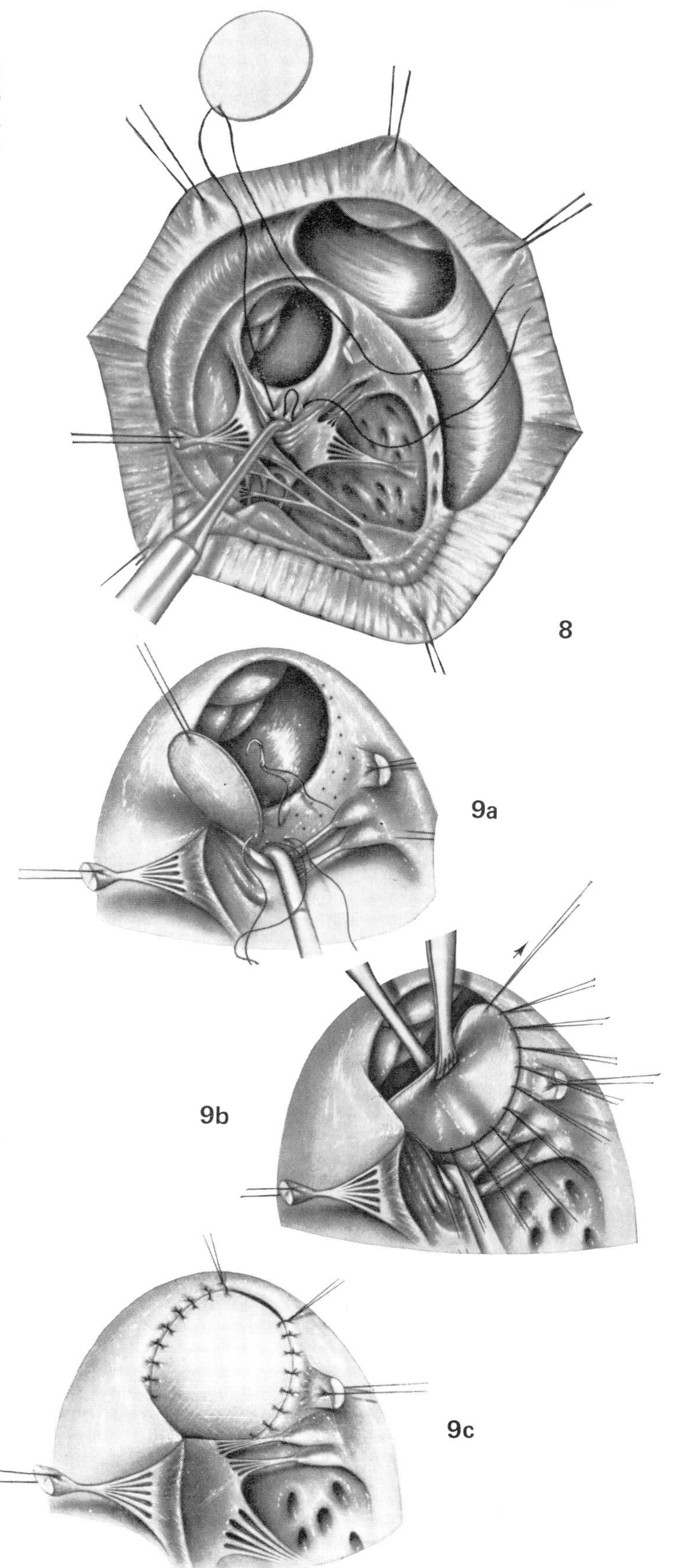

RIGHT VENTRICULAR OUTFLOW TRACT RECONSTRUCTION

In approximately 40–60 per cent of patients it will be necessary to widen the right ventricular outflow tract. This may be due to: (*a*) extreme anterior position of the infundibular septum (*b*) a small pulmonary valve annulus (*c*) stenosis or hypoplasia of the main pulmonary artery and /or the right and left pulmonary arteries. In such cases, the initial longitudinal incision in the infundibulum of the right ventricle can now be extended as necessary.

10

Extreme anterior position of the infundibular septum

Even when the infundibular septum and the septal and parietal insertions have been reduced in size by excision, when the heart is tonic the infundibular septum sometimes protrudes into the outflow path of the right ventricular infundibulum. If in this case the pulmonary valve annulus and the main pulmonary artery are of satisfactory size, then a gusset of pericardium is inlaid in the ventriculotomy site, thus increasing the volume of the right ventricular infundibulum. The gusset does not cross the pulmonary valve annulus.

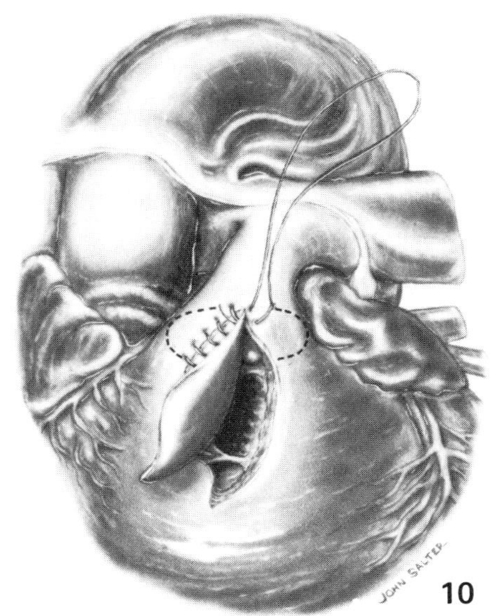

10

11, 12 & 13

Anterior position of infundibular septum with hypoplasia of pulmonary valve annulus and main pulmonary artery

When this triad of abnormalities exists the whole of the right ventricular outflow tract must be enlarged by a gusset of pericardium. Alternatively, a section of an aortic valve homograft tailored into a monocusp can be used, thus preserving a competent pulmonary valve mechanism. At present there is no evidence to suggest that pulmonary incompetence has a deleterious effect on right ventricular function.

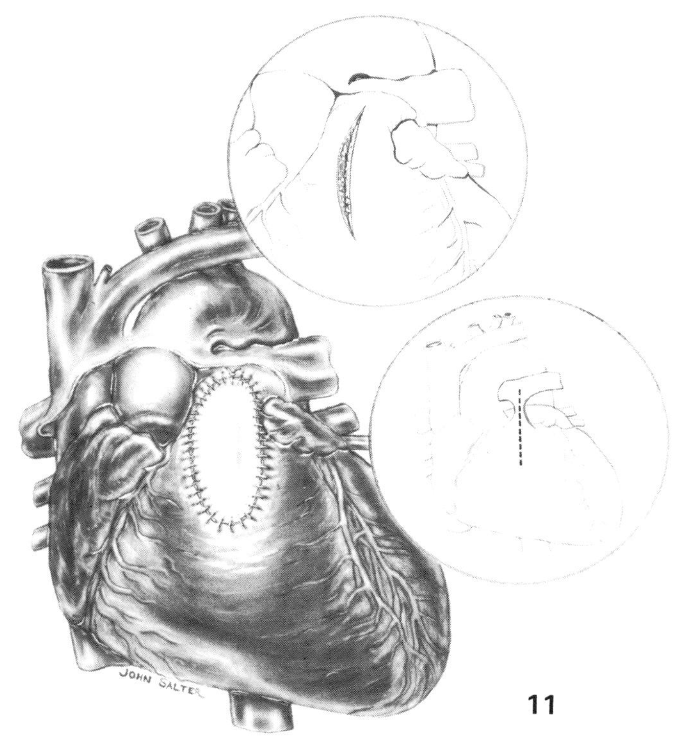

11

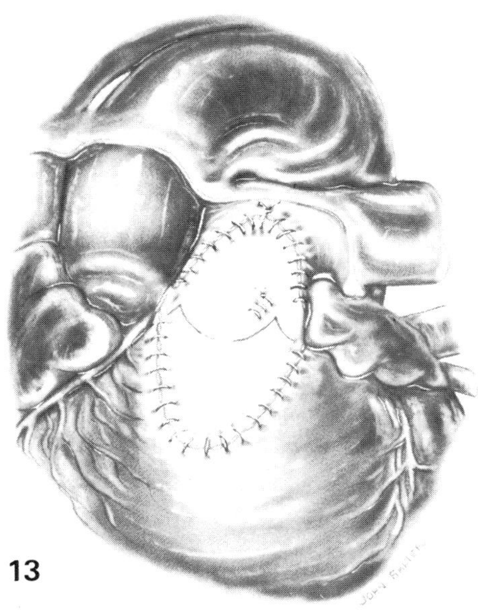

13

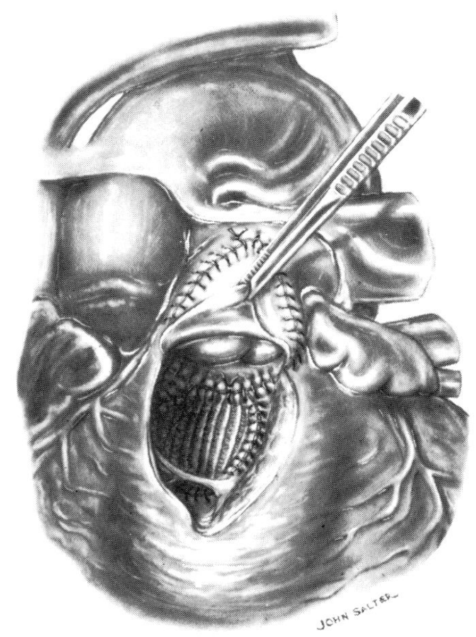

12

14

Coronary artery anomalies in tetralogy of Fallot

In 2 per cent of patients the left anterior descending coronary artery may either arise or receive a major contribution from the right coronary artery. In this case, the anomalous coronary artery crosses the right ventricular outflow tract. In these hearts relief of right ventricular outflow tract obstruction by extending the longitudinal incision in the right ventricular infundibulum is precluded because of the danger of damaging this critical coronary artery.

The coronary artery can be dissected free of the myocardium, and a gusset placed posterior to the vessel. An alternative method is to bypass the anomalous coronary artery by the insertion of a right ventricular-pulmonary artery external tube conduit, containing a valve.

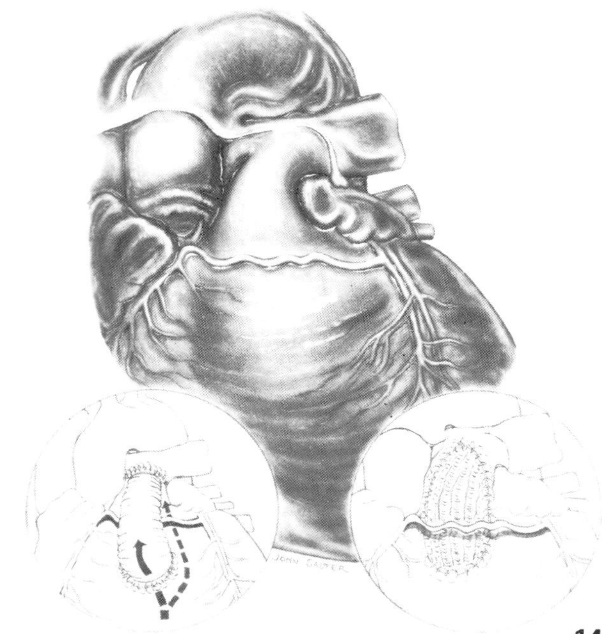

14

POSTOPERATIVE CARE

Following the operation the patient is returned from the operating theatre to the cardiac intensive care unit, where his condition is managed by personnel specifically trained in postoperative care of cardiac patients. The patient is ventilated by a volume-cycled artificial ventilator, until his cardiorespiratory state is stable and he is fully conscious with evidence of a satisfactory cardiac output. Only then will artificial ventilation be discontinued and the endotracheal tube be removed.

Systemic arterial pressure, mean right atrial pressure, mean left atrial pressure, urinary output and central and peripheral temperature are monitored every 15 min. Observation of these criteria will provide evidence of his cardiorespiratory status. When possible, cardiac output and cardiac index should be monitored.

Drainage of blood from the chest drains is observed carefully, and fluid replacement with whole blood or volume expander is replaced in equal volumes. Observation of the left and right atrial pressures, together with the blood pressure, urinary output and temperature gradient gives guidance to the administration of volume to maintain an adequate ventricular filling pressure in both the left and right ventricles.

Excessive drainage from the mediastinal and pericardial chest drains is an indication for re-operation to secure further haemostasis.

Administration of intravenous fluids (5 per cent dextrose with or without potassium chloride supplement) is at the rate of 500 ml/m^2 of body surface on the day of surgery, and 750 ml/m^2 of body surface area on the first postoperative day.

Cardiac action can be manipulated by means of cardiotonic drugs (Digoxin and/or isoprenaline sulphate) or by beta adrenergic blocking agents which have both a myocardial action and a direct action on the systemic vascular resistance—for example, isoprenaline sulphate, salbutamol sulphate. When a low cardiac output state exists, provided there is evidence of satisfactory ventricular filling, and that the patient is not hypovolaemic, then myocardial action must be assisted by pharmacological means.

Progressive ambulation is begun on the third postoperative day, and the patient is usually discharged from hospital on the twelfth postoperative day.

References

Anderson, R. H., Wilkinson, J. L., Arnold, R., Becker, A. E. and Lubkiewicz, K. (1974). 'Morphogenesis of bulboventricular malformations. II Observations on malformed hearts.' *Br. Heart J.* **36**, 948

Kirklin, J. W. and Karp, R. (1970). *The Tetralogy of Fallot from a Surgical Viewpoint.* Philadelphia: Saunders

[*In this Chapter on Complete Intracardiac Repair of Fallot's Tetralogy illustrations 2, 6, 7, 10–14 were drawn by Mr. J. Salter; illustration 1 was drawn by Mr. J. Desley; illustrations 3–5 were drawn by Mr. R. Drake and illustrations 8 and 9 were drawn by Mr. J. M. Hutcheson.*]

The Rashkind Procedure and Blalock - Hanlon Operation for Transposition of the Great Arteries

Eoin Aberdeen, F.R.C.S., F.A.C.S.
Director of Cardiovascular Surgery,
The Children's Hospital of Newark, New Jersey

PRE - OPERATIVE

Indications

Any infant born with transposed great arteries (TGA) cannot survive unless there is some intercommunication between the independent systemic and pulmonary circulations. A patent foramen ovale supplies this for a short period after birth but usually becomes too small. A large interatrial defect is the most effective means of allowing the two circulations to mix, because a two-way ebb and flow can occur in each cardiac cycle. A ventricular septal defect is less effective in allowing mixing of the two circulations and is also associated with the early development of pulmonary vascular obstructive disease. The operative creation of an atrial defect in the first months of life has been replaced by the closed technique of balloon septostomy, first described by Rashkind. However, this technique may not be effective after the first months of life when the atrial septum becomes thicker. Creation of an atrial septal defect can sometimes be part of a successful palliative operation in tricuspid atresia and some complex types of malposition of the great arteries.

RASHKIND PROCEDURE

The technique of atrial septostomy, first described by Rashkind and Miller in 1966, has rapidly found an important and widely used place in infant cardiology. The value is two-fold: not only does the technique create an atrial septal defect with an acceptably low risk rate, but it also allows the palliative procedure to be done at the time of the initial diagnosis, so that there is the least possible delay in the treatment of even the very ill infant.

1

Equipment

The essential piece of apparatus is the balloon catheter. The balloon is fixed in a subterminal position to a double-lumen catheter. Pressures can be recorded beyond the balloon even when the balloon is firmly inflated.

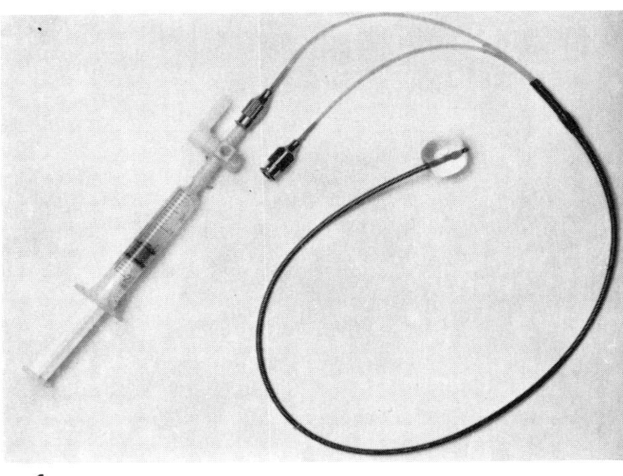

1

Method

Cardiac catheterization must be performed to give a complete diagnosis. When this has been achieved, the balloon catheter, with the balloon collapsed, is introduced into the long saphenous vein near its junction with the femoral vein in the groin, and passed up the femoral vein and inferior vena cava to the right atrium. The catheter is then manipulated through the foramen ovale and the position of the catheter tip is checked by pressure and oxygen recordings and by x-ray.

When the position of the catheter in the left atrium is confirmed, the balloon is inflated by injecting radio-opaque liquid down the catheter. Initially the balloon is inflated with 2 ml of liquid; the catheter is then jerked sharply through the atrial septum. The balloon is pulled down to, but not into, the inferior vena cava.

Rashkind emphasizes the value of a big jerk on the end of the catheter.

2&3

After one passage through the foramen ovale, the catheter is re-introduced into the left atrium and inflated with a further 0·5 ml of radio-opaque liquid and the catheter again sharply jerked back into the right atrium. This manoeuvre is repeated with the addition of 0·5 ml of radio-opaque liquid on each occasion. When the balloon contains 3 ml of liquid the manoeuvre is repeated until no further resistance is felt. Usually this has created an adequate atrial septal defect. The effect of this defect can immediately be measured by repeating the diagnostic catheterization studies. Angiocardiography with injections into left and right ventricles is usually performed at the time of first catheterization, unless the infant is extremely ill. If pulmonary consolidation and congestion are severe, full intensive care is required, with artificial ventilation via a nasotracheal tube.

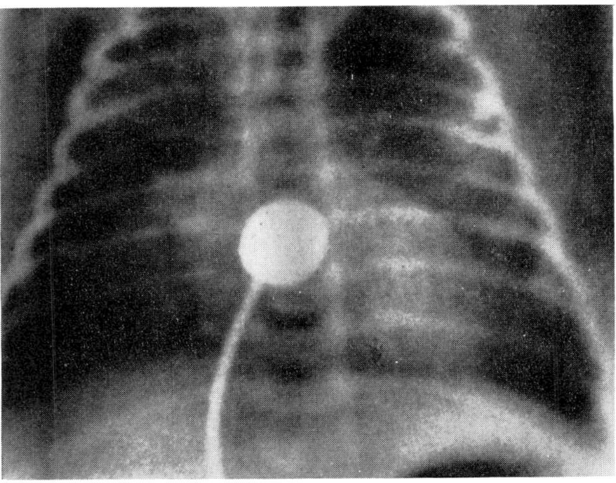

2

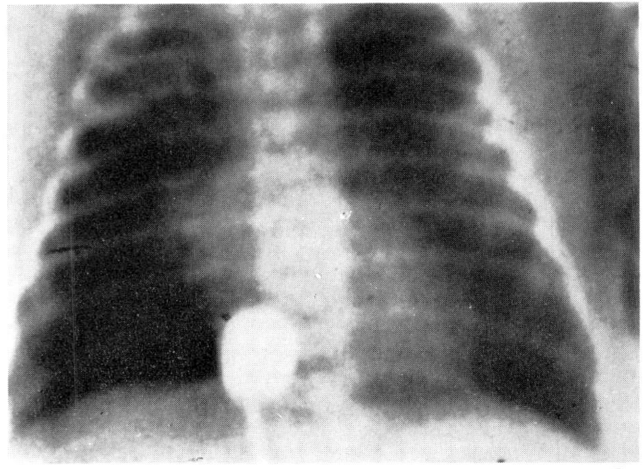

3

BLALOCK-HANLON OPERATION

Special equipment

Special paediatric cardiovascular clamps of the modified Satinsky pattern, including Cooley's infant clamp, are necessary. The fine teeth of the clamp should be relatively atraumatic, because the atrial wall has been torn by sharp toothed clamps.

Pre-operative investigations

An accurate assessment both of the abnormal anatomy and the haemodynamics is essential before operation. Cardiac catheterization with sampling from all chambers including the pulmonary artery is necessary, as is angiocardiography with injection into both right and left ventricles. In infants with transposition of the great arteries the presence of a large ventricular septal defect must also be determined or excluded, so the need for pulmonary artery constriction (banding) can be determined (*see* Chapter on Pulmonary Artery Constriction', pages 69–75).

Anaesthesia

Halothane or endotracheal nitrous oxide and oxygen with muscle relaxants are preferred.

THE OPERATION

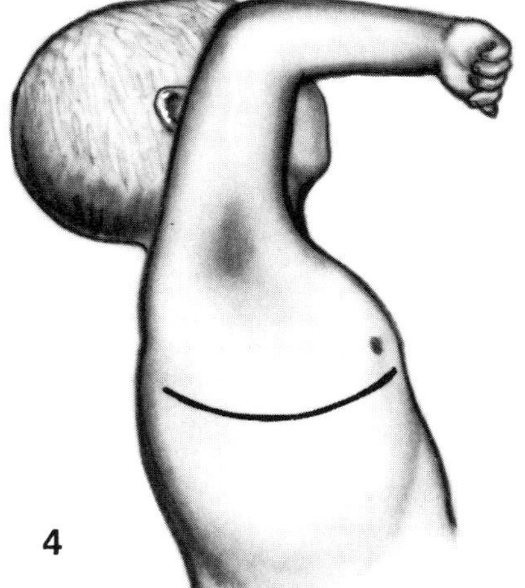
4

4

The incision

A right lateral thoracotomy is made through the full length of the fifth interspace. The skin incision in a girl can be placed slightly lower than shown in the illustration, so that it later lies in the submammary groove. The incision should be kept almost horizontal posteriorly. In an infant it is not necessary to curve the incision superiorly and posteriorly around the scapula because this leaves an unsightly scar.

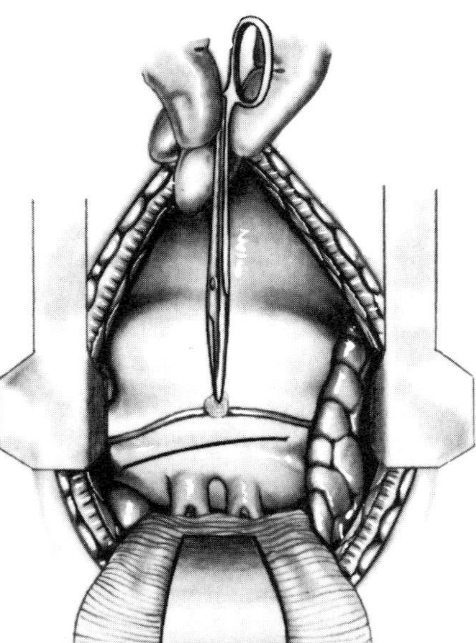
5

5

Mobilizing the phrenic nerve

The phrenic nerve usually lies close to the hilum of the right lung in the position where it is desired to incise the pericardium. It can be gently stroked forward with a moist gauze swab so that the incision can be made in the desired place and the phrenic nerve removed from the likelihood of injury.

6

Pericardial incision

A liberal incision over 4 or 5 cm is made in the pericardium in front of the right pulmonary veins, and overlying the interatrial groove. Inferiorly the incision can be carried posteriorly to the level of the inferior vena cava.

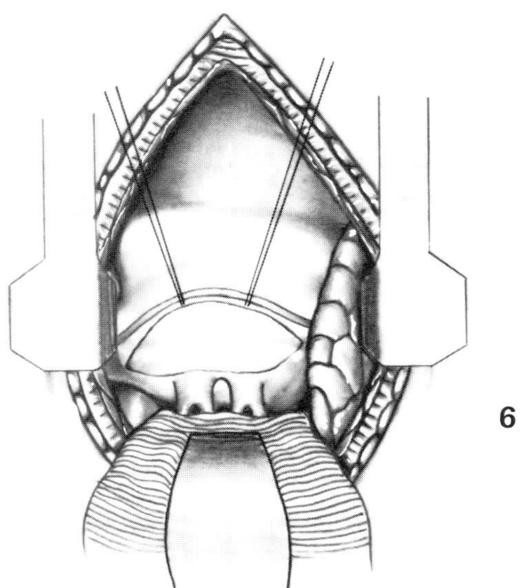

6

7

Placement of snares and partial occlusion clamp

Dissection is made around the right pulmonary artery and around the upper and lower right pulmonary veins, and a plaited silk ligature (No. 3) is passed around each vessel and held in a snare cut from a 5 cm length of 8 Ch catheter. A partial occlusion clamp is placed with one jaw behind the right pulmonary veins and one jaw in front. The final positioning of the clamp before closure is assisted if the atrial wall is grasped with a forceps at the region of the interatrial groove inferiorly, and this is drawn to the right. It is important that a reasonable amount (at least 1 cm) of right atrium should be included by the clamp. The sequence is to close the pulmonary artery snare first, and to help empty the right lung of blood by manual compression, the pulmonary vein snares are then tightened and the partial occlusion clamp is closed. If the operating room staff are unfamiliar with this operative technique it is wise to have several practice runs of the moves to be made in the next 2 or 3 min. Technically this is a challenging operation. It is one of the most imaginative operations in surgery and can change in seconds from a smooth surgical cadenza to a bloody disaster if the operator is not in complete command. Should the heart slow markedly when the clamp is applied the clamp and snares should be released promptly. Another attempt to place the snares and clamp can be made after a few minutes often without further heart slowing.

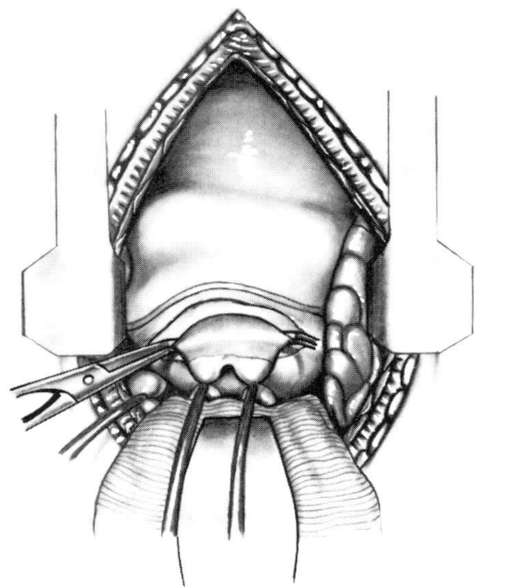

7

8

Incising the atria

The incision is first made into the right atrium parallel with the interatrial groove and about 3 mm to the patient's left of this groove. Recognition of the intimal lining of the right atrium is essential. The incision should not be made too long, but should be confined to about 12 – 15 mm. Exposure can be aided if the assistant grasps the cut atrial edge with a fine haemostat (rather than the stay stitch shown here). A second incision is made to the patient's right, and posteriorly to the interatrial groove, to open into the left atrium. This incision is made exactly where the pulmonary vein joins the left atrium. Dissection into the atrial septum can easily occur and can confuse the operator. Again, recognition of the intimal lining of the left atrium is important and the first indication that the left atrium has been opened is the appearance of a small amount of bright red blood. A narrow-tipped sucker is essential to see this clearly.

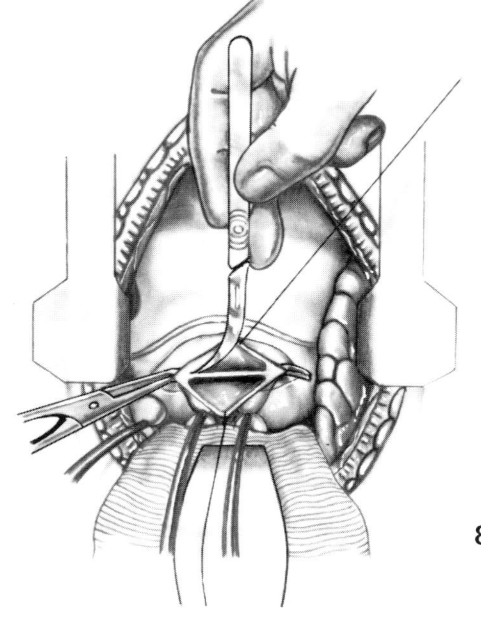

8

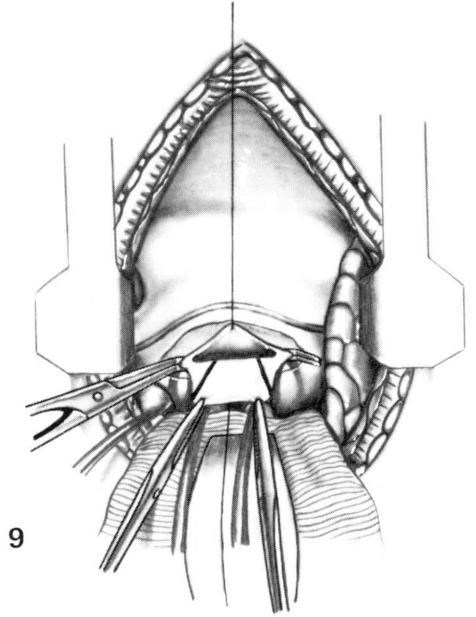

9

9

Excising the atrial septum

The aim is to remove a segment of atrial septum measuring about 10 – 12 mm × 10 – 15 mm. It is important not to try to remove a very large piece of septum as this increases the technical risks and is unnecessary. The free edge of the atrial septum is grasped with two or three straight mosquito forceps and parallel incisions are made above and below these forceps.

10 & 11

Drawing the atrial septum from the heart

An extra portion of the atrial septum can be removed at this stage by gently releasing the partial occlusion clamp and, at the same time, pulling out the portion of atrial septum grasped by the haemostats. In this way an extra 5 – 7 mm of atrial septum can be withdrawn from the wound.

Often when this segment is being excised it is found that the foramen ovale is cut into and forms part of the edge of the new defect.

12

Closure of atrial incision

A second partial occlusion clamp, which is smaller than the one already in position is now applied so that the edges of the atrial incision are clamped together. The posterior partial occlusion clamp is then released and the snares on the pulmonary veins are released and, finally, the snare on the right pulmonary artery. Usually the cuff of atrial wall protruding through the clamp is not sufficient to make suturing of the atrial incision easy, and therefore the large partial occlusion clamp is placed from the anterior approach, immediately underneath the smaller clamp. The smaller clamp is removed leaving a larger cuff of tissue available for suturing. Care must be taken to avoid obstructing the right upper pulmonary vein when applying this second clamp. The value of this clamping technique is that it reduces the time during which the right lung is excluded from the circulation; the total duration of clamping is usually between 2 and 3 min, and very unusually should exceed 3 min. In this brief period it is very rare for the heart action to deteriorate significantly.

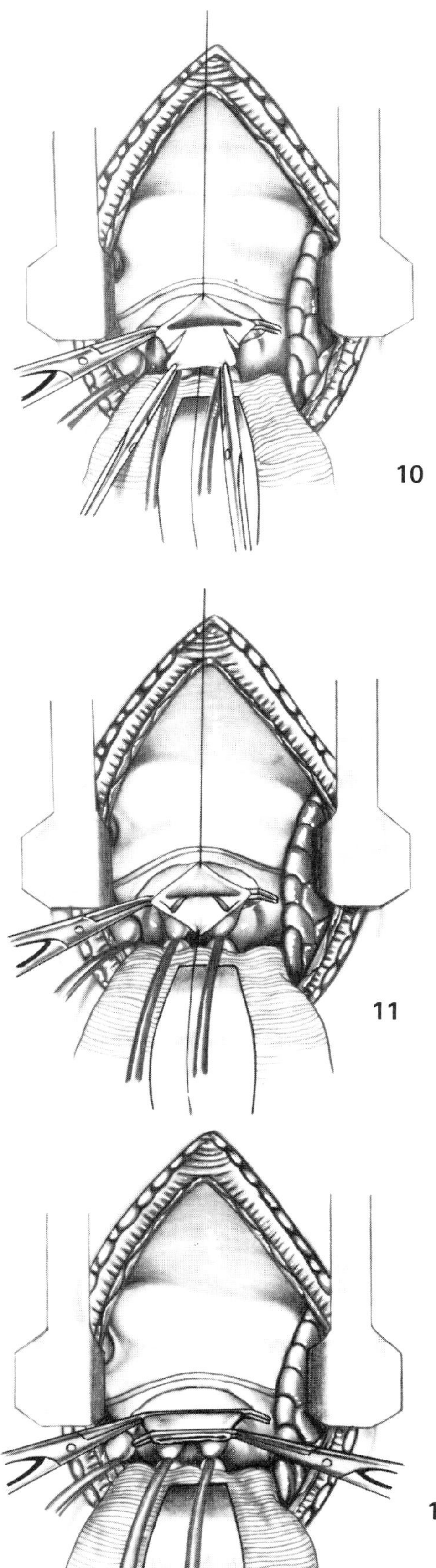

13

Suture of atrial incision

The cut edges of the atrial incision are closed with continuous 5/0 suture.

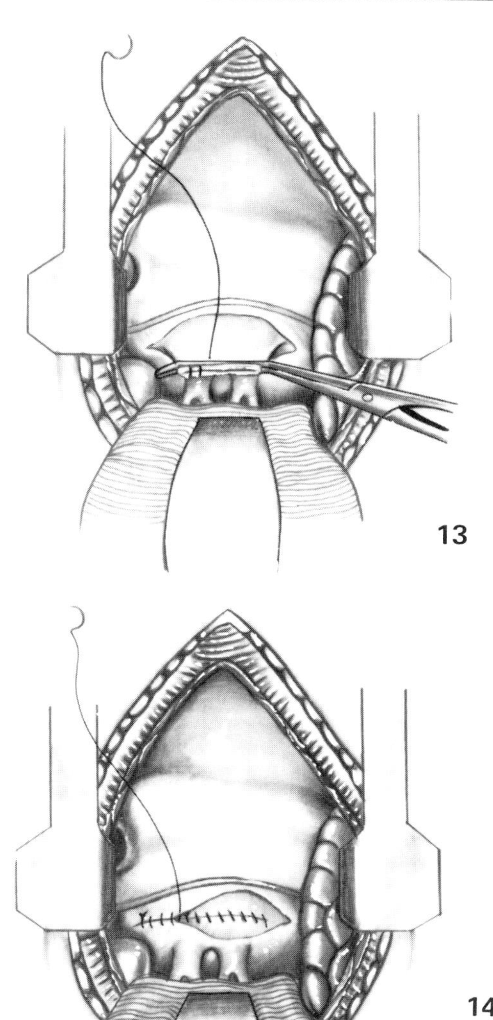

14

Closure of pericardial cavity

When complete haemostasis of the atrial incision has been achieved, and any blood in the pericardial cavity has been gently sucked away, the pericardial incision is closed with continuous 5/0 or 6/0 suture, except for a small opening left at either end of this incision for drainage.

Wound closure

The thoracotomy wound is closed with three pericostal chromic catgut sutures (No. 1) and the muscles closed with continuous 3/0 chromic catgut. Subcutaneous tissues are approximated with continuous 4/0 chromic catgut, and the skin closed with continuous subcuticular 5/0 clear nylon suture. A drain tube is always placed in the right pleural cavity attached to an underwater seal drainage bottle.

POSTOPERATIVE CARE AND COMPLICATIONS

Problems of cardiac function are unusual after this operation. The principal postoperative complications are pulmonary. If the infant has been referred before pulmonary consolidation has occurred then the postoperative period may be quite uneventful and the child may be sent home a week after operation, or a few days after balloon septostomy. Sometimes, however, considerable lung consolidation has occurred and this may tax the resources of any intensive care unit, and is almost the only cause of death after this operation in recent years.

Widespread lung consolidation and collapse will be associated with a high P_{CO_2} and metabolic acidosis. Nasotracheal intubation and artificial ventilation support become necessary, together with the correction of the metabolic acidosis.

Provided that blood is not spilt into the pericardial cavity and care is taken not to put gauze swabs into the pericardial cavity, there need be no pericardial adhesions postoperatively except over the site of the atrial incision. Thus, later performance of a Mustard operation is not made more difficult.

Results and prognosis

When children are operated on after the age of 3 months the survival rate is about 95 per cent. In the first 6 weeks of life there is a much higher surgical risk and it is these children especially that the atrial septostomy, using the balloon catheter technique of Rashkind, is preferable

References

Blalock, A. and Hanlon, C. R. (1950). 'Surgical treatment of complete transposition of aorta and pulmonary artery.' *Surgery Gynec. Obstet.* **90,** 1

Rashkind, W. J. and Miller, W. W. (1966). 'Creation of an atrial septal defect without thoracotomy. A palliative approach to complete transposition of the great arteries.' *J. Am. med. Ass.* **196,** 991

[*The illustrations for this Chapter on The Rashkind Procedure and Blalock-Hanlon Operation for Transposition of the Great Arteries were drawn by Mr. G. Lyth.*]

Mustard's Operation for Transposition of the Great Arteries

Jaroslav Stark, M. D.
Consultant Cardiothoracic Surgeon, The Hospital for Sick Children,
Great Ormond Street, London

PRE-OPERATIVE

Introduction

The natural history of infants with transposition of the great arteries is unfavourable. Without treatment 85 per cent die before their first birthday. The milestones in the treatment of patients with transposition of the great arteries were atrial septectomy (*see* page 108) and the re-arrangement of venous inflow within the atria (Senning, 1959; Mustard, 1964).

Diagnosis

A complete cardiological investigation is mandatory. This includes the measurement of pressures and sampling for oxygen saturation in all chambers of the heart and great vessels. Oxygen consumption can be measured and pulmonary and systemic blood flow calculated. It is important to calculate the pulmonary arteriolar resistance. Angiocardiograhy and echocardiography help to diagnose accurately additional cardiac malformations.

Indications

At the present time, all children with transpositon of the great arteries can be offered surgical treatment. Those with atrial septal defect or previous balloon atrial septostomy are operated on with a low risk at the age of 6 – 12 months. Should balloon atrial septostomy prove ineffective, the author prefers an early Mustard operation to septectomy. Patients with transposition of the great arteries and ventricular septal defect should be operated on before the age of 6 months because they develop early pulmonary vascular disease. If the pulmonary arteriolar resistance is higher than eight units/m^2, Mustard's operation can still be performed, provided the ventricular septal defect is left open – 'palliative Mustard' (Lindesmith *et al.*, 1972).

Anaesthesia

Infants under 15 kg are premedicated with 0·075 ml 'Pethidine Co.' (1 ml contains Pethidine 25 mg, chlorpromazine 6·25 mg and promethazine 6·25 mg) /kg body weight and 0·2 – 0·3 mg atropine, intramuscularly, 45 min before operation. Those over 15 kg receive Omnopon (papaveretum) 0·4 mg/kg, and scopolamine (hyoscine) 0·008 mg/kg, 1 – 1·5 hr before the operation. The patient is induced with cyclopropane and paralyzed with succinylcholine. Anaesthesia is continued with nitrous oxide and oxygen supplemented by intravenous morphine.

THE OPERATION

1

Insertion of monitoring devices

An arterial cannula is inserted percutaneously into a radial artery (*1*). When this is not successful in a small infant, a radial or brachial artery is exposed and the cannula inserted under direct vision. It is secured by a skin stitch and connected to a monitoring device. Two venous lines are required: one for the transfusion and one for monitoring the central venous pressure (*2, 3*). The author prefers an internal or external jugular vein for monitoring. A cephalic vein or a vein on the dorsum of the hand is usually adequate for transfusion. (*2*). Two temperature probes (*4, 5*) (oesophageal and nasopharyngeal), ECG electrodes (*6*) and a urinary catheter (*7*) are put in place.

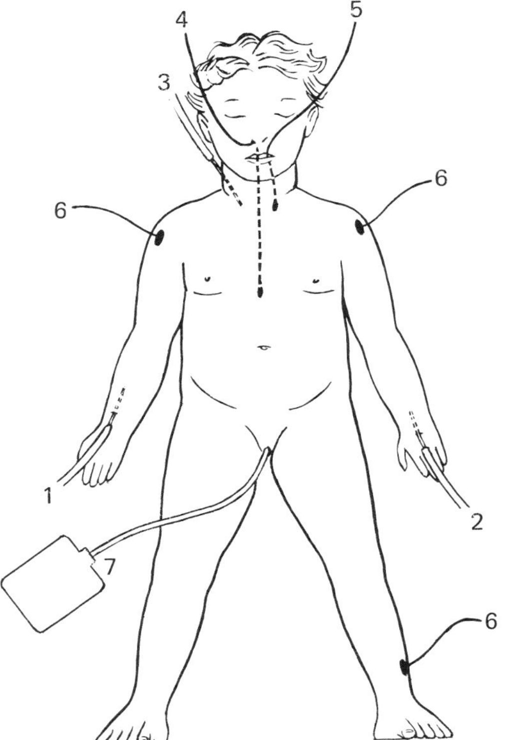

1

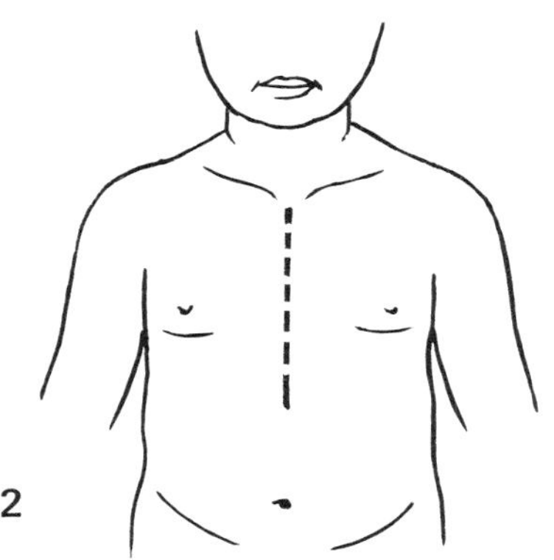

2

2

The incision

The patient is operated on in the supine position. The skin incision extends from the upper end of the sternum to approximately 4 cm below the xiphoid. The sternum is opened with an electric saw. The anterior surface of the pericardium is cleaned by sharp (scissors) and blunt (moist swab) dissection. The thymic lobes are dissected and freed from the pericardium. The pleura is pushed to each side and care is taken not to open either pleural space.

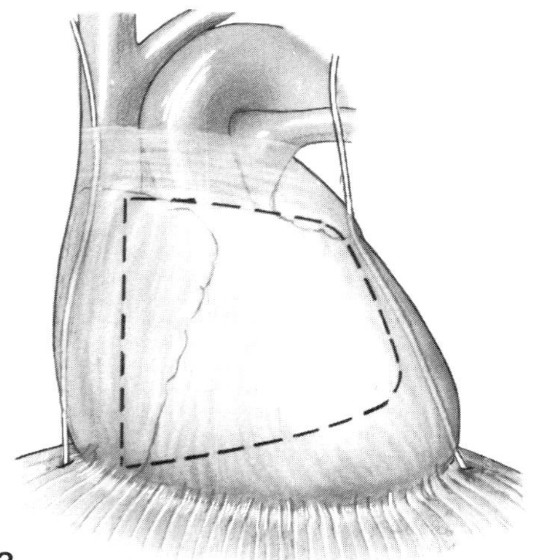

3

3

Pericardial patch

The pericardium is incised vertically on the right side parallel with the phrenic nerve and about 15 – 20 mm in front of it. Stay-stitches are placed at the upper and lower ends. Incisions are then continued to the left, across the heart. An adequate pocket of pericardium should be left at the apex of the heart, otherwise, this dislocates easily. If a previous intrapericardial operation has been performed, dissection of the pericardium may be tedious and the pericardium may not be suitable for the baffle. In this situation, the author uses a 'weaveknit' patch (Thackeray's No. MT 44).

4&5

Calculating the size of the patch

We use the technique described by Brom. The flat diameter of the superior vena cava and inferior vena cava is measured. The patch is then cut according to these measurements before the heart is opened. A to B is the distance between the left upper and lower pulmonary veins. It is not measured, but estimated at about 1 cm for a 1 year old child. It can be a few millimetres shorter for a neonate and about 1·5 cm for a 3 – 4 year old. E to D is, in practice, twice the flat diameter of the superior vena cava and D–F is twice the flat diameter of the inferior vena cava.

$$C–D = \frac{(ED) + (DF)}{2}$$

The angle is about 30°. The legs of the patch are trimmed to the appropriate length when the patch is being inserted. These measurements are helpful, but adjustments are sometimes necessary because the anatomy of each atrium differs slightly.

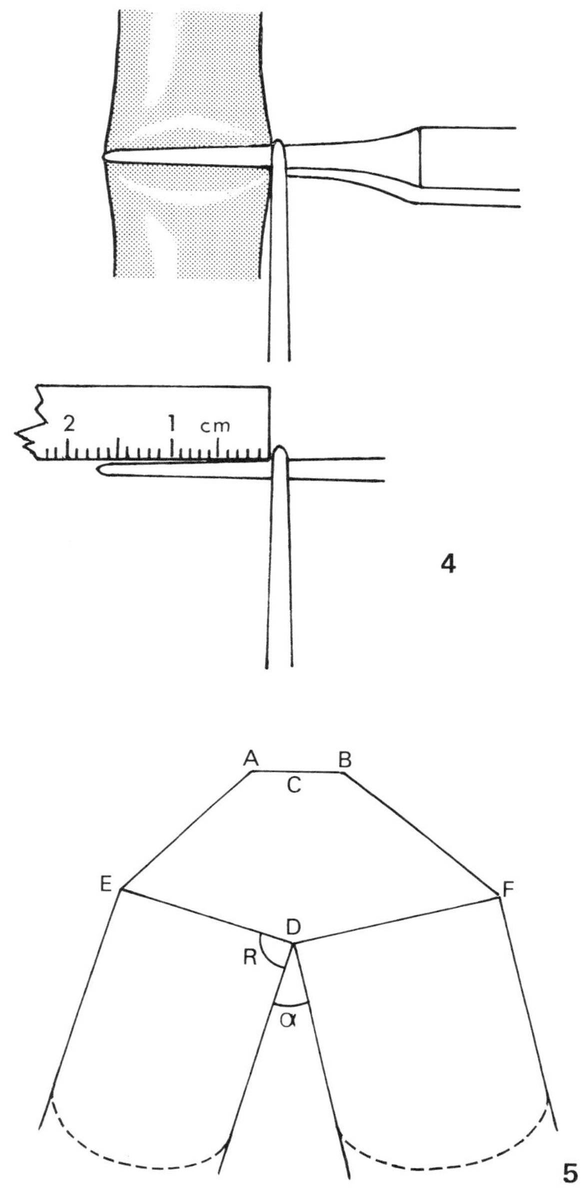

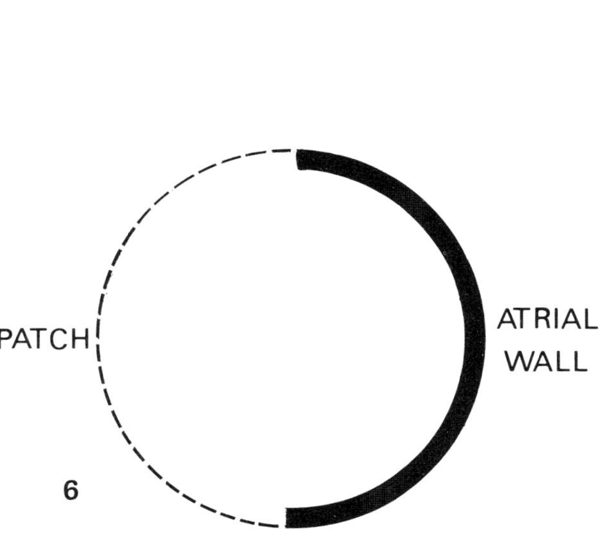

6

The fundamental reason for these measurements is to construct adequate pathways without excessive ballooning of the patch. In due course, when the pericardium shrinks, the atrial wall should form at least 40 – 50 per cent of the circumference of the pathway.

7

Dissection of inferior and superior venae cavae

The pericardium is freed from the lower portion of the superior vena cava. Care must be taken not to injure the phrenic nerve especially with diathermy. A purse-string suture is then placed directly on the superior vena cava, starting about 15 mm above its junction with the right atrium. It should be more oblong than circular so as to avoid superior vena caval constriction when it is tied. The inferior vena cava cannulation site lies posteriorly at the junction of the right atrium with the inferior vena cava. Intracardiac pressures are then measured and heparin is given.

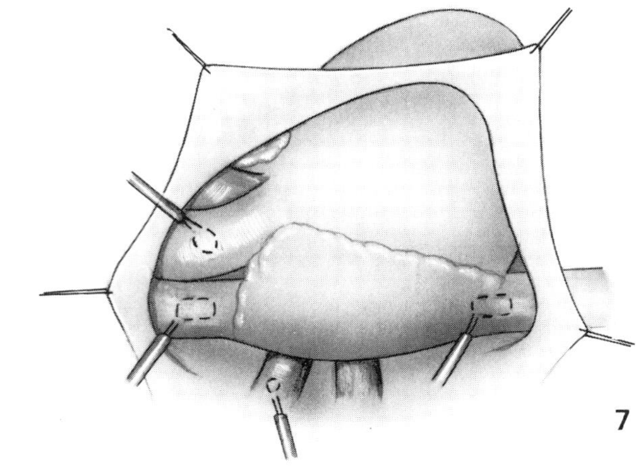

7

Left atrial line

A left atrial line is inserted through a purse-string stitch placed on the right upper pulmonary vein. A PVC cannula is inserted through a needle. It is then fixed with a second purse-string suture and tied to the pericardium about 1 – 3 cm from the heart. The left atrial line is then brought through the skin to the left of the mid-line using a different needle. It is connected to a monitoring system using a Touhey connector.

8

Aortic and caval cannulation

Standard aortic cannulation with a right-angled metal cannula is used. For caval cannulation, a technique avoiding partial occlusion clamps is preferred. Fine artery forceps grasp the atrial wall within the purse-string suture (*A*). An incision is made (*B*) and enlarged with another artery forceps (*C*). A right-angled Rygg cannula (*D*) is then inserted without difficulty. The purse-string suture is tightened and secured to the cannula (*E*). The inferior vena cava is cannulated in the same way.

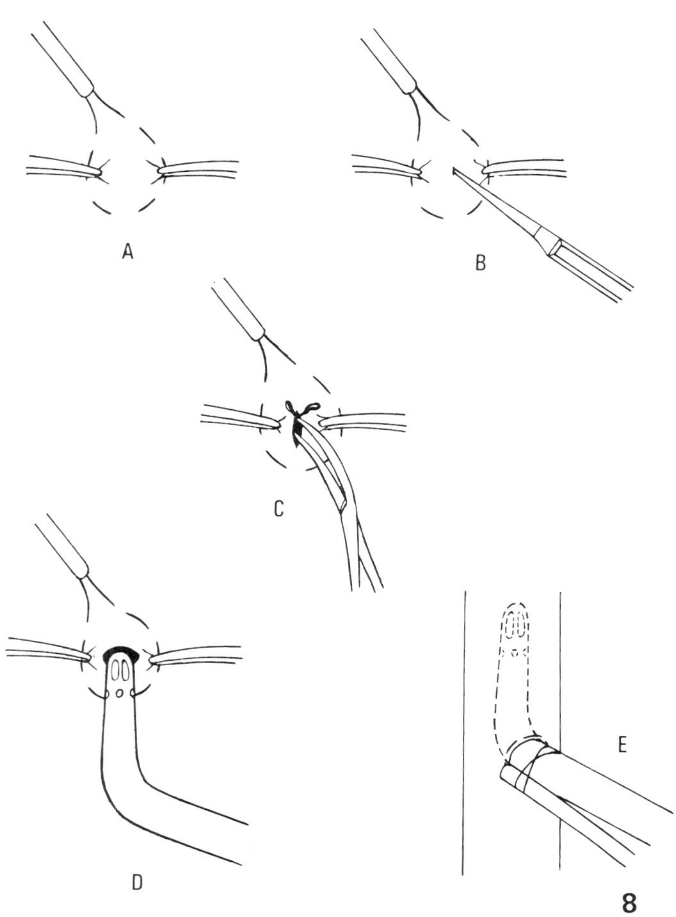

8

9

Cardiopulmonary bypass

Care is taken not to let any air into the right atrium during cannulation because the tricuspid valve is the systemic atrioventricular valve. A vent is inserted into the uppermost part of the right ventricle through a small purse-string suture. In infants, a coronary artery cannula or a small feeding tube provides an adequate vent. When the calculated flow is achieved (2·4 l/m^2/min), the caval snares are tightened and ventilation discontinued. The lungs are inflated during perfusion at a pressure of 5 cm of water. The perfusate is cooled at 25°C and, at this temperature, the aorta is cross-clamped. The right atrium is opened and a small retractor inserted. The incision is then extended upwards towards the right atrial appendage and downwards towards the inferior vena caval cannula. It should not run too close to the cannula so as to avoid distortion of the baffle during subsequent closure of the atriotomy.

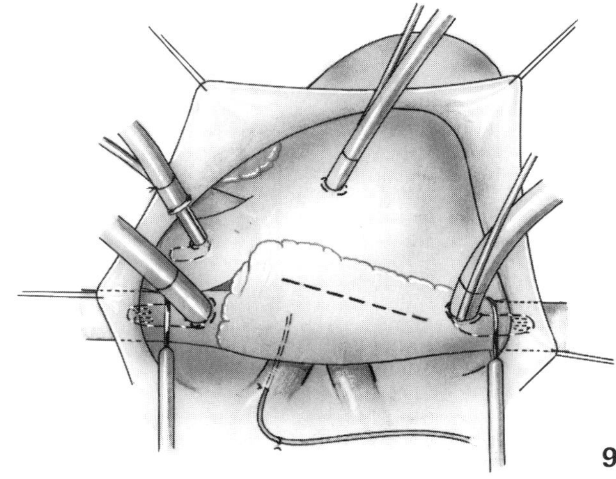

9

10

Atrial stay sutures

Stay sutures are placed anteriorly close to the tricuspid valve and posteriorly on the crista terminalis. These bring both atrial cavities into view without excessive use of retractors.

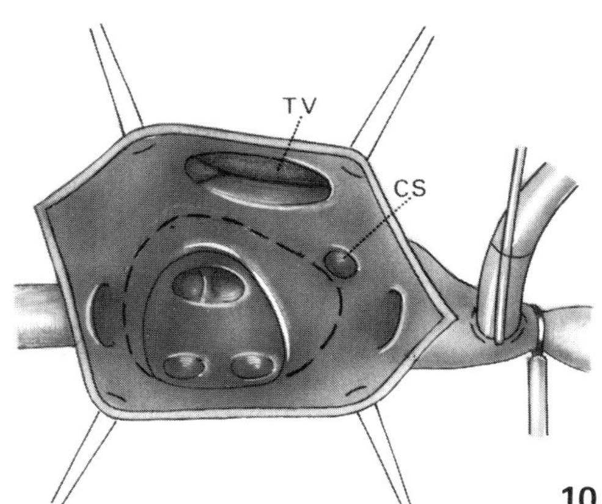

10

Excision of the atrial septum

After careful inspection of the right atrium, tricuspid valve, atrial septal defect, left atrium and orifices of all pulmonary veins, the remnant of the atrial septum is excised. It is carefully detached from the lateral and superior wall of the atrium. Care must be taken not to cut through the wall of the atrium. This can happen, but if recognized and repaired properly, is of no great consequence.

11

Suture of raw surfaces in the atrium and cutback of the coronary sinus

The raw surfaces remaining after the excision of the atrial septum are oversewn with a continuous stitch. The coronary sinus can be cut back to the left atrium towards the base of the left atrial appendage. Alternatively, it can be left intact and the baffle sutured to its posterior rim.

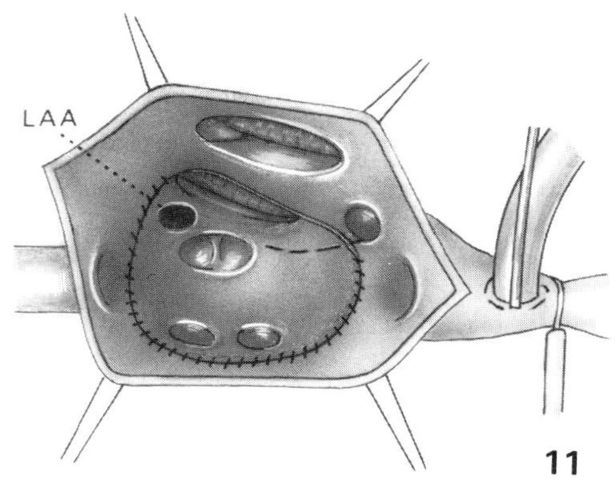

11

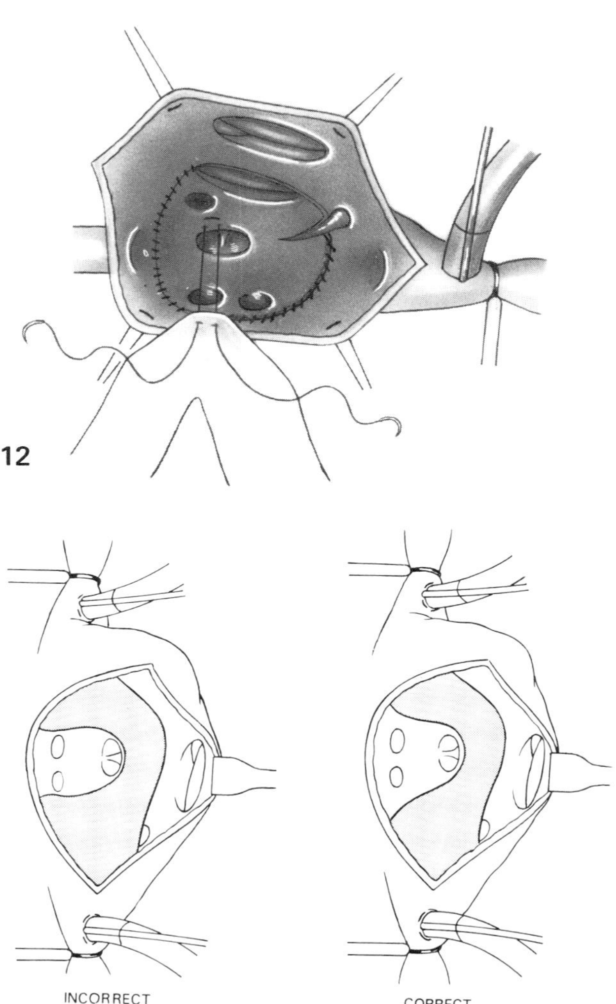

12

13

12&13

Placement of pericardial baffle

A double-needled suture of 5/0 (Ethiflex or Prolene) is used. It starts at the point 'C' on the patch, which is attached between the left pulmonary veins and the base of the left atrial appendage. The suture line then runs superiorly around the orifice of the pulmonary veins, then across the posterior wall of the left atrium towards the upper margin of the right upper pulmonary vein. The lower part of the patch encircles the lower left pulmonary vein and runs across to between the right lower pulmonary vein and the orifice of the inferior vena cava. Care is taken not to bring the two suture lines too close together on the lateral wall of the right atrium, because a constricting ring may thus be formed.

14

The anterior part of the baffle

Point 'D' on the baffle is then sutured with a second double-needled stitch to the remnant of the atrial septum. The suture line continues upwards and then around the superior vena cava to construct a wide superior vena caval pathway. If the trabeculations here are numerous, the suture is brought through the wall of the right atrium as a continuous mattress stitch to avoid leaks behind the trabeculations.

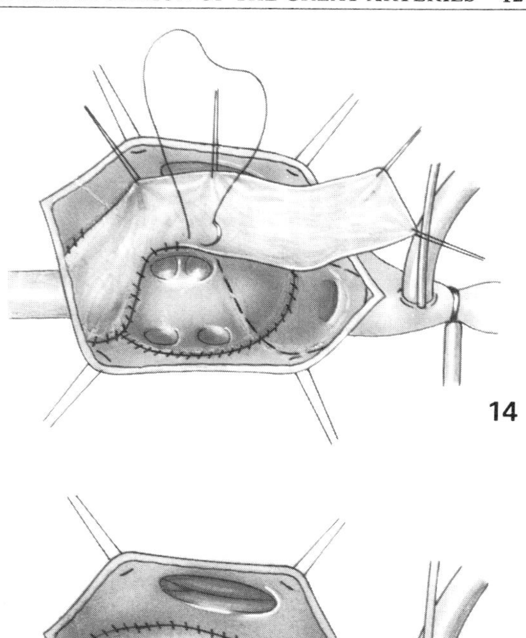

14

15

The lower part of the baffle

The lower part of the baffle is sutured to the cut edge of the septum, then through the floor of the coronary sinus. The length of the patch is trimmed for both the superior vena cava and the inferior vena cava to allow adequate ballooning; the two pathways should not meet when filled with blood. The completed patch is shown.

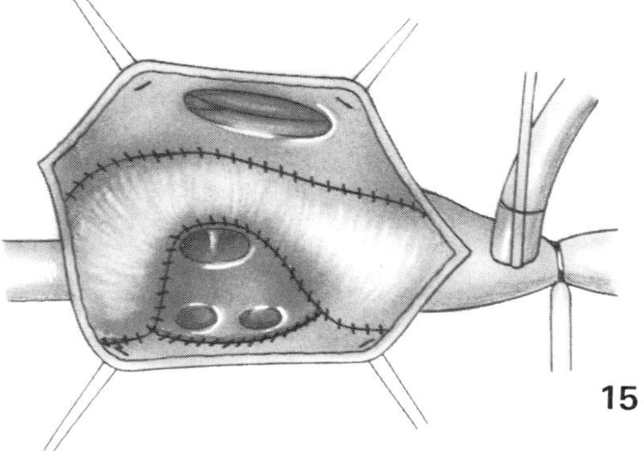

15

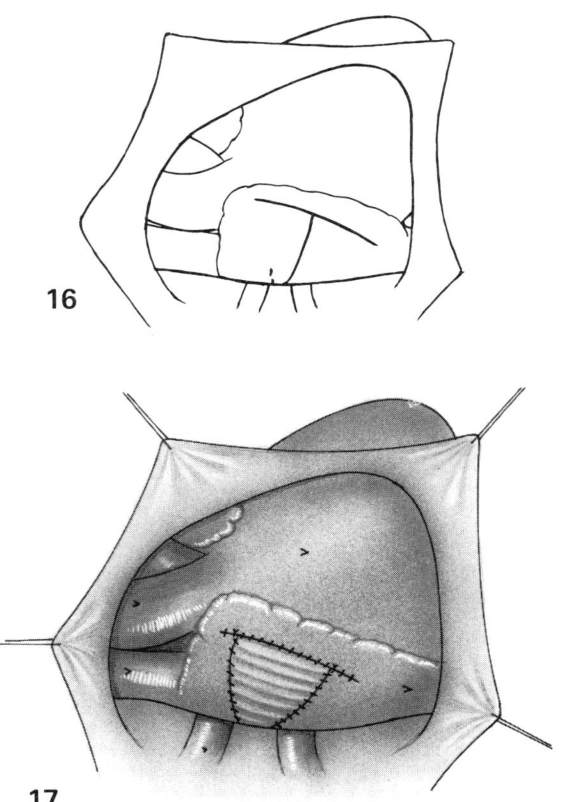

16

17

16 & 17

Enlargement of the pulmonary venous atrium

When the distance between the superior and inferior venae cavae is short, or when after insertion of the baffle, there is uncertainty as to whether the new pulmonary venous atrium is of sufficient size, the author prefers to enlarge it with an outside patch. This is mainly done in infants under the age of 3 months. An incision from about the middle of the atriotomy runs down between the upper and lower pulmonary veins, and extends another 4 – 5 cm towards the posterior aspect of the left atrium. An oval patch of Dacron is then stitched in place with Prolene sutures. This separates the upper and lower pulmonary veins and enlarges the pulmonary venous atrium. The corrugations of the patch should run parallel with the superior and inferior venae cavae.

Atrial closure and termination of bypass

The patient is rewarmed and the atriotomy is closed with a running stitch of Prolene. Prior to completion of the suture line, the heart is electrically fibrillated and an aortic needle vent inserted through a purse-string suture. Caval snares are released and all air evacuated while the heart cannot eject. When the fibrillator is removed, the heart usually resumes sinus rhythm spontaneously. If not, it is defibrillated and then the right ventricular vent and aortic needle are removed. A raised pressure in the pulmonary venous atrium (LA) is advantageous at this stage. One should avoid over-distension of the heart, but a negative atrial pressure is also hazardous, as air can be sucked into the heart through the needle holes. Perfusion is gradually discontinued at a left atrial pressure of 10 – 12 mmHg.

Removal of the cannulae

The superior vena caval cannula is removed and the purse-string suture tied. A right atrial (systemic venous atrial) monitoring line can be inserted through the inferior vena caval cannulation site, using the same technique as described for the left atrial line insertion. Transfusion is completed from the oxygenator to achieve the desired left atrial pressure. The arterial cannula is removed and protamine given. Both aortic purse-string sutures are tied. Bleeding points are carefully checked, atrial and ventricular pacemaker wires are inserted and pericardial and mediastinal drains put in place.

POSTOPERATIVE CARE

All patients are intubated with a nasotracheal tube and ventilated on a volume cycled respirator. On return to the intensive care unit, the fractional concentration of oxygen in the inspired gases is gradually decreased to 40 per cent. The patient is then placed in the headbox or an oxygen tent, breathing 60 per cent oxygen. If the PaO_2 remains over 70 and $PaCO_2$ under 50 mmHg, and the patient's breathing is not laboured, he can be extubated. This is usually achieved within 12 – 24 hr. Infants may be weaned off the respirator using a constant positive airway pressure system.

The atrial lines are usually removed the following morning and mediastinal and pericardial drains 1 – 2 hr later – to prevent collection of blood should any bleeding occur after the removal of the atrial lines. If cardiac output is inadequate, the same criteria as for patients with other congenital heart lesions are applied, i.e. the preload is increased by transfusion of blood or plasma depending on the haematocrit. If the systemic vascular resistance is high, Largactil, Rogitine or nitroprusside can be used. If inotropic support is required, the author prefers dopamine (5 – 10 μg/kg/min) to isoprenaline or adrenaline (0·1 – 0·2 μg/kg/min).

Complications

Obstruction of the caval pathways or pulmonary venous obstruction can occur. In the author's experience, it is rare when the pericardium is cut into the trouser shape described earlier. Various arrhythmias can occur both early and late in the postoperative period. Care must be taken to avoid injury to the sino-atrial and the atrioventricular nodes during all stages of the operation. Occasionally severe tricuspid incompetence requires valve replacement.

Results and prognosis

Our operative mortality for patients with transposition of the great arteries without additional lesions is around 5 per cent. So far, long-term results are satisfying (Champsaur, 1973; Clarkson, 1976; Stark, 1974; Taylor, 1977).

Re-operation

Obstruction of the pulmonary veins should be treated surgically. Isolated narrowing or even complete obstruction of the superior vena cava often does not require treatment because if the azygos vein remains patent, and the inferior vena caval channel is adequate patients may not show any symptoms of obstruction. If symptoms persist the superior vena caval channel is enlarged with a patch. For all re-operations in patients with transposition of the great arteries the author prefers a right thoracotomy through the fifth intercostal space, extending it across the sternum if necessary. Cannulation of the superior and inferior venae cavae is easier; the aorta is usually anterior and right-sided and thus easily reached from this approach. As the operation is performed in the right atrium, one can avoid dissection underneath the sternum where the right ventricle and the coronary arteries are no longer protected by pericardium.

ADDITIONAL LESIONS

Patent ductus arteriosus

If a patent ductus arteriosus causes severe heart failure early in infancy, it is ligated through a left thoracotomy. If it is patent at the time of the Mustard operation, an anterior approach is used.

Coarctation of the aorta

This is preferably resected prior to correction through a left thoracotomy (*see* Chapter on 'Coarctation of the Aorta', pages 43–49).

Ventricular septal defect

Pulmonary artery banding is offered in the first month or two (*see* Chapter on 'Pulmonary Artery Constriction', pages 69–75). In older children a ventricular septal defect may be closed through the tricuspid valve. A short high incision in the right ventricle or a left ventriculotomy provide an alternative approach to a ventricular septal defect in patients with transposition of the great arteries (*see* Chapter on 'Ventricular Septal Defect', pages 64–68).

Left ventricular outflow tract obstruction

Pulmonary valve stenosis can be easily relieved by valvotomy. Severe fibromuscular obstruction is sometimes difficult to relieve as is the obstruction caused by an abnormal mitral valve. A conduit from the left ventricle to the pulmonary artery may bypass this obstruction (Singh, 1976). If the ventricular septal defect and left ventricular outflow tract obstruction are associated with transposition of the great arteries, a Rastelli operation is the treatment of choice (*see* Chapter on 'Rastelli Operation', pages 130–135).

References

Champsaur, G. L., Sokol, D. M., Trusler, G. A. and Mustard, W. T. (1973). 'Repair of transposition of the great arteries in 123 pediatric patients. Early and long-term results.' *Circulation* **47**, 1032

Clarkson, P. M., Neutze, J. M., Barratt-Boyes, B. G. and Brandt, P. W. (1976). 'Late postoperative hemodynamic results and cineangiocardiographic findings after Mustard's atrial baffle repair for transposition of the great arteries.' *Circulation* **53**, 525

Lindesmith, G. G., Stiles, Q. R., Tucker, B. L., Gallaher, M. E., Stanton, R. E. and Meyer, B. W. (1972). 'The Mustard operation as a palliative procedure.' *J. thorac. cardiovasc. Surg.* **63**, 75

Mustard, W. T. (1964). 'Successful two-stage correction of transposition of the great vessels.' *Surgery* **55**, 469

Senning, A. (1959). 'Surgical correction of transposition of the great vessels.' *Surgery* **45**, 966

Singh, A. K., Stark, J. and Taylor, J. F. N. (1976). 'Left ventricle to pulmonary artery conduit in treatment of transposition of the great arteries, restrictive ventricular septal defect and acquired pulmonary atresia.' *Br. Heart J.* **38**, 1213

Stark, J., de Leval, M. R., Waterston, D. J., Graham, G. R. and Bonham-Carter, R. E. (1974). 'Corrective surgery of transposition of the great arteries in the first year of life. Results in 63 infants.' *J. thorac. cardiovasc. Surg.* **67**, 673

Taylor, J. F. N., Schmitz, J. P., Graham, G. R. and Stark, J. (1977). 'Late results of Mustard's operation for transposition of the great arteries.' *Br. Heart J.* **39**, 353 (Abstract)

[*The illustrations for this Chapter on Transposition of the Great Arteries. Mustard's Operation were drawn by Mr. F. Price.*]

The Senning I Operation in the Treatment of Transposition of the Great Arteries

A. G. Brom, M.D.
Professor of Thoracic Surgery, University Hospital, Leiden

INTRODUCTION

It may be that, in the near future, arterial switch will become the treatment of choice in transposition of the great arteries (Baffes, 1961; Jatene, 1976; Ross and Yacoub, 1976). However, inflow correction by the Mustard or Senning operation are still the most widely used procedures. It is difficult to decide which of these two procedures is better. The differences between the two operations include.

(*1*) The use of a large patch in the Mustard procedure, compared to a small one (slightly larger for a Blalock-Hanlon operation) in the Senning procedure. This should preserve the ability of the atria to grow.

(*2*) The crossing of blood flows takes place at the level of the former atrial septum in the Mustard procedure, whereas in the Senning procedure additional space, outside the heart, is used for this crossing. Furthermore, the shape and size of the intra-atrial baffle used in the Mustard operation has to be determined with great accuracy to avoid obstruction of the systemic or pulmonary veins. In contrast, in the Senning operation, this problem is virtually eliminated because of the design of the operation and the fact that the heart itself determines the size of the baffle.

(*3*) The atrial function is probably better after the Senning operation, as the new right atrium can contract relatively normally while the left contracts against a yielding right atrium. This is in contrast to the contraction of both right and left atria in the Mustard procedure which occurs against the still, immobile prosthetic patch.

(*4*) Injury to the sinus node or its artery is more difficult to avoid in the Senning than in the Mustard operation. However, our experience, to date, has shown that arrhythmia is very uncommon after the Senning operation.

(*5*) The Senning operation is probably more difficult technically, but with increasing experience this can be overcome.

We believe that the Senning operation is the more obvious solution to inflow correction than the Mustard procedure.

PRINCIPLES

The principles of the Senning operation are the same as those of the Mustard procedure.

(*1*) A new right wall for the new 'right' atrium has to be formed. In the Mustard operation this is done via the mid-portion of the patch, whereas in the Senning operation it is done via the remnants of the atrial septum and that part of the former right atrium that is localized behind the crista terminalis.

(*2*) The blood from the two venae cavae has to be guided to the left ventricle without obstruction. In the Mustard operation this is done via the 'legs' of the patch, whereas in the Senning operation it is done via two tubes fashioned from the same dorsal part of the right atrium.

(*3*) The blood from the left pulmonary veins has to join the blood from the right pulmonary veins, without obstruction, behind the new right atrium and flow to the right ventricle via a common opening. In the Mustard operation this is effected along the right lateral aspect of the patch *within* the heart, whereas in the Senning operation it is done along the posterior aspect of the old atrial septum and laterally to the right of the venae cavae along the *outside* of the heart.

(*4*) Avoidance of any direct trauma to the sino-atrial node, its artery and the atrioventricular node.

THE OPERATION

1

The incision

Median sternotomy.

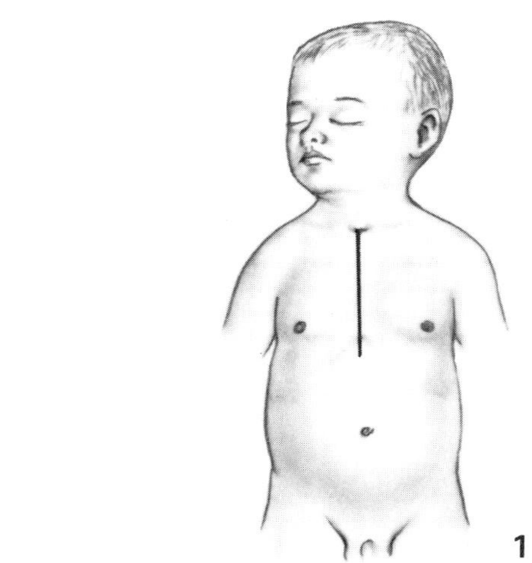

1

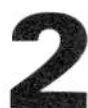

Preparation for bypass

In younger children (below 1 year of age) surface cooling to a nasopharyngeal temperature of 28°C is used. A cannula is then inserted in the right atrium for venous return, and another in the ascending aorta for perfusion. The body temperature is reduced to 20°C by core cooling. In older children, during cooling, the venae cavae are cannulated as far as possible from the heart. Venous return then takes place through the venae cavae cannulae.

Atrial incision

An incision (A–B) is made in the right atrium a few millimetres ventral to the terminal crest. The sinoatrial node is located in the crest and this site should not be touched with instruments during this procedure. The incision extends over a distance equal to approximately three-quarters of that between the venae cavae. At a later stage the incision is extended in the direction of the lateral end of the valve of the inferior vena cava (Eustachian valve).

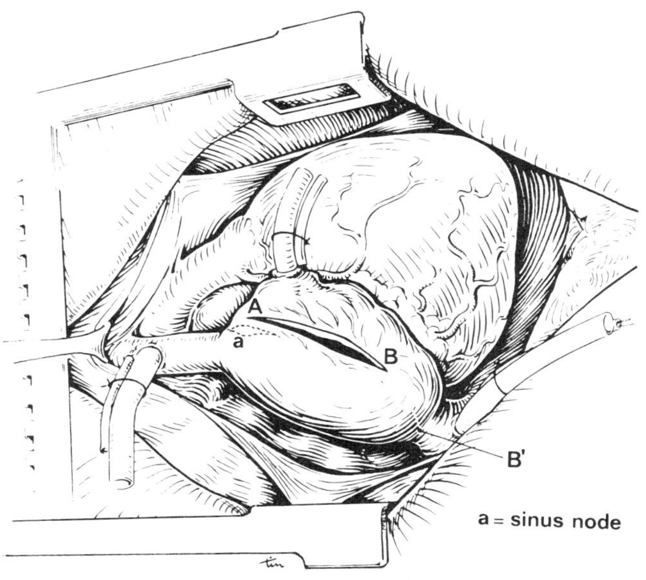

2

3

Mobilization of the atrial septum and formation of a flap

After opening the right atrium the septum is carefully inspected. Following a balloon septostomy only the fossa ovalis is missing. However, after a Blalock-Hanlon procedure the septum is largely absent. In either case a trapeziform roof must be constructed to be sutured above the left pulmonary veins (comparable to the trapeziform mid-portion of the Mustard patch). After a Rashkind procedure the incision is started in the foramen ovale and extended parallel to the tricuspid valve ring in a caudocranial direction for a distance of about 7 mm (C D). From point D the incision extends to the junction of the superior vena cava with the atrial septum (E). The same is repeated for the inferior vena cava, starting at the lower corner of the fossa ovalis. At this site, tissue is sometimes absent making the incision (F G) unnecessary. The atrial wall is re-endothelialized by a few interrupted sutures. The resulting flap has nearly always the same dimension in infants aged 6–12 months. Its base is formed by the atrial wall between the two venae cavae, about 3 cm in length. Its height is about 2 cm. The dimension of the pulmonary veins are then measured with Hegar's dilators (usually size 6 or 8 mm) which indicate that the distance above the two left pulmonary veins is about 1·5–2 cm. The length of the top side of the trapeziform, therefore, has to be the same length. This is achieved by using a small patch, very slightly larger, to allow for the suture line. After a Blalock-Hanlon operation the absent atrial septum is replaced by a trapeziform Dacron patch to achieve the same dimensions, mentioned above, for the atrial septal flap.

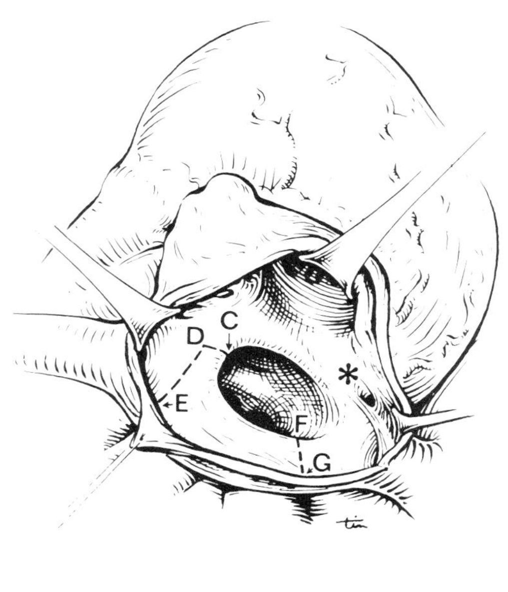

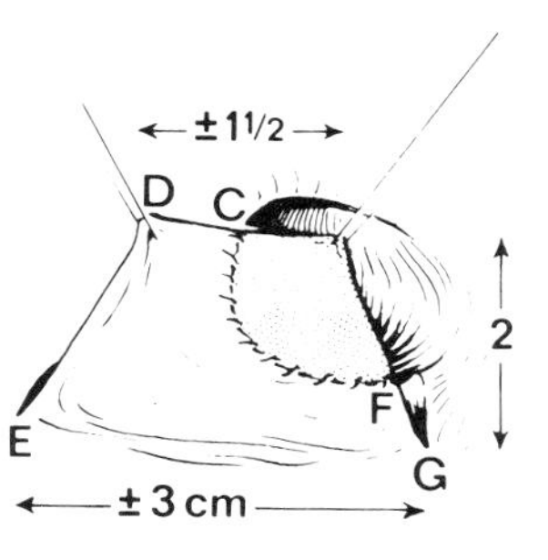

3

* coronary sinus

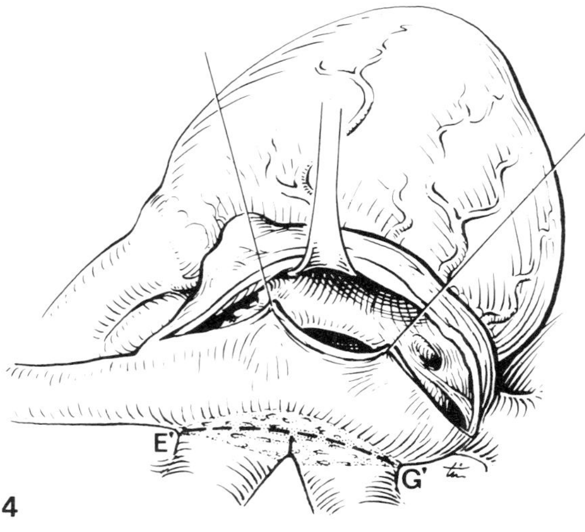

4

4

Formation of a left atrial outlet

The interatrial groove is dissected in front of the right pulmonary veins thus slightly separating the two atria. The left atrium is then opened by a craniocaudal incision as close to the mid-line as possible (E′, G′). These two points, situated on the outside of the heart, correspond to points E and G (mentioned earlier) inside the heart. The length of the left atrial incision is, therefore, likewise about 3 cm. The left atrial outlet is further enlarged by a small transverse incision between the two pulmonary veins.

5

Fixing the atrial septal flap inside the left atrium

The atrial septal flap (like the central part of the patch in the Mustard procedure) is sutured in front of the left pulmonary veins and along the posterior wall of the left atrium.

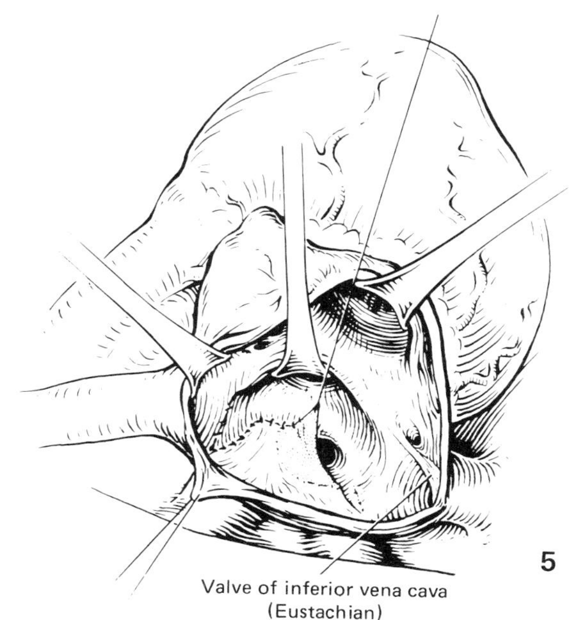

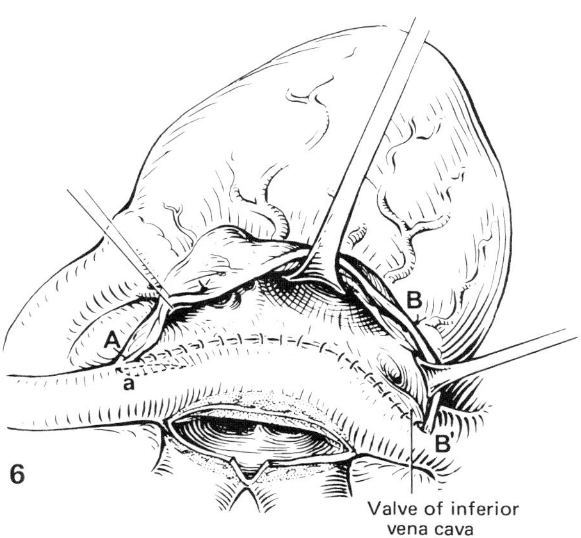

6

Creation of a new right atrium

A cannula is passed through the left atrial appendage and directed into the inferior vena cava, to replace the inferior vena caval cannula, if present. This provides a clear view of the inferior vena caval valve (Eustachian valve) which indicates the ventral boundary of the inferior vena cava. The original right atrial incision is now extended to the lateral end of the Eustachian valve (B′). The posterior part of the right atrial wall is then sutured to the atrial septal remnant between the atrioventricular valves making use caudally of the Eustachian valve. Cranially the sutures are placed in the endocardial layers of the atrial wall to avoid the sino-atrial node which is located immediately below the epicardium.

7

Creation of a new left atrium (i.e. joining the pulmonary venous chamber to the tricuspid valve)

The ventral part of the lateral right atrial wall is sutured to the right border of the left atrial incision (E′, G′). This suture line extends over both venae cavae (AE′ and B′ and G′). Both these distances are approximately 1·5 cm in length. The central part of the suture line is approximately 3 cm in length. The same length must be available in the border of the right atrial wall. Cranially and caudally there should be sufficient length to cross the superior and inferior venae cavae. In our experience the border of the anterior segment of the lateral atrial wall (AB′) is always about 7 cm in length, thus supplying adequate length. When suturing over the superior vena cava, this should be done using superficial bites, thus avoiding the atrioventricular node. The central part of the suture line is performed using interrupted silk sutures to allow for growth. If the diameter of one of the pulmonary veins corresponds to Hegar's size 8 mm dilator, then the space behind the trapeziform should pass a Hegar dilator size 12 mm and the space between the lateral wall of the new right atrium and the right side of the left atrial incision (E′, G′) should correspond to at least size 17 mm Hegar dilator. These measurements are achieved if the length of the left atrial incision (E′, G′) is slightly longer than 3 cm.

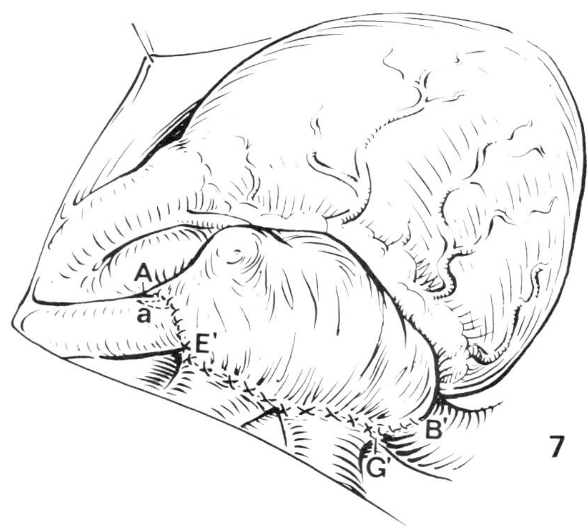

7

POSTOPERATIVE CARE

The postoperative management of small children is more difficult and as important as the operation itself. The patient returns to the recovery room still intubated but if possible breathing spontaneously. If, after 1 or 2 hr, respiration is adequate the tube is taken out otherwise ventilation using a volume controlled respirator is maintained until the next morning. In small infants it is desirable to remove the endotracheal tube as soon as possible as it constitutes a hazard (risk of blockage and atelectasis). Soon after return from theatre an x-ray picture is taken to check expansion of the lungs and the position of the endotracheal tube. During the postoperative period the following parameters are monitored: blood loss, electrocardiogram, arterial pressure, venous pressure, urine output, blood gases and electrolytes. Any early signs of low cardiac output, such as high venous pressure, low venous oxygen saturation, diminishing urine output, is treated by small doses (3–5 μg/min/kg) of dopamine. Digitalis is also started early (0·02 mg/kg). The same drug is also used for treatment of tachycardia. The amount of intravenous fluids administered is limited to approximately 2 ml/kg/hr. Urine output should be greater than 1 ml/kg/hr, (urine output is nearly always high during the first hours after extracorporeal circulation. This has no connection with the diuresis which occurs later). If diuresis diminishes, frusemide (1–2 mg/kg) is given. However, mostly these patients do very well and need little support.

References

Baffes, T. G., Ketola, F. H. and Tatooles, C. J. (1961). 'Transfer of coronary ostia by 'triangulation' in transposition of the great vessels and anomalous coronary arteries.' *Dis. Chest* **39**, 648

Geldof, W. C. and Aytug, Z. (1975). 'Chirurgische correctie van transpositie der grote vaten; een modificatie van de Mustard-techniek.' In *Thoraxchirurgie Leiden van 1950 tot 1975*, p. 187

Janse, M. J. and Anderson, R. H. (1974). 'Specialized internodal atrial pathways – fact or fiction?' *Europ. J. Cardiol.* **2**, 117

Jatene, A. D., Fontes, V. F., Paulista, P. P., Souza, L. C. B., Neger, F., Galantier, M. and Sousa, J. E. M. R. (1976). 'Anatomic correction of transposition of the great vessels.' *J. thorac. cardiovasc. Surg.* **72**, 364

Quaegebeur, J. M., Rohmer, J. and Brom, A. G. (1977). 'Revival of the Senning operation in the treatment of transposition of the great arteries. Preliminary report on recent experience. *Thorax* **32**, 517

Ross, D., Rickards, A. and Somerville, J. (1976). 'Transposition of the great arteries: logical anatomical arterial correction.' *Br. med. J.* **1**, 1109

Senning, A. (1959). 'Surgical correction of transposition of the great vessels.' *Surgery* **45**, 966

Yacoub, M. H., Radley-Smith, R. and Hilton, C. J. (1976). 'Anatomical correction of complete transposition of the great arteries and ventricular septal defect in infancy.' *Br. med. J.* **1**, 1112

[*The illustrations for this Chapter on the Senning I Operation in the Treatment of Transposition of the Great Arteries were drawn by J. Tinkelenberg.*]

The Rastelli Operation

Jaroslav Stark, M.D.
Consultant Cardiothoracic Surgeon, The Hospital for Sick Children, Great Ormond Street, London

INTRODUCTION

Correction of transposition of the great arteries plus ventricular septal defect and left ventricular outflow tract obstruction used to carry a risk of about 50 per cent. The high mortality was mainly due to the difficulty of relieving the left ventricular outflow tract obstruction adequately without injury to the adjacent structures such as the mitral valve and the bundle of His. The high risk of this operation was in contrast with a low mortality rate in the Mustard operation for children with 'uncomplicated' transposition of the great arteries. The prognosis has improved since Rastelli proposed his ingenious technique of anatomical correction (Rastelli, 1969).

Diagnosis

Complete cardiac catheterization and angiocardiography are essential. The size and position of the ventricular septal defect and the size of the main pulmonary artery are important. Additional lesions, such as patent ductus arteriosus, large bronchial collaterals or patency of previous shunts have to be diagnosed with certainty.

Indications

Severe cyanosis, polycythaemia and/or cyanotic spells are indications for the operation. If symptoms occur in infancy a systemic pulmonary shunt is the treatment of choice. We prefer a Blalock-Taussig shunt on the side opposite to the aortic arch (*see* Chapter on 'Blalock-Taussig Operation', pages 85–88). A Rastelli operation is better deferred until the age of 3–4 years. At this age, an adult size homo- or heterograft can be used. Although the progress after a shunt operation is usually satisfactory, we believe that correction should not be delayed beyond the age of 7–8 years.

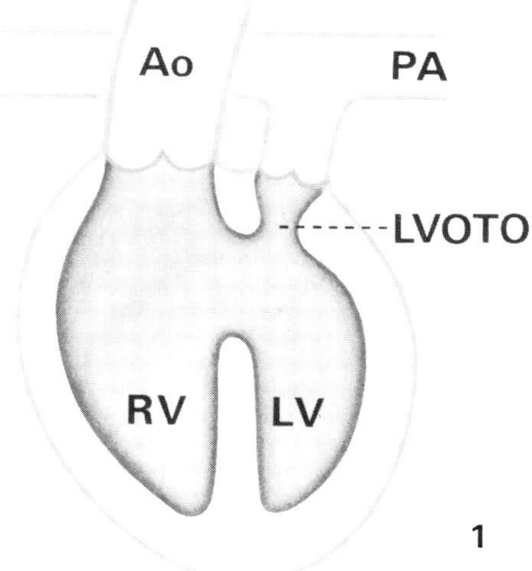

1

1, 2 & 3

The principle of the operation is shown in *Illustrations 1–3*. Left ventricular outflow tract obstruction is not resected and the ventricular septal defect is not closed, but the left ventricle is connected to the aorta using a large intraventricular patch (*see Illustration 2*). Exit from the left ventricle to the pulmonary artery is closed by transection of the pulmonary artery and suture. Currently we prefer to suture the pulmonary valve through the ventricular septal defect and then ligate the pulmonary artery just above the valve. The continuity between the right ventricle and the pulmonary artery is then established using a valved conduit (*see Illustration 3*).

Anaesthesia

Premedication and anaesthesia are as used for other open heart procedures in children.

Cannulation and perfusion

The aorta is cannulated higher than usual or the external iliac artery is used for arterial return. The pulmonary artery and aorta are completely dissected. This is particularly important when there are adhesions after previous operations. Dissection should be completed before the patient is heparinized. Intracardiac pressures are measured and a left atrial line inserted.

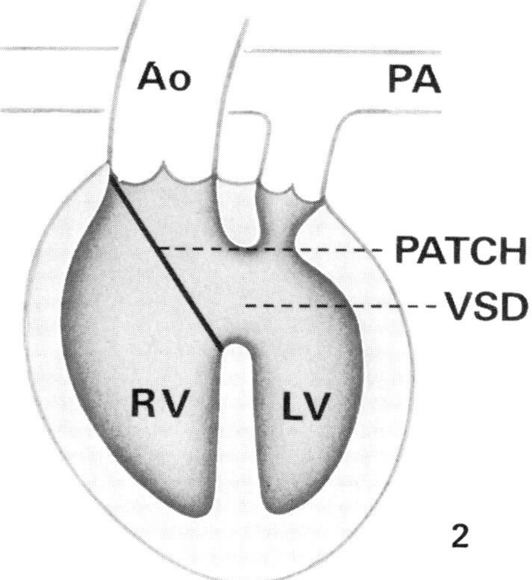

2

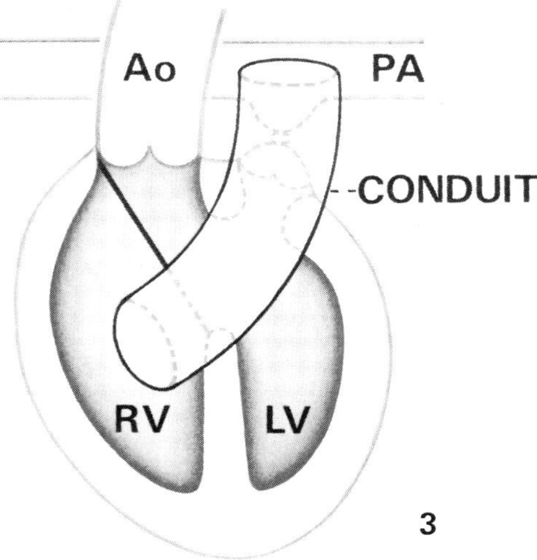

3

4

The superior vena cava is cannulated through the right atrial appendage and the inferior vena cava at the right atrium/inferior vena caval junction. A vent is inserted into the apex of the left ventricle, the perfusate is cooled to 25°C and the aorta cross-clamped. The right atrium is first opened and the atrial and ventricular anatomy assessed. If an atrial septal defect (natural or previous Blalock-Hanlon septectomy) is present, it is closed (*see* Chapter on 'Atrial Septal Defect', pages 54–59). Another vent is then introduced through the right atrium to the right ventricle and the right atriotomy is partially closed. A right ventriculotomy is then performed. It is a vertical or oblique incision in the direction of the main pulmonary artery. The position of the papillary muscle is checked through the tricuspid valve before the ventriculotomy is performed. The author does not excise a button of myocardium to prepare for the anastomosis with the conduit. If the anterior right ventricular wall is excessively thick, it is thinned near the edges of the ventriculotomy.

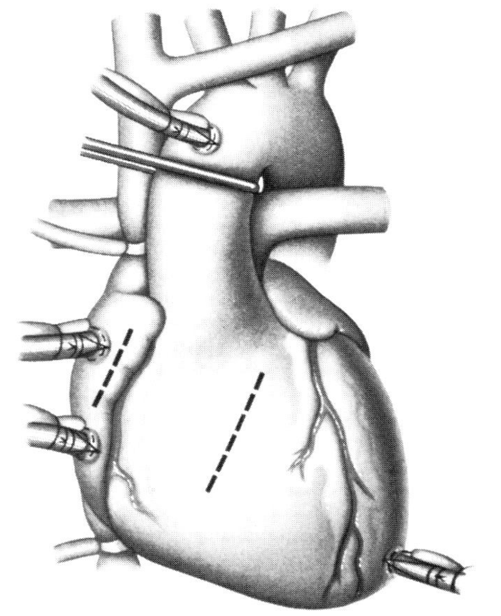
4

5,6&7

When it is established that the left ventricle can be connected to the aorta through the ventricular septal defect the pulmonary valve (PV) is inspected through the ventricular septal defect and carefully stitched with 4/0 Prolene. The main pulmonary artery is then doubly ligated just outside the heart. In this way transection of the pulmonary artery can be avoided.

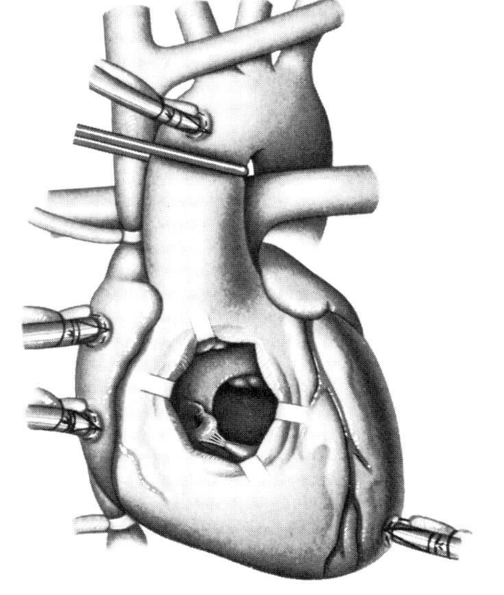
5

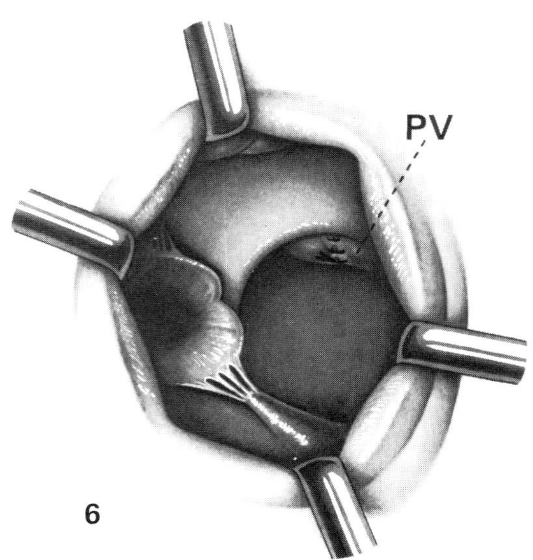

6

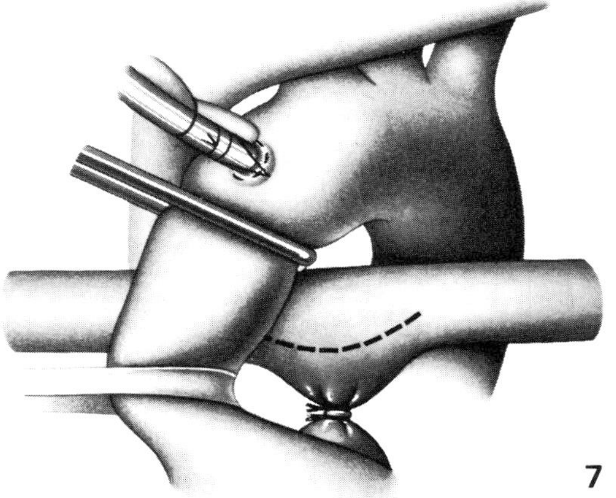
7

8

If it is decided to divide the pulmonary artery the ventricular end is oversewn with a continuous mattress stitch and then over-and-over Prolene stitches. This suture line must be meticulous because it is very difficult to deal with any leaks once the conduit is inserted.

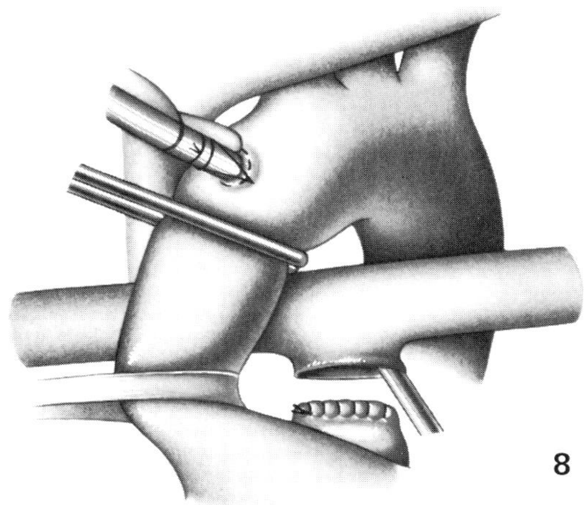

8

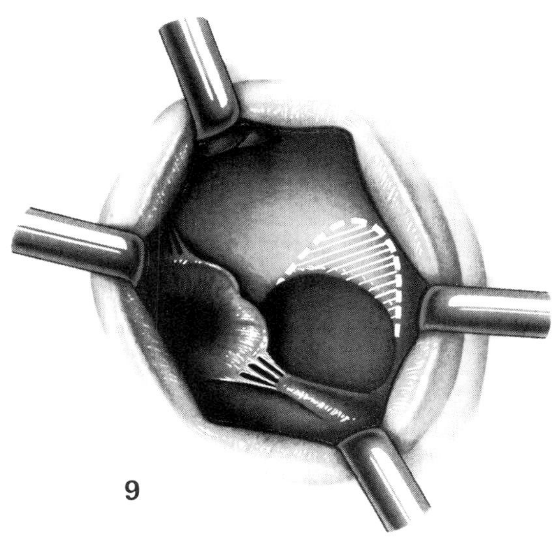

9

9

The ventricular septal defect is checked and if it is smaller than the aortic valve ring, it is enlarged in the lateral superior margin. Either a simple incision or an excision of a wedge of the muscle is used.

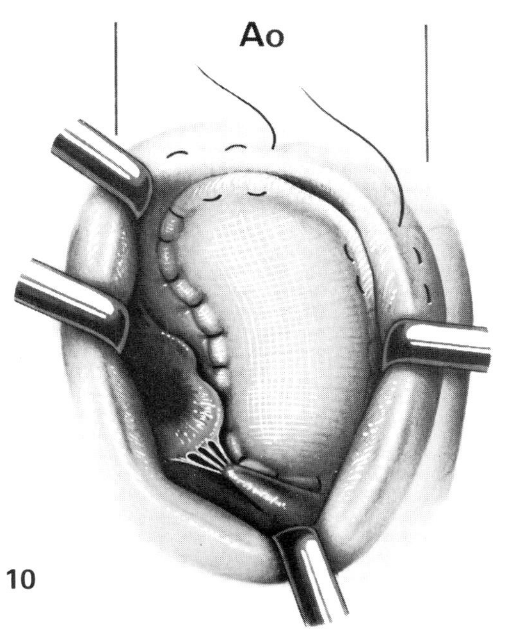

10

10

The length and width of the channel from the left ventricle to the aorta is then measured and a generous patch of Dacron velour is prepared. The suture line of the patch is started from the lower corner of the ventricular septal defect close to the tricuspid valve. On the left side it runs around the ventricular septal defect and up to the anterior wall of the right ventricle and the edge of the ventriculotomy. On the other side, the suture line runs to the right of the aortic valve ring and again up to the edge of the ventriculotomy. At present the author uses a stitch of 4/0 Prolene which may be re-inforced with several mattress stitches of 3/0 silk buttressed with Teflon pledgets.

Anteriorly, the last three to four stitches are not tied to keep the access to the aortic valve free. This is important because each time the aortic clamp is removed, great care is exercised to make the aortic valve incompetent to avoid coronary air embolization.

11

The pulmonary artery is opened. This can be done either longitudinally or the incision can be extended both to the left and right pulmonary arteries. A valved conduit is stitched to the pulmonary artery using a continuous 5/0 Prolene stitch. A posterior anastomosis is first performed starting from the left side. A sucker or sump is left in the right pulmonary artery during this procedure. If the pulmonary return is excessive, the left pulmonary artery is temporarily clamped. The valve is placed distally close to the pulmonary artery. In this position, it is protected by the ascending aorta and compression of the valve is avoided. An aortic homograft with the anterior cusp of the mitral valve is preferred by some surgeons. Another choice is a heterograft in a Dacron tube (Hancock); its availability in various sizes is its major advantage. Currently we use a homograft extended towards the right ventricle with a piece of woven Dacron tube. The largest conduit which will fit the pulmonary artery is selected. After the age of 3 years, at least a 22 mm valve can usually be used. The conduit is preclotted to improve the haemostasis at the time of coming off bypass.

The anterior part of the anastomosis is completed with the second needle of the Prolene suture.

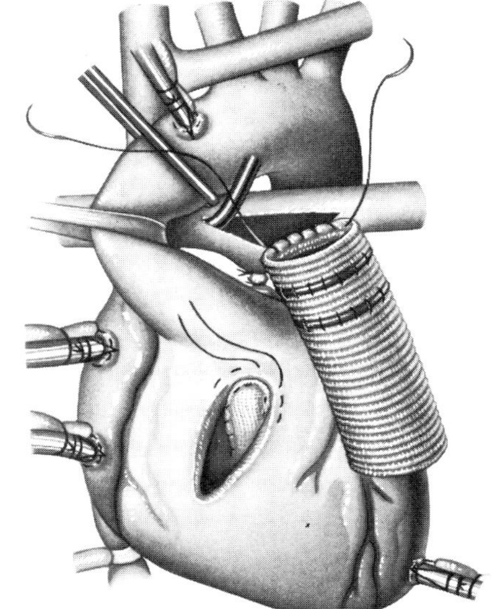

11

12 & 13

The aortic clamp is removed and the last stitches on the ventricular septal defect patch are tied. The length of the conduit is assessed on the beating heart and the conduit is trimmed. The proximal anastomosis is performed using 4/0 Prolene on a large needle. The upper part of the conduit is sutured to the edge of the intraventricular patch. The completed conduit is illustrated.

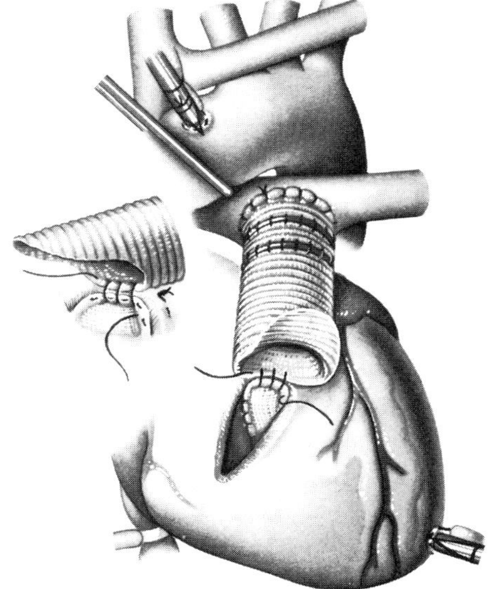

12

Termination of perfusion

When the patient is completely rewarmed, the heart is fibrillated and air removed from the left ventricle, right ventricle and aorta. The superior and inferior vena caval snares are released and the fibrillator disconnected. Left ventricular and right ventricular vents are removed and the right atrial suture line completed. If the heart does not defibrillate spontaneously, a d.c. shock is used. Perfusion is reduced keeping left atrial pressure at 13–15 mmHg. Bleeding points are checked and when the blood pressure is adequate and blood gases within normal limits, perfusion is terminated. Intracardiac pressures are measured before the cannulae are removed from the heart. Transfusion is completed and protamine given. Pacemaker wires and drains are inserted and the sternotomy closed in a routine manner.

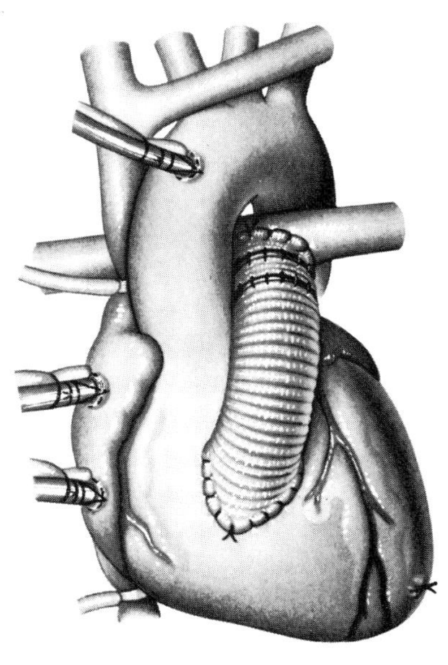

13

POSTOPERATIVE CARE

This does not differ from the care given to other patients with congenital heart lesions.

Complications

Numerous suture lines and a long conduit increase the risk of postoperative bleeding and tamponade. Haemostasis must therefore be meticulous. Preclotting of the conduit is helpful. Compression of the conduit by the sternum occurred in earlier years in several series; this can be avoided by placing the conduit away from the mid-line so that it does not cross the mid-line. It is usually placed to the left of the aorta (*see Illustration 13*). Residual ventricular septal defect, pseudo-aneurysm of the right ventricle, stenosis of the conduit, obstruction between the left ventricle and aorta, and late infections have been described (Merin and McGoon, 1973; Marcelletti *et al.*, 1976; Jacobs, de Leval and Stark, 1974; Daenen, de Leval and Stark, 1976). The long-term fate of the valve and the conduit will have to be evaluated. So far, the homograft aorta with the aortic valve which was irradiated and deep-frozen seems to be the less suitable conduit.

Results

The current operative mortality reported in two series was 8 and 15 per cent (Marcelletti *et al.*, 1976; Daenen, de Leval and Stark, 1976).

References

Daenen, W., de Leval, M. and Stark, J. (1976). 'Transposition of the great arteries, ventricular septal defect and left ventricular outflow tract obstruction. Results of 23 Rastelli operations.' *Br. Heart J.* **38,** 878 (Abstract)

Jacobs, T., de Leval, M. and Stark, J. (1974). 'False aneurysm of right ventricle after Rastelli operation for transposition of the great arteries, ventricular septal defect and pulmonary stenosis.' *J. thorac. cardiovasc. Surg.* **67,** 543

Marcelletti, C., Mair, D. D., McGoon, D. C., Wallace, R. B. and Danielson, G. K. (1976). 'The Rastelli operation for transposition of the great arteries: Early and late results.' *J. thorac. cardiovasc. Surg.* **72,** 427

Merin, G. and McGoon, D. C. (1973). 'Reoperation after insertion of aortic homograft as a right ventricular outflow tract.' *Ann. thorac. Surg.* **16,** 122

Rastelli, G. C. (1969). 'A new approach to the "anatomic" repair of transposition of the great arteries.' *Mayo Clin. Proc.* **44,** 1

[*The illustrations for this Chapter on The Rastelli Operation were drawn by Mr. M. J. Courtney.*]

Anatomical Correction of Transposition of the Great Arteries

Magdi H. Yacoub, F.R.C.S.
Consultant Cardiac Surgeon, Harefield Hospital, Middlesex and National Heart Hospital, London

PRE-OPERATIVE

Indications

Anatomical correction of transposition of the great arteries is the logical and most direct approach for the treatment of this condition. Delay in applying this operation has been due to the technical difficulties of transposing the coronary ostia at a very young age, and the fact that the posterior ventricle should be capable of supporting the systemic circulation immediately after operation. Although these difficulties have been largely solved the operation is still not widely used and should be attempted only in specialized centres with wide experience in open heart surgery in infants and children. The operation can be performed as a one-stage procedure only in patients with additional defects which maintain a high peak systolic pressure in the posterior ventricle (at least two-thirds that of the systemic pressure), such as large ventricular septal defects, persistent ductus arteriosus and subpulmonary stenosis. In the absence of one of these lesions (as in the majority of patients), regression of fetal pulmonary vasculature leads to a fall in pulmonary vascular resistance and systolic posterior ventricular pressure with rapid diminution in left ventricular mass. It is estimated that after the first week or two of life approximately 50 per cent of the infants, with transposition of the great arteries and intact inter-ventricular septum, will have left ventricles incapable of sustaining systemic arterial pressure. In these patients it is possible to redevelop the posterior ventricle by banding the pulmonary artery in combination with an aortopulmonary shunt proximal to the band (Yacoub, Radley-Smith and Maclaurin, 1977). The band should be adjusted to produce a pressure at or just below systemic level proximally and a distal systolic pulmonary artery pressure of about 25–30 mmHg. Although the overall effect of this first-stage operation is probably a reduction in actual pulmonary flow, cyanosis may improve due to enhanced 'mixing' across the atrial septal defect thus increasing the 'effective pulmonary flow'. It is believed that the first-stage operation should preferably be performed during the first few weeks of life before diminution in the left ventricular mass is advanced. The definitive operation ideally should be performed during the first year of life before the development of irreversible pulmonary vascular disease and to have the greatest impact on the natural history of the disease.

THE OPERATION

1

The incision

Median sternotomy.

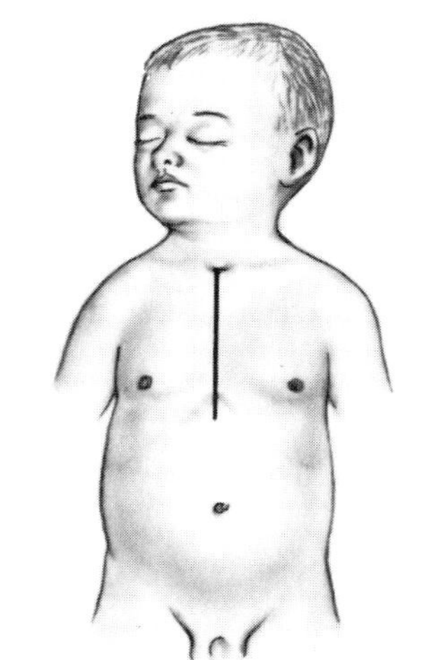

1

2

Preparation for bypass

The position and relative size of the great arteries, as well as the site of origin and exact distribution of the coronary arteries is determined. All four chambers are inspected and pressures recorded. If the ventricular peak systolic pressure is lower than two-thirds that of the anterior ventricle, the patient is considered unsuitable for anatomical correction. A cannula is inserted into the ascending aorta for arterial return. The superior and inferior venae cavae are separately cannulated through the right atrial wall. The patient is then cooled to a nasopharyngeal temperature of 18°C.

Marking the site for transfer of the coronary ostia

Before transecting either vessel it is important to identify two points on the posterior vessel for future positioning of the coronary ostia without kinking. These points are marked by two small 6/0 sutures placed in the adventitia of the posterior vessel.

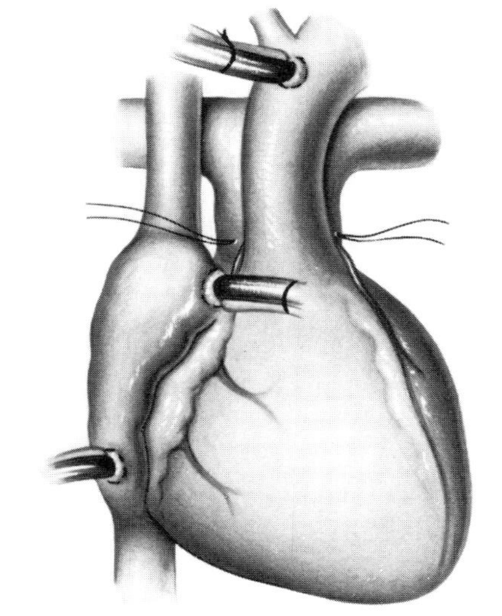

2

3

Mobilization of aorta and pulmonary arteries

The two great arteries are separated by dividing the pericardial reflection and areolar tissue between them, starting from the level of the top of the commissures of the pulmonary artery and extending to the level of the ductus or ligamentum arteriosum. If the latter is patent, it is ligated and divided.

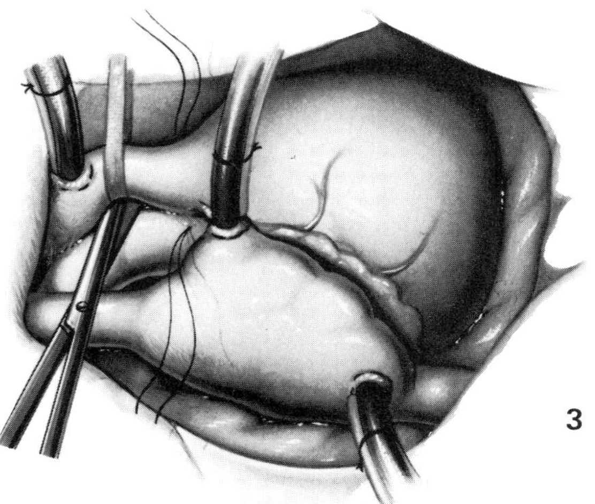

3

4

Inspection of the pulmonary valve and left ventricular outflow

The pulmonary valve is inspected through a transverse incision in the pulmonary artery at the level chosen for transecting the two great arteries (3 mm above the top of the aortic sinuses of Valsalva) and only patients with a normal tricuspid pulmonary valve and essentially normal left ventricular outflow tract are considered suitable for anatomical correction. The presence of pulmonary valve stenosis, bicuspid pulmonary valve or severe deformity of the left ventricular outflow are considered to be contraindications to anatomical correction. (Instead, a Rastelli procedure or inflow correction is performed.)

Mild to moderate subpulmonary stenosis, due to a fibrous diaphragm, can be corrected by resecting the diaphragm through the pulmonary valve.

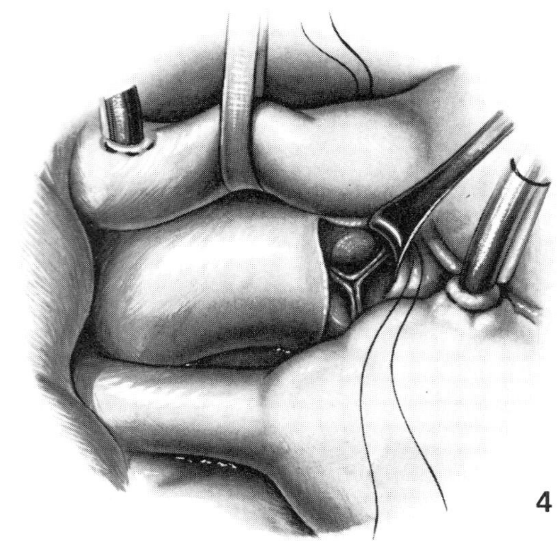

4

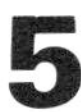

Transection of the aorta and pulmonary arteries

The aorta is clamped just below the aortic cannula and both great vessels are transected about 3 mm above the level of the superior border of the aortic sinuses of Valsalva.

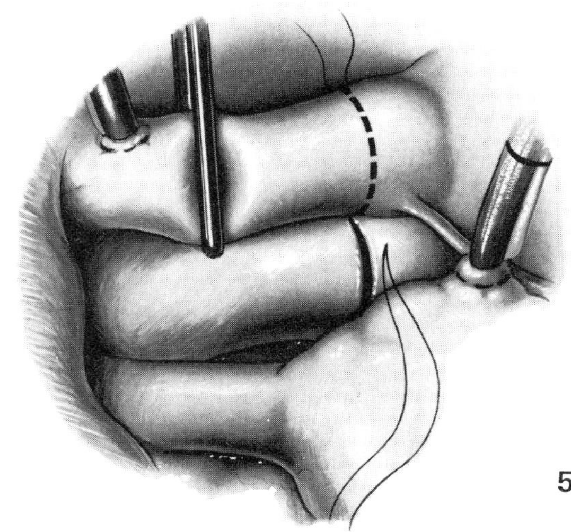

5

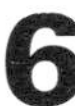

Identification of coronary anatomy

The position of the coronary ostia and their relation to the sinuses of Valsalva of the aortic and pulmonary valves is determined. In addition, the course and mode of branching of the proximal 4 mm of each artery is carefully inspected. In transposition the aortic valve has one anterior and two posterior sinuses of Valsalva, while the pulmonary valve has two anterior and one posterior sinus.

Most commonly, the right and left coronary arteries arise from the right and left posterior sinuses respectively (type A). Occasionally both arteries arise either by a common trunk, or by two orifices adjoining each other, very closely related to the commissure between the two posterior cusps (types B and C). Occasionally the right coronary artery gives rise to the circumflex branch which passes behind the pulmonary artery (the posterior vessel) to reach the atrioventricular groove (type D).

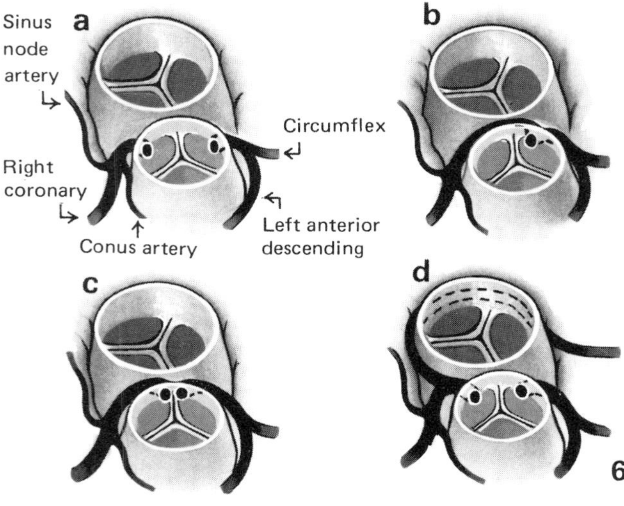

6

Transferring the coronary arteries to the posterior vessel

The technique used depends on the type of coronary anatomy.

Transferring type A coronary vessels to the posterior vessel

7

Mobilization of coronary ostia

The ostia are mobilized with a 2 mm rim of aortic wall, starting at the edge of the transected aortic wall. The proximal 3 mm of each coronary artery are then mobilized to avoid undue tension, torsion, or kinking of the main vessel or one of its branches.

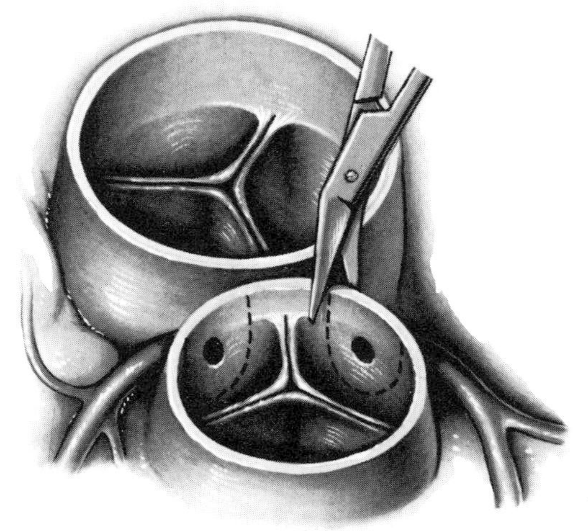

7

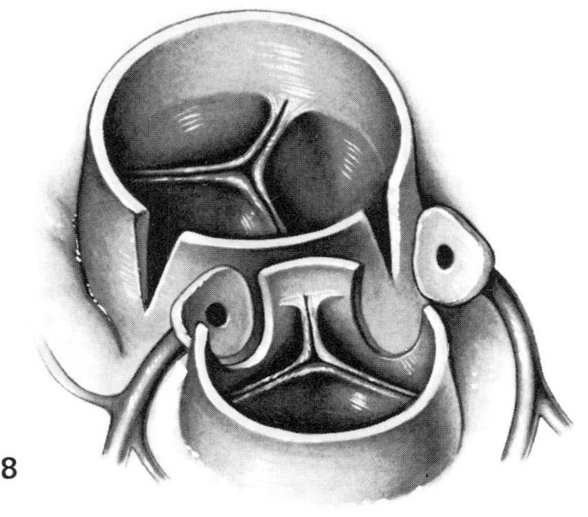

8

8

Preparation of posterior vessel for coronary anastomosis

A vertical incision at a right angle to the transected pulmonary arterial wall is then made at the marked preselected point.

9

Coronary anastomosis

The coronary transfer is completed by suturing the rim of aortic wall to the pulmonary arterial wall using a continuous 6/0 Ticron suture for approximately half of the circumference and interrupted for the remaining half to allow future growth. Before starting the anastomosis special care is taken to avoid any axial torsion or kinking of the vessel.

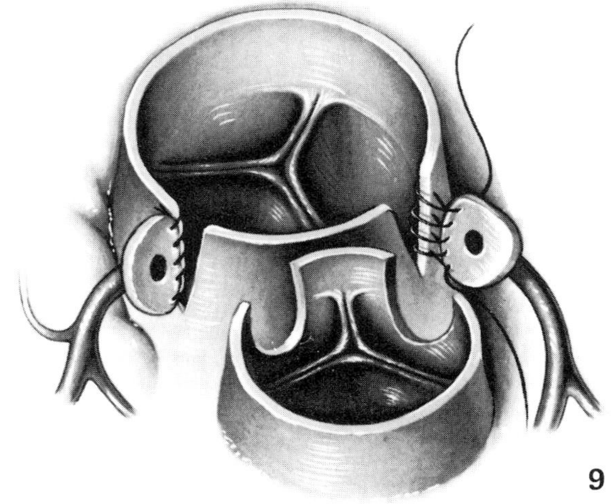

9

Transferring other types of coronary vessels

In patients with types B, C or D the use of the above technique can result in serious kinking of one or more of the coronary arteries. For this purpose a different method is used.

10

Incising the aortic wall around the coronary ostium or ostia

The aortic wall is cut in a semicircular fashion 2 mm from the rim of the ostia. Slight mobilization of the resulting disc is then performed.

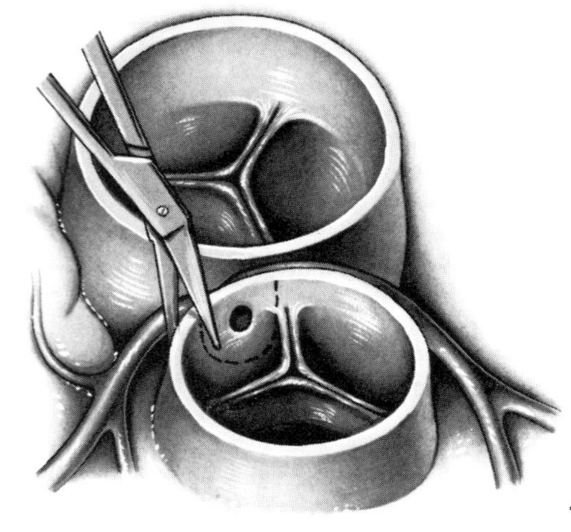

10

11

Anastomosis of upper border of coronary ostium to edge of pulmonary artery

The straight upper margin of the rim of aortic wall around the coronary ostium or ostia is anastomosed to the adjoining edge of the transected pulmonary artery.

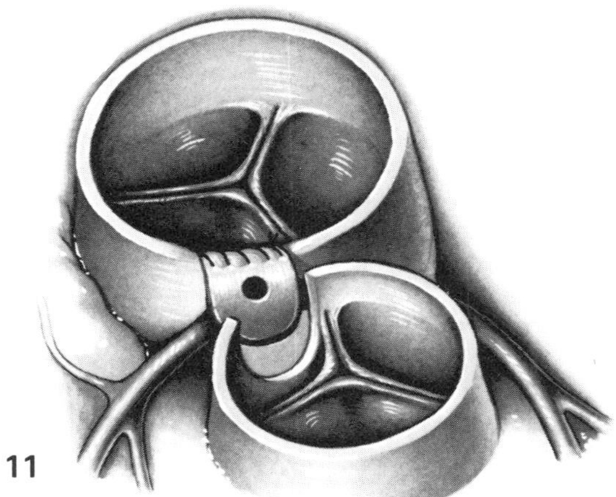

11

12 & 13

Completing the coronary anastomosis

The distal end of the transected aorta is cut obliquely with a longer lip anteriorly. This is anastomosed to the remaining part of the circumference of the aortic wall around the coronary ostium.

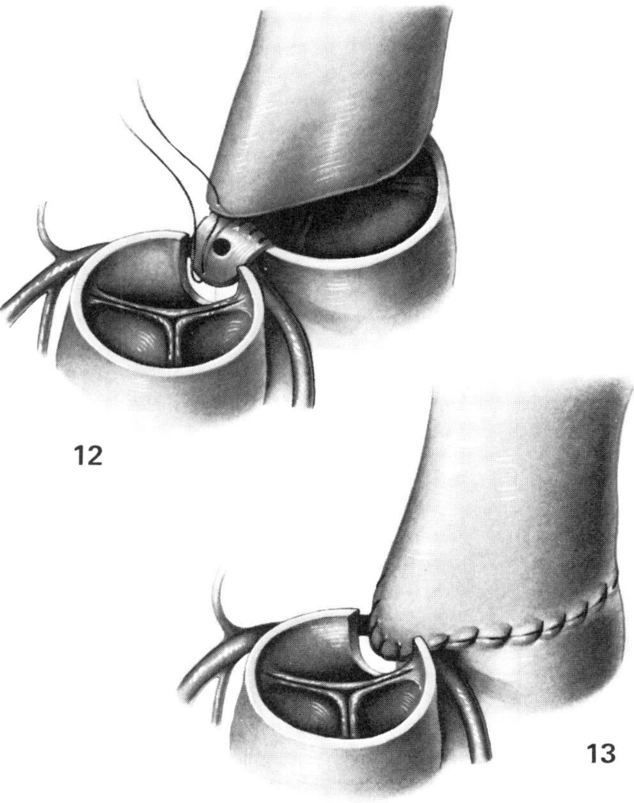

12

13

14

Anastomosis of distal aorta to proximal pulmonary artery

The small distal end of the aorta is matched to the much larger proximal pulmonary artery by cutting the former obliquely or by using a triangular patch of autogenous pulmonary artery to enlarge the lumen of the distal aorta. The two vessels are anastomosed using continuous 5/0 sutures for half of the circumference and interrupted sutures for the remaining half.

The aortic clamp is then released, thus allowing perfusion of the coronary arteries.

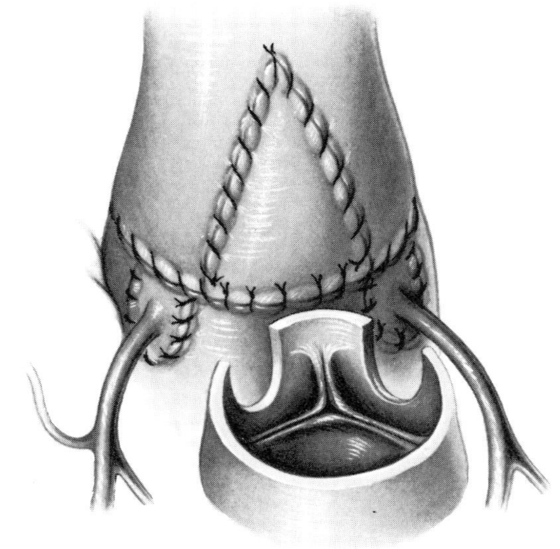

14

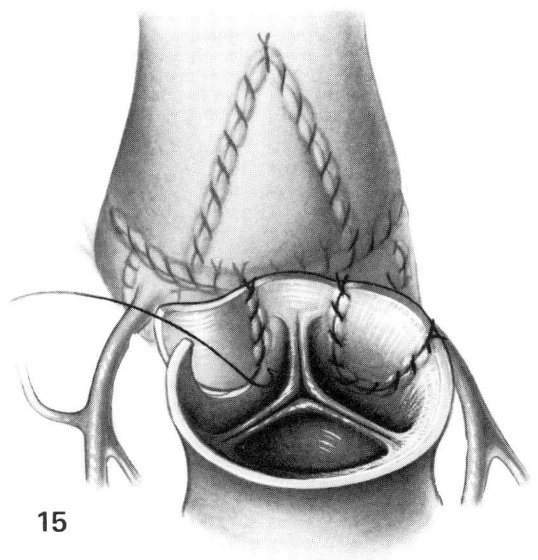

15

15

Reconstruction of the aortic root

Following transfer of type A coronary ostia, two large defects are produced in the two posterior sinuses of the anterior vessel (aorta). These are repaired by inserting two semicircular patches of autogenous pericardium or preserved homologous dura mater. The size of the patch should be approximately twice the size of the defect, thus enlarging the diameter of the proximal aorta to match the size of the distal pulmonary artery.

16

Bridging the gap between proximal aorta and distal pulmonary artery

The anteriorly placed transected proximal aorta is usually separated from the posteriorly placed distal pulmonary artery by a long distance which precludes direst anastomosis without undue tension or pressure on the coronary arteries. For this purpose a segment of woven Dacron graft (16–24 mm in diameter) is anastomosed to the distal pulmonary artery using 5/0 Mersilene sutures and positioned on the right side of the newly reconstructed ascending aorta. The graft is then trimmed and anastomosed to the proximal aorta using 5/0 sutures.

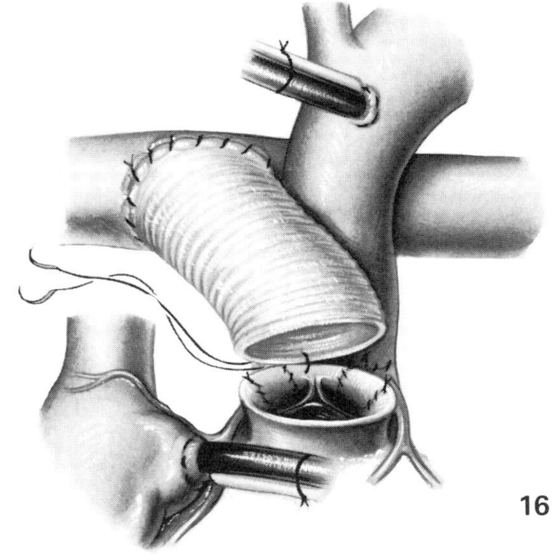

16

17

Closure of atrial septal defect

The atrial septal defect is closed through a longitudinal atriotomy, using a patch of autogenous pericardium or homologous preserved dura mater, fixed in place by 5/0 Mersilene sutures.

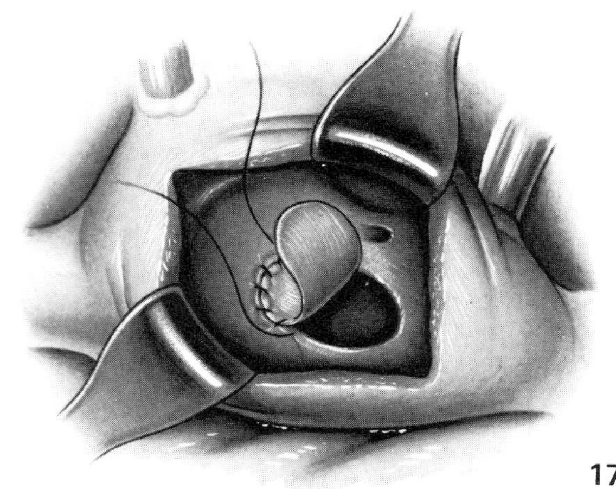

17

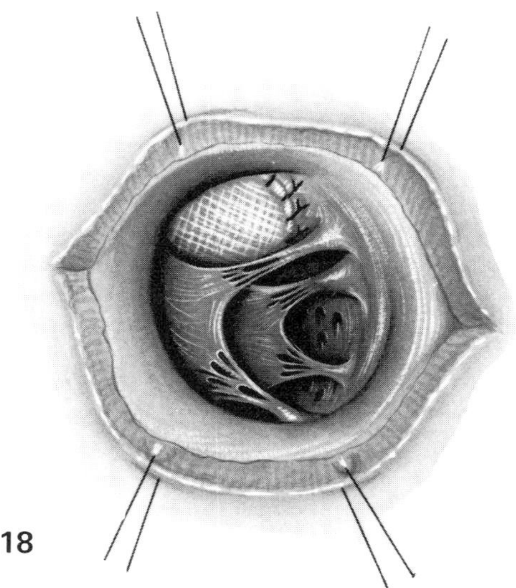

18

18

Closure of ventricular septal defect

Ventricular septal defect, if present, is then closed through a transverse ventriculotomy using a Dacron patch fixed in place by interrupted and continuous 5/0 sutures.

Decannulation and closure of chest

The child is rewarmed to a nasopharyngeal temperature of 36°C and bypass discontinued. The left atrial pressure is continually monitored. When cardiac action and rhythm are stable the perfusion cannulae are removed and haemostasis is secured. The pericardium is left open and drainage tubes inserted in the pericardium and mediastinum. The chest is then closed in layers.

POSTOPERATIVE CARE

The child is nursed in the intensive care unit for approximately 48 hr. Artificial ventilation, through an endotracheal tube, is continued for several hours until the cardiac output is judged to be stable for 2 hr and the chest film and results of blood gas analysis are satisfactory. The following parameters are monitored:

Pulse, blood pressure, electrocardiogram, central venous pressure, left atrial pressure, rectal (central) and toe (peripheral) temperatures, urinary output and blood drainage.

In patients who had a peak systolic left ventricular pressure lower than systemic pre-operatively, an afterload reducing agent, e.g. phenoxybenzamine, is used for the first 48 hr. Any sign of a low cardiac output state, e.g. fall in peripheral temperature, low urinary output, poor peripheral perfusion, fall in blood pressure, is treated by increasing preload by plasma or blood transfusion, depending on the result of the packed cell volume at the time and not allowing the mean left atrial pressure to rise above 18 mmHg, or inotropic agents (such as dopamine or isoprenaline) administered as a slow drip. Intravenous clear fluids, in the form of one-fifth normal dextrose saline, is limited to 2 ml/kg/hr. Blood sugar is measured every 3 hr and any tendency to hypoglycaemia is corrected by administering 5–15 ml of 50 per cent dextrose.

Reference

Yacoub, M. H., Radley-Smith, R. and Maclaurin, R. (1977). 'Two-stage operation for anatomical correction of the great arteries with intact interventricular septum.' *Lancet* **1**, 1275

[*The illustrations for this Chapter on Anatomical Correction of Transposition of the Great Arteries were drawn by Mr. M. J. Courtney.*]

Pulmonary Atresia. Reconstruction with Aortic Homograft

Donald N. Ross, F.R.C.S.
Consultant Surgeon, Guy's Hospital, London;
Senior Surgeon, National Heart Hospital, London

and

John R. W. Keates, F.R.C.S.
Formerly, Senior Lecturer, Cardiothoracic Institute, University of London;
Consultant Cardiothoracic Surgeon, King's College Hospital, London

PRE-OPERATIVE

Pathological anatomy

The most important consideration in the operation for correction of pulmonary atresia is the presence, size and connections of the pulmonary arteries.

1,2&3

Relatively normally sized pulmonary arteries may fill from:

(*a*) patent ductus arteriosus (pseudotruncus) (*Illustration 1*);

(*b*) ascending aorta via one or two orifices (truncus arteriosus types I, II and III) (*Illustration 2*);

(*c*) large aortopulmonary collateral vessels often arising from the upper part of the descending aorta (bronchial arteries) (truncus arteriosus type IV) (*Illustration 3*).

Alternatively the left and right pulmonary arteries may be underdeveloped and may not supply all parts of the lungs.

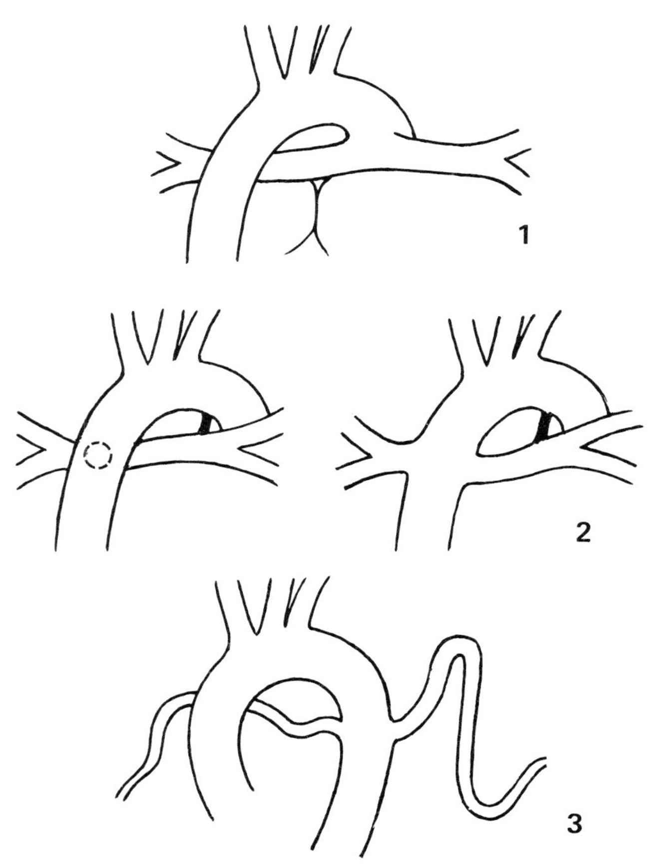

Indications and contra-indications to correction

All patients with this condition should have operative repair unless there is a contra-indication. The main contra-indication is the absence of recognizable arteries going to the right lung and left lung. Another is a marked rise in pulmonary vascular resistance.

THE OPERATION

4

Preparation of patient

A median sternotomy is used. When a large ductus arteriosus is present it is dissected out and a loose ligature passed around it. Any particularly large aortopulmonary collateral vessels or previous Blalock anastomoses are also loosely snared. Cardiopulmonary bypass is then instituted using caval cannulae and returning the blood to the aorta. The ligatures previously placed are then tied. Mild hypothermia (30°C) is used.

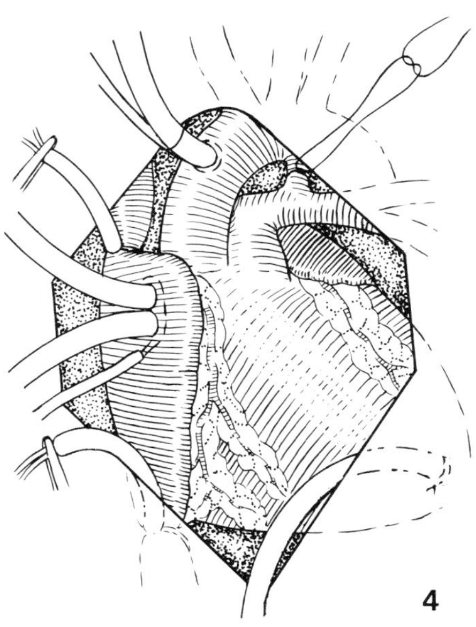

4

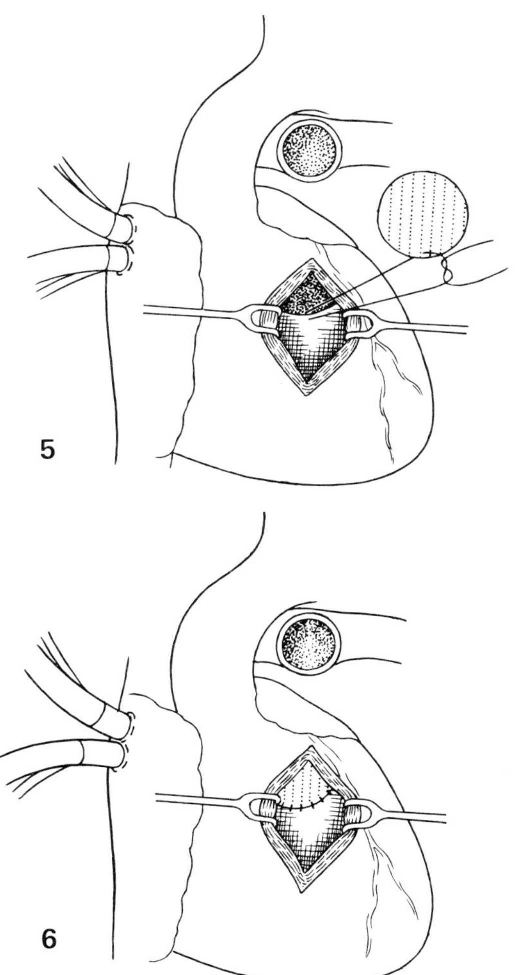

5

6

5&6

Repair of ventricular septal defect

A vertical right ventriculotomy is made. The defect is identified and closed with a knitted prosthetic patch using a continuous suture re-inforced with multiple interrupted sutures avoiding the trigone and adjoining edge of the defect where lies the bundle of His. The aorta is cross-clamped briefly during this procedure to allow a dry and still operating field.

7&8

Insertion of aortic homograft

The pulmonary artery is identified and opened. An aortic homograft is prepared by ligating the coronary artery stumps and trimming to size.

The right ventriculotomy is extended by excising a portion of the ventricular wall. The distal anastomosis is made first with a 4/0 continuous suture starting posteriorly. The proximal anastomosis is then fashioned in a similar way using a piece of woven Dacron to help close the ventriculotomy.

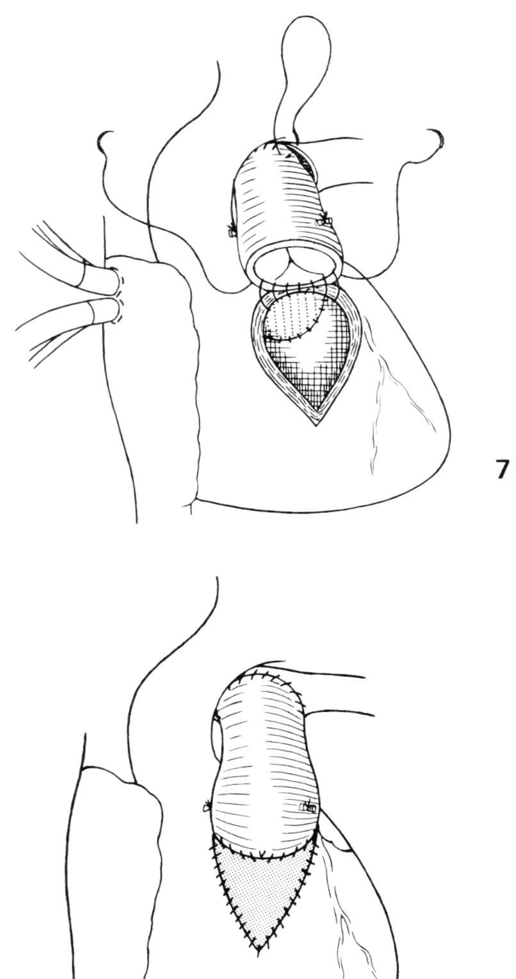

Completing the operation

Ventricular fibrillation is used to prevent ejection as all air is evacuated from the chambers and pulmonary veins by aspiration. Sinus rhythm is produced by a d.c. shock. The heart is then weaned off bypass, monitoring the atrial pressures. Even in the absence of any periods of heart-block during the operation temporary pacing electrodes are usually left *in situ*.

Poor-risk group

A certain number of patients come into this category on the basis of poor pulmonary artery anatomy. They are dependent on their large aortopulmonary blood vessels for an adequate pulmonary blood flow. In these patients the collaterals are not tied at the time of operation.

Hypothermia to 24°C is utilized so that the pump flow may be reduced during the operation, thus preventing troublesome back-bleeding from the pulmonary arteries during the construction of the conduit. In these patients it is hoped that the true pulmonary arteries will enlarge to accommodate the increased blood flow so that the collateral vessels may be ligated at a later date.

POSTOPERATIVE CARE AND COMPLICATIONS

This proceeds along conventional lines of intensive care. Left atrial pressure measurement is useful in regulating optimal blood volume replacement.

Complications

The two commonest complications seen after this operation are operative haemorrhage and low cardiac output. The haemorrhage is that often seen with serious congenital cyanotic disease and is due to both a primary and secondary haemostatic defect. It is treated with transfusion of fresh blood and fresh frozen plasma.

The low cardiac output is associated with a combination of right ventricular failure and abnormally high pulmonary vascular resistance. It is a common cause of death in the poor-risk patients. Care should be taken to avoid residual stenosis at the distal anastomosis.

[*The illustrations for this Chapter on Pulmonary Atresia. Reconstruction with Aortic Homograft were drawn by Mr. F. Price.*]

Persistent Truncus Arteriosus

Marc de Leval, M.D.
Consultant Cardiothoracic Surgeon, The Hospital for Sick Children, Great Ormond Street, London

Incidence and definition

Persistent truncus arteriosus is a rare condition which accounts for less than 3 per cent of all congenital heart defects. It is characterized by: (*1*) the presence of a single arterial trunk emerging from the bases of both ventricles by way of a single semilunar valve; (*2*) a high ventricular septal defect subjacent to the valve; and (*3*) the pulmonary arteries taking origin from the truncus and in Type III, the right and left pulmonary pulmonary trunk connects the left and right pulmonary arteries to the truncus. In Type II, the arteries originate from a common orifice of the truncus and in Type III, the right and left pulmonary arteries originate separately from the lateral aspect of the truncus. Patients with Collett and Edwards Type IV truncus arteriosus in whom the lungs are supplied by way of systemic arteries should be grouped with patients having pulmonary atresia (*see* Chapter on 'Pulmonary Atresia Reconstruction with Aortic Homograft', pages 144–146).

Natural history

The median age of death reported in autopsy series varies from a few weeks to a few months. Congestive heart failure, secondary to large pulmonary blood flow with or without associated truncal valve regurgitation, is a major cause of death in early infancy. Progressive pulmonary vascular obstructive disease is likely to occur in patients who survive beyond the age of 1 year.

Indications for surgery

Banding of the pulmonary artery (or arteries) as a palliative treatment of heart failure in young infants carries a very high mortality and there is now a tendency to consider performing complete repair even in infancy when the patient is in intractable congestive heart failure. In older patients, surgical repair should be undertaken before irreversible pulmonary vascular obstructive disease develops, and probably before the age of 2 years.

Pre-operative investigations

Complete cardiac catheterization and angiocardiography are necessary to delineate the exact anatomy and to evaluate the haemodynamic status. The latter includes an assessment of the pulmonary arteriolar resistance and of the competence of the truncal valve.

Anaesthesia

Premedication and anaesthesia are similar to that used for other congenital heart defects.

THE OPERATION

Cannulation and perfusion

The heart is approached through a mid-line sternotomy, the anatomy defined and the aorta and the pulmonary arteries are dissected free.

1

The ascending aorta is cannulated if there is enough room above the origin of the pulmonary artery (or arteries). If not, the oxygenated blood is returned through an iliac artery. The venae cavae are cannulated in the usual fashion and the left ventricle is vented through its apex.

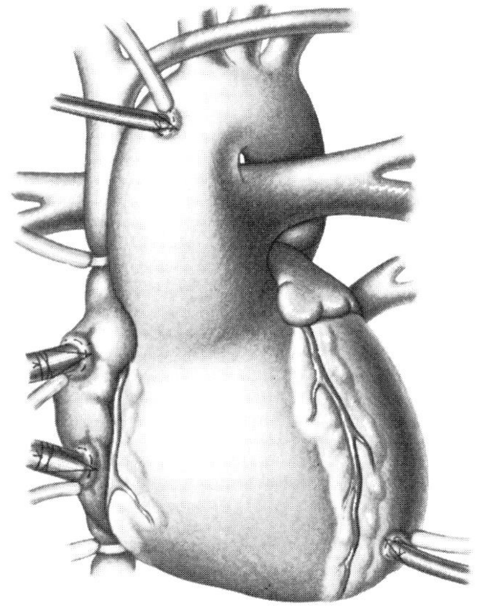

1

Total cardiopulmonary bypass at 2·4 litres/min/m^2 is instituted with the whole body perfusate cooled to 22° – 25°C. The repair is performed with intermittent cross-clamping of the aorta, releasing the clamp for a 3–5 min period every 15–20 min. During the cooling period before the aorta is clamped, when the contractions of the heart become less effective, flooding the lungs and overloading the left ventricle must be avoided. This can be achieved simply with a clamp on the pulmonary artery (or arteries) as soon as cardiopulmonary bypass is instituted. For young infants, the technique of deep hypothermia and circulatory arrest has proved very useful. The technique is described in the Chapter on 'Total Anomalous Pulmonary Venous Drainage', pages 76–84. If more time than the safe duration of circulatory arrest is necessary to complete the repair, venous cannulae are introduced into the venae cavae through the opened right atrium and the rest of the operation is performed on cardiopulmonary bypass.

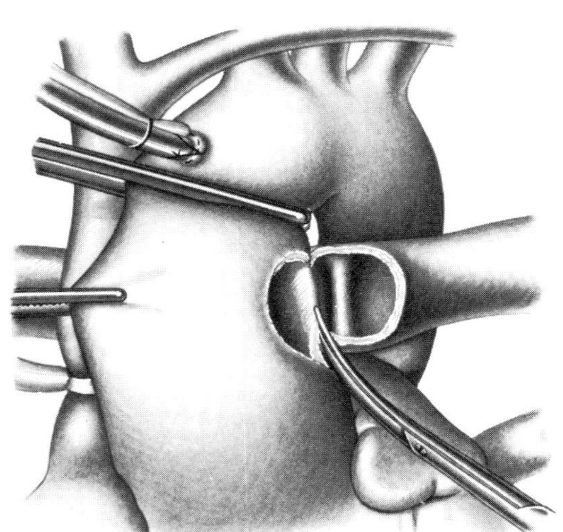

2

Surgical repair

2

First, the pulmonary arteries are excised from the truncus. If they originate from two separate orifices, they are cut out with a piece of aortic wall. During the separation of the pulmonary arteries, one must avoid any damage to the left coronary artery, the ostium of which can be closely related to the pulmonary artery orifice.

3

The defect formed in the back of the truncus is then closed usually by direct suture in a transverse direction with a continuous mattress suture re-inforced with a continuous running suture. If the defect is too large a patch closure might be indicated.

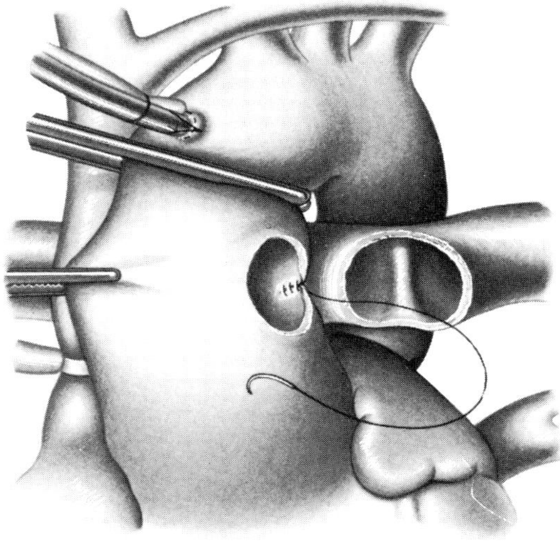

3

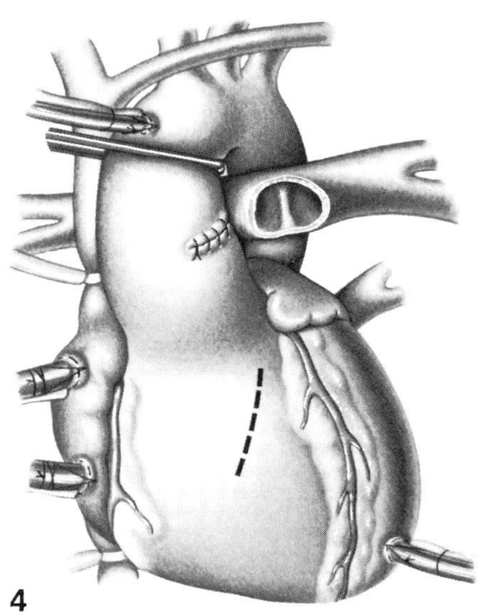

4

4

A vertical ventriculotomy is then performed in the anterior wall of the right ventricle at a sufficient distance from the level of the truncal valve and the left anterior descending coronary artery. The aortic clamp is then released for the first time. A right-angled clamp is inserted via the ventriculotomy to keep the truncal valve open until air is evacuated from the aortic root by blood.

5

The ventricular septal defect is typically located immediately beneath the cusps of the truncal valve and does not extend posteriorly to the tricuspid valve annulus, leaving an excellent rim of septum well away from the usual location of the bundle of His.

The ventricular septal defect is closed with a Dacron patch so that the left ventricle empties into the aorta. Interrupted or continuous sutures are placed along the edge of the defect inferiorly, and superiorly the patch is attached to the deep margin of the upper part of the ventriculotomy. The last stitches are untied in order to maintain access to the truncal valve while the aorta remains clamped.

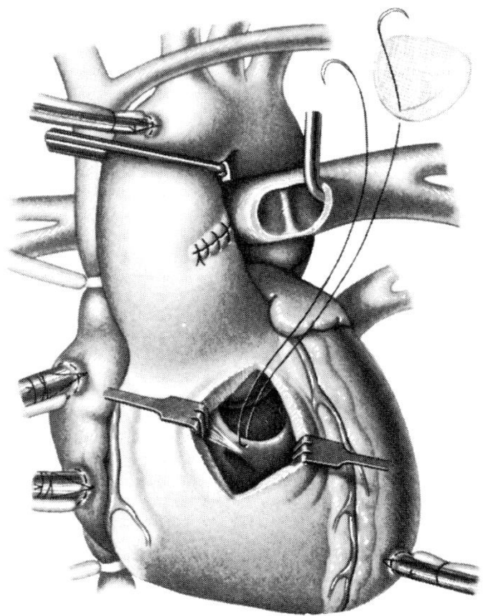

5

6

Next, a valved conduit is attached to the pulmonary arteries. The bronchial blood flow can usually be retrieved by a sump sucker placed in the pulmonary artery orifice. If the anastomosis is hampered by too much blood returning to the operative field, overwhelming the removal capacity of the suckers, the cardiopulmonary bypass flow can be temporarily reduced and a clamp can be usefully applied on one or both pulmonary arteries. Good exposure can be obtained by placing the conduit along the left border of the heart into the pericardial sac, while completing the posterior aspect of the anastomosis. The sump sucker can then be positioned in the pulmonary artery through the conduit while suturing anteriorly. Rewarming of the perfusate is begun at the completion of the anastomosis and the aortic clamp is released for the final time.

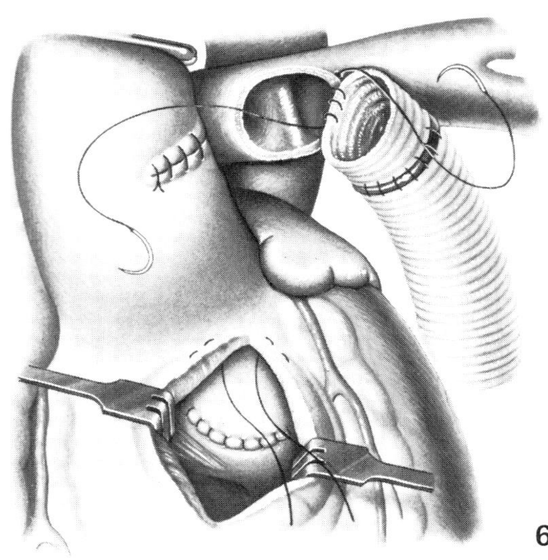
6

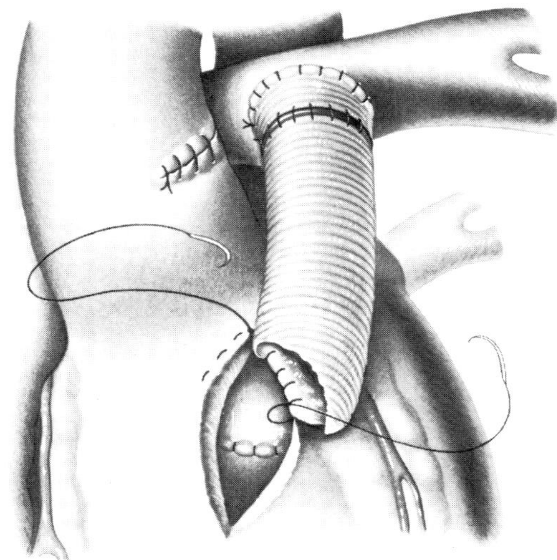
7

7

The last stitches of the ventricular septal defect are now tied and the proximal end of the conduit is anastomosed to the margins of the ventriculotomy to terminate the repair.

8

At the present time we are using either a Dacron conduit bearing a Porcine semilunar valve prepared and preserved in gluteraldehyde, or a fresh antibiotic homograft which may be advantageous particularly in small infants in whom a larger size conduit can be interposed between the right ventricle and the pulmonary artery.

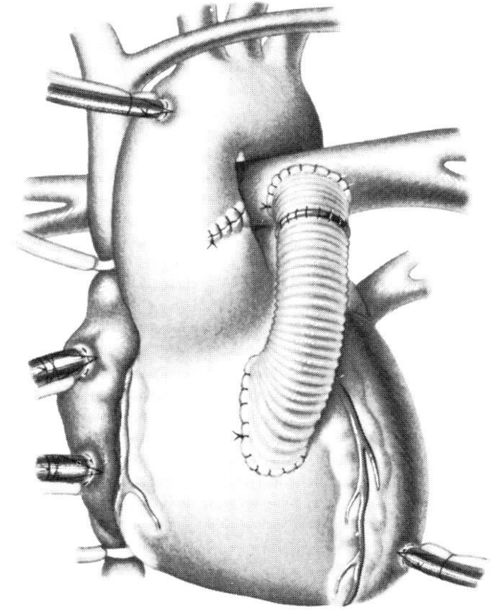
8

RESULTS

Published results of large series of truncus arteriosus deal mainly with patients operated on after the age of 2 years. The current operative mortality is approximately 20–25 per cent in that age group. The late results are less good in patients with significant pre-operative truncal valve regurgitation and/or obstructive pulmonary vascular disease. Although only a few results of complete repair in infancy have been published, we are very encouraged by our early experience with these patients.

References

McGoon, D. C., Rastelli, G. C. and Ongley, P. A. (1968). 'An operation for the correction of truncus arteriosus'. *J. Am. med. Ass.* **205**, 69

Singh, A. K., de Leval, M. and Stark, J. (1975). 'Total correction of Type I truncus arteriosus in a 6 month-old infant.' *Br. Heart J.* **37**, 1314

Singh, A. K., de Leval, M. R., Pincott, J. and Stark, J. (1976). 'Pulmonary artery banding for truncus arteriosus in the first year of life.' *Circulation* **54**, (Suppl III), 17

Wallace, R. B., Rastelli, G. C., Ongley, P. A., Titus, J. L. and McGoon, D. C. (1969). 'Complete repair of truncus arteriosus defects.' *J. thorac. cardiovasc. Surg.* **57**, 95

[*The illustrations for this Chapter on Persistent Truncus Arteriosus were drawn by Mr. M. J. Courtney.*]

Tricuspid Atresia

F. Fontan, M.D.
Professor of Cardiac Surgery, University of Bordeaux;
Surgeon to the Hôpital du Tondu, Bordeaux

PRE-OPERATIVE

Palliative operations for tricuspid atresia can improve the clinical status of the patient but they do not eliminate the mixing of venous and arterial blood. In 1968 an operation was developed which completely overcomes this mixing. The principle of the operation is to redirect the entire caval return into the lungs, having closed all septal defects. This is not an anatomical correction, but rather a physiological restoration of blood flow in which all shunts are eliminated. A similar technique can be used for patients with primitive ventricle and pulmonary stenosis.

Indications

Two different techniques may be used to correct tricuspid atresia depending upon the anatomy.

(*1*) If there are normally related great arteries with the pulmonary artery (PA) arising from the outlet chamber, a non-valved Dacron conduit is used from the right atrium (RA) to the outlet chamber of the right ventricle (RV) preserving the patient's own pulmonary valve.

(*2*) If there are transposed great arteries with the aorta arising from the outlet chamber a valved conduit, usually an antibiotic sterilized aortic homograft, is used to connect the right atrial appendage to the pulmonary arteries.

Selection for surgery

Only patients who fulfill a rigid set of criteria obtained from pre-operative cardiac catheterization and angiography are accepted for operation.

(*1*) There should be a normal sized or large right atrium with no right-sided atrioventricular (tricuspid) valve.

(*2*) The pulmonary arteries should be of normal size.

(*3*) In patients who are being considered for an atrioventricular conduit, the pulmonary valve ring should be of normal size – at least 75 per cent of the diameter of the aortic valve.

(*4*) The pulmonary vascular resistance should be normal, i.e. less than 4 units/m^2.

(*5*) Left ventricular function should be normal with an ejection fraction of at least 50 per cent.

Patients between 4–14 years of age appear to be most suitable for this technique.

Anaesthesia

The standard technique for cardiac surgery is employed with the exception that the patient should be allowed to breathe spontaneously at the end of the operation. This permits early postoperative extubation and avoids positive pressure ventilation which inhibits systemic venous return. The patient's status is better as soon as he is breathing spontaneously.

Position of patient

The patient lies supine – arterial and venous cannulae are inserted to enable the blood pressure to be monitored and fluids to be administered.

THE OPERATION

ATRIOVENTRICULAR CONDUIT OPERATION

1

A median sternotomy is performed and extracorporeal circulation established. An atriotomy through the right atrial appendage and a ventriculotomy in the outlet chamber of the right ventricle are performed to inspect the anatomy of the heart and to exclude unexpected contra-indications to operation such as a single atrium or a small pulmonary valve ring.

In order to interfere as little as possible with the anatomy and function of the atrium and to reduce the risk of atrial dysrhythmia certain precautions are taken.

(*1*) The cavae are cannulated directly.

(*2*) The atriotomy and conduit anastomosis is made from the right atrial appendage and not the atrium itself – thus preserving the atrial muscle and its arterial supply. The atrial septal defect is closed through the incision in the atrial appendage which is opened near its crista and this will be used for subsequent anastomosis to the conduit.

(*3*) The Eustachian valve is preserved.

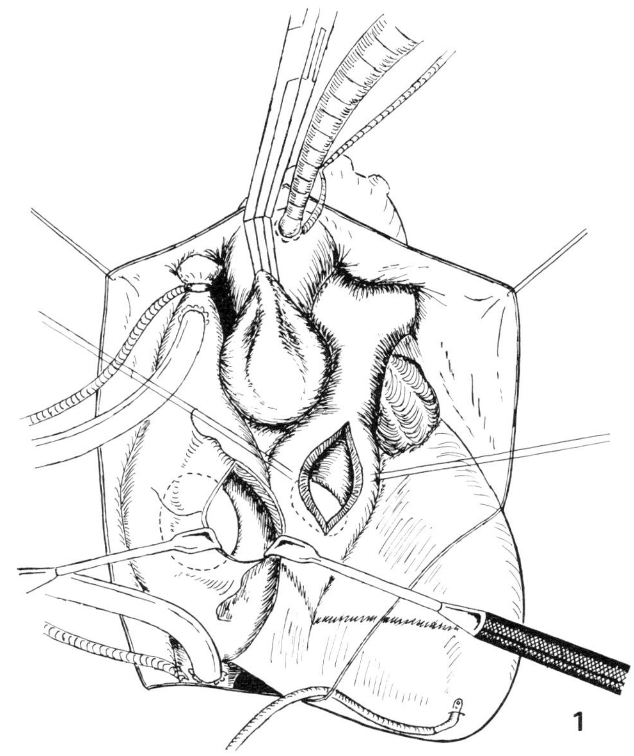
1

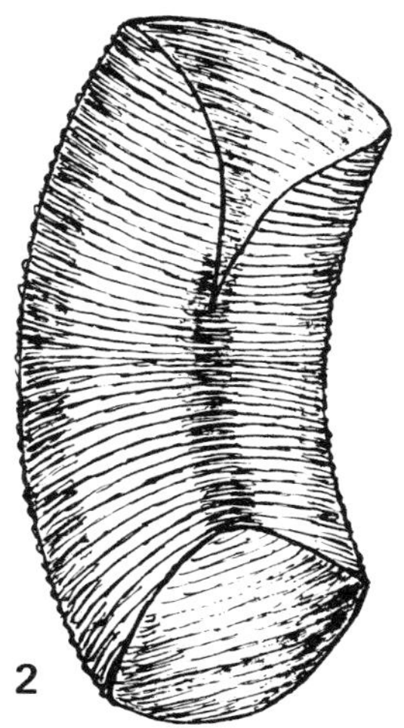
2

Preparation of the woven Dacron conduit

2

Before operation the conduit is cut at both ends. A 20 mm conduit should be used for children under 5 years old and 22–24 mm conduit for older patients. The ventricular end is cut more obliquely in a racquet shape so that there is the widest possible communication between it and the ventriculotomy. Before going on bypass the conduit is preclotted with the patient's blood to minimize the risks of postoperative bleeding.

3a&b

The right outlet chamber is approached through a high vertical ventriculotomy 1 cm below the pulmonary valve ring – avoiding the coronary arteries and also the veins if they are large.

If the outlet chamber is small and difficult to identify, the pulmonary artery can be opened and a probe passed through the pulmonary valve to facilitate the correct siting of the ventriculotomy.

The ventricular septal defect is closed with interrupted sutures buttressed by Teflon pledgets if it is small (*Illustration 3a*) or with a patch if it is large (*Illustration 3b*). In order to prevent atrioventricular block the sutures should be placed on the right side of the septum in all cases – even if two defects are present.

3a

3b

4

The atrial septal defect is closed with a Dacron patch and continuous sutures. The distal anastomosis between the Dacron conduit and the outlet chamber is performed with a continuous 5/0 Prolene suture. With the heart beating a careful inspection of the atrial septum and the patch is then made to exclude leaks around the suture line of the patch and other small defects in the atrial septum which may occur in its lower part.

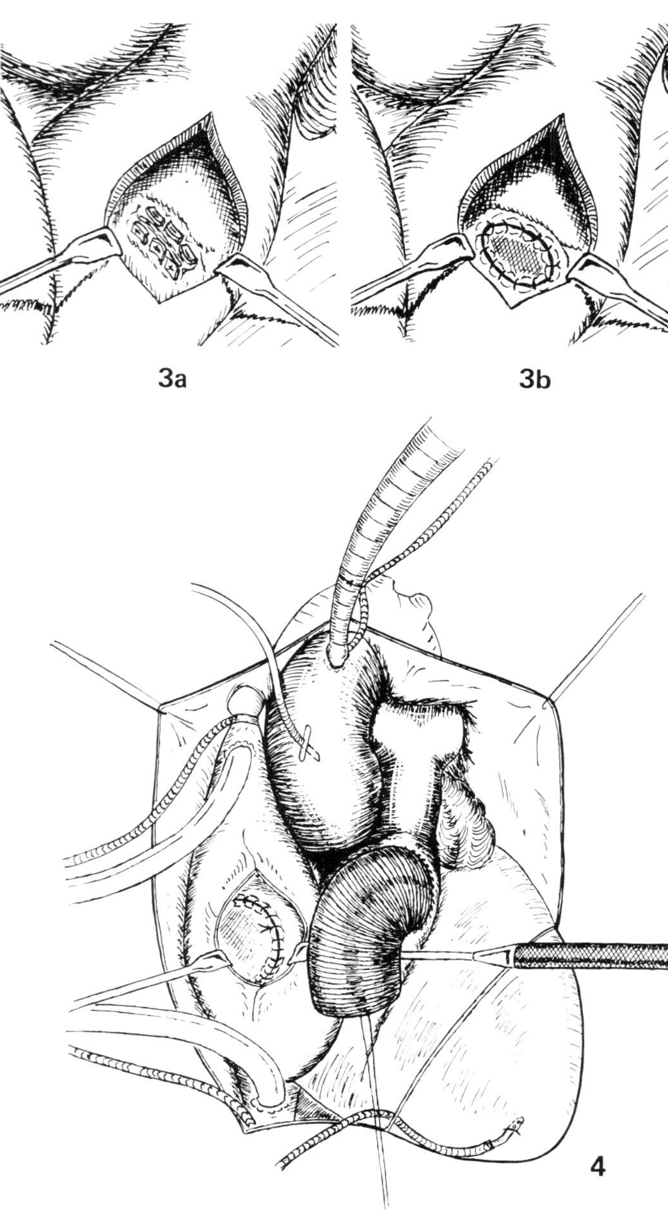

4

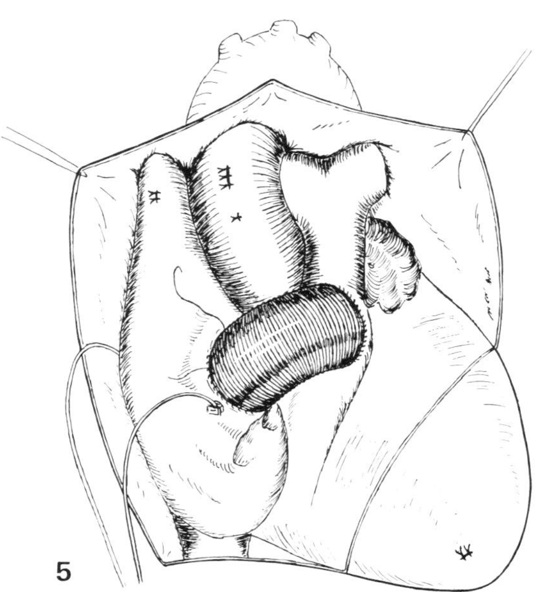

5

5

The proximal anastomosis between the Dacron conduit and the right atrial appendage is now made – again using a continuous 5/0 Prolene suture. All the suture lines are then checked.

Right and left atrial lines are inserted for postoperative monitoring. Bypass is discontinued as soon as the haemodynamic state is stable with a systemic pressure at or above 100 mmHg, a right atrial pressure between 12 and 18 mmHg and left atrial pressure between 8 and 12 mmHg.

ATRIOPULMONARY CONDUIT

A median sternotomy is again performed. In this instance an antibiotic sterilized aortic valve homograft is used as the conduit between the right atrium and the right and main pulmonary arteries.

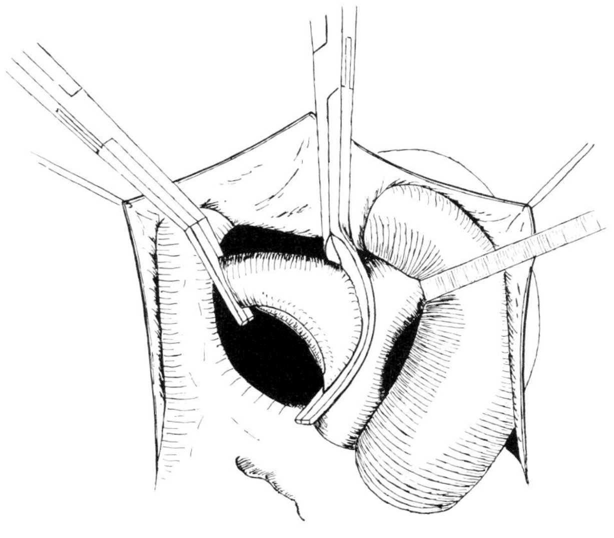

6a

6a&b

The distal anastomosis between the homograft and the pulmonary arteries is constructed first, preferably before placing the patient on bypass. A clamp is placed on the side of the main pulmonary artery occluding the right pulmonary artery with a second clamp on the distal right pulmonary artery. Care is taken not to occlude the main pulmonary artery and left pulmonary artery completely so that the blood supply to the lungs is not jeopardized when the patient is not on bypass. An incision is made in the main pulmonary artery, and right pulmonary artery as shown in the illustration and the anastomosis performed with 5/0 Prolene continuous sutures. The clamps are then released and the suture line inspected. The position of the aortic valve homograft must be checked to ensure that it fits well, not only at the distal anastomosis but also at the proximal anastomosis which will be constructed later.

Some people prefer, or find it easier, to do this part of the operation with the patient on bypass.

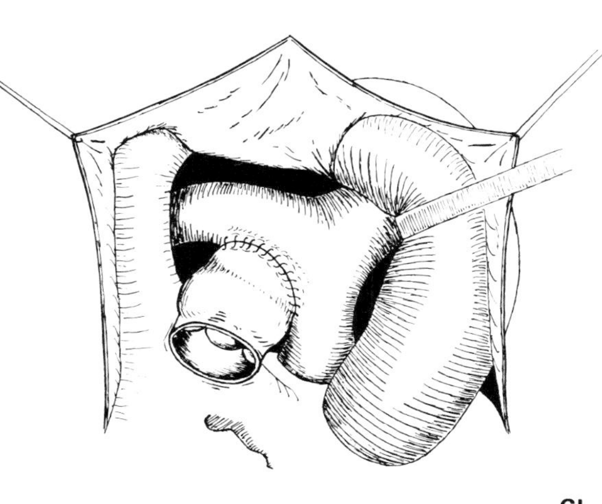

6b

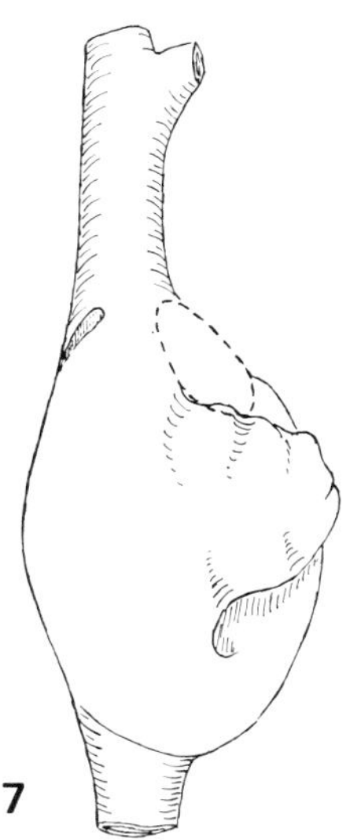

7

7

Illustrated here is a convenient site for the right atriotomy and proximal anastomosis. It is usually between the superior vena cava and the appendage but more or less on the appendage. Care must be taken to avoid the sinus node (at the junction of superior vena cava and right atrium) and to preserve its blood supply.

8

The right atriotomy is then performed with the patient on bypass, and the atrial septal defect closed with a patch. With the heart beating the suture line and the atrial septum are then checked as described previously.

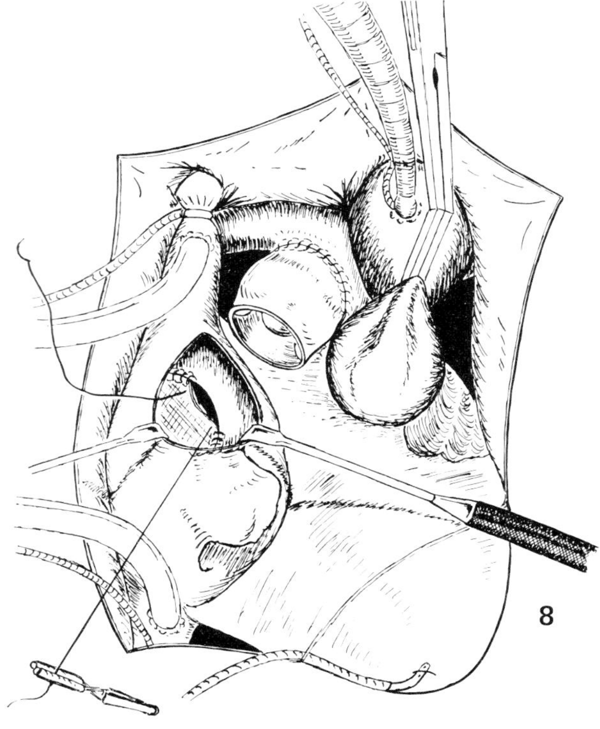
8

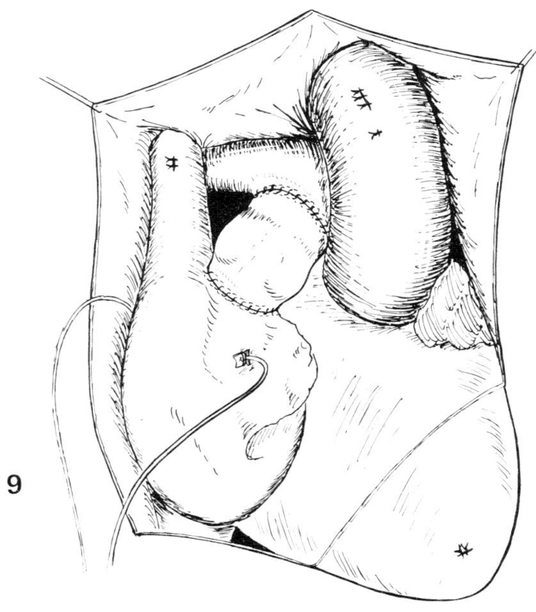
9

9

Finally, the proximal anastomosis is performed, again using a continuous 5/0 Prolene suture. The main pulmonary artery is transected proximal to the attached conduit and each end oversewn. All suture lines are checked and bypass discontinued. Right and left atrial lines are inserted for monitoring.

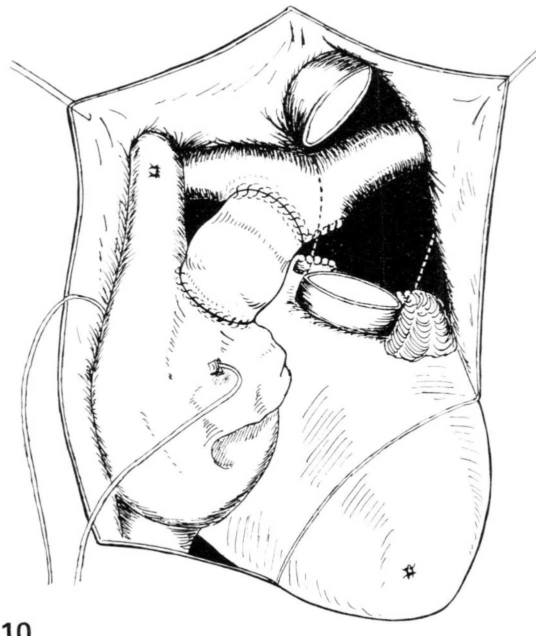
10

10

In this illustration the aorta is omitted to show the method of transection of the main pulmonary artery and the suture lines on the proximal and distal ends of this vessel.

Closure

Before closing the sternum a check must be made that it does not compress the conduit. If it does, the posterior 'table' of the sternum should be resected in front of the conduit. The pericardium is left widely open. Mediastinal and pericardial drainage tubes are inserted – one above and one below the conduit. The right pleura is drained as right pleural effusions frequently develop in the immediate postoperative period.

POSTOPERATIVE CARE

The patient is placed in the head-up (45°) feet-up (30°) position to facilitate systemic venous return and thus pulmonary artery perfusion. The patient should be allowed to breathe spontaneously as soon as possible (*see* Anaesthesia, page 152) and extubated as soon as the blood gases, clinical and haemodynamic state allow. Monitoring of the atrial and arterial pressures is important. These should be maintained at the same level as at the end of bypass. Because of the frequent pooling of fluid in the extravascular spaces (pleural effusions, ascites, oedema and hepatomegaly) in the immediate postoperative period, additional blood, plasma and intravenous fluid may be required. Diuretics may be helpful but digitalis is rarely necessary. This postoperative syndrome usually disappears within a few days.

RESULTS

The long-term results are excellent within the limits of the present follow-up (9 years). The importance of careful patient selection and full assessment of the anatomical and haemodynamic data pre-operatively and at the time of surgery cannot be minimized. As always, careful attention to surgical principles and technical details is essential if the best results are to be obtained.

[*The illustrations for this Chapter on Tricuspid Atresia were drawn by Dr. C. Deville.*]

Closed Mitral Valvotomy

J. R. Belcher, M.S., F.R.C.S.
Surgeon, London Chest Hospital; Thoracic Surgeon, The Middlesex Hospital;
Consulting Thoracic Surgeon, North West Thames Regional Health Authority

PRE - OPERATIVE

MITRAL VALVE DISEASE

Mitral stenosis, mitral incompetence and the common mixed lesions are all amenable to surgical correction. The treatment of pure mitral stenosis and restenosis remains closed valvotomy. Open operation must be used for pure incompetence and is being used increasingly for the mixed lesions, and for heavily calcified valves. However in view of the late results of mitral valve replacement, every effort should be made to conserve the valve wherever possible.

MITRAL STENOSIS

Indications

All patients with simple mitral stenosis, or stenosis associated with trivial incompetence, who have symptoms, including embolic phenomena, should be considered for closed mitral valvotomy whatever their age. Not only should it be suggested for first operations, but also for second or even third ones if pure stenosis is present.

The operative mortality is less than 3 per cent and the short- and long-term results are excellent.

Pre-operative preparation

If digitalis is already being given, it should be continued up to the time of the operation; if not, it should be started a few days before surgery, for although the drug does not prevent fibrillation, it does prevent tachycardia.

Atropine should be avoided as a premedication, as the cardiac output may be reduced by the tachycardia it produces; pethidine is preferable. If the patient is orthopnoeic it is essential that he should remain in an upright position while being taken to the theatre.

Position of patient

The patient lies on his right side on a chest rest, the head and the pelvis are securely anchored to the table by wide straps so that he may be rolled slightly backwards when the chest is opened. The left arm is held above and in front of the patient's face to draw the scapula up as far as possible.

Anaesthesia

It is essential that a technique should be used which allows a considerable degree of collapse of the left lung in order that it may not be obtrusive during the intracardiac manipulations.

THE OPERATION

1

Incision

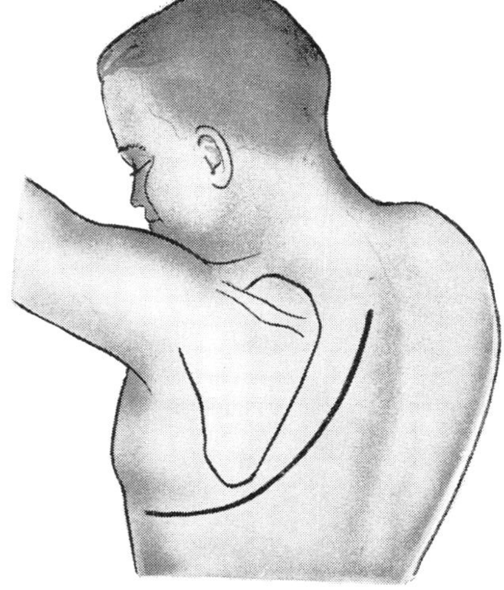

A long posterolateral incision is made from 4 cm from the mid-line posteriorly to the anterior axillary line. The trapezius and the rhomboid muscles are partially divided, and the latissimus dorsi is completely cut; the incision is then carried down through the serratus anterior, after the periosteum has been stripped from the upper border of the sixth rib. The pleural space is entered through the fifth interspace. The ribs are spread apart and held in that position by a self-retaining retractor.

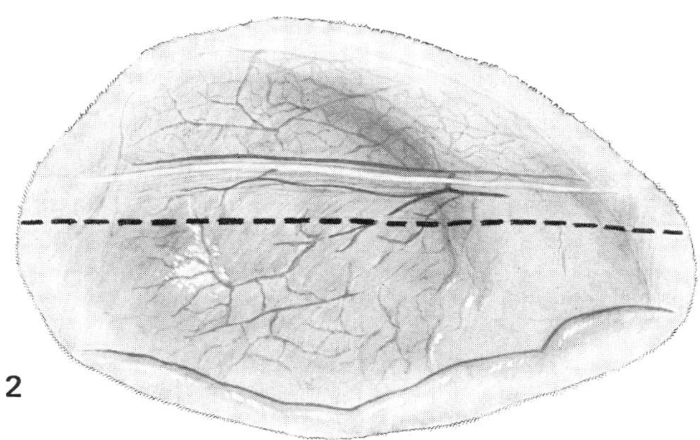

2

2

Opening the pericardium

The lung is retracted backwards and an incision is made in the pericardium behind the phrenic nerve and parallel with it. This incision should extend from the upper edge of the pulmonary artery almost to the diaphragm. Two long curved forceps are applied to the posterior edge of the incision to act as retractors and to hold the lung out of the way; a stitch is passed through the anterior edge and through an adjacent intercostal muscle to hold the pericardium forwards during manipulations.

3

Amputation of the atrial appendage

A special non-crushing clamp is applied to the base of the appendage, care being taken not to include the coronary sinus. The tip of the appendage is amputated in such a way that the resulting lumen will just admit the second interphalangeal joint of the index finger.

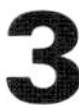

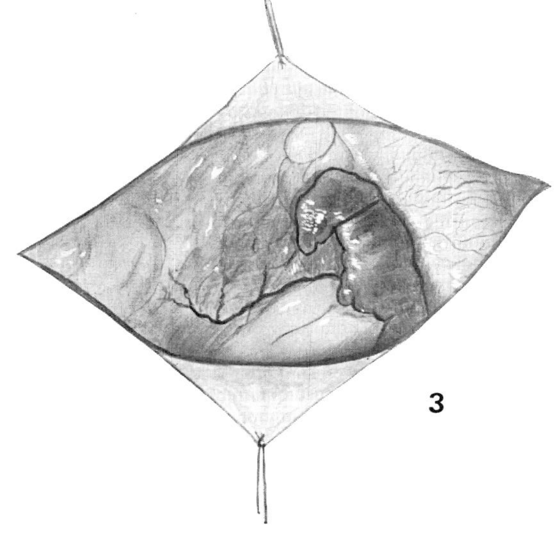

3

4

Disposal of thrombi

The clamp is momentarily released to allow any loose thrombi to be washed out. The index finger is then insinuated through the appendage into the cavity of the atrium, and the clamp is removed. If the patient is fibrillating, if there is a history of previous embolism, or, more particularly, if thrombi which cannot be flushed out are still present in the appendage, the anaesthetist should be asked to compress the carotid arteries in the neck during the insertion of the finger. If this is done any dislocated pieces of clot will be much less liable to reach the cerebral vessels. Similarly if the valve is heavily calcified, carotid compression should be undertaken during the manipulation of the valve, as 'calcium emboli' might otherwise cause cerebral damage.

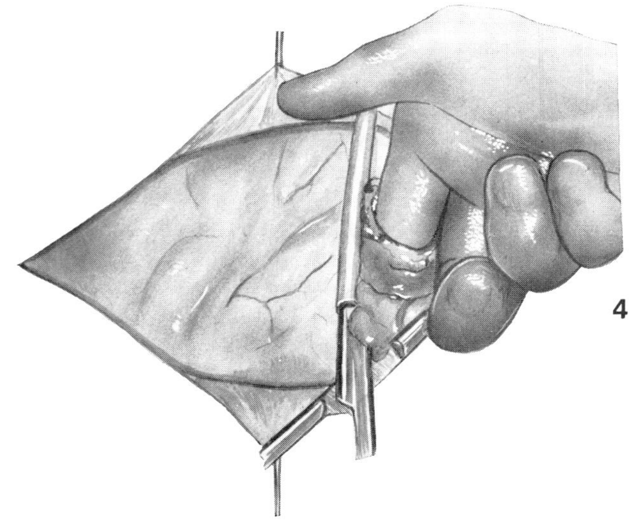

4

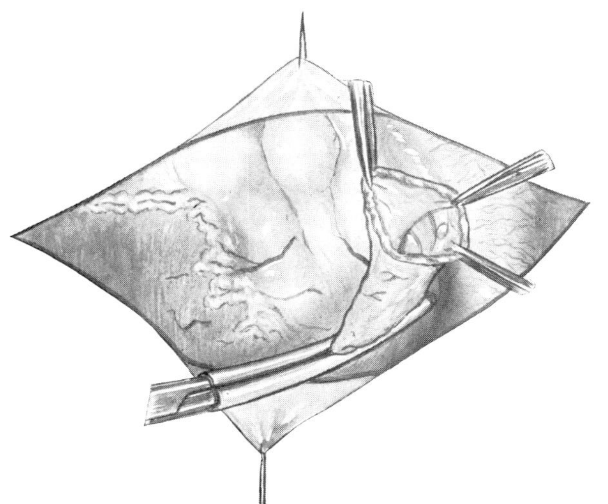

5

Commissurotomy

The valve is palpated and diagnosis of simple mitral stenosis or restenosis is confirmed. The finger is thrust through the mitral orifice, and pressure is exerted first in the direction of the posteromedial commissure and then towards the anterolateral one. Occasionally, complete division of the commissures may be achieved in this way. More usually the transventricular dilator has to be used.

6

Transventricular dilatation

A stab incision is made near the apex of the left ventricle with the right index finger still in the cavity of the left atrium. A 6 mm sound is passed through this incision into the cavity of the left ventricle; it is then withdrawn and the Tubbs' dilator is passed down the track which it has made. The dilator is then passed through the mitral orifice from below, being guided by the finger in the left atrium. When it is certain that the blades are in the valve orifice and that their shoulders are well inside the left ventricle, it is opened until the outsides of the blades are 3·5 cm apart (this must be measured and adjusted with the 'stop' screw before the instrument is inserted). If it is felt that the commissurotomy is complete, the instrument is closed and withdrawn; if not, it may be opened again and the commissures may be further opened with the finger; alternatively, the 'stop' screw may be adjusted to allow wider separation of the blades so that the commissurotomy may be completed.

The instrument is then withdrawn, an assessment of the commissurotomy and any residual incompetence is made, and the finger is withdrawn from the left atrium, a clamp being applied across the base of the appendage.

The stab wound in the ventricle which has been controlled by light finger pressure is sewn with one or two 0/0 Mersilene sutures which include the whole thickness of the ventricular wall, and the knots are tied lightly to avoid 'cutting' the myocardium. Slight haemorrhage may continue, but it soon stops with gentle pressure.

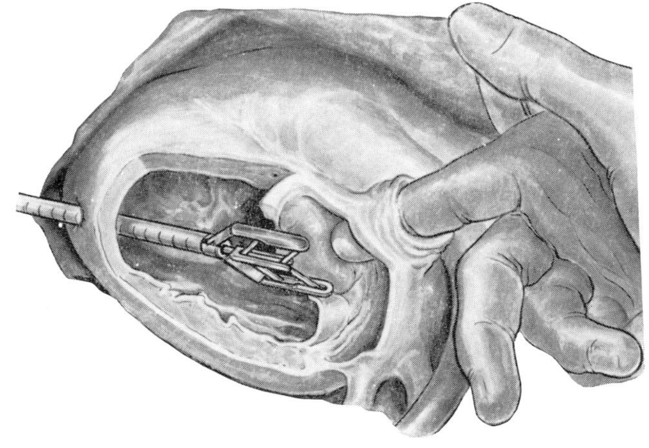

6

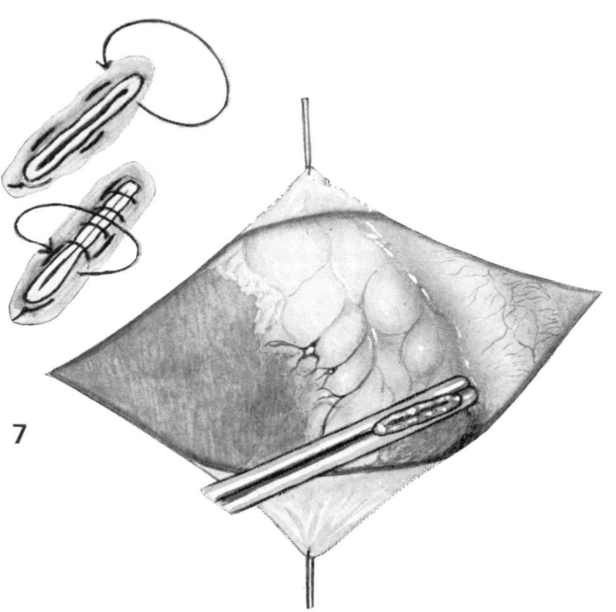

7

7

Suture of the appendage

The clamp is re-applied to the appendage and two stout ligatures are tied proximal to the clamp. Redundant appendage is then removed, but a good 'cuff' must be left distal to the ligatures.

Alternatively, the appendage may be oversewn as illustrated.

8

Suture of the pericardium

The pericardium is sewn with interrupted sutures, leaving gaps at the upper and lower ends of the incision to allow drainage.

A tube is inserted through a stab incision in the tenth intercostal space. The wound is sewn in layers.

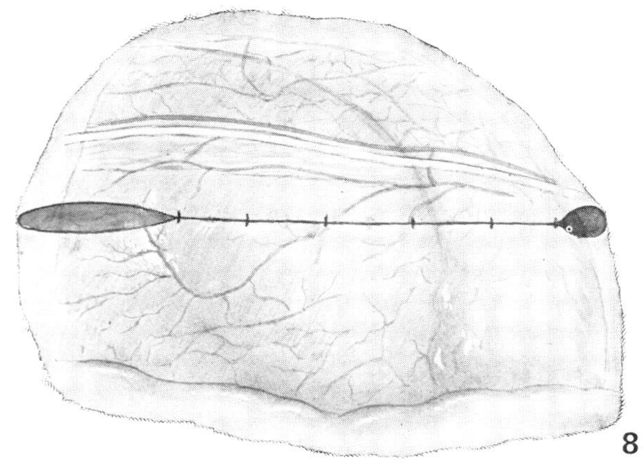

8

9

Approach to the valve via the atrial wall

When the appendage is fibrosed and too small to admit the finger, or when it has been amputated during a previous valvotomy, or when it is full of clot, the approach must be made directly through the atrial wall. A purse-string suture of 0/0 Mersilene is inserted. The ring included by the suture must be larger than the diameter of the index finger at the second interphalangeal joint. The ends of the Mersilene are drawn through a Rumel tourniquet and are controlled by an assistant. An incision through the atrial muscle is made with a tenotomy knife and the orifice is then enlarged with a long artery (Roberts') forceps great care being taken not to cut the purse-string suture in the process. The finger is inserted through the incision and the valvotomy is carried out in the manner already described, haemorrhage being controlled by the tightening of the purse-string suture. When the operation has been completed the finger is removed and the purse-string suture is tied tightly. Further interrupted stitches are inserted if necessary and the wound is closed in the usual way.

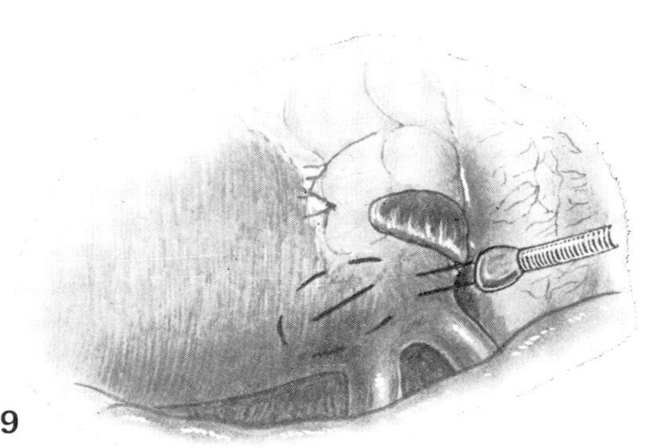

9

POSTOPERATIVE CARE AND COMPLICATIONS

The drainage tube is removed between 24 and 48 hr after the operation unless a quantity of blood is still being discharged through it at the end of this period. Where digitalis was being administered before the operation it is continued with the dosage unaltered.

A radiograph is taken on the day after the operation, and if atelectasis, a pneumothorax, or a large pleural effusion is present, appropriate treatment should be instituted.

Cerebral and peripheral embolism

Cerebral and peripheral embolism are the major hazards of mitral valvotomy. Peripheral emboli should be treated on their merits; an aortic saddle embolus should almost always be treated surgically.

Haemorrhage

Occasionally persistent leakage of blood may occur from the atrial appendage or the wall of the ventricle. Should this happen it is essential to keep the drainage tube clear and to give sufficient blood by transfusion to keep pace with the loss. If the blood loss becomes severe, thoracotomy should be undertaken. The leak in the suture line may then be oversewn.

Atrial fibrillation

This is a frequent sequel to mitral valvotomy. When it occurs the rate should be controlled with digitalis, but no attempt should be made to restore normal rhythm until at least the tenth day after the operation. Possible causes of the arrhythmia such as pleural effusion or atelectasis should be dealt with as they arise. Conversion to sinus rhythm can then usually be achieved, with external d.c. counter-shock and is likely to be maintained if the patient was in sinus rhythm before operation.

Postvalvotomy syndrome

The cause of postvalvotomy syndrome is uncertain, the treatment is symptomatic, and the prognosis is good. The symptoms and signs are malaise, precordial pain, fever, tachycardia, and to a variable extent congestive cardiac failure. Radiologically there may be an increase in the pleural effusion, or a pericardial effusion.

Some or all these symptoms and signs may appear at any time between the first few days and the third week after the operation; their severity may vary widely. The syndrome usually persists for several days, but it almost invariably settles with symptomatic treatment.

[*The illustrations for this Chapter on Mitral Valvotomy were drawn by Mr. F. Price.*]

Open Mitral Valvotomy

Magdi H. Yacoub, F.R.C.S.
Consultant Cardiac Surgeon, Harefield Hospital, Middlesex and National Heart Hospital, London

PRE-OPERATIVE

Indications

Open mitral valvotomy is indicated in patients with severe symptomatic mitral stenosis, or moderate mitral stenosis with a history of systemic embolism. The presence of additional mitral regurgitation or calcification are not contra-indications to open mitral valvotomy. Compared to closed valvotomy, the open operation has the advantages of:

(*1*) achieving full opening of the commissures;

(*2*) removal of calcium from the cusps;

(*3*) more extensive mobilization of the subvalvar mechanism;

(*4*) repair of mitral regurgitation;

(*5*) removal of any clot from the left atrium.

However, for this operation to be applied effectively, it is essential to have a well-established open heart unit with a large experience in perfusion techniques. All patients with severe mitral stenosis awaiting operation for more than 2 weeks should be anticoagulated.

THE OPERATION

1

The incision

Median sternotomy is used, with division of the sternum using a mechanical saw. In patients who have had previous operations through a similar incision, the pericardium and right ventricle are carefully dissected off the posterior aspect of the sternum before using a spreader.

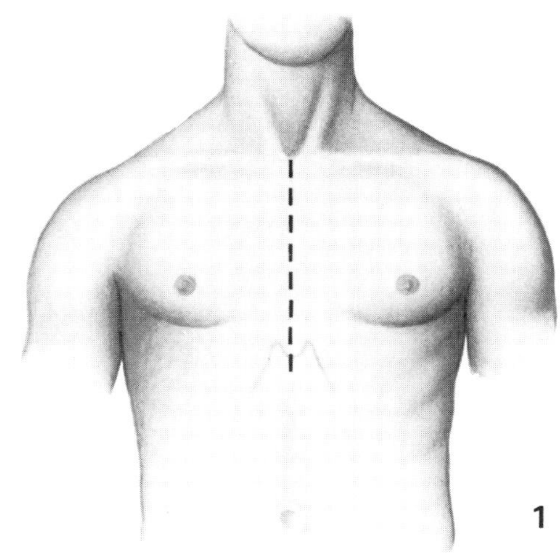

1

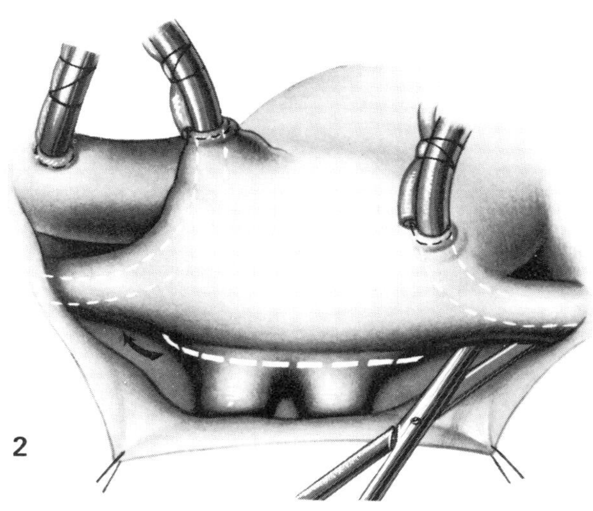

2

2

Preparation for cardiopulmonary bypass

All four chambers are inspected and pressures recorded. A cannula is inserted in the ascending aorta for arterial return. The superior and inferior venae cavae are separately cannulated through the right atrial wall. To facilitate retraction the lateral aspect of the superior vena cava and the posterior aspect of the inferior vena cava are separated from the pericardium.

Left atrial incision

The ascending aorta is clamped and the left atrium opened by an incision which starts in the right upper pulmonary vein immediately behind the interatrial groove and extends upwards towards the roof of the left atrium and downwards into the oblique sinus, behind the pericardial reflection, avoiding the thin-walled inferior pulmonary vein.

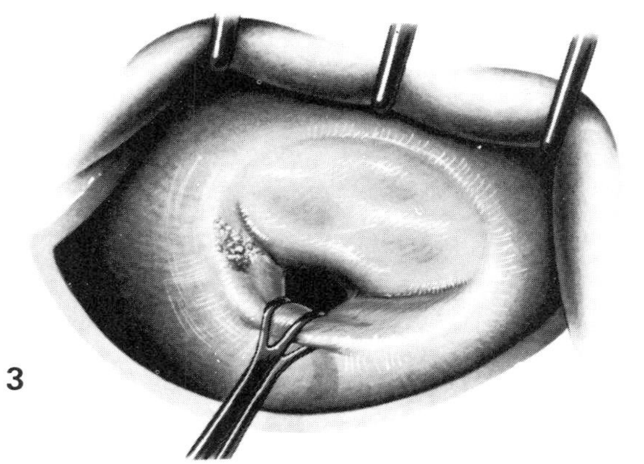

3

3

Inspection of the mitral valve

Any clots in the left atrial cavity or appendage are removed by a process of decortication. The mitral valve is brought into view by retracting the atrial septum and pulling on the mid-point of the posterior cusp using a non-traumatic long Allis forceps. The fused commissures are accurately identified.

4

Incision of fused commissures

The commissures are divided sharply to the ring using a sawing movement if necessary. The incision is started at the mitral orifice and extended towards the right and left fibrous trigones. The direction of the knife should be at right angles to the surface of the cusp to avoid injuring chordae attaching either cusp to the papillary muscle.

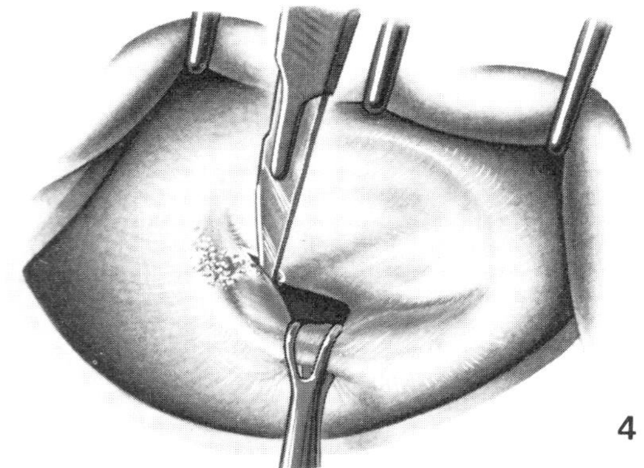

4

5

Removal of calcium

All calcium on the surface or in the substance of either cusp is removed using a sharp rongeur. This can be achieved in most cases without producing defects in the cusps. However, if this occurs the defects should be repaired by direct suture or by inserting small patches of pericardium or preserved dura mater.

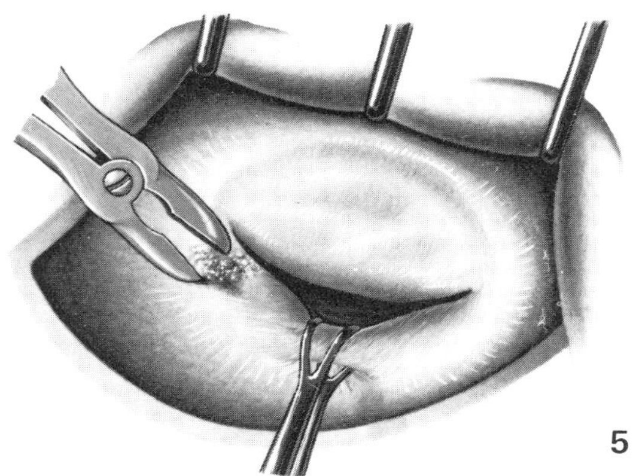

5

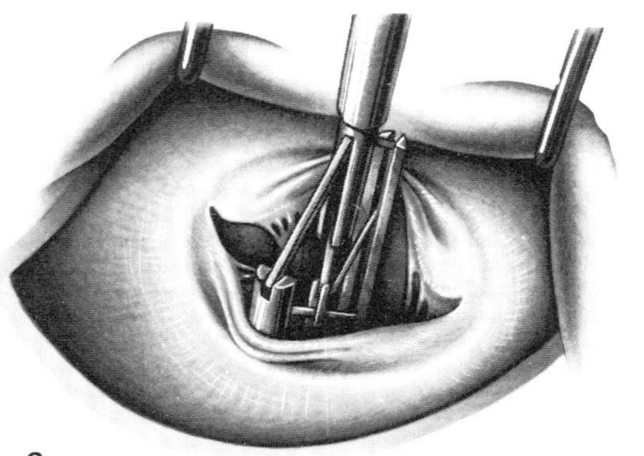

6a

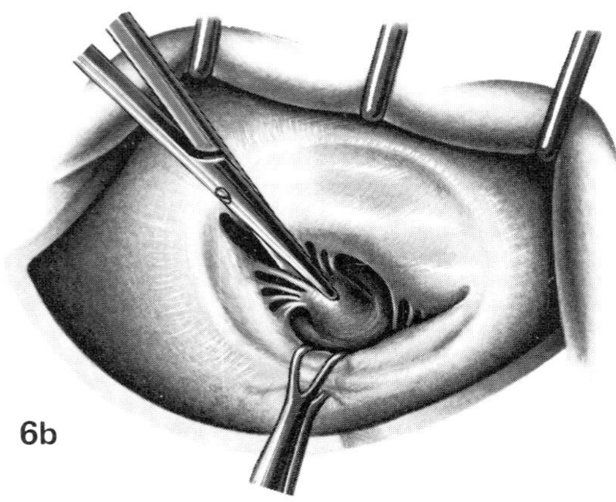

6b

6a&b

Mobilization of subvalvar apparatus

(*a*) The subvalvar apparatus is mobilized using a Tubb expanding dilator set at 3·8 cm and placed at right angles to the axis of the commissures. If need be the dilator can be used more than once using progressively larger settings.

(*b*) The valve is inspected again by traction on the posterior cusp. If the fused heads of the papillary muscle are judged to be limiting the mobility of the cusps, the plane of cleavage developed by the dilator is extended by sharp dissection into the left ventricle, thus separating the components of the papillary muscle.

7

Testing mitral valve competence

The mitral valve is tested under controlled dynamic conditions using two cannulae (each measuring 4 mm in diameter) connected to the arterial line by a Y-piece. One cannula is used to perfuse the aortic root for approximately 2–3 min until vigorous ventricular contraction is achieved. The second cannula is then used to perfuse the left ventricle retrogradely, and the mitral valve is inspected through the left atrium. The peak systolic pressure to which the mitral valve is subjected, measured through a needle inserted into the aortic root, should be adjusted to be in the physiological range by altering the amount of blood injected into the apex of the left ventricle. The extent and cause of any residual mitral regurgitation is identified.

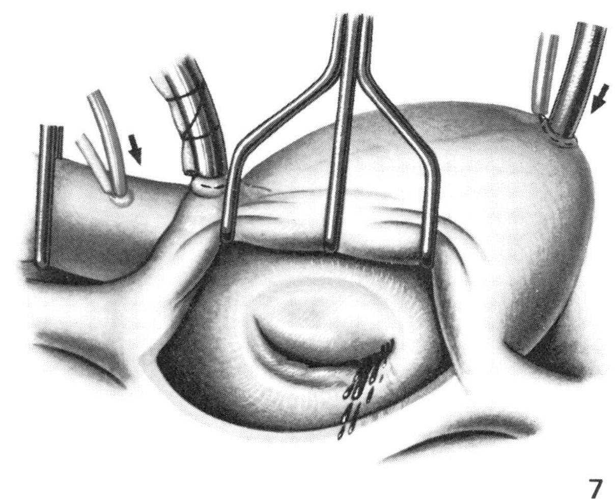

7

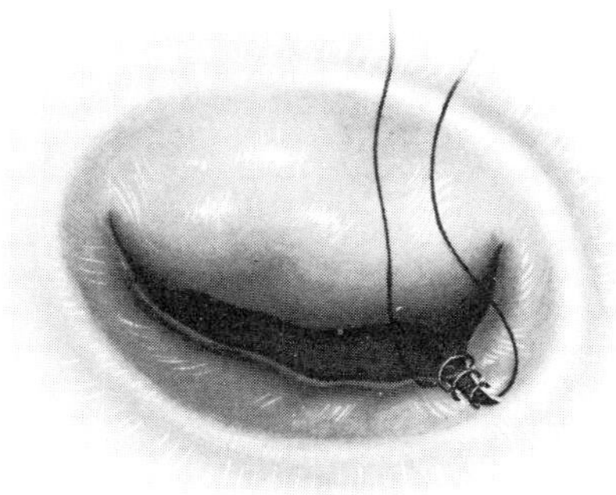

8a

8a&b

Repair of residual regurgitation

Residual regurgitation may be due to a tear in one cusp produced during a previous closed operation or during mobilization of the valve. The tear is repaired by direct suture using 4/0 Mersilene and the valve tested again.

More commonly regurgitation is produced by sagging of the posterior cusp which can be repaired by one or more 2/0 Mersilene mattress sutures starting at a fibrous trigone (right or left, depending on the site of regurgitation) and used to elevate the posterior cusp by shortening its annular attachment. Small autogenous pericardial pledgets are used to reinforce these sutures and prevent them from cutting through the annulus.

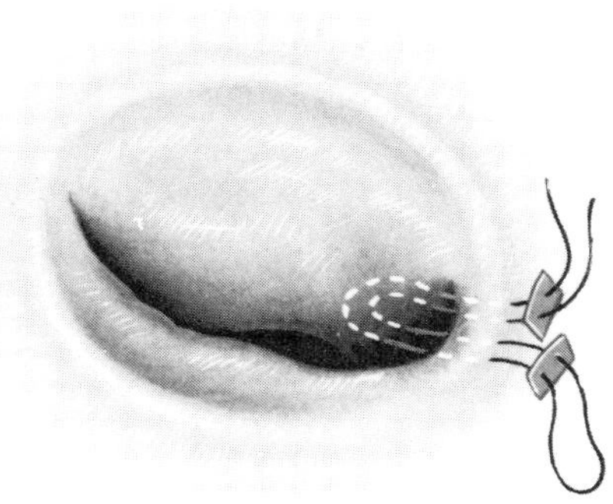

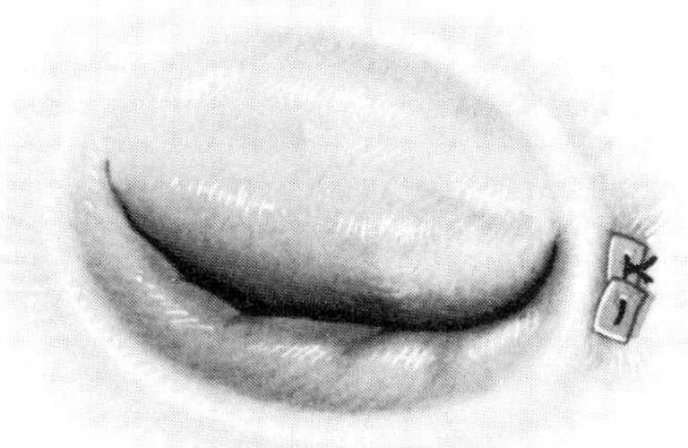

8b

9

Closure

After ensuring competence of the valve, the left ventricle is decompressed through a vent inserted into the apex. Coronary perfusion is continued through the cannula in the aortic root and the left atrial incision is closed using 3/0 sutures. After removing air from the left side of the heart, the cannula inserted in the root of the aorta is removed and the aortic clamp is released.

Supportive bypass is continued for a period of approximately 5 min to allow the left ventricular myocardium to recover from the effects of ischaemia and stretching produced by valvotomy and testing for competence. After that, bypass is discontinued and left atrial pressure measured to ensure good junction of the mitral valve and recovery of the myocardium.

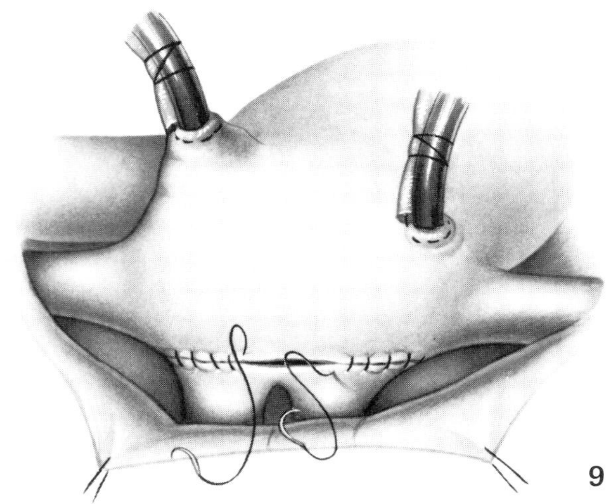

9

POSTOPERATIVE CARE

As for Homograft Replacement of the Mitral Valve (*see* page 190).

[*The illustrations for this Chapter on Open Mitral Valvotomy were drawn by Mr. M. J. Courtney.*]

Mitral Valve Reconstructive Surgery

Alain Carpentier, M.D.
Professor of Cardiac Surgery, Hôpital Broussais, University of Paris

INTRODUCTION

Where possible mitral valve repair is preferred to prosthetic replacement for the following reasons:

(*1*) it reduces the risk of thrombo-embolism;

(*2*) it avoids the need for long-term anticoagulation;

(*3*) it eliminates the risks associated with mechanical valve failure.

The method, however, has been criticised because it has been stated that the technique is more complicated, requires a longer bypass time and the functional result is less predictable. Such criticisms are no longer valid. Recent progress in myocardial protection and extracorporeal circulation allows for more sophisticated surgical techniques which are associated with a high degree of predictability and stable long-term results. The additional effort on the part of the surgeon to acquire the necessary experience is rewarded by the improved quality of life given to the patient.

CLASSIFICATION

The disease may affect several structures either valvar (annulus, leaflet tissue, commissures) and/or subvalvar (chordae tendinae, papillary muscles).

Mitral insufficiency

Type I

Without subvalvar lesions. Annulus dilatation-deformation, leaflet perforation or tear, leaflet shrinkage.

Type II

With subvalvar lesions: Leaflet prolapse
(*a*) Ruptured chordae
(*b*) Elongated chordae
(*c*) Ruptured papillary muscle.

Type III

With subvalvar lesions: Restricted leaflet motion. Commissural fusion, chordal retraction, chordal fusion, calcification.

Mitral stenosis

Type I

Without subvalvar lesions. Commissural fusion, leaflet thickening, calcification.

Type II

With subvalvar lesions. Chordal retraction, chordal fusion, chordal hypertrophy, calcification.

The type of valve lesions can be assessed by the results of the following investigations:

(*1*) physical examination;
(*2*) echocardiography with image intensification to identify valve calcification;
(*3*) echocardiography to demonstrate leaflet motion;
(*4*) angiocardiography to assess orifice size, leaflet motion and regurgitation;
(*5*) catheterization to measure the pressure gradient and calculate the orifice area.

INDICATIONS FOR MITRAL VALVE REPAIR

Mitral insufficiency

If the pre-operative assessment suggests that the valve is suitable for repair, rather than replacement, the decision to operate may be taken as soon as possible after the onset of atrial fibrillation. An early correction of mitral incompetence is more likely to be followed by successful conversion to sinus rhythm and thus avoid the need for anticoagulants.

Repair is more likely to be feasible in Type I and Type II mitral insufficiency in the absence of recent myocardial infarction or acute endocarditis. In Type III mitral insufficiency, the probability of successful valve repair is only 20 – 40 per cent. It is, therefore, preferable to delay operation until the patient's symptoms are severe with progressive increase in heart size.

In children, as atrial fibrillation is exceptional even in advanced disease, the indications for mitral valve repair are based on repeated episodes of heart failure or significant increase in heart size. The probability of successful valve repair in children is 90 per cent.

Mitral stenosis

Established mitral stenosis alone usually merits early surgical relief; again operation should not be deferred after the onset of atrial fibrillation. Pulmonary oedema and systemic embolization are additional urgent indications. Long-standing disease and the presence of calcification make the valve less suitable for reconstruction.

THE OPERATION

The incision

A mid-line sternal splitting incision is preferred. On exploring the heart, increased pulmonary artery pressure, atrial fibrillation, enlarged left atrium with a systolic thrill are common findings in mitral insufficiency.

A small left atrium may be found in mitral stenosis raising the question of the appropriate approach to the valve.

An enlarged right atrium suggests associated tricuspid valve disease but there are false right atrial enlargements due to distension by a very large left atrium. They can be recognized by intra-atrial palpation.

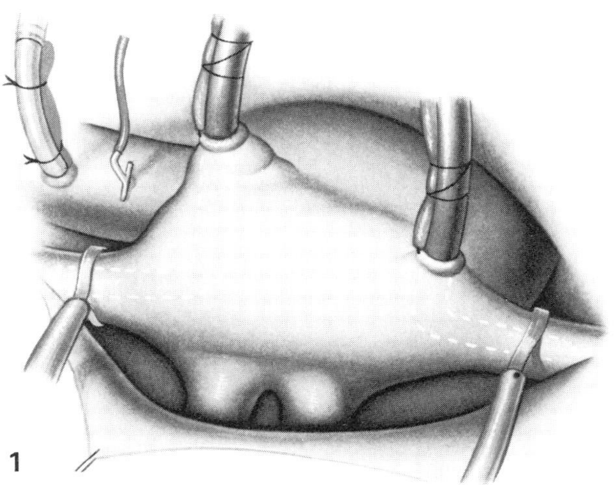
1

1

Cardiopulmonary bypass

The venae cavae are cannulated separately and surrounded by tapes. A plastic cannula is inserted into the ascending aorta just below the innominate artery. A needle for removing air and preventing air embolism is also inserted into the ascending aorta 1 cm below the aortic cannula. This needle is connected to suction. The patient is cooled to 31°C. Exposure of the mitral valve apparatus is facilitated by periods of aortic cross-clamping which renders the heart flaccid. The aortic clamp is positioned between the aortic cannula and the aortic needle. Cross-clamping periods should never exceed 12 min. Every 12 min, the aortic clamp is released for 2 min after suction has been established through the aortic needle; at the same time the mitral valve is prevented from closing to further diminish the risk of air embolism.

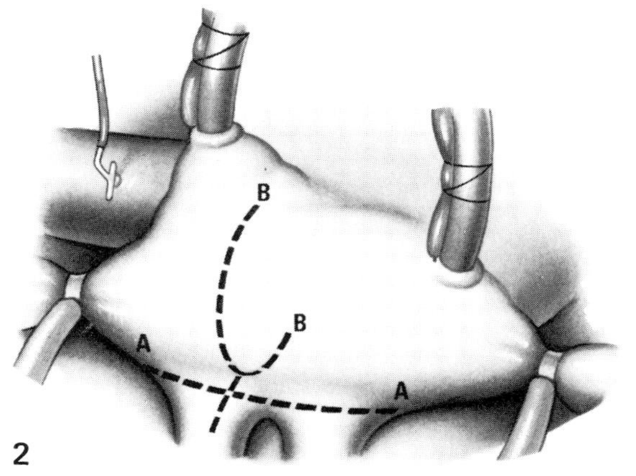

2

2

Left atrial incision

The incision is carried out between the posterior interatrial groove and the pulmonary veins (AA). A bi-atrial transeptal incision is preferred when the left atrium is small: both atria are opened from the right atrial appendage in the direction of the right superior pulmonary vein. The septum is incised forwards towards the aorta (BB).

3

Exposure and exploration of the mitral valve

Occasionally pericardial adhesions must be divided in order to mobilize the heart and to facilitate the exposure of the subvalvar apparatus. Two medium-sized Leriche retractors are used to expose the mitral valve. To facilitate exposure of the anterior papillary muscle, a swab may be placed in the pericardial cavity at the apex of the heart. To improve access to the posterior papillary muscle, a swab is placed between the pericardium and the diaphragmatic surface of the heart.

Each structure of the mitral apparatus must be systematically and critically inspected: annulus, leaflets, commissures, chordae tendinae and papillary muscles.

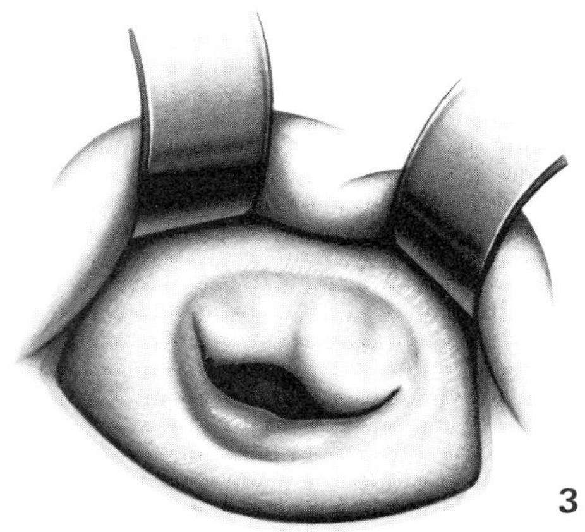

3

Repair of annulus deformation

The lesions

In the normal mitral valve, the transverse diameter of the annulus exceeds the anteroposterior.

4

The annulus is deformed when its transverse diameter TT is found to be smaller than the antero-posterior diameter (AP). The deformity may be symmetrical OB = OC or asymmetrical OB ≠ OC. A dilatation of the orifice is usually associated with the deformation. The dilatation affects the mural leaflet and the commissures but not the anterior leaflet portion of the annulus.

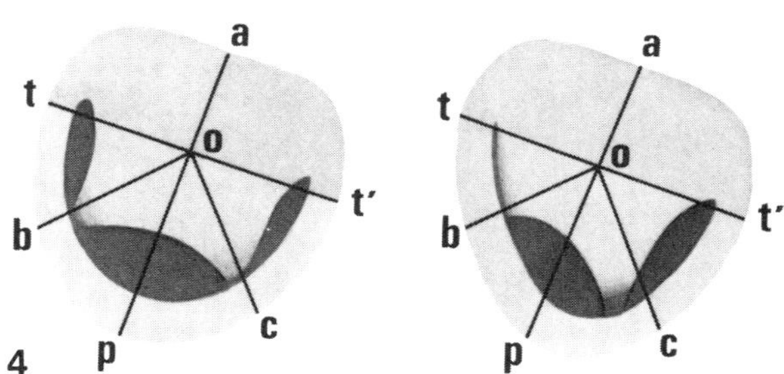

4

Annulus remodelling

5

Annulus remodelling by a prosthetic ring, contrary to annulus narrowing by commissure plication or circular sutures, restores the normal shape and therefore the normal function of the valve. Ring selection is based on measurement of the base of the aortic leaflet which is not affected by dilatation. One pilot suture is placed at each commissure and the distance between these two points is measured using obturators specifically designed for this purpose. The appropriate-sized prosthetic ring is then selected.

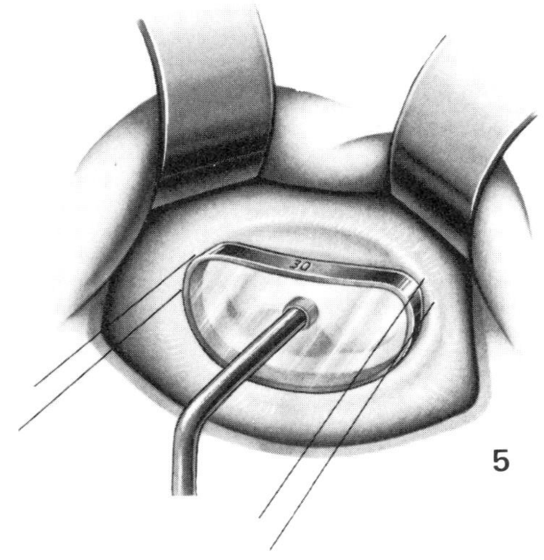

5

6

Fifteen sutures are placed through the annulus around the whole periphery of the mitral ring. These sutures are evenly and equally spaced between the base of the aortic leaflet and the corresponding portion of the prosthetic ring. Elsewhere spacing of sutures is so arranged as to achieve remodelling of the natural valve ring to conform to the size and shape of the prosthesis. If there is an asymmetric dilatation of the annulus with a predominant enlargement of one commissure, the distribution of the sutures must obviously be adapted: the spacing of the sutures must be especially reduced in the corresponding area of the prosthetic ring.

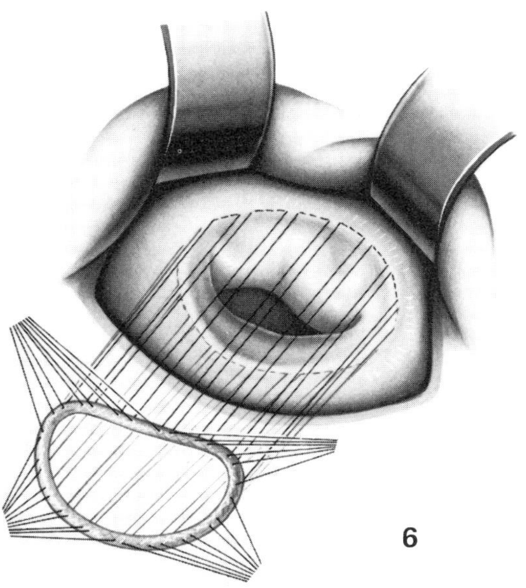

6

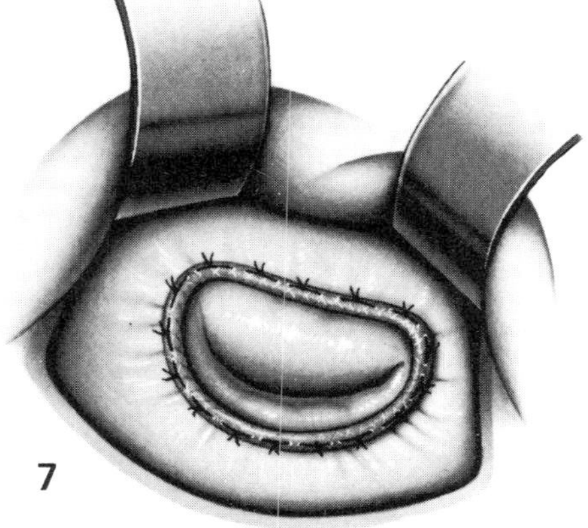

7

7

This is then slid into position and the sutures tied, thus repositioning the different annular structures without reducing the normal orifice area or affecting leaflet motion.

Repair of leaflet perforation

The lesions

Leaflet perforation is the result of bacterial endocarditis and may involve either the anterior or the posterior leaflet. Valve repair should not be attempted in the presence of active infection.

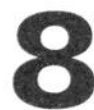

The repair

Mural leaflet perforations are treated by leaflet resection and repair of the resulting gap using interrupted stitches (5/0 Prolene). Anterior leaflet perforations may be treated by oval resection and suture-closure if the hole is less than 5 mm in diameter. Larger holes should be closed using a pericardial patch.

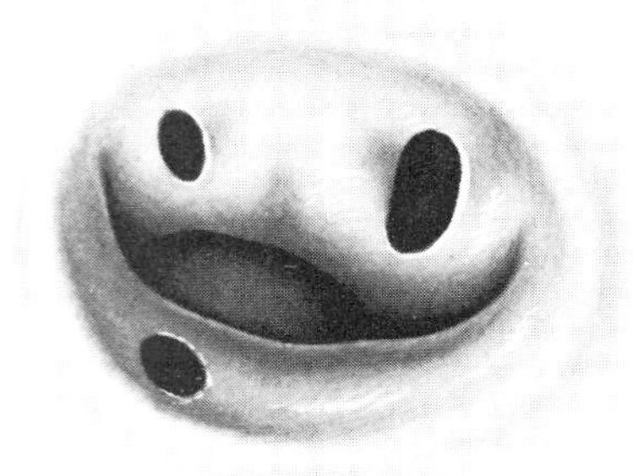

8

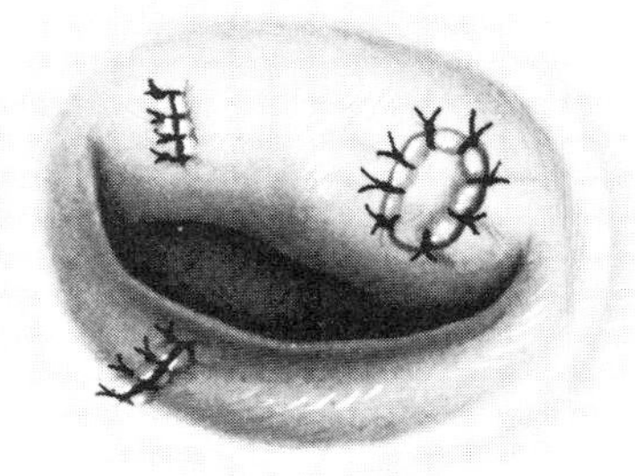

Repair of leaflet prolapse

The lesions

A leaflet prolapse must be systematically searched for in all cases of mitral insufficiency by using the following manoeuvre: the leaflet is pulled towards the atrium using a nerve hook. Prolapse is present if the free edge of the leaflet over-rides the plane of the orifice. This may result from ruptured chordae, chordal elongation or a ruptured papillary muscle.

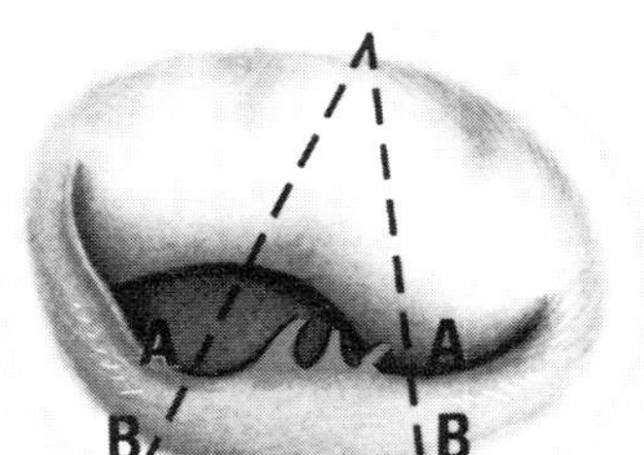

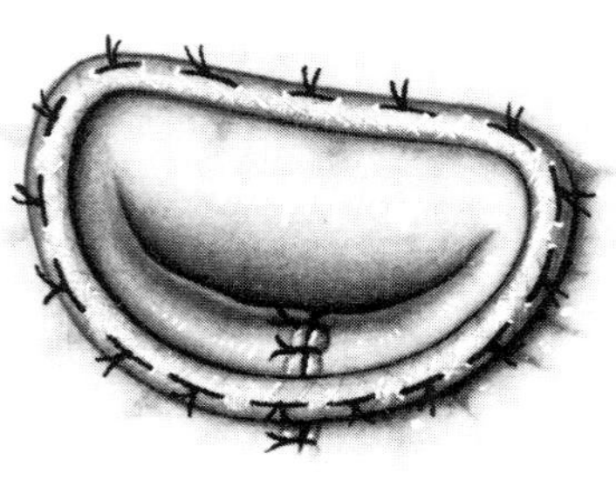

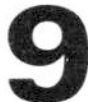

Repair of ruptured chordae

Two guy sutures are placed around the normal chordae at the limits of the prolapsed part of the leaflet (AA). The distance between these two chordae is projected down to the annulus (BB), so that a square or rectangle is formed which corresponds to the prolapsed portion of the leaflet. This tissue is removed. A 'U' suture is placed into the annulus in order to approximate the free edges of the leaflet which are then sutured using interrupted 5/0 Prolene sutures. Such a quadrangular resection seems preferable to the usual triangular plication or resection as it avoids excess tension on the free edge of the leaflet. A prosthetic ring is placed to re-inforce the repair and to remodel the annulus. A valve replacement is necessary if the rupture affects more than one-third of the mural leaflet or the main chordae of the aortic leaflet.

Repair of chordal elongation

Chordal elongation was not recognized for a long time and was responsible for many residual insufficiencies following valve repair.

10

As with ruptured chordae, chordal elongation of the mural leaflet is treated by quadrangular resection of the prolapsed part the leaflet and subsequent suture-closure. Elongation of two or three chordae of the anterior leaflet is treated by a 'sliding plasty' of the corresponding papillary muscle. The portion of the papillary muscle corresponding to the elongated chordae is split longitudinally and is resutured at a lower level. The length of the sliding displacement (CC) should correspond to the excess length of the chordae, which is judged by the degree of the leaflet over-riding.

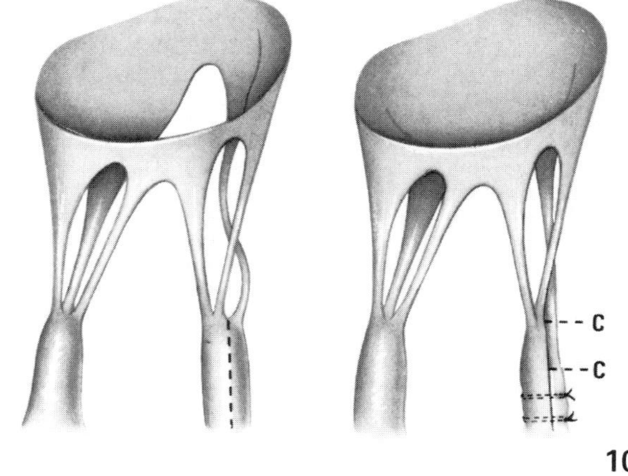

10

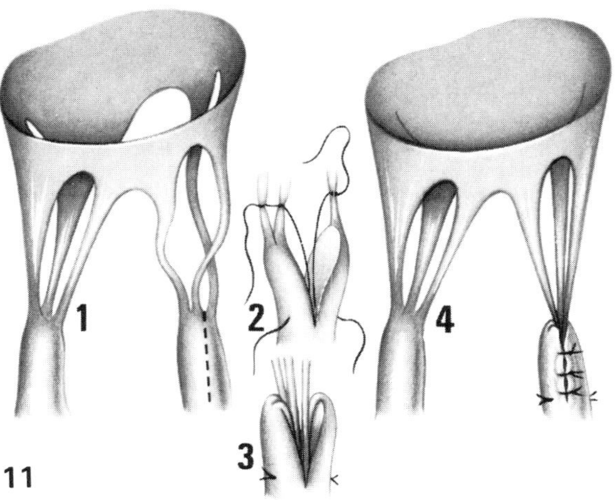

11

11

If all of the chordae arising from a papillary muscle are elongated, a *shortening plasty of the chordae* should be performed. The tip of the papillary muscle is incised longitudinally (*1*). A stay suture is passed through or tied around the chordae at a distance from the tip of the papillary muscle equal to half of the excess length of the chordae (*2*). This suture is then passed through the papillary muscle at the base of the cleft in order to bury the excess length of the chordae (*3*). The papillary muscle is then closed around the buried portion of the chordae (*4*).

Repair of restricted leaflet motion

The lesions

The motion of the leaflet may be restricted by commissure fusion, short chordae, hypertrophied chordae, fused chordae and/or leaflet thickening. The secondary and basal chordae, those which are respectively inserted on the inferior surface and at the base of the leaflets, are often thick and hypertrophied and responsible, at least in part, for the leaflet thickening.

12

The repair

The mobilization of the leaflet may be achieved by a commissurotomy, the resection of the secondary chordae and the fenestration of the fused chordae by resecting a triangular portion of fibrous tissue. On rare occasions, the leaflet can be thinned by removing excess fibrous tissue.

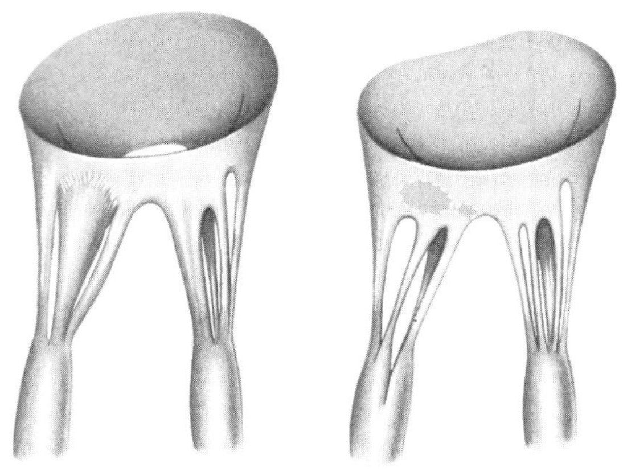

12

Repair of valvar stenosis

13

The lesions

Fusion of the commissures may be classified into three grades according to the severity of the lesions.

Grade I corresponds to partial fusion of the commissures with preservation of normal commissural chordae.

Grade II corresponds to complete fusion of the commissures with a well-defined border between the anterior and the mural leaflets.

Grade III corresponds to complete fusion of the commissures with no delineation between the anterior and posterior leaflets.

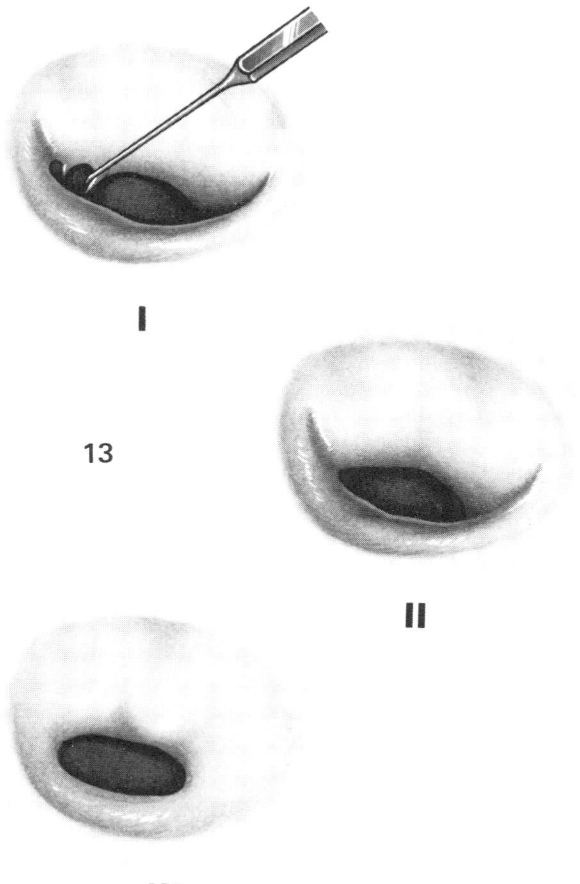

13

The repair

In Grades I and II stenosis, commissurotomy is easily performed and should not extend to closer than 3 mm of the annulus.

In Grade III, it is difficult to determine the correct site for commissurotomy. The direction of the commissures lies parallel to a line joining the attachment of the main chordae of the anterior leaflet to the fibrous trigone. A curvilinear incision should be commenced 2 mm posterior to this line near the trigone and extended towards the fused commissural chordae.

Repair of subvalvar stenosis

The lesions

Subvalvar stenosis is the result of chordal hypertrophy, chordal fusion, chordal shortening and/or adhesion of papillary muscles to leaflet tissue.

14

The repair

Release of subvalvar stenosis is difficult. Splitting the chordae and the papillary muscles is not sufficient and is followed by rapid refusion. The secondary and basal chordae should be resected. The primary chordae, those arising from the free edge of the leaflet, are fenestrated by resection of a triangular portion of fibrous tissue which can be extented to the papillary muscle.

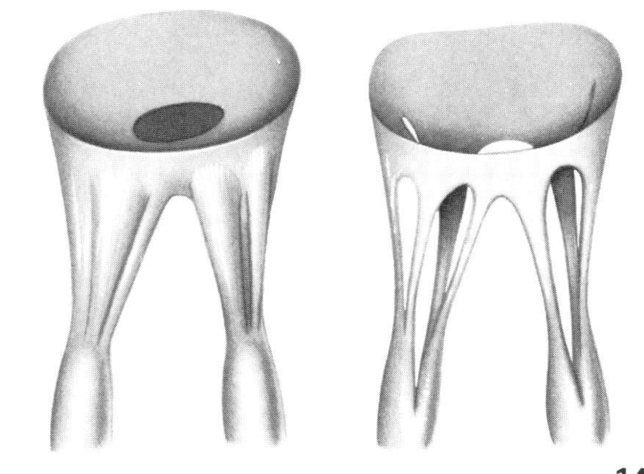

14

15

Practical steps and control of the repair

In almost every case of mitral valve disease, there are several distinct abnormalities which should be separately assessed and then treated. The sequence to follow in the correction of these lesions is as follows: commissurotomy, quadrangular leaflet resection, repair of subvalvar lesions, suture of leaflet edges, annulus remodelling.

The competence of the valve is now tested on a beating heart. The aorta is cross-clamped. Suction is established through the needle in the ascending aorta in order to prevent air embolism to the coronary arteries. Saline is injected into the left ventricle under pressure from a 250 ml bulb syringe or through a ventricular line. If the competence of the valve is satisfactory, a tube is placed into the ventricle through the valve orifice and the atrium is closed. The tube is removed after the air has been removed and the heart function proven to be satisfactory.

15

POSTOPERATIVE CARE

The patient is nursed in an intensive care unit for 24–48 hr, being ventilated using an endotracheal tube for the first 12 hr.

Anticoagulants are started as soon as significant pericardial drainage has ceased and there is no other evidence of major bleeding, often within 6 hr. Anticoagulation should be maintained for 2 months in all patients, at which time it can be discontinued in patients in sinus rhythm. In the remaining patients, electrical cardioversion should be attempted 2 – 4 months postoperatively. If sinus rhythm is established and maintained anticoagulants may now be stopped.

Anticoagulation may be discontinued after 6 months in patients with irreversible atrial fibrillation if the atrium is only moderately enlarged.

[*The illustrations for this Chapter on Mitral Valve Reconstructive Surgery were drawn by Mr. M. J. Courtney.*]

Prosthetic Replacement of the Mitral Valve

D. B. Clarke, F.R.C.S.
Consultant Cardiothoracic Surgeon,
The Queen Elizabeth Hospital, Birmingham

INTRODUCTION

Although there remains some controversy regarding the respective merits of biological and prosthetic substitutes for the diseased mitral valve, many surgeons elect to use the latter because of their proven long-term reliability, ease of insertion and ready availability.

Unfortunately, the danger of embolism must be accepted; this is reduced but not entirely abolished by anticoagulant therapy, which in turn has its hazards and inconveniences.

Many varieties of prosthesis are available; none bear any resemblance to the natural mitral valve but are an engineer's compromise, determined by the nature of metals and plastics which are available. Inevitably, the haemodynamic performance must be inferior to the natural valve but this does not detract from striking benefits which valve replacement confers on the patient crippled by mitral valve disease.

Because of the drawbacks outlined above, valve replacement is usually reserved for the severely symptomatic patient or for those patients shown to have dangerously abnormal intracardiac pressures when studied at cardiac catheterization. In experienced hands an operative mortality in the region of 5 per cent can be anticipated, with a further late mortality which can be in part attributed to systemic embolism. The incidence of this complication varies with different prostheses and reflects the efficacy of anticoagulant control. Most valves produce about four to eight episodes per 100 years of patient use.

About 80 per cent of patients who survive surgery are alive five years later.

Prosthetic valves currently in general use may be of the caged ball type (Starr-Edwards, Smeloff-Cutter, de Bakey-Surgitool and Braunwald-Cutter valves are examples), or the low profile caged disc valve may be preferred as it occupies little space in the ventricle. The Beall and Cooley–Cutter prostheses represent typical examples of the many valves of this pattern which are available.

Tilting disc valves are enjoying wide popularity at present. The Björk-Shiley prosthesis is illustrated in this section. Animal valves which have been chemically modified by immersion in gluteraldehyde and then mounted on frames are properly referred to as bioprostheses. The Hancock porcine valve has been shown to be mechanically sound after 4 years of clinical use and it is remarkably free from embolic complications even though anticoagulants are not employed.

An accurate estimation of valve and myocardial function will have been provided by cardiac catheter and cineangiographic studies.

Pre-operative preparation

Culture of the throat, nose, skin and hair will reveal sources of bacterial contamination which are eradicated by nasal antibiotic creams, shampoos and medicated baths. Dental sepsis is treated well in advance of the operation.

Digoxin is discontinued 48 hr prior to surgery, and, if the patient's general condition permits, diuretic therapy is stopped. Potassium replacement must be continued and serum potassium levels are closely monitored during and after surgery. Failure to maintain normal potassium levels is the commonest reason for abnormalities of rhythm and death at these times.

THE OPERATION

The patient lies supine, with arms at the sides. A urethral catheter is passed, cannulae are inserted into the radial artery and the superior vena cava by way of the internal jugular vein in order to record systemic arterial and central venous pressures. Body temperature is recorded by a thermistor probe in the oesophagus. A reliable, free-running intravenous infusion is essential.

The surgeon stands on the patient's right side and the heart is approached through a median sternotomy, as described on page 8. The self-retaining retractor is inserted so that its blades lie within the pericardium. As it is opened, the pericardial edges are compressed against the sternum and the heart is elevated on a cradle of pericardium.

Palpation of the tricuspid valve by a finger inserted through the right atrial appendage, together with observation of the venous pressure trace and reference to the cardiac catheter findings, will enable the surgeon to decide whether associated tricuspid incompetence is present and severe enough to require correction.

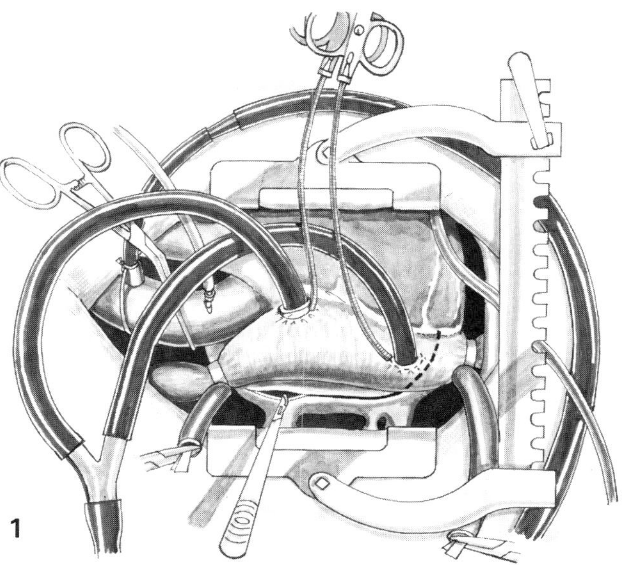

1

1

Preparation for cardiopulmonary bypass

The aorta and venae cavae are encircled with tapes. The patient is heparinized and an arterial cannula is inserted high in the ascending aorta. Palpation confirms that its tip lies in the aortic arch. Venous cannulae are inserted, one through the right atrial appendage, and the other through a purse-string suture close to the inferior vena cava.

The disposition of cannulae to permit unobstructed access to the left atrium is shown.

The approach to the mitral valve

Cardiopulmonary bypass is commenced and the patient is cooled to between 27°–30°C.

A vent drain is inserted through the apex of the left ventricle.

The aorta is clamped and the left atrium is incised at the level of the superior pulmonary vein. The incision is extended downwards and curves behind the inferior vena cava towards the back of the heart. Superiorly, the incision is extended to the level of the junction of the superior vena cava with the right atrium.

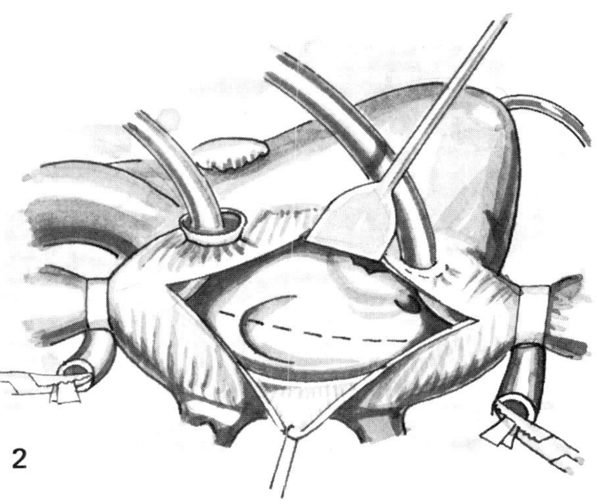

2

2

If repair or replacement of the tricuspid valve is necessary, the right atrium is incised vertically, taking care to avoid dividing the crista terminalis, which contains an important conduction pathway.

The left atrium is entered by a second incision in the interatrial septum, through the fossa ovalis.

3

A left atrial retractor is inserted and the mitral valve is exposed. Loose thrombus is carefully removed, ensuring that no fragments drop into the pulmonary veins. Organized thrombus can usually be peeled from the atrial wall.

Visualization may be difficult if the left atrium is small, but a pack behind the apex of the heart may displace the valve into view. Optimal operating conditions are afforded if the aorta is clamped and the heart is cold and relaxed. Thirty minutes of ischaemia are tolerated without damage to the myocardium; additional protection is conferred by cooling the patient prior to clamping the aorta and by frequent irrigation of the pericardium and the interior of the heart with saline cooled to 4°C. This technique of myocardial preservation has proved satisfactory in the author's hands. Some surgeons prefer to perfuse the coronary arteries.

If the intracardiac procedure is likely to be difficult or prolonged the aortic cross-clamp should be released at 15-min intervals in order to permit coronary perfusion for periods of 3–4 min. A needle in the aortic root is essential to remove air which has passed through the aortic valve; pressure on the origin of the right coronary artery reduces the risk of air passing into this vessel when the aortic clamp is released.

A stout traction suture is inserted into the anterior leaflet of the mitral valve.

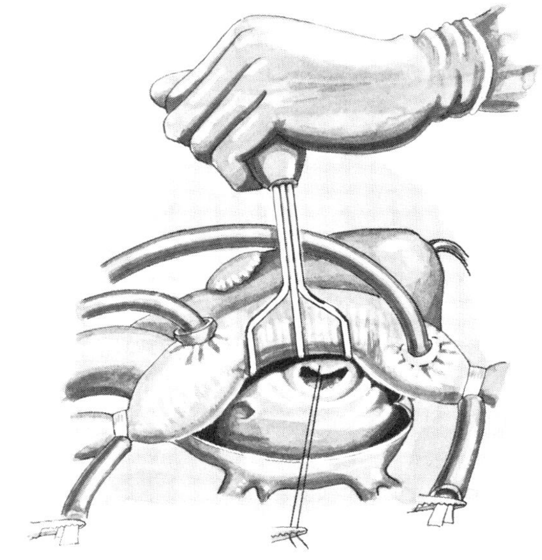
3

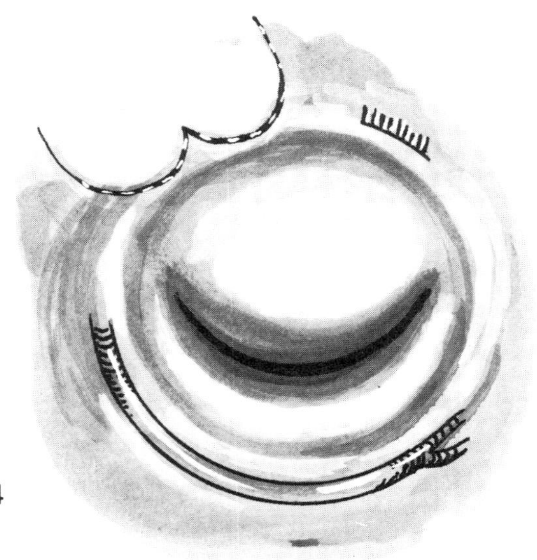
4

4

Excision of the mitral valve

The important anatomical relationships are shown. The aortic valve and the circumflex coronary artery are in close proximity and may be injured. The bundle of His (shaded area) is less intimately related and is seldom damaged.

5

Excision is commenced by an incision in the anterior leaflet which is extended circumferentially by either the knife or scissors. A rim of valve leaflet is left attached to the annulus. If the valve is regarded as a clock face a traction suture is inserted at 12 o'clock through the annulus.

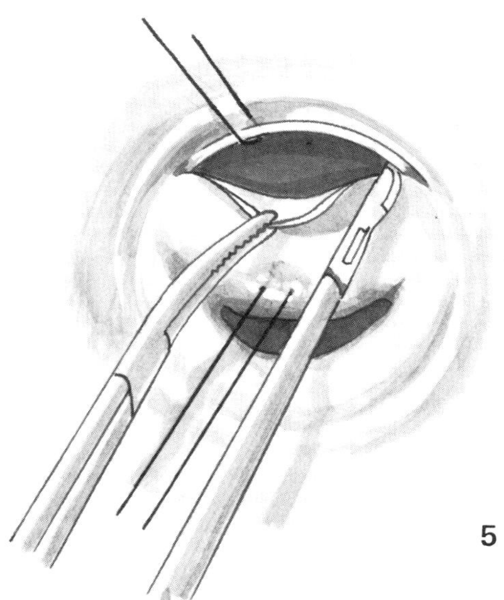

5

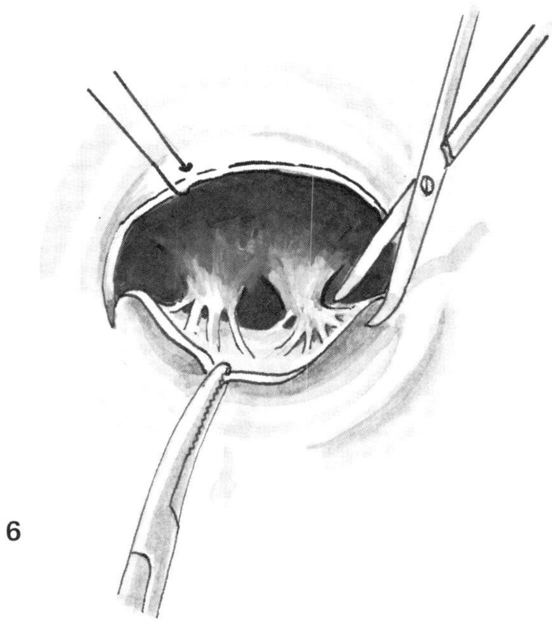

6

6

Traction on the valve by long artery forceps facilitates excision. As the circumferential incision reaches 3 and 9 o'clock the papillary muscles come into view.

7

A long curved artery forceps is passed behind the papillary muscles in turn and each is divided close to its tip. This prevents inadvertent injury to the posterior wall of the left ventricle.

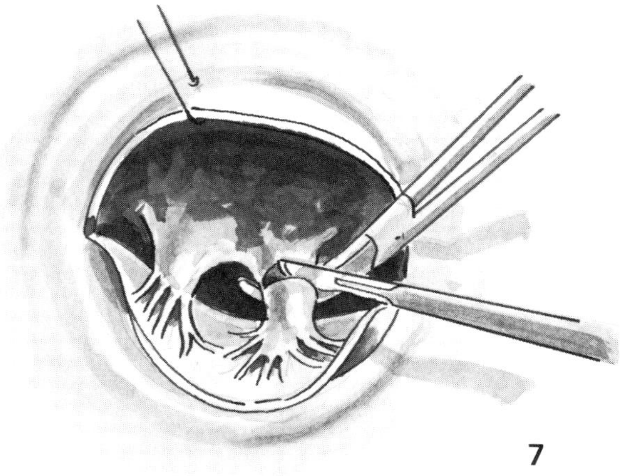

7

8

The valve can now be everted into the atrium and the short chordae tendinae which are attached to the posterior leaflet can be displayed and divided under vision.

Finally the posterior leaflet is excised taking great care not to allow the line of excision to encroach on the atrioventricular junction. Calcific deposits in the annulus are common in this region and are best removed with pituitary rongeurs or blunt dissection after the valve has been excised.

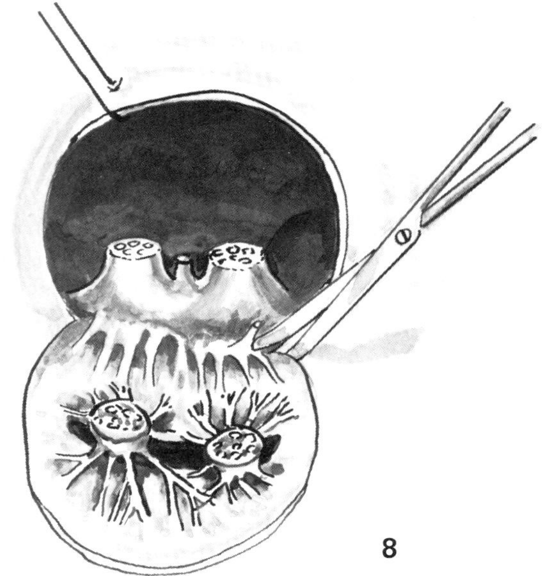

8

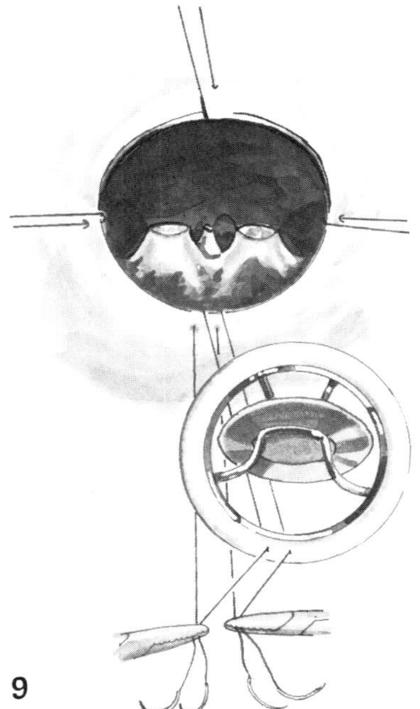

9

Insertion of the prosthesis

9

Further traction sutures are inserted at 3 and 9 o'clock. The diameter of the annulus is measured with valve sizers and an appropriate valve is selected. Handling of the valve is reduced to a minimum. It is recommended that the Björk valve be mounted on the special holder. The strut assembly rotates within the sewing ring to permit adjustment of orientation after the prosthesis has been sewn in place. A preliminary twist at this time will ensure that this adjustment can be achieved with minimum force.

The prosthesis is orientated so that its larger orifice is directed posteriorly and two sutures are inserted through the valve annulus at 6 o'clock. These are passed through the sewing ring of the prosthesis as shown.

10

It is generally possible to use a continuous suture technique, which is as secure as the interrupted suture method but much simpler and quicker. Contra-indications to this technique are described below.

The prosthesis is lowered into place so that most of its circumference is displaced into the cavity of the left ventricle, and the two 6 o'clock sutures are tied. Suturing commences, with the needle being passed first through the annulus and then through the sewing ring of the prosthesis. The assistant retracts on the appropriate stay suture and 'follows' the valve suture with tension in a radial direction. This is a key manoeuvre which draws the valve annulus into the field of vision as suturing progresses.

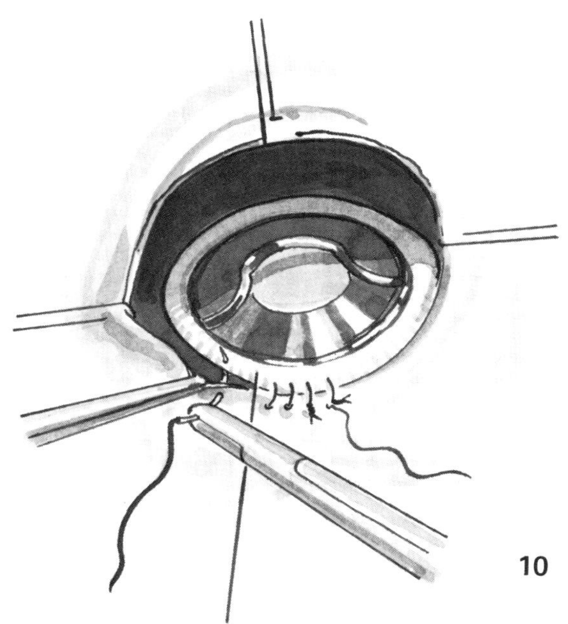

10

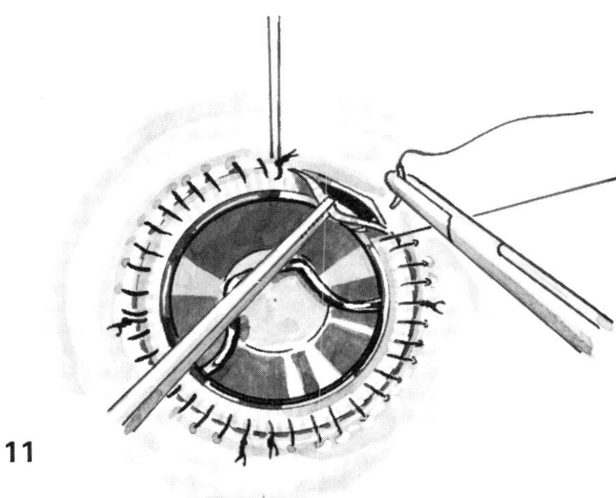

11

11

When one half of the prosthesis has been sutured in place, the 12 o'clock stay stitch is passed through the sewing ring of the prosthesis and tied to the running suture. The other half of the suture line is now completed. Ability to use a needle in either the orthodox or reversed position on the needle holder greatly facilitates the procedure.

Finally, the remaining stay sutures are passed through the annulus and tied.

12

An interrupted suture technique is indicated if the annulus is calcified or subject to myxomatous degeneration as in the 'floppy valve' syndrome. It is advisable if the annulus is of normal consistency and valve replacement is undertaken for subvalvar incompetence due to papillary muscle infarction. Interrupted mattress sutures, buttressed with pledgets of Teflon felt, are passed through the annulus and then through the sewing ring of the valve, which is mounted on a holder. When all sutures have been placed, the valve is lowered into position and the sutures are tied.

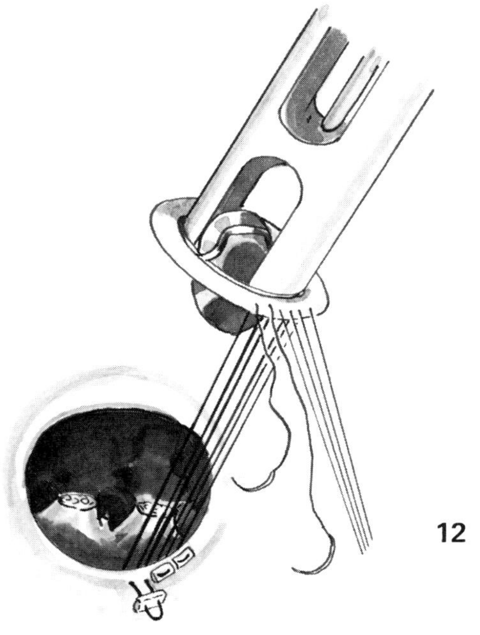

12

13

If the atrial appendage contains clot, it is prudent to excise it. If the orifice is closed with a running suture from within the atrium, superficial bites must be taken to avoid damaging the left coronary artery. A catheter is passed through the valve to render it incompetent and hence prevent premature ejection. The atriotomy is closed with two running sutures.

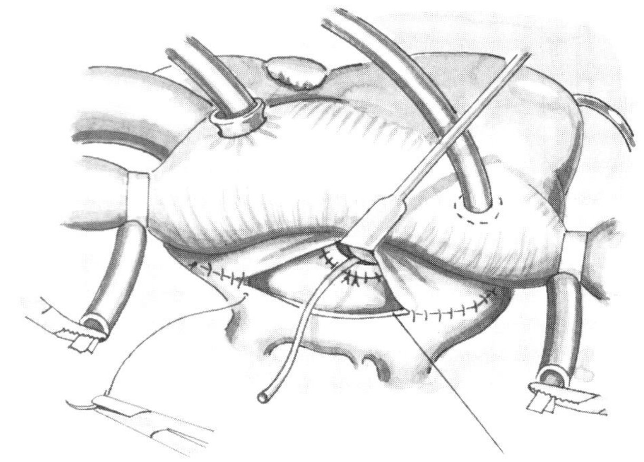

13

14

Every precaution must be taken to eliminate air from the chambers of the heart before ejection occurs. The following sequence of actions is best carried out before the aortic cross-clamp is removed.

The head of the table is lowered, so that air will tend to collect in the aortic root. The aortic air vent needle and left ventricular vent are attached to suction and the apex of the heart is elevated, so that bubbles will rise to the highest point and be evacuated by the vent.

Blood is allowed to fill the heart slowly and the ventricles are squeezed in order to dislodge any bubbles which may be trapped. The lungs are inflated to expel blood and any entrapped air from the pulmonary veins.

The left atrial appendage is invaginated with a finger.

Finally, the left atrium, left atrial appendage and pulmonary veins are aspirated with a syringe and needle. The cross-clamp is now removed from the aorta and the heart is defibrillated. Once vigorous ventricular contraction is restored, assisted by inotropic drugs when necessary, cardiopulmonary bypass is discontinued. Cannulae are removed and heparin is reversed with protamine. Once haemostasis is assured, drainage tubes are placed in the pericardium and retrosternal space. Temporary pacing electrodes are sutured to the right atrium and right ventricle. The wound is closed.

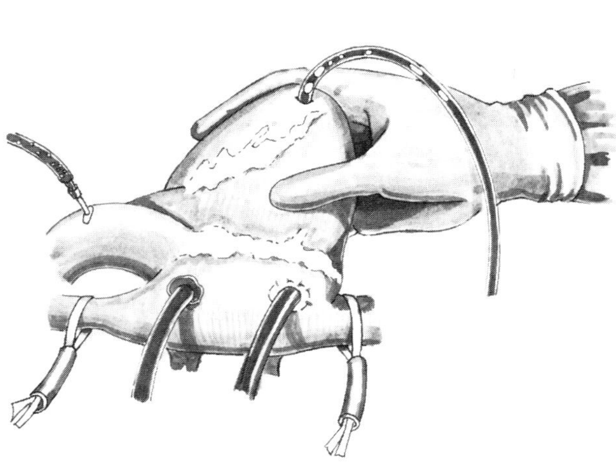

14

POSTOPERATIVE CARE AND COMPLICATIONS

In addition to the maintenance of blood volume and ventilation, which is standard care after all cardiac surgery, special problems may arise in these patients, who may have suffered from rheumatic heart disease for many years. Prolonged diuretic therapy and the electrolyte shifts consequent upon cardiopulmonary bypass may lead to profound hypokalaemia in the postoperative period. This will precipitate dangerous and sometimes fatal rhythm disturbances. Potassium chloride is given as a slow intravenous infusion, with additional increments as dictated by frequent estimations of the serum potassium. Digoxin should be given in small doses (0·0625 mg) and then only when rapid atrial fibrillation has to be treated. Nodal rhythm and bradycardia respond to pacing.

A flagging cardiac output is improved by infusion of isoprenaline (1–2 mg in 500 ml). Fluid intake is restricted and urine output maintained at 30 ml/hr or more, with the aid of diuretics where necessary. Mechanical ventilation can usually be discontinued on the first postoperative day, and anticoagulant therapy is commenced. This must be continued for life. Broad-spectrum antibiotics are used to cover the operation and the subsequent 5 days, but prolonged antibiotic therapy without a specific indication is inadvisable as infective endocarditis due to resistant bacteria or fungi may result.

[*The illustrations for this Chapter on Prosthetic Replacement of the Mitral Valve were drawn by the Author.*]

Homograft Replacement of the Mitral Valve

Magdi H. Yacoub, F.R.C.S.
Consultant Cardiac Surgeon, Harefield Hospital, Middlesex and
National Heart Hospital, London

PRE-OPERATIVE

Indications

Mitral valve replacement is indicated in patients with severe symptomatic mitral valve disease in whom valve-conserving procedures are judged not to be feasible. With increasing experience in applying restorative operations for the treatment of mitral stenosis and/or regurgitation, the number of patients requiring replacement should constitute approximately 15–25 per cent of all patients undergoing operations on the mitral valve. The choice of valve substitute may influence the survival as well as the quality of life after valve replacement. At present there is no agreement as to what constitutes the best available mitral valve substitute.

Aortic valve homografts offer the advantages of almost complete freedom from thrombo-embolic complication and haemolysis, and do not require long-term anticoagulation. There is, however, some concern about the durability of homografts. The available evidence suggests that the early and long-term function of the homograft depends, to a large extent, on the methods of sterilization, storage and insertion. These should have minimal effect on the physical and biological properties of the grafts and should guarantee optimal functional conditions by avoiding distortion, preserving the sinuses of Valsalva, and allowing the different components of the homograft to change in shape during the different phases of the cardiac cycle.

THE OPERATION

1

The incision

Median sternotomy is used, with division of the sternum using a mechanical saw. In patients who have had previous operations through a similar incision, the pericardium and right ventricle are carefully dissected off the posterior aspect of the sternum before using a spreader. A piece of pericardium, measuring approximately 8 cm in diameter is then excised.

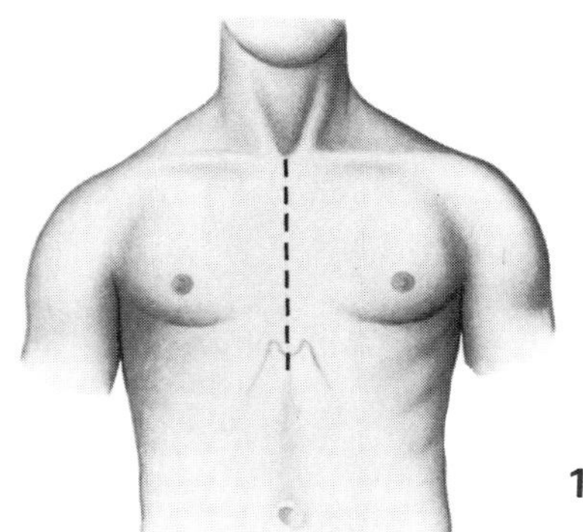

1

2

Preparation of the homograft

Homografts are obtained from routine postmortem material, sterilized by antibiotics and stored in tissue culture medium. The largest available aortic homograft (2·4–3 cm in diameter) is selected. The graft is trimmed in a circular fashion 1 mm above the top of the commissures at one end and 1 mm below the lowest point of the attachment of the cusps at the other. The coronary ostia are sutured, and the valve fixed inside a segment of woven Dacron tube (35 mm in diameter) measuring about 4 cm in length, which has a collar of two-way stretch Dacron previously sutured to it. The 'ventricular' end of the graft is sutured to the tube by a continuous 5/0 taper cut Mersilene suture, taking care not to evert the attachment of the right coronary cusp. The Dacron collar is then covered by autogenous pericardium. The width of the collar depends on the size of the left atrium and should be trimmed accordingly.

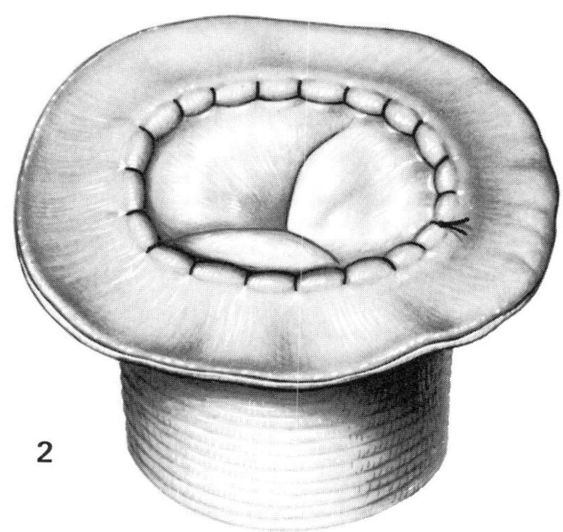

2

3

Preparation for cardiopulmonary bypass

All four chambers are inspected and pressures recorded. A cannula is inserted in the ascending aorta for arterial return. The superior and inferior venae cavae are separately cannulated through the right atrial wall. To facilitate retraction the lateral aspect of the superior vena cava and the posterior aspect of the inferior vena cava are separated from the pericardium.

Left atrial incision

The ascending aorta is clamped and the left atrium opened by an incision which starts in the right upper pulmonary vein immediately behind the interatrial groove and extends upwards towards the roof of the left atrium and downwards into the oblique sinus, behind the pericardial reflection, avoiding the thin-walled inferior pulmonary vein.

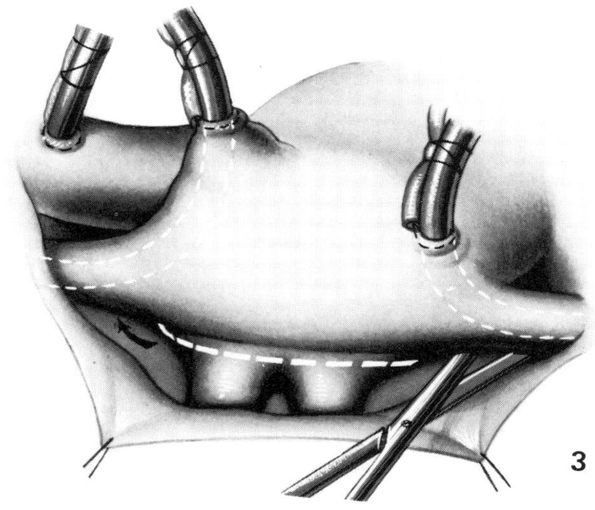

3

Excision of the mitral valve

4a

The mitral valve is brought into view by retraction on the interatrial septum and pulling on the posterior cusp using volsellum forceps. Excision is started by incising the anterior cusp 2 mm distal to its junction with the left atrial wall, which is well defined. The incision is extended in both directions around the areas of the commissures.

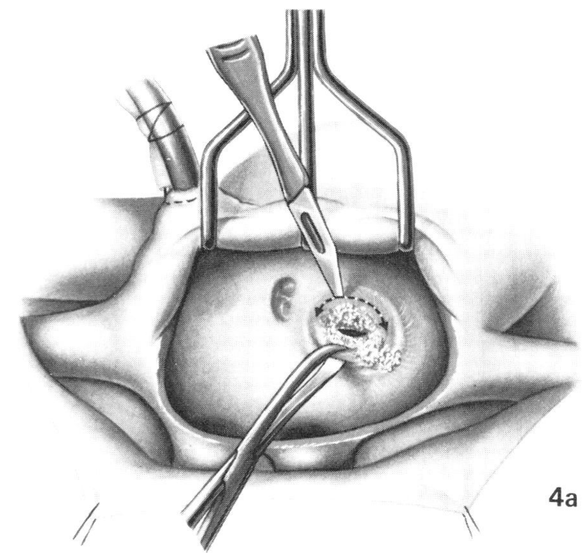

4a

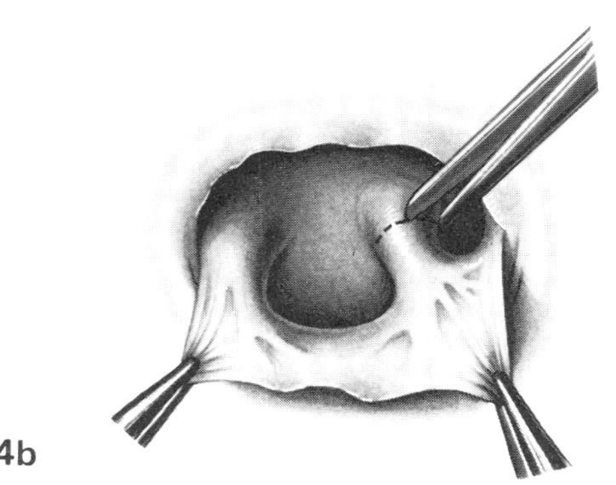

4b

4b

Traction on the cut edge of the anterior cusp brings the attachment of the papillary muscles into view. Both papillary muscles are then divided near their bases, taking care not to include parts of the surrounding free ventricular wall.

4c

Further traction on the valve brings into view the junction between the posterior cusp and ventricular myocardium which is always well defined and easy to identify, in contrast to the junction between the atrial aspect of the posterior cusp and left atrial wall. Excision of the mitral valve is completed by incising the posterior cusp 2 mm distal to its ventricular attachment. Any remnants of calcification of the mitral annulus are carefully removed.

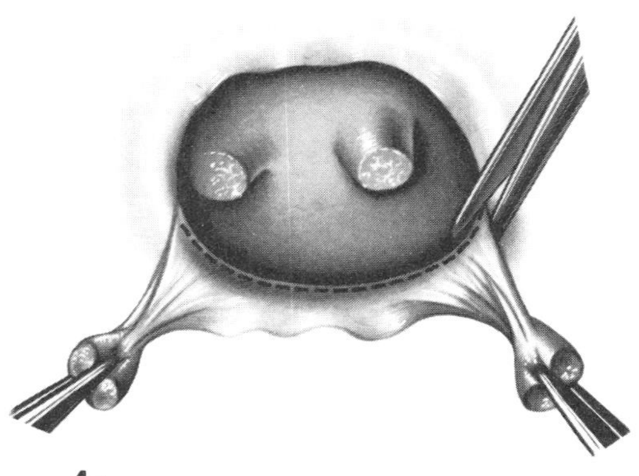

4c

Myocardial protection

Continuous coronary perfusion at 30°C is preferred. This is achieved by releasing the aortic clamp after excising the valve. A vent is placed in the apex of the left ventricle to keep its cavity free of blood. The heart is allowed to beat until the valve is lowered into the atrium, when the ventricles are fibrillated electrically. If aortic regurgitation is excessive the aorta is opened and the coronary arteries are cannulated and perfused.

Valve insertion

5a

The first suture line

This consists of a series of interrupted everting mattress sutures (2/0 Mersilene or Ethiflex) placed in the mitral annulus with the loop on the atrial side of the remnants of the cusps. The sutures are then passed through the aortic wall of the homograft and surrounding Dacron sleeve.

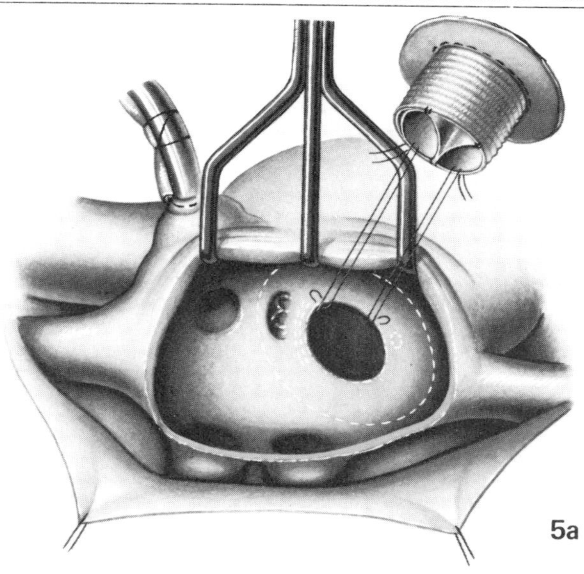

5a

5b

Positioning of the valve

The heart is fibrillated.

The valve is then lowered into the left atrium and sutures are tied. The edge of the homograft is compressed between the everted mitral annulus and Dacron sleeve.

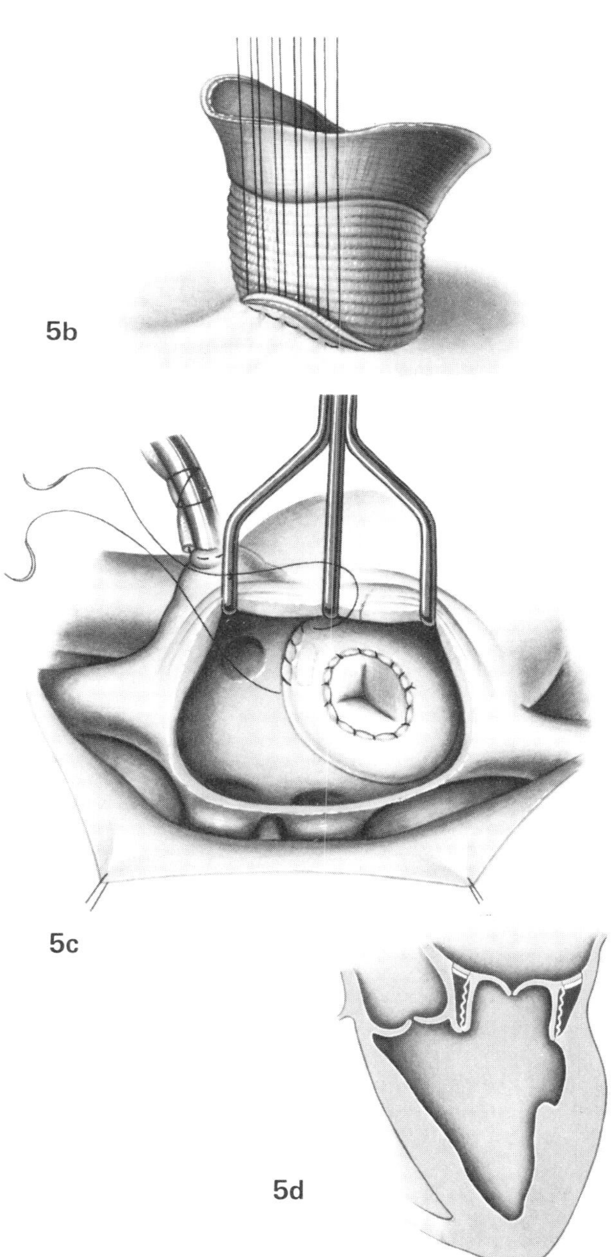

5b

5c

5d

5c & d

Upper suture line

Special care is taken to ensure absence of any torsion between the upper and lower suture lines. The pericardial and Dacron collars are fixed to the left atrial wall using continuous 3/0 Mersilene sutures, starting at the ridge between the left pulmonary veins and the left atrial appendage and passing upwards to the roof of the atrium on to the atrial septum in one direction and on the posterior wall towards the septum in the other. This suture line excludes the knots of the first suture line, all prosthetic material and the cavity of the left atrial appendage from the circulation.

6

Closure

The left atrium is closed using 2/0 sutures. During this period the left ventricle is decompressed by suction through the vent. A finger should be passed through the homograft to avoid injury to the cusps. Trapped air in the left side of the heart is removed and the heart defibrillated. A 5–10 min period of supportive bypass is utilized to ensure vigorous contraction of the heart with return of the ST segment to the prebypass shape. Bypass is then discontinued. Heparin is then reversed and haemostasis secured. Before closing the chest, drainage tubes are inserted in the pericardium and mediastinum and attached to suction.

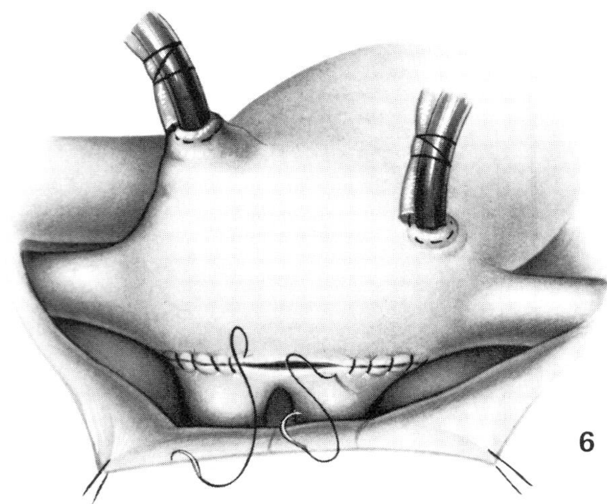

6

POSTOPERATIVE CARE

The patient is nursed in an intensive care unit. Mechanical ventilation is continued until the patient is fully awake with quarter hourly recording of blood loss, blood pressure, central venous pressure, pulse rate, urinary output, central (rectal) and peripheral (toe) temperature. The electrocardiogram is continuously monitored. Potassium and arterial gas measurements are repeatedly measured to maintain normal values. Any drop in cardiac output is treated at an early stage by correcting hypovolaemia or administering inotropic drugs. Mechanical ventilation is continued for several hours until the following criteria are satisfied.

(*1*) Patient is fully conscious and co-operative.

(*2*) Absence of excessive blood drainage (more than 50 ml/hr).

(*3*) Steady normal cardiac output with warm periphery and good urinary output.

(*4*) Radiographic evidence of clear lung fields.

(*5*) Satisfactory arterial blood gas values.

The patient is then disconnected from the ventilator and allowed to breath spontaneously through the endotracheal tube with an oxygen mask. If all the above criteria are maintained, the tube is removed. Anticoagulants are not used in the early or late postoperative period unless there is a specific indication such as removal of clot from the left atrium, deep vein thrombosis or persistent low cardiac output state for several days delaying ambulation. Prophylactic antibiotics are used for 5 days postoperatively.

[*The illustrations for this Chapter on Homograft Replacement of the Mitral Valve were drawn by Mr. M. J. Courtney.*]

Prosthetic Replacement of the Aortic Valve

Albert Starr, M.D., F.A.C.S.
Professor of Surgery and Chief of Thoracic Surgery,
University of Oregon Medical School, Portland, Oregon

PRE - OPERATIVE

Indications

Aortic valve replacement is employed as the treatment of choice in patients with considerable and progressive disability in whom a reparative operation is not possible. It is required in the overwhelming majority of patients with symptomatic calcific aortic stenosis, combined aortic stenosis and regurgitation and pure regurgitant lesions regardless of aetiology. Aortic commissurotomy is reserved for patients with flexible leaflets free of calcification as seen in infancy or childhood. Repair of aortic regurgitation is rarely possible but may be successful in some instances of prolapse of an otherwise normal valve as may occur in acute aortic root dissection or in ventricular septal defect.

The severity of symptoms when brought to medical attention varies widely and considerable judgement must be exercised in the selection of the appropriate time for operation given the presence of anatomically significant aortic valve disease. For patients with significant disability due to angina or left heart failure, prompt surgery is advised. Patients with syncope only, even if functionally well in between attacks, are also accepted for operative consideration. Patients with haemodynamically significant aortic regurgitation may remain symptom-free for a considerable period but such patients are accepted for operation if cardiomegaly is severe and progressive. It is now well established that the late results are poor in patients with massive cardiomegaly, with death occurring frequently from arrhythmia or progressive congestive failure.

Another indication for aortic valve replacement is compromised performance of a previously placed prosthesis due to thrombotic stenosis, thrombotic interference with motion of the ball or disc, multiple embolic complications, infection, major perivalvular leak or variance of the ball or disc from mechanical wear, chemical change or both.

Contra-indications

Advanced age, marked elevation of pulmonary vascular resistance, multiple valve involvement, aortic aneurysm, heart-block or other conduction abnormalities and intractable congestive failure do not contra-indicate operation. Patients with concomitant coronary artery disease are accepted for operation and all significant lesions are treated with aortocoronary bypass at the time of valve replacement. However, advanced coronary disease may preclude operation if, as a result of previous infarction, there is irretrievable loss of left ventricular function. The presence of severe chronic renal disease in patients suitable for renal transplantation or a chronic dialysis programme does not preclude valve replacement. Of course, operation is not recommended in the presence of uncorrectable non-cardiac disease, the prognosis of which is so poor that the valvular disease is of no consequence to the patient. Acute endocarditis is usually a contra-indication to operation, the treatment being primarily medical. However, operation may be recommended even before the infection is under control under the following indications:

(*1*) severe heart failure,

(*2*) septic embolism,

(*3*) the development of conduction abnormality suggesting spreading infection at the base of the aortic leaflets.

Pre-operative

While not essential to the management of all cases, cardiac catheterization with haemodynamic studies is of value in marginal clinical situations in defining the need for operation and in providing an objective basis for postoperative comparison. In patients over 35 years of age, coronary arteriography is the single most important pre-operative study. At the same study, supravalvular aortography is helpful for the delineation of aneurysms and an assessment of the size of the aortic root.

Once the decision is made in favour of operation, the following plan is put into action. Smoking is completely forbidden. Foci of infection around the teeth, paranasal sinuses and genito-urinary tract are cleared by appropriate therapy. The staphylococcal carrier state is eradicated by instillation of antibiotic ointment into the nasal vestibule and by daily bath and shampoo with medicated soap. Diuretic medication is discontinued shortly before surgery to avoid pre-operative sodium and potassium depletion. Potassium chloride is administered orally or if necessary parenterally to maintain a normal level in the blood. Digitalis is usually discontinued the day prior to operation. The patient is shaved on the morning of operation and a urinary catheter is placed.

Anaesthesia

A radial artery catheter and two venous catheters are placed in an upper extremity together with needle electrodes for continuous electrocardiographic monitoring. A doppler probe may be substituted for radial artery cannulation. Anaesthesia is induced with an intravenous barbiturate and relaxant and the patient rapidly intubated. Anaesthesia is maintained by a nitrous oxide-relaxant-analgesic mixture, or by light Fluothane. Isoproterenol (isoprenaline hydrochloride), dopamine or lidocaine (lignocaine) may be required in very ill patients prior to cardiopulmonary bypass because of bradycardia, hypotension or myocardial irritability. In such patients, pump support should be obtained as soon as possible and meticulous haemostasis deferred until closure. If Fluothane is used during extracorporeal circulation, it is discontinued prior to removal of the patient from pump support because of its myocardial depressant effect. After perfusion, anaesthesia can usually be maintained with 50 per cent nitrous oxide relaxants and hyperventilation.

Position of patient

The patient lies supine with arms at the sides, and the surgeon stands at the patient's right side. The entire chest, abdomen and upper thighs are exposed, bacteriologically prepared and covered with adhesive transparent plastic before towelling. Body temperature is recorded by a thermistor in the oesophagus. Should aortocoronary bypass graft be indicated, both legs are included in the operative field, down to the ankles, and supported in external rotation in the frog-kick position.

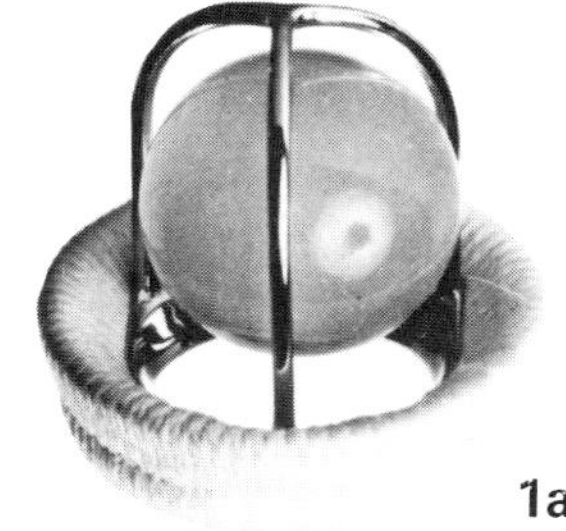

1a

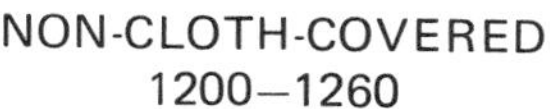

NON-CLOTH-COVERED
1200–1260

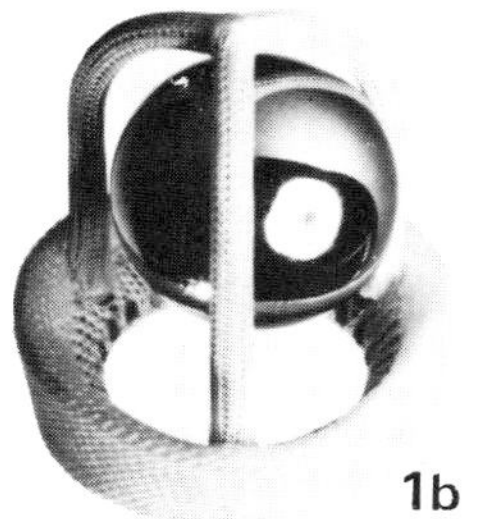

1b

CLOTH-COVERED
2310–2320

1,2&3

Choice of prosthesis

The most widely accepted choices for aortic valve replacement are prostheses made entirely of artificial materials (mechanical valves) or prostheses fabricated in part of biological material (bioprostheses). Mechanical valves include the non-cloth-covered caged-ball valve (*Illustration 1a*), the cloth-covered ball valve (*Illustration 1b*), the non-overlapping tilting disc valve (*Illustration 2a*) and the overlapping pivoting disc valve (*Illustration 2b*). Bioprostheses in current use are primarily frame-mounted gluteraldehyde-preserved, porcine aortic valves (*Illustration 3*). Frame-mounted dura-mater, gluteraldehyde-preserved bovine pericardium and living homografts have also been employed in limited clinical series.

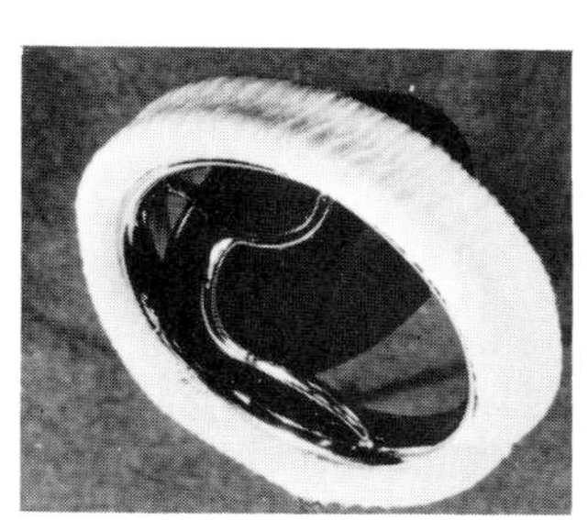

2a

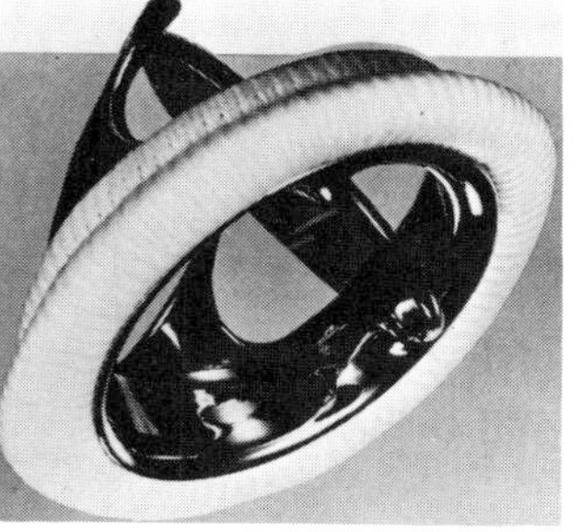

2b

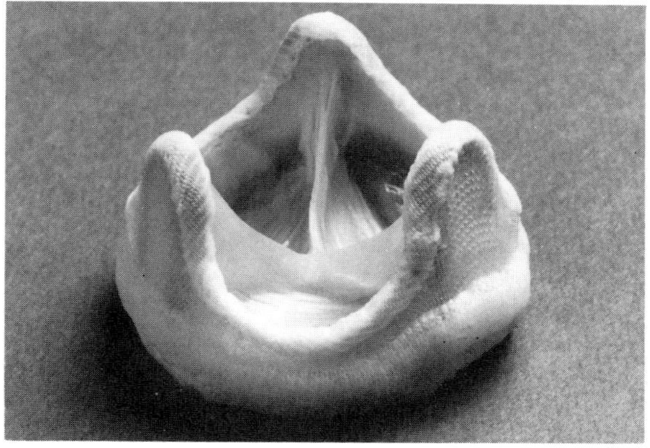

3

Apart from unstented living aortic homografts, also currently employed in limited series of patients, the operative technique of aortic valve replacement is very much the same regardless of valve type selected. Each has a cloth margin to allow implantation using a suture technique. Since all, appropriately sized, are haemodynamically acceptable, it is unlikely that the selection of valve type would influence the immediate risk of operation. However, valve type may play a significant role in late morbidity and mortality and the gathering of such information is currently underway.

THE OPERATION

The incision

A vertical mid-line incision is made beginning at the suprasternal notch and extending downwards to a point mid-way between the xiphoid and umbilicus. The periosteum over the sternum is divided with a coagulating current and the entire sternum cut with an oscillating saw. Both pleural reflections are wiped laterally and the thymus is divided in the mid-line up to the innominate vein and separated from the pericardium. The pericardium is then opened in the mid-line and sutured to the skin towels.

Exploration of the heart

The heart is inspected for chamber and great vessel size and palpated for thrills. Pressure measurements are made from the left atrium, right atrium and right ventricle. A purse-string suture is placed around the right atrial appendage and the tricuspid valve palpated.

Preparation for cardiopulmonary bypass

The aorta is separated from the pulmonary artery and surrounded by tape in preparation for cross-clamping. The patient is then heparinized and cannulated, using appropriately sized venous catheters through the right atrial appendage and a plastic cannula inserted directly into the ascending aorta.

Preparation of the heart for entry

With the onset of cardiopulmonary bypass, the pericardial reflection between the inferior vena cava and the right inferior pulmonary vein is divided and a tape passed around the inferior vena cava. If tricuspid surgery is necessary, another tape is passed around the superior vena cava. If exposure of the mitral valve is required, the posterior interatrial groove is developed by sharp dissection. The patient is cooled to 30°C.

Exposure of the aortic valve

For isolated aortic valve replacement, a left ventricular vent is placed, the aorta is cross-clamped, the heart electrically fibrillated and iced Ringer's solution added to the pericardium. A transverse incision is made approximately 2 cm above the origin of the right coronary artery. The left ventricular vent is placed on suction. However, when mitral replacement is required, the left heart is vented through the mitral prosthesis via the left atrial incision.

4,5&6

Replacement

The aortic valve is excised making a smooth bed for the prosthesis (*Illustration 4*). Calcium extending down onto the outflow tract portion of the mitral valve is removed. Calcific deposits entering the septum beneath the right cusp are not pried loose but are cut flush with the septum. The aortic root and annulus are measured with obturators corresponding to different sized prostheses. Double-needle interrupted sutures of Teflon-impregnated Dacron are placed through the zone of leaflet attachment (*Illustration 5*) and then through the cloth margin of the prosthesis with the ventricular needle close to the metallic portion and the aortic needle close to the free margin of the cloth (*Illustration 6 insert A*). At 15 min of cross-clamping, coronary catheters are placed in the left and right coronary ostia. The cold Ringer's solution is removed from the pericardium and the heart defibrillated. If all the sutures have not yet been placed in the aortic root, this portion of the operation is completed with the heart beating. The remaining sutures are then systematically placed through the cloth margin of the prosthesis. The valve is then passed down into place and the sutures tied and cut (*Illustration 6, insert B*).

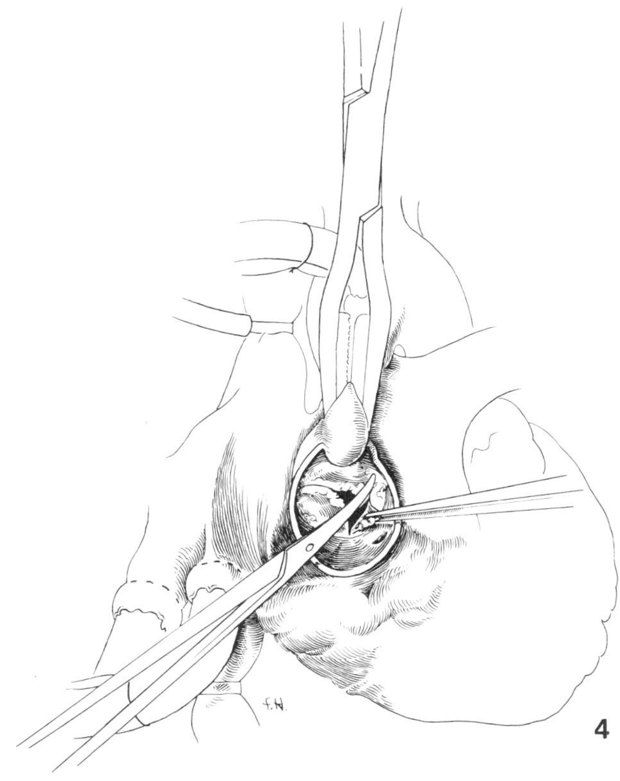

4

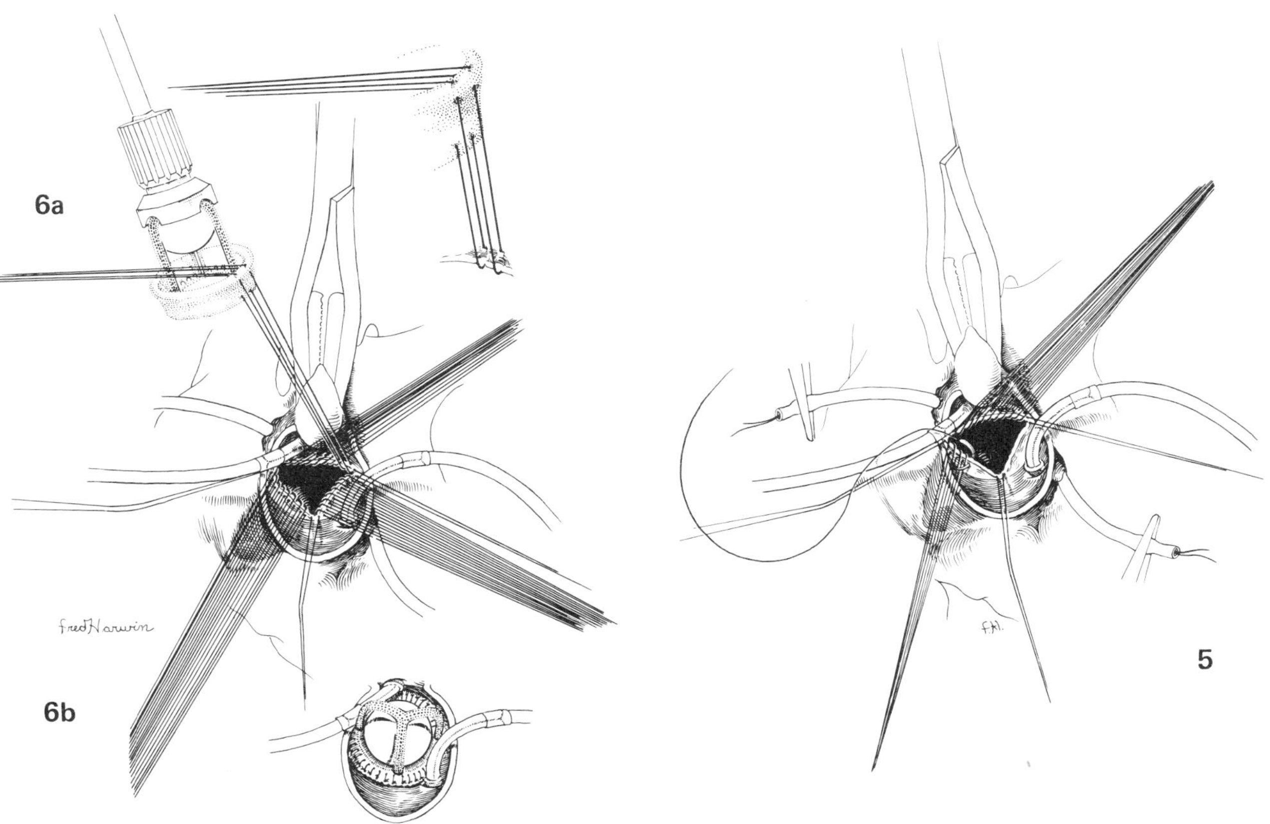

5

Aortic closure

The aortotomy incision is partially closed while the heart continues to beat. Just prior to complete closure the coronary cannulae are removed and the heart electrically fibrillated. Following aortic closure the apex is elevated and the heart massaged with the lungs inflated intermittently to expel air through the apical vent. The heart is then defibrillated, the vent catheter removed when a satisfactory rhythm returns. The patient is removed from cardiopulmonary bypass.

Myocardial protection

The technique described above consists of a transient period of aortic cross-clamping without coronary perfusion but with the heart protected by irrigation of the pericardium with iced Ringer's solution. The remainder of the operation is done with coronary perfusion at 30°–32°C, 300–500 ml/min flow, and the heart beating. There are alternate approaches which provide equally satisfactory initial results. These include *(1)* the use of myocardial cooling alone by continuous irrigation of the pericardium with iced Ringer's solution, *(2)* the use of cardioplegic solution injected into the aortic root or coronary arteries with or without local hypothermia, or *(3)* the combination of intermittent cold perfusion and cold pericardial irrigation.

POSTOPERATIVE CARE

The patient is returned to the cardiac surgical recovery room with equipment for continuous monitoring of the electrocardiogram, arterial and venous pressure and, in seriously ill patients, left atrial pressure as well. Chest tubes are placed to water seal drainage and blood replacement is given as necessary with attention to the level of both systemic venous and pulmonary venous pressure. Digitalis is administered with care as indicated. Intravenous potassium chloride is given both during and after bypass in the operating room as well as in large amounts postoperatively to replace urinary losses and maintain a normal serum potassium. In the very ill patients, isoproterenol (isoprenaline hydrochloride) may be required to increase myocardial rate and contractility or Dopamine may be required to maintain adequate levels of arterial pressure. Intra-aortic balloon pumping is used without hesitation in low output states unresponsive to pharmacological management. Frequent ventricular ectopic beats are usually managed by atrial pacing when possible or by ventricular pacing in the presence of chronic atrial fibrillation. Patients who are unable to follow the atrial pacer will respond well to ventricular pacing but the cardiac output is usually 20–30 per cent less than with atrial pacing.

The patient is kept at bedrest for 2 or 3 days and is discharged from the hospital during the second or third postoperative week. Long-term anticoagulant treatment is started on the third postoperative day and maintained indefinitely in patients with mechanical valves unless strongly contra-indicated. The patient is allowed to return to work of a sedentary nature within 2 or 3 months after operation and to active physical labour within 6 months following operation.

[*The illustrations for this Chapter on Prosthetic Replacement of the Aortic Valve were drawn by Mr. F. Harwin.*]

Homograft Aortic Valve Replacement

Donald N. Ross, F.R.C.S.
Consultant Surgeon, Guy's Hospital, London;
Senior Surgeon, National Heart Hospital, London

and

John R. W. Keates, F.R.C.S.
Formerly, Senior Lecturer, Cardiothoracic Institute, London;
Consultant Cardiothoracic Surgeon, King's College Hospital, London

PRE-OPERATIVE

Indications

Aortic valve replacement, especially in certain categories:

(*a*) young patients;
(*b*) patients with a relatively small aortic ring;
(*c*) patients with concomitant supramembranous ventricular septal defect;
(*d*) those patients in whom anticoagulants are contra-indicated;
(*e*) where emergency operation is indicated in the presence of endocarditis.

Collection, sterilization and storage

Valves are collected at autopsy up to 48 hr after death. They are dissected out of the heart along with the ascending aorta and freed of muscle and fascia.

They are then carefully measured with obturators to the nearest millimetre and are packed and stored in a nutrient medium containing antibiotics and antifungal agents. Storage is at room temperature for 24 hr and then at 4°C. Bacteriological checks on portions of the aortic wall are performed. These have shown consistent sterility after 24 hr at room temperature in nutrient antibiotic solution.

THE OPERATION

1

Exposure

A median sternotomy is used. Cardiopulmonary bypass with moderate hypothermia (30°C) is instituted using a right atrial basket and returning the blood via a cannula in the ascending aorta. The left ventricle is vented and the aorta cross-clamped. A curved vertical incision is used to expose the aortic valve. Coronary perfusion is set up with the heart maintained in normal rhythm and the aortic valve is excised and the aortic ring carefully measured.

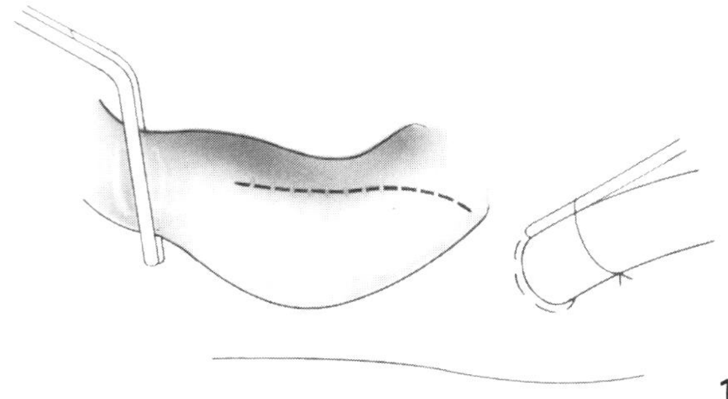
1

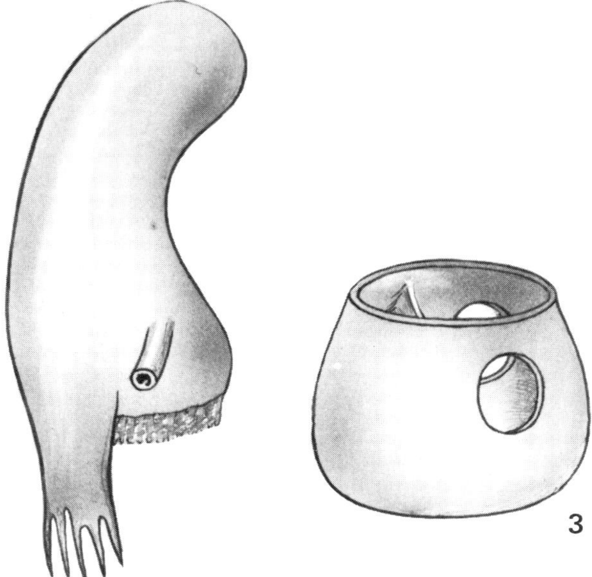
2 3

2&3

Preparation of the graft

A suitably sized aortic homograft valve is rinsed in normal saline and trimmed. The homograft aorta is transected 3 mm above the upper limit of the commissures. The muscle and anterior cusp of the mitral valve are trimmed to leave a 3 mm horizontal border below the cusps to take sutures. The coronary ostia are excised leaving side holes in the graft approximately 8 mm in diameter.

4&5

The lower suture line is then located using three double-needled 4/0 sutures placed through the corresponding parts of the patient and graft valve rings at the nadir of the three cusps. These sutures are then tied and the graft is turned downwards inside-out to allow completion of the inferior suture line. The graft is then returned to its normal upright position. The three commissures of the homograft are located on the patient's aortic wall and sutured there with 3/0 mattress sutures passed through the whole thickness of the aortic wall. It is important that these sutures be correctly placed in line with the patient's commissures and under slight tension to ensure competence of the valve.

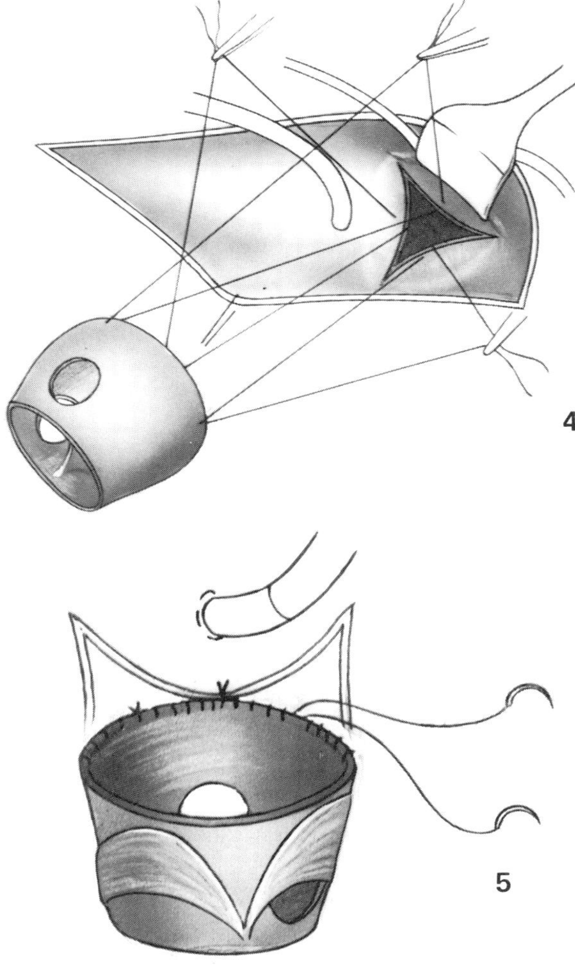

4

5

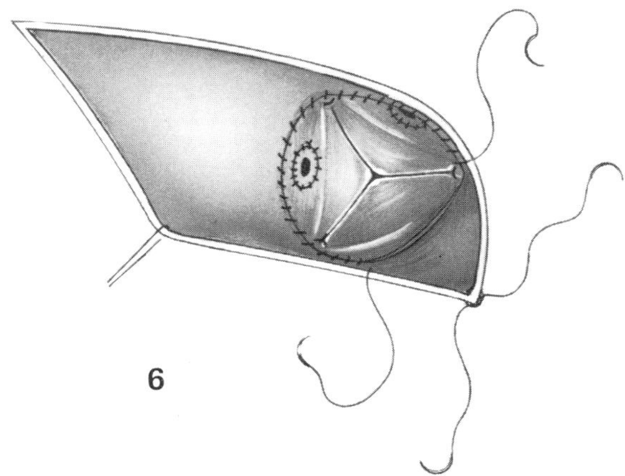

6

6

Finally the coronary orifices are sewn in place using continuous 4/0 sutures (the coronary cannulae are removed temporarily for this procedure), and the upper suture line is completed with 4/0 continuous sutures.

7

Closure

Closure of the aortotomy is effected with a 3/0 suture incorporating the non-coronary sinus of the homograft. With the heart fibrillating all air is evacuated from the ascending aorta and left ventricle. Air is aspirated from the left atrial appendage and right superior pulmonary vein.

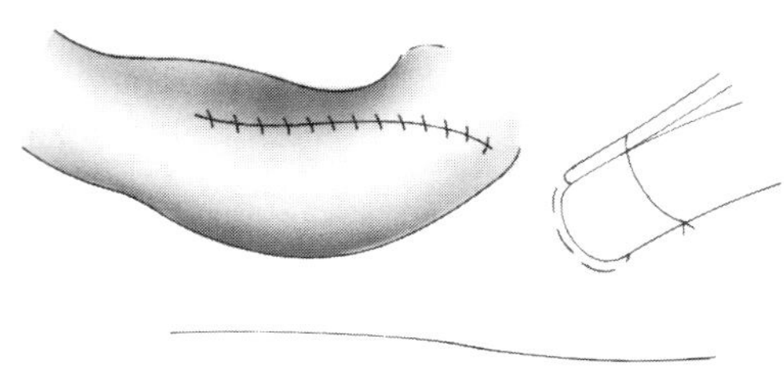

7

POSTOPERATIVE CARE

Routine postoperative care in an intensive care unit includes careful monitoring of physiological variables and correction of significant abnormalities. There are no special features applicable to aortic homografts.

Antibiotics are prescribed for 2 days. No anticoagulants are needed. It is wise to use antibiotics to cover dental treatment and other possible bacteraemic episodes indefinitely.

[*The illustrations for this Chapter on Homograft Aortic Valve Replacement were drawn by Mr. F. Price.*]

Surgery for Coronary Artery Disease

J. E. C. Wright, F.R.C.S.
Consultant Cardiothoracic Surgeon, London Chest Hospital, and Southend-on-Sea Hospital Group

AORTOCORONARY SAPHENOUS VEIN BYPASS GRAFT OPERATION

Operations directed at restoring an adequate blood supply to myocardium rendered ischaemic as a result of coronary artery disease have been described and performed for over 40 years. The operation to be described here has supplanted the earlier procedures almost entirely. It was first performed in 1967 and depends on three factors for its success. The first is the ability of Cardiologists to obtain detailed pictures of the anatomy of the coronary circulation by means of selective coronary angiography. Examination of these pictures reveals the presence of coronary artery occlusion or stenosis. A stenosis of greater than 50 per cent is thought to be significant, i.e. to require a bypass graft. The graft will be inserted beyond the narrow area, the site being determined at operation, bearing in mind the information derived from the angiogram. The second factor is the use of autogenous saphenous vein as a bypass conduit. It is readily available, satisfactory to work with and appears to last well for many years in its new role. The final factor is the use of standard cardiopulmonary bypass techniques during the operation.

1

The first step in the operation is to obtain a length of saphenous vein. The lower leg is preferred, since being of small diameter, there is less discrepancy compared to the size of the coronary artery. Each graft will require approximately 10–15 cm of vein. A continuous incision is made over the vein, which may be marked out prior to operation using a skin pencil if this is thought necessary.

The side branches are ligated close to the vein, to avoid potential sites of thrombosis. Great care is taken to avoid unnecessary handling of the vein itself as intimal damage may occur. The vein having been removed, the leg incision is closed and the leg firmly bandaged, starting from the foot, to prevent haemorrhage. The distal end of the vein is carefully marked with a fine suture. This is to ensure that the graft, which must be reversed because of the venous valves, is correctly orientated. The marked end is the aortic end. Prior to use the vein is tested by filling it with the patient's blood from a syringe, and any leaks are repaired. Blood is preferred to saline, which may damage the intima. To prevent drying of the vein it is kept immersed in blood until required.

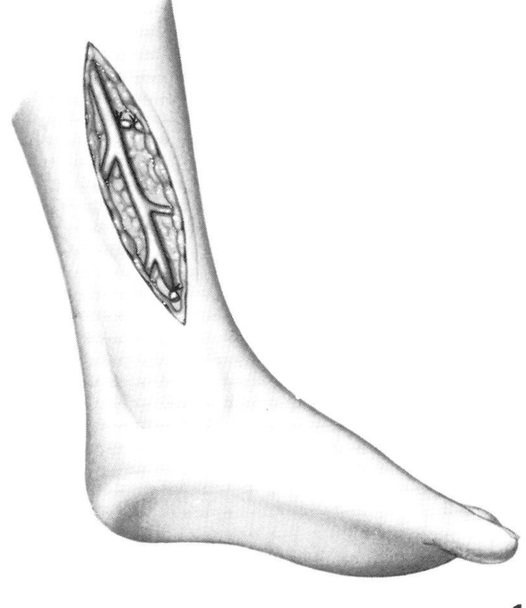

1

2

The chest is opened through a median sternotomy in all cases. Preparations are made for cardiopulmonary bypass in the usual way. Two caval cannulae are used if the circumflex is to be grafted to ensure adequate venous return when the heart is dislocated. A single right atrial basket may be employed for grafts to the right coronary or left anterior descending coronary artery.

On total bypass, the body temperature is allowed to drift down slowly to 32°C. This provides an added safety margin during any subsequent period of ischaemic arrest. Rewarming to 36°C is commenced near to the end of the bypass period. No vent is necessary for simple vein graft procedures. However, until sufficient experience is obtained, it may be safer to use a left ventricular vent. If a vent is used, careful degassing of the heart will be necessary at the end of bypass before the heart is allowed to beat. The heart is now electrically fibrillated, but the electrode is removed once fibrillation is achieved.

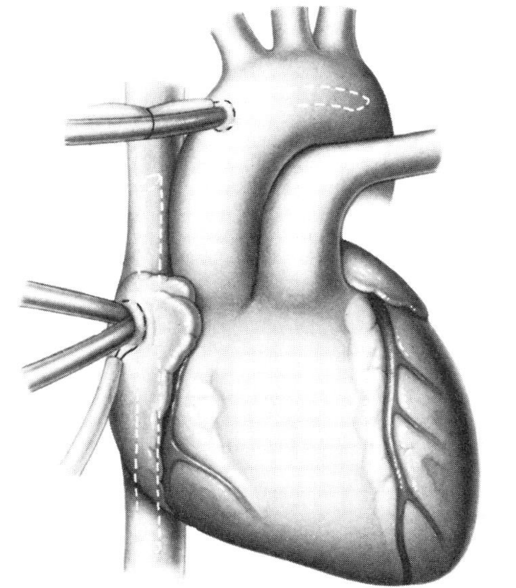

2

Access

The left anterior descending coronary artery is easy to isolate, since it lies on the front surface of the heart. All that is necessary is to place one or two packs behind the heart to lift it forward. It is usually readily visible, but may sometimes lie deep in fat or even muscle and in these cases it must first be exposed by dissection with the heart fibrillating.

3a

The right coronary is most conveniently approached just before it divides to give rise to the posterior descending. It is still of maximum diameter at this point, for simple vein grafting, and if endarterectomy is required, cores can be removed from both the posterior descending and the left ventricular branches. This region is on the base of the heart. Once again, two or three packs are placed behind the heart, and the assistant retracts the apex upwards exposing the base. Sometimes, the posterior descending is grafted directly, but it is often of a much smaller diameter.

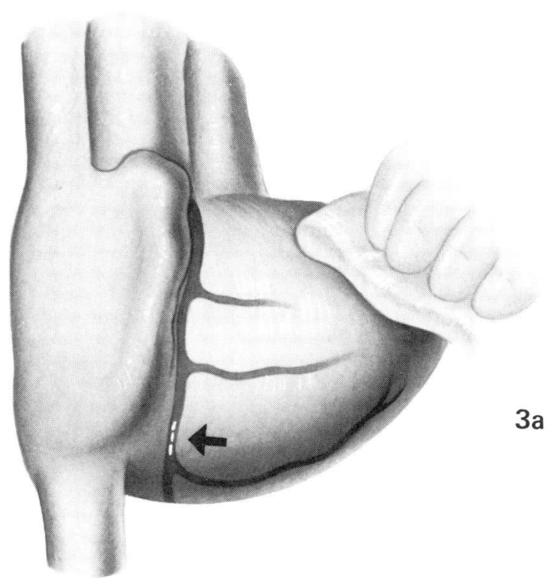
3a

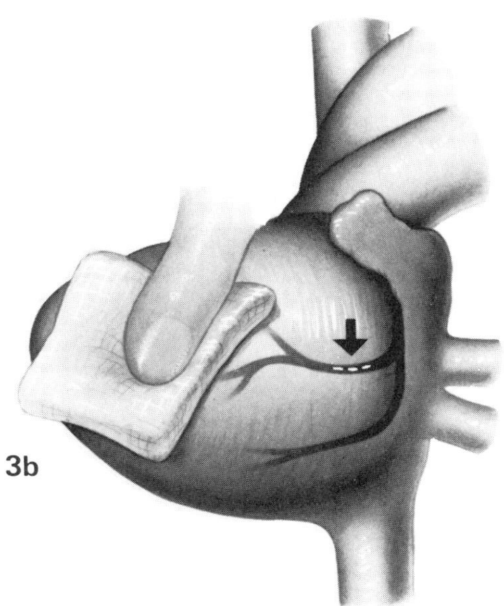
3b

3b

The most difficult vessel to isolate is the circumflex. The operating table is rotated towards the surgeon. The assistant places his right thumb over the left ventricle pushing it towards the surgeon. Cross-clamping is usually required to prevent cardiac distension. The main left circumflex lies deep in the atrioventricular groove and is not usually opened. The lateral branches of the circumflex are of sufficient size to permit grafting and these are usually selected.

4

The coronary artery is isolated at a convenient point, just distal to the diseased portion, as judged from the coronary angiogram and direct inspection. Snares of 0 Prolene are placed around the artery above and below the anastomotic site to stabilize the vessel and to stop the coronary blood flow, thus allowing clear vision.

Stay stitches are placed close to the point of incision, to open the vessel and allow for easier suturing. A vertical incision, 1 cm long, is made in the artery.

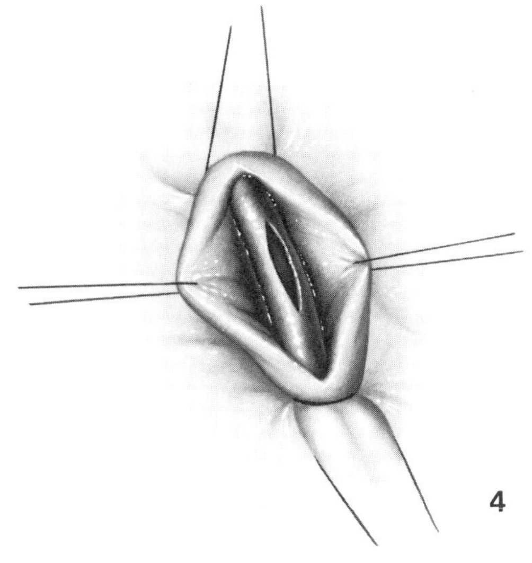
4

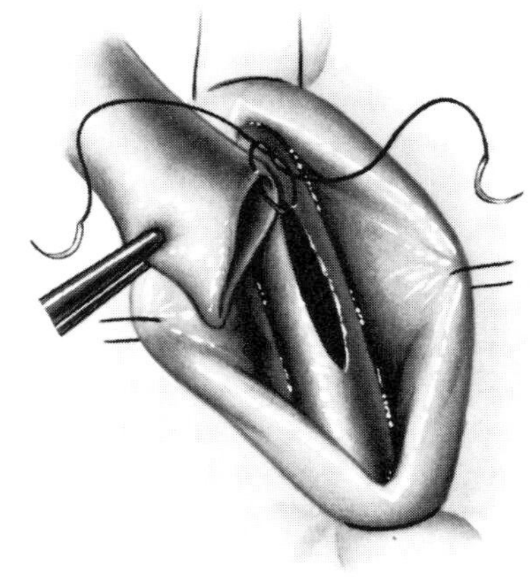

5a

5a,b&c

The end of the length of vein is now cut obliquely to correspond to the length of incision in the artery. If there is any bleeding obscuring the site of anastomosis, cross-clamping the aorta will produce a dry field and the clamp may be safely left on for up to 15 min. The end of the vein is now joined to the artery using 6/0 Prolene double-ended sutures.

A single bite is taken at the heel first, passing through a minimum of tissue only. This is now tied down, and a continuous suture run half way down each side. The needle is always passed from inside the artery to the outside, to minimize the risk of dislodging any atheromatous plaques. A second suture is now used to fix the tip of the vein and used to complete the anastomosis.

A probe is passed up and down to test the patency of the anastomosis before the final knot is tied. If the probe will not pass, the anastomosis must be revised, or there is a possibility of infarction subsequent to coronary obstruction.

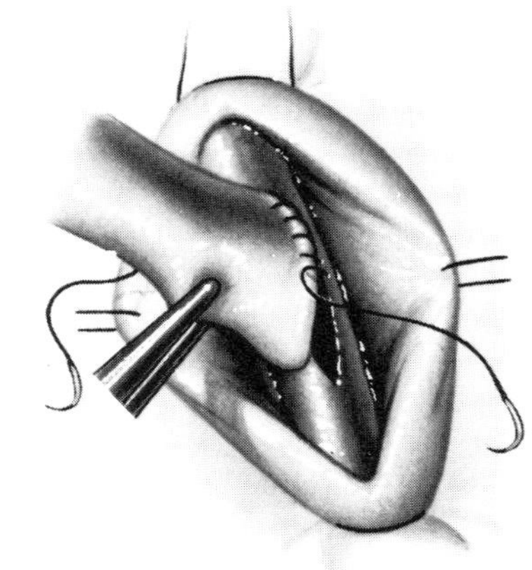

5b

The heart is now allowed to beat, defibrillating if necessary. The venous return to the pump oxygenator is temporarily occluded to allow the heart to refill, and thus assume a more normal size. The vein is now cut to an appropriate length. While the top end is being joined to the aorta, the myocardium will recover from any ischaemia incurred while the lower anastomosis was completed.

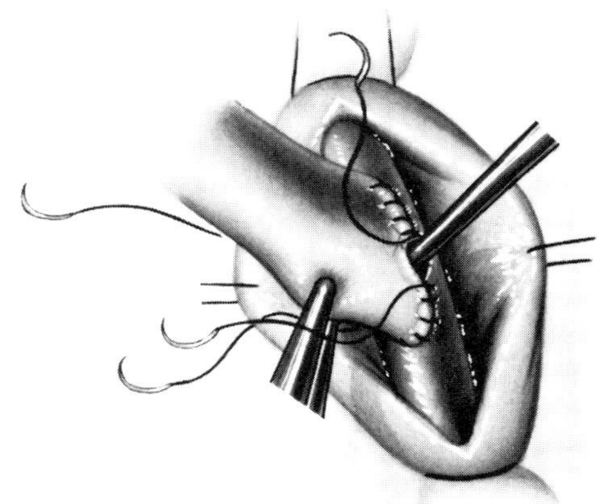

5c

6&7

The end of the vein is cut obliquely. A side clamp is placed on the ascending aorta and a disc of aortic wall is removed from the isolated portion of the aorta. The aortotomy is made using a bone rongeur as a punch, to remove a 5 mm disc of aortic wall. A vein is joined to the aortotomy using a 5/0 double-ended Prolene suture. A series of stitches is taken leaving loops 3–4 cm long. About half the anastomosis is completed in this fashion before the vein is pulled down. It is completed as a running stitch. Before releasing the bulldog clip, a needle hole is made in the vein graft to allow trapped air to escape.

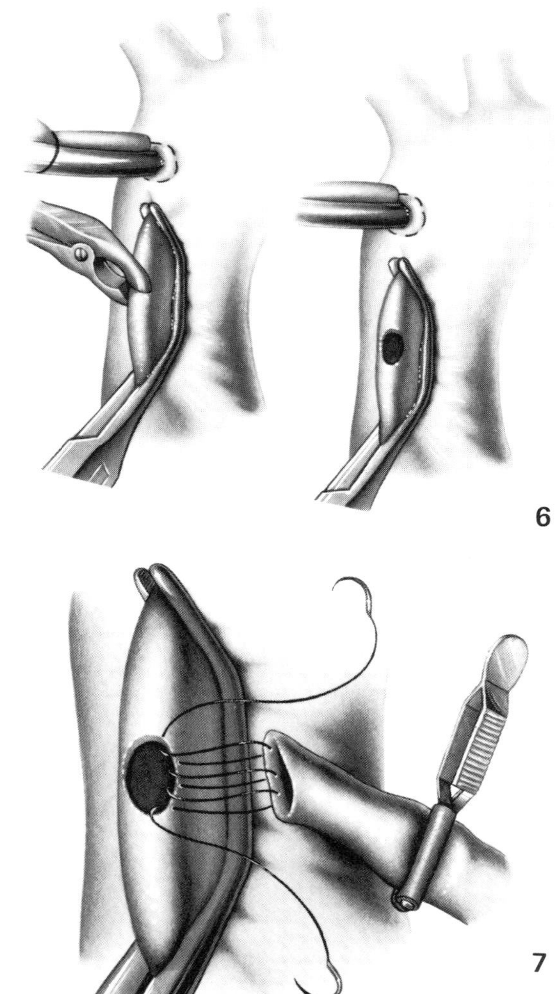

6

7

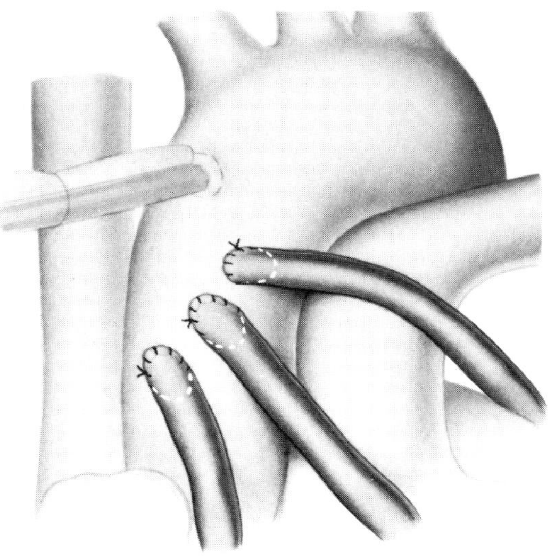

8

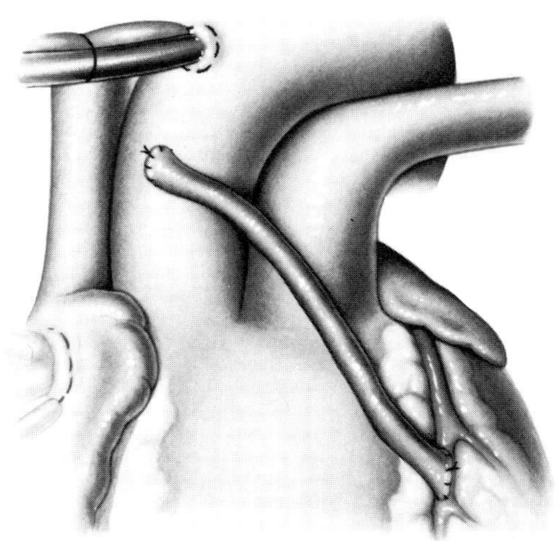

9

8&9

For multiple grafts, the process is now repeated. It is important that the aortic anastomosis be correctly orientated. Grafts to the circumflex approach the aorta from the left side, across the pulmonary artery. The heel of the vein should therefore be positioned to the left side of the aortic orifice. Failure to do this will lead to kinking of the graft. The grafts to the right coronary and left anterior descending approach more obliquely as in the illustration. The proximal anastomosis may be completed either on or off bypass.

10&11

If the coronary artery is diffusely diseased, rather than the more usual isolated proximal disease, then an endarterectomy is necessary. This procedure is commonly employed on the right coronary but may also be safely applied to the anterior descending and circumflex. It is pointless and potentially dangerous to graft directly to a heavily diseased vessel as occlusion and infarction often follow.

The artery is isolated as before with snares. The vertical incision reveals not the lumen of the vessel, but a core of atheroma. The core is easily separated through a plane of cleavage in the media of the vessel. A blunt probe is used for this, usually a MacDonald's dissector. By traction on the core, and with careful use of the dissector, the core can be extracted. Two or three centimetres are removed from the proximal artery, the core then being cut off. The most proximal atheroma is left *in situ*. The distal core is carefully removed totally, unblocking the distal divisions. Long cores of atheroma can be removed in this way. Cross-clamping is always employed to provide ideal operation conditions.

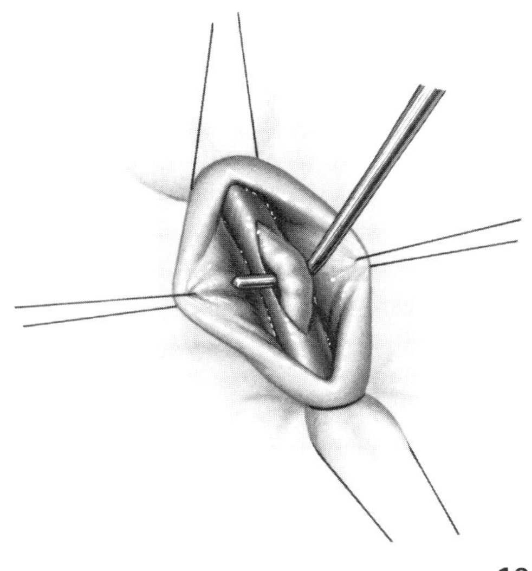

10

The resultant endarterectomized vessel is thin-walled, but will take stitches satisfactorily. The incision is now used for anastomosis of a vein graft in all cases, and this is completed as before. It is particularly important to ensure that a probe passes easily through the endarterectomized portion, thus excluding flap formation at the distal point of separation of the atheroma core.

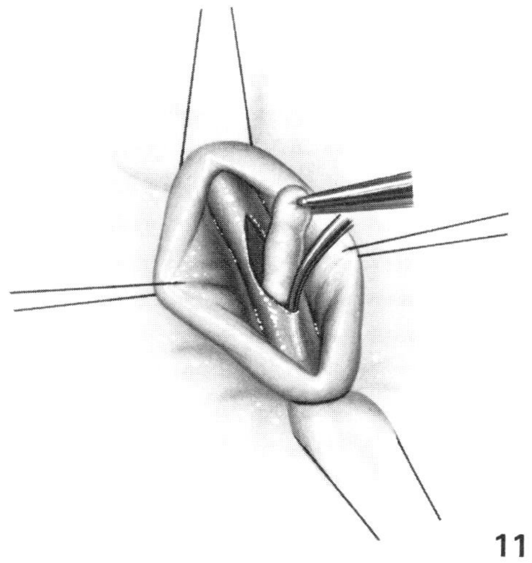

11

VEIN GRAFTING IN ASSOCIATION WITH VALVE REPLACEMENT

The most important consideration for procedures involving vein grafting plus valve replacement is to avoid ischaemic damage occurring as a consequence of the coronary artery disease, while the valve is being operated upon.

In general, if the coronary stenosis is 70 per cent or less the risk of ischaemic damage occurring is minimal and the valve may be dealt with as usual. The vein grafts are completed following this. If the coronary artery stenosis is greater than 70 per cent, or of course completely occluded, then revascularization should be completed before the valve is replaced. This eliminates the risk of ischaemic damage while the valve is being operated upon.

For mitral valve replacement, where the aortic valve is intact, a routine vein graft is performed and at once joined to the aorta. The mitral valve may then be dealt with safely.

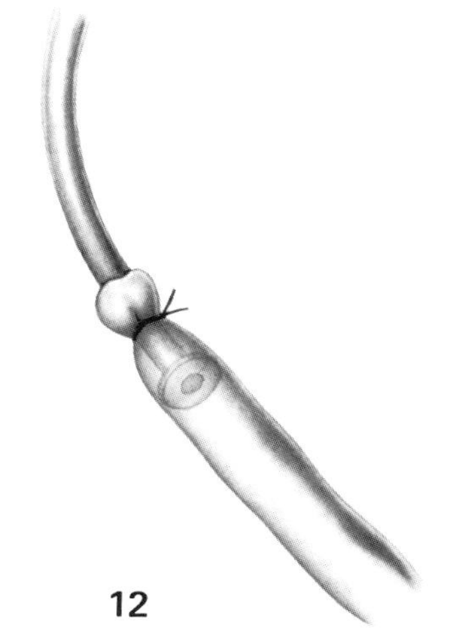

12

12 & 13

If the aortic valve is diseased, the procedure is more complex. In the presence of aortic regurgitation the aortic cross-clamp is applied to prevent distension of the ventricle by the reflux of blood. For a single graft the distal end is completed during a period of ischaemic arrest. This period should not exceed 15–20 min. The aorta is then opened to expose the aortic valve. The aortotomy should be made in such a way to allow adequate space later for insertion of the top ends of the vein grafts to the aorta. Occasionally, if the aorta is very long, one or two grafts may be joined to the aorta high up and still allow room for application of the cross-clamp and an aortotomy. Both coronaries are perfused as usual, using individual coronary cannulae. The vein grafts, if not already anastomosed to the aorta above the clamp, are now perfused using separate cannulae taken as side arms from the coronary lines. Thus, all coronaries will receive an adequate blood supply. If more than one graft is to be performed, it is safer to open the aorta first and perfuse the coronary arteries in the normal way. Following this, the distal anastomoses are completed in succession, each graft being perfused separately. After valve insertion, the aorta is closed, any remaining anastomoses are completed and bypass is then discontinued. (The final appearance of the aorta is illustrated.)

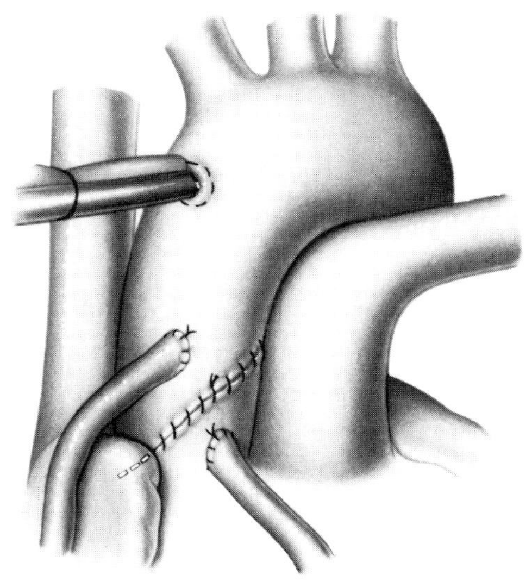

13

RESECTION OF LEFT VENTRICULAR ANEURYSM

The usual consequence of a myocardial infarction is the development of an area of scarring in the wall of the ventricle. In a very small proportion of cases, the scar tissue stretches, leading to the formation of an aneurysm. If this is large enough, it may move paradoxically and thus lead to left ventricular failure. Occasionally, clot, which often forms in such an aneurysm, may embolize.

The approach is similar to that already described. A standard median sternotomy is used, and cardiopulmonary bypass instituted. A single atrial basket, with aortic return, is usually employed.

As a result of the transmural infarction, adhesions are invariably present between the aneurysm and the pericardium. To avoid dislodging thrombus present in the aneurysm, the adhesions are divided when on cardiopulmonary bypass, and the aorta is cross-clamped. Thus the risks of per-operative embolism are reduced.

14

Once mobilized, a vent is inserted into the scarred area. Suction on the vent leads to collapse of the aneurysm, and this helps to demonstrate the area to be excised.

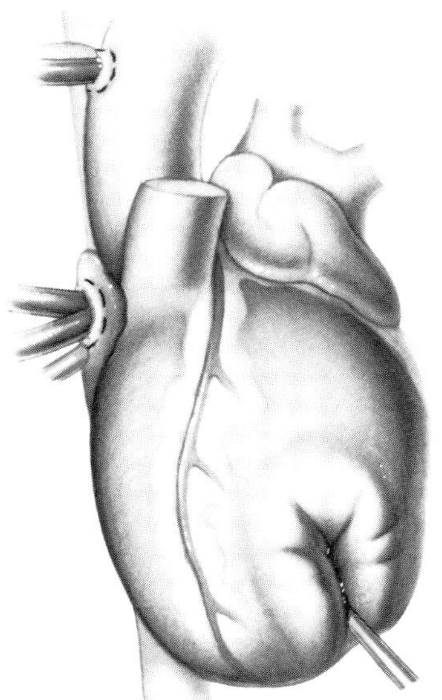

14

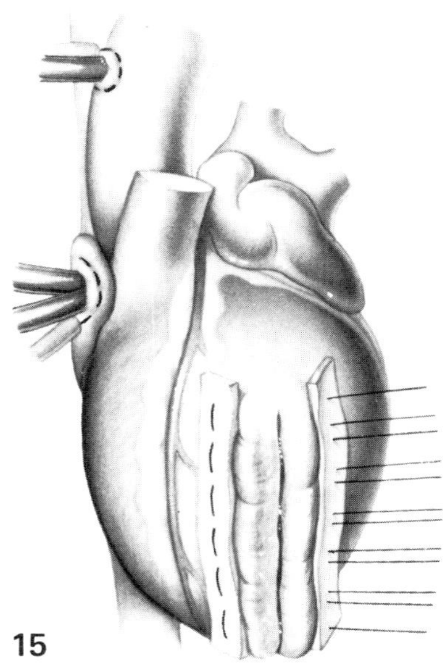

15

15

The thin wall of the aneurysm is now opened and any clot removed with care. The dead tissue is cut away leaving a 1 cm piece of scar tissue. The demarcation between scar and viable muscle is usually easy to see. The colour change from white to pink is clearly defined, and at the same point the thinned scar passes into normal thick myocardium. The 1 cm piece is left to facilitate stitching. Teflon buttressing, as shown, is only necessary if the aneurysm is recent and the scar tissue weak. Once the row of interrupted mattress sutures has been completed, a continuous 2/0 Prolene suture is inserted. The mattress sutures provide strength and the continuous stitch provides haemostasis. Careful degassing is of course required.

REPAIR OF ISCHAEMIC VENTRICULAR SEPTAL DEFECT

The blood supply of the interventricular septum comes mostly from the septal branches of the left anterior descending artery. In addition, a little is derived from the posterior descending artery. Ischaemic ventricular septal defects are, therefore, related to occlusion of the anterior descending coronary artery and usually lie anteriorly, close to the junction of the septum with the anterior wall of the heart.

If the septum ruptures, it does so within hours or days of infarction before the dead muscle can be replaced by scar tissue. At this stage of development, the edges of the ventricular septal defect are soft and friable thus taking stitches poorly. If the condition of the patient allows, it is better to close the defect after 4–6 weeks to allow the edges to become firmer.

A standard approach is made and cardiopulmonary bypass established using two caval cannulae.

16

The left ventricle is opened through the infarct, similar to the incision for a left ventricular aneurysm. The ventricular septal defect will be seen easily. The edges of the fault are trimmed, and if the defect is small, it can be closed as shown, incorporating the two edges of the infarct and the ventricular septal defect together. If the defect is large, then a patch must be inserted to avoid undue tension. Teflon or Dacron material is suitable.

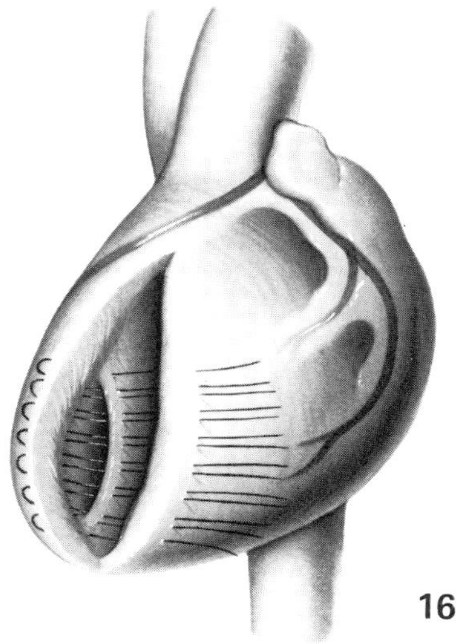

16

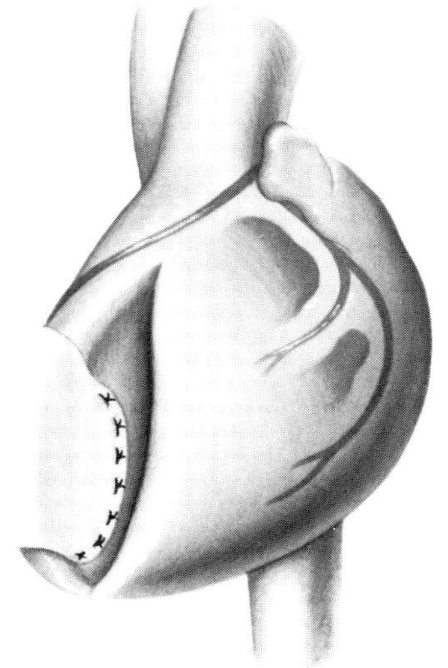

17

17

The patch is firstly fixed to the edge of the ventricular septal defect, and then brought out through the incision. The edges of the infarct are sutured as for an aneurysm but now incorporating the free edge of the patch. If the edges of the ventricular septal defect are soft, then buttressing will be required to stop the the stitches cutting out.

POSTOPERATIVE CARE FOLLOWING VEIN GRAFT PROCEDURES

Prior to chest closure, two drainage tubes are inserted. One is passed into the back of the pericardial cavity, and the other anteriorly to lie behind the sternum. These are connected to drainage bottles on gentle suction, of approximately 15 cm of water. Haemorrhage of more then 200 ml/hr, except in the first hour, usually indicates the need for re-exploration. The commonest cause for bleeding is failure to secure the vein side branches adequately.

The patient is ventilated artificially following operation until he is fully awake and able to breathe adequately spontaneously. It is often convenient to leave the patient ventilated and sedated overnight, and discontinue ventilation the following morning.

The heart rate and rhythm are monitored continuously using a videoscope display. Ventricular ectopic beats are common, and are usually due to low serum potassium, which should be kept between 4 and 5 mmol/litre. Atrial fibrillation is often seen and should be treated as usual by digitalization. Spontaneous reversion to sinus rhythm is the rule.

The blood pressure is best monitored by using a radial artery cannula (usually inserted before operation) connected to a pressure transducer with visual display. Low pressure may be corrected by use of beta adrenergic stimulation drugs such as isoprenaline, given by slow intravenous infusion.

The central venous pressure is monitored using a right atrial cannula, usually inserted percutaneously into the internal jugular vein. The usual venous pressure is between 5–10 mm of water, but varies from patient to patient. Blood infusion is determined principally by observing the central venous pressure.

In some patients, particularly if the left ventricular function was impaired by previous myocardial infarction, a state of low cardiac output follows operation. There is no doubt that this should be treated not by beta adrenergic stimulation, but by intra-aortic balloon pumping, which can increase cardiac output and reduce the ventricular load at the same time. Balloon counter pulsation should be started as soon as the condition is suspected, and continued for as long as necessary: often 2 or 3 days.

Finally, anticoagulants are commenced 24 hr after the chest drains are removed. The main reason for their use is to prevent leg vein thrombosis. They may be stopped after 3 months.

[*The illustrations for this Chapter on Surgery for Coronary Artery Disease were drawn by Mr. M. J. Courtney.*]

Aneurysms of the Aorta

B. B. Milstein, F.R.C.S.
Consultant Cardiothoracic Surgeon, Addenbrooke's Hospital and Papworth Hospital, Cambridge

PRE - OPERATIVE

Fusiform or saccular aneurysms occur in the ascending aorta, arch, and descending thoracic aorta. The majority are due to atherosclerosis. Other causes are syphilis, trauma, cystic medial necrosis, coarctation of the aorta and aortitis. Aneurysmal dilatation of the ascending aorta is often associated with aortic regurgitation from dilatation of the aortic valve ring.

Dissecting aneurysms start in the ascending or descending aorta, and may extend proximally or distally, resulting in occlusion of major aortic branches, aortic regurgitation, or rupture into the pleural or pericardial cavities.

Indications and contra-indications

The prognosis for patients with thoracic aortic aneurysms is difficult to determine. The greatest danger is of rupture, which occurs in 20–30 per cent, and when symptoms develop the life expectancy is usually not more than 6–18 months. On the other hand about half of untreated patients with these aneurysms die from other manifestations of atherosclerotic cardiovascular disease.

The operative mortality for these conditions is high, partly because of the magnitude of the operation but also because of the influence of associated conditions such as hypertension, ischaemic heart disease and renal and cerebral atherosclerosis. Commonly the patients are elderly, and the presence of chronic bronchitis and emphysema adds a further hazard.

This high mortality, even in experienced hands, means that careful consideration should be given to every patient before surgical treatment is advised. If the patient is symptomless and elderly, and the aneurysm is not enlarging, surgical treatment may not be advised. The location of the aneurysm is also an important factor. Operative mortality is lowest for procedures on the descending aorta and highest for those on the arch. The risk of rupture of the untreated aneurysm follows the same order.

Surgical treatment is imperative when the aneurysm is enlarging, or producing ill-effects from pressure or from erosion of adjacent structures. Intractable pain from erosion of vertebrae, ribs or sternum, venous obstruction and complications from tracheal or bronchial obstruction represent absolute indications. When there is haemoptysis from leakage into the lung or haematemesis from oesophageal erosion, urgent surgical treatment is essential.

Pre-operative management

Patients should be admitted to hospital a week before the operation. A full assessment is carried out including high-quality aortography in two planes. Particular attention should be paid to the state of the bronchi. Smoking must be prohibited, and breathing exercises and coughing practice started. The bronchial secretions are examined for pathogenic bacteria. If the patient has purulent bronchitis, a course of appropriate antibiotic treatment is prescribed. In any case, a 3-day course of prophylactic penicillin, cloxacillin and gentamicin is started immediately before the operation.

Special techniques

Clamping and opening of the thoracic aorta produces specific problems which have to be overcome by the use of special methods. The problems involved are the prevention of ischaemic damage to the brain, spinal cord, kidneys and myocardium, and the prevention of air embolism. The brain may be protected by separate perfusion of the cerebral vessels, or by the use of hypothermia. Renal and spinal cord protection can be achieved by creating a bypass around the occluded segment of descending aorta either from the left atrium to the femoral artery or from ascending to descending aorta using a heparin bonded shunt. The latter method avoids the problems associated with systemic heparinization. Unfortunately, paraplegia occurs occasionally irrespective of the method of prophylaxis used. Recent experience shows that if the time of cross-clamping can be limited to 30–45 min, and hypotension is avoided at all times, the incidence of paraplegia is no greater than when a shunt is used.

Myocardial protection is provided by normothermic or hypothermic coronary perfusion, or, as we prefer, by topical hypothermia in which the pericardium and ventricular cavity are flooded with ice-cold Hartmann's solution.

The prevention of air embolism involves careful filling of the aorta and its branches with blood by progressive release of the clamps, with the patient in the head-down position.

Immediate postoperative haemorrhage is a major hazard in aortic reconstruction. Bleeding can result in exsanguination or the need for massive blood transfusion, which brings additional problems. The source of bleeding may be the suture lines, porous grafts, or the large raw area at the site of dissection. A further cause is the derangement of the blood clotting mechanism from loss of fibrinogen and platelets after prolonged cardiopulmonary bypass and failure to completely neutralize heparin at the end of the procedure.

Woven grafts of Dacron or Teflon should be used, and it is wise to preclot these. Suture lines may be re-inforced with strips of Teflon felt, if necessary both on the outside and inside of the aorta where the wall seems unduly friable. As soon as the protamine has been given, a transfusion of fresh blood is started, and blood components should be available in the theatre for administration if repeated tests for coagulation factors show any abnormality.

Damage to the lung by retraction can be avoided and exposure improved by selective inflation using a Carlens endobronchial tube. Significant pulmonary arteriovenous shunting occurs after the operation, and therefore positive pressure ventilation with a high oxygen concentration is necessary in the first 24–48 hr.

THE OPERATIONS

ANEURYSMS OF ASCENDING AORTA
(Saccular or fusiform)

Saccular aneurysms

Saccular aneurysms are best dealt with by lateral aortorrhaphy. A median sternotomy gives excellent exposure. If the aneurysm is adherent to or eroding the anterior chest wall it is likely to rupture while this incision is being made. Under such circumstances the best procedure is to induce deep hypothermia by perfusion of cold blood from femoral vein to artery and then to arrest the circulation completely for a short time while the incision is being made. A bilateral transverse thoracotomy may permit a safer dissection of the aneurysm in these cases.

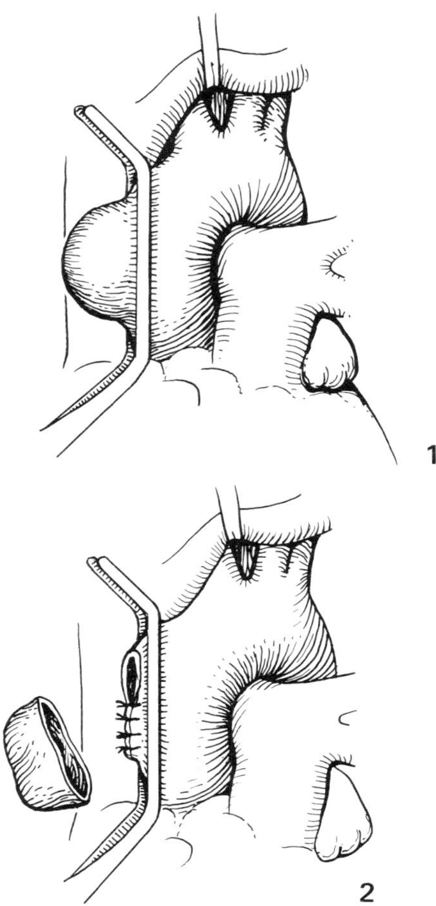

1&2

The neck of the sac is now isolated and a clamp placed across it. If the circulation has not been arrested it may be advisable to induce hypotension for a short period at this time. The neck of the aneurysm is divided, leaving a portion of it attached to the aorta for suturing. The opening in the side of the aorta is closed with a series of mattress sutures of 2/0 polypropylene, and the repair completed with a continuous suture approximating the edges.

The contents of the aneurysmal sac are removed and the accessible part of the sac itself excised. However, it should not be removed from the superior vena cava or the right pulmonary artery because it may be densely adherent to these structures and there is grave risk of injuring them.

Fusiform aneurysms

Total cardiopulmonary bypass

Fusiform aneurysms of the ascending aorta, such as are found in Marfan's syndrome and rheumatoid disease, require the use of total cardiopulmonary bypass. After the chest has been opened the patient is heparinized and venous catheters are introduced into both venae cavae from the right atrium. It is not wise to use a single catheter draining the right atrium, as the superior vena cava may be stretched flat over the aneurysm; and when blood is drained from the right atrium the vena cava may become completely obstructed. Arterial blood is returned to the body via a cannula in the femoral artery.

3

Cardiopulmonary bypass is started and the body cooled to 30°C. A vent is placed in the left ventricle through the apex and a thermistor tip inserted into the ventricular septum. The aorta is clamped just proximal to the innominate artery. We prefer topical cooling of the heart for myocardial protection. At this stage Hartmann's solution at 4°C is infused into the pericardial space and the excess removed by suction.

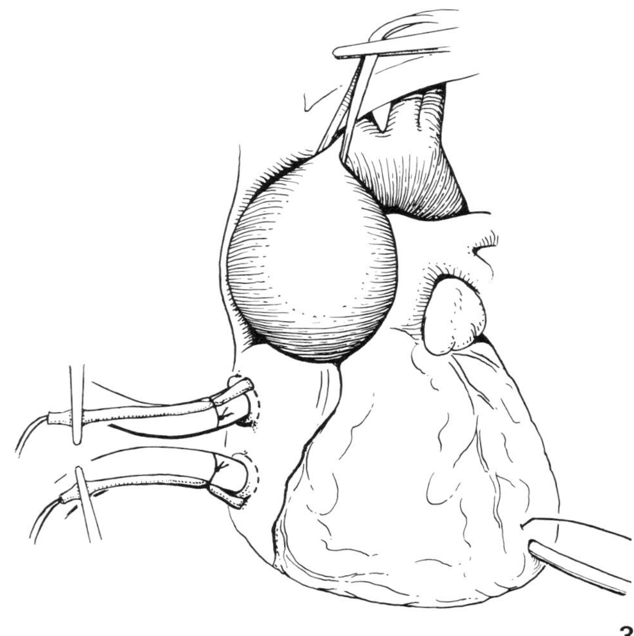

3

4

Dissection of aneurysm

The anterior wall of the aneurysm is now cautiously incised, and with care a plane can be found just external to the intima which permits freeing of the whole interior of the sac, with its contained clot, without entering the lumen.

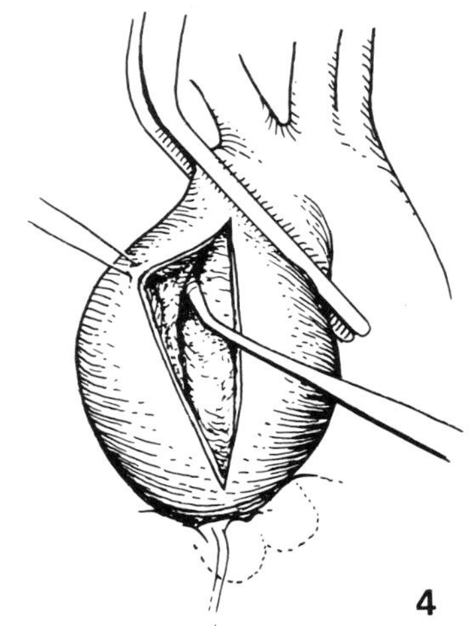

4

Placing of catheters

This inner layer is divided just above the aortic valve, and just proximal to the distal clamp.

The ventricular vent is now clamped, and the interior of the left ventricle repeatedly irrigated with ice-cold Hartmann's solution. The myocardial temperature falls to 10°–15°C.

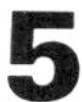

If coronary perfusion is chosen as the method of myocardial protection, perfusion catheters from the arterial line of the heart-lung machine are fixed in both coronary orifices as soon as the ostia are exposed.

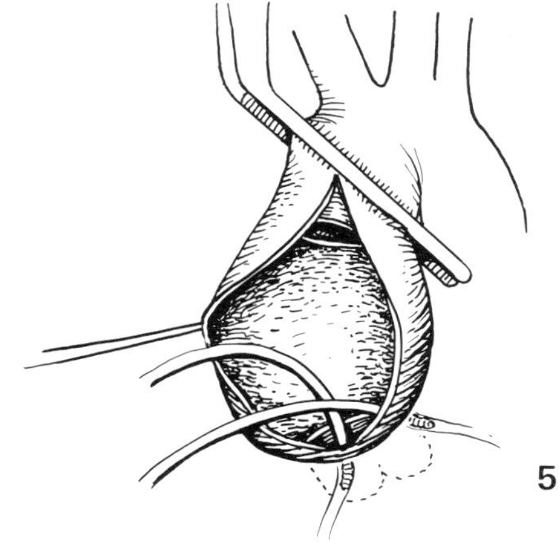

5

Transection of aorta

It may be fairly simple to transect the whole thickness of the aorta at each end of the aneurysm. If this appears to be dangerous because of adherence to adjacent structures, especially the main and right pulmonary arteries, it should not be attempted. In such cases a fold of the whole thickness of the aortic wall can be invaginated from within and used to suture to the prosthetic graft.

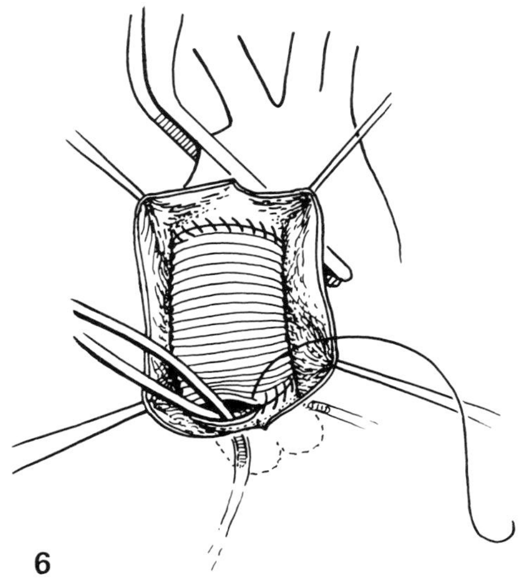

6

6

Insertion of graft

A preclotted woven Dacron graft is sutured first to the proximal end of the aorta. A continuous suture of 3/0 polyethylene is used. The distal anastomosis is now carried out. Pericardial cooling is stopped at this stage. If coronary cannulae have been utilized, they are now removed. The heart is filled with blood by occluding the left ventricular vent and the venous drainage catheters. The air in the left ventricle and aorta must be completely removed at this stage, through the remaining gap in the suture line and through the left ventricular vent site. The aortic clamp is removed and the heart is defibrillated.

7

Closure

If the graft has been preclotted in the patient's own blood (before heparinization) the bleeding through it is short-lived and can easily be controlled. As soon as possible the cardiopulmonary bypass is discontinued. The circulating heparin is neutralized with the appropriate dose of protamine sulphate and complete haemostasis can now be achieved. The redundant part of the sac is cut away, but a portion is preserved and sutured over the graft. This diminishes bleeding from the graft, the cut edges of the sac and the bed of the aneurysm. The incision can now be closed with drainage of the opened pleural cavities and with two or three drains in the pericardial sac and the anterior mediastinum. No attempt is made to close the pericardium as this may favour the development of cardiac tamponade. The cut edges of the sternum should be approximated with five or six braided Dacron sutures.

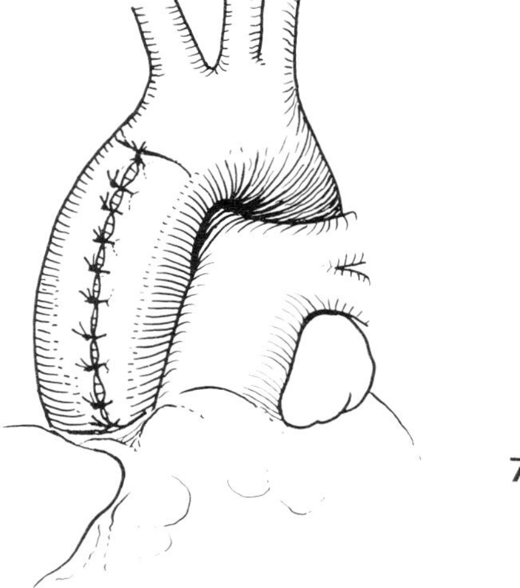

7

Aneurysms of the ascending aorta frequently cause dilatation of the aortic valve ring, leading to serious aortic regurgitation. This combination is usually found when the cause is rheumatoid or Marfan's disease. In such cases, the aortic valve must be replaced as well as the ascending aorta, and the origins of the coronary arteries have to be transposed to the aortic graft.

8

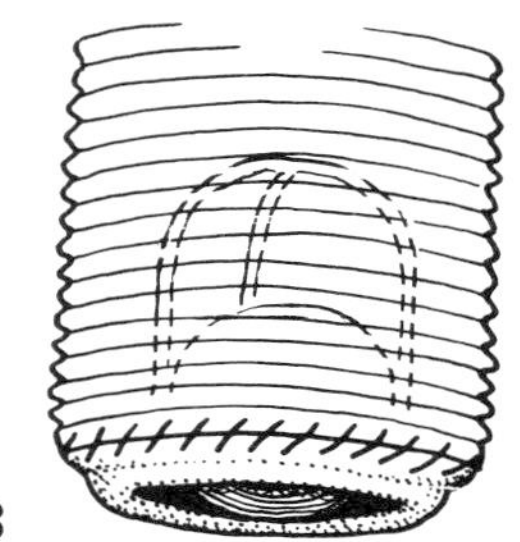

8

The initial steps are as described in *Illustrations 3–5*. A large Starr-Edwards valve is then inserted inside a 30–35 mm woven Dacron tubular graft which has been previously clotted in the patient's blood. The edge of the graft is sutured to the upper rim of the valve sewing ring with a continuous suture of 2/0 Mersilene. If coronary perfusion is to be used, it is helpful to remove the ball from the cage before the suturing.

The valve is then fixed to the aortic valve ring with a series of interrupted 2/0 Mersilene sutures (*see* Chapter on 'Prosthetic Replacement of the Aortic Valve', pages 191–196).

9,10 & 11

A side hole 1 cm in diameter is then cut out of the graft opposite the left coronary orifice. Using a double-armed 4/0 polypropylene suture, the edges of this opening are attached to the margins of the left coronary orifice, starting in the middle of the posterior or right side of the opening. When the anastomosis is half-completed, the left coronary cannula is clamped, removed, passed down through the distal open end of the aortic graft, through the side hole, and into the coronary orifice. Coronary perfusion is restarted, and the anastomosis completed. The right coronary artery anastomosis is carried out in a similar manner, taking care to avoid tension on the aortic graft, which might result in tearing of the aortic wall adjacent to the coronary orifices.

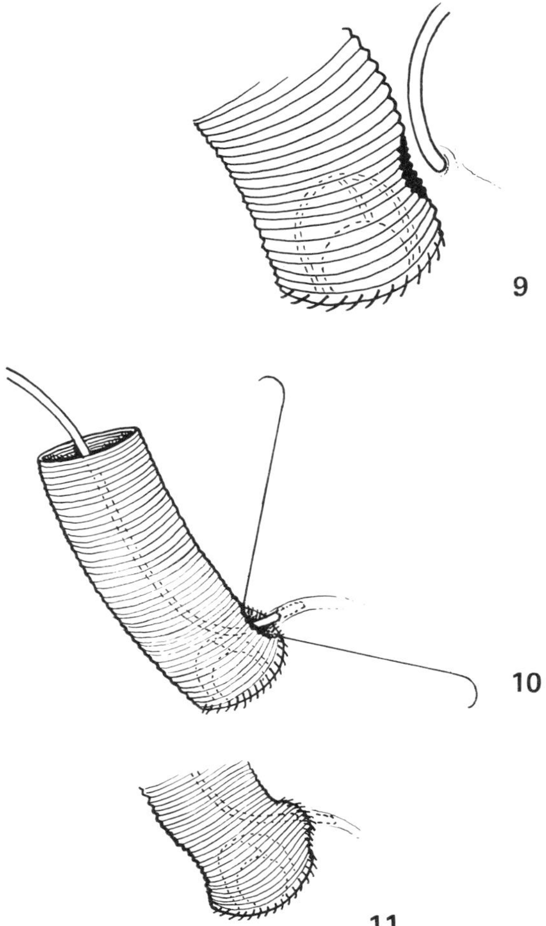

12

12

The aortic graft is now trimmed to the correct length, and anastomosed to the distal aorta with 3/0 polypropylene, using the end of the aorta if it can be easily transected. If not the anastomosis is made to the interior of the distal end of the sac, the posterior layer being made first. The coronary cannulae are removed before the anastomosis is completed. The remaining steps of the operation are described in *Illustrations 6* and *7*.

If hypothermia is used for myocardial protection, the problems associated with coronary cannulation are avoided, and there is also less damage to blood components as a result of coronary suction.

ANEURYSMS OF AORTIC ARCH

The operative approach to these aneurysms must be determined by their position and type. In the case of saccular aneurysms a high right or left posterolateral thoracotomy may give the best approach when a lateral aneurysmorrhaphy is proposed. If the aneurysm is a fusiform one involving the whole aortic arch, or is a very large saccular one, or when there are multiple saccular aneurysms, a median sternotomy which may be combined with a unilateral or bilateral anterior thoracotomy, or with an extension upwards along the anterior border of the left sternomastoid, will give a very wide exposure. The technique for lateral aortorrhaphy has already been described. In some of these cases, instead of a direct suture of the defect in the aortic wall it may be preferable to insert a gusset of preclotted woven Dacron arterial substitute.

Resection of the aortic arch

Fusiform aneurysms of the aortic arch necessitate a difficult and hazardous operation. Surgical treatment involves total resection of the aortic arch, although preservation of a cuff of the aorta from which the major branches arise is usually possible. The operation is carried out through a median sternotomy, extended if necessary.

Two methods of approach to the problem will be described. The first utilizes multiple cannulation and perfusion for protection of the brain and myocardium. The second approach is to provide this protection by means of deep hypothermia.

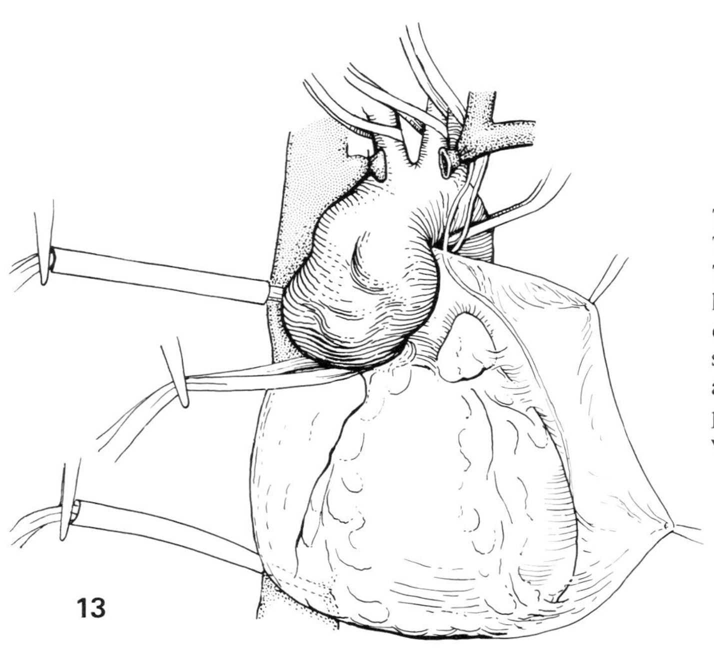

13

13

The pericardium is incised vertically in the mid-line. The innominate vein is doubly ligated and divided. The aortic arch, the three major branches to the head, and the ascending aorta are exposed, dissected out, and encircled with tapes. The descending aorta is similarly treated after retracting the lung forwards and downwards. The vagus, recurrent laryngeal and phrenic nerves are dissected out and preserved. The venae cavae are encircled with tapes.

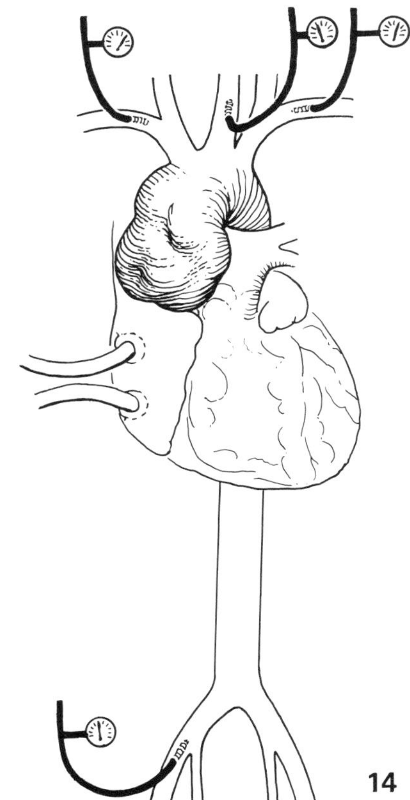

14

14 & 15

Perfusion technique

After whole body heparinization, the superior and inferior venae cavae and one femoral artery are cannulated and connected to the heart-lung machine. The right axillary artery is then exposed and an angled Bentall cannula inserted for retrograde perfusion of the right vertebral and right common carotid arteries. The left axillary artery is similarly cannulated for perfusion of the left vertebral artery. Cardiopulmonary bypass is now started and the nasopharyngeal temperature lowered to 25°C. A cannula is inserted into the left common carotid artery above the aneurysm. If this proves impossible because of the extent of the pathological process, the artery can be exposed in the neck, or it can be perfused via its orifice when the aorta has been opened. A left ventricular vent is inserted. The major aortic branches and the descending aorta are clamped, the ascending aorta is opened, and cannulae are inserted into both coronary orifices.

Although it is possible to establish this system with a single arterial pump, there is a real danger of cerebral overperfusion. It is preferable, therefore, to use separate pumps for each cannulation, monitoring flow and pressure in each arterial line.

Appropriate flow rates are:

R. axillary artery	600–800 ml/min
L. axillary artery	400 ml/min
L. common carotid artery	500 ml/min
L. coronary artery	150–200 ml/min
R. coronary artery	80–150 ml/min

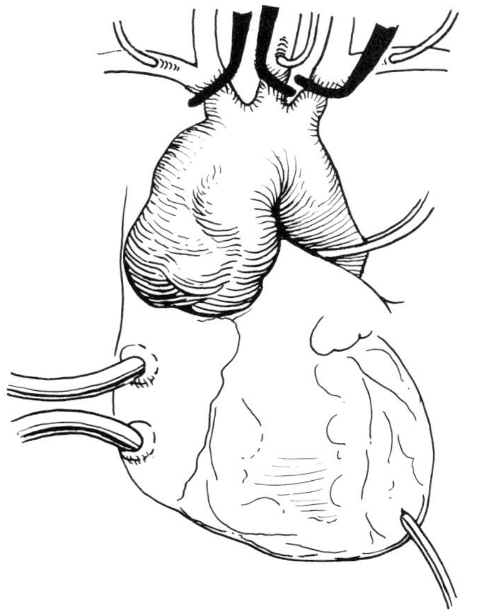

15

16

The aneurysm is excised, preserving a cuff of aorta around the origin of the brachiocephalic arteries. Parts of the sac which are densely adherent are left *in situ*. A preclotted woven Dacron graft is sutured to the cut end of the descending aorta with a double-armed 3/0 polypropylene suture. This suture line can be buttressed with a 1 cm strip of Teflon felt to avoid bleeding from stitch holes.

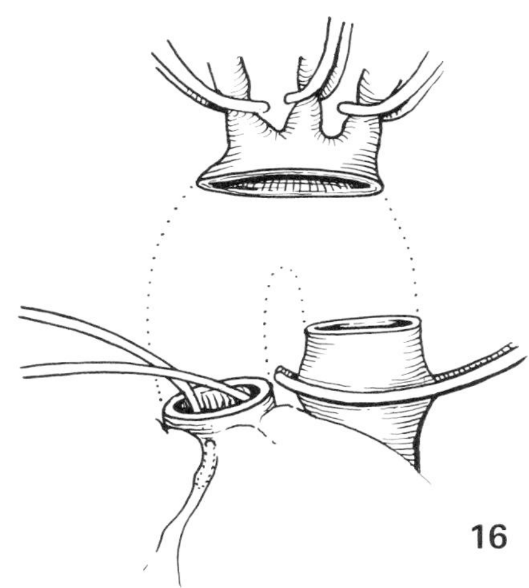
16

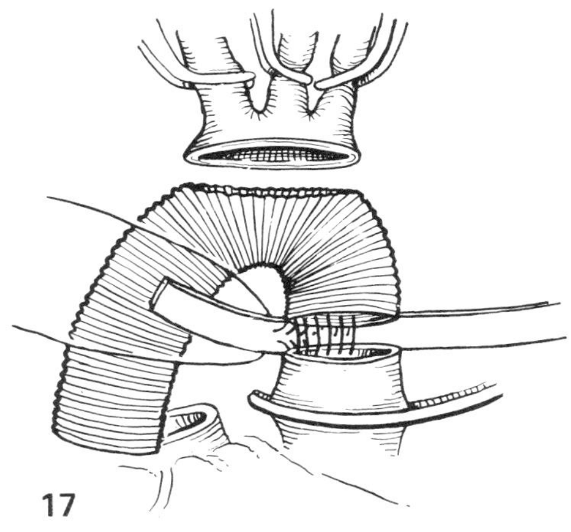
17

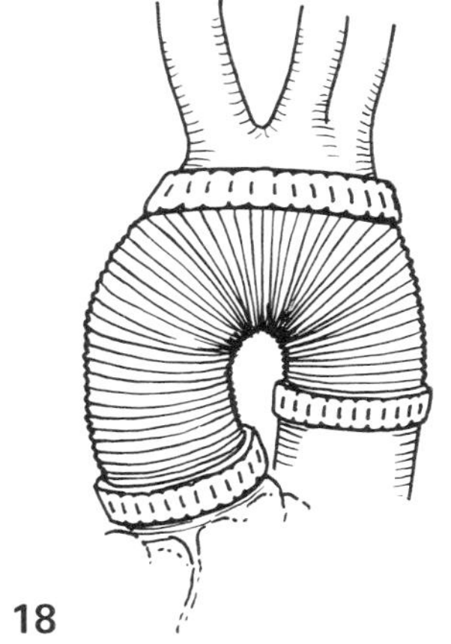
18

17 & 18

An ellipse is excised from the upper margin of the graft, and the aortic cuff containing the origin of the great vessels is sutured to this opening, using the same suture material and a felt buttress. The interior of the graft is now flushed out to remove any solid particles. Finally the proximal end of the graft is sutured to the divided ascending aorta. When this anastomosis is two-thirds completed, the patient is tilted head downwards and the distal aortic clamp is momentarily released to fill the graft with blood. The clamps on the aortic branches are removed and these vessels are milked so as to displace any trapped air into the graft. A clamp is now placed across the proximal end of the graft and the proximal anastomosis completed. Air is aspirated from the highest point of the graft and from the left ventricular vent before the clamp is removed. The coronary cannulae are removed before inserting the final sutures.

In some cases it may be preferable to leave the whole aneurysm *in situ*, opening the anterior wall widely and performing all the suturing from within. The sac can then be closed over the completed repair, thus leaving a much smaller raw area and so diminishing the problem of haemorrhage after termination of bypass.

19

Rewarming starts at a suitable stage in the operation which will ensure that the temperature has reached 37°C when the anastomoses have been completed. The heart is defibrillated as soon as vigorous fibrillation is seen. A careful search is made for bleeding from the suture lines. Any leaks are controlled with mattress sutures tied over Teflon felt pledgets. The bypass is now discontinued and the arterial and atrial cannulae are removed. Protamine is given to reverse the action of heparin, and a transfusion of fresh whole blood is started. Bleeding is controlled initially by packing and subsequently by treatment of individual bleeding points. If clotting appears defective, a sample of blood is examined for deficiency of individual clotting factors, and appropriate treatment with platelet-rich plasma or fibrinogen is instituted.

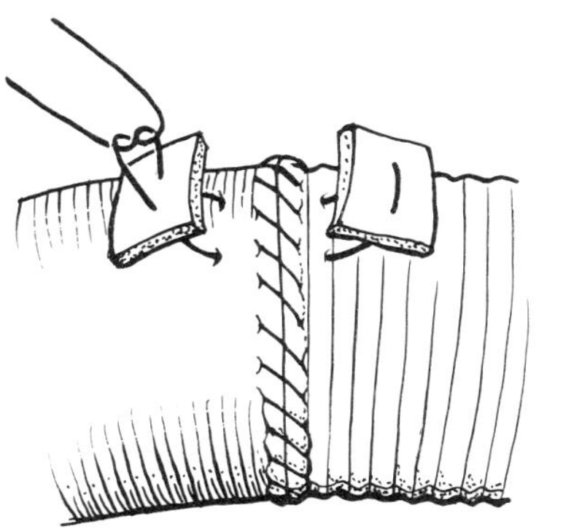

19

Deep hypothermia technique

After cardiopulmonary bypass has been established, the nasopharyngeal temperature is lowered to 12°C. The flow rate of the bypass is now reduced to 100 ml/min and the aortic branches are clamped. It is unnecessary to mobilize or clamp the descending aorta. The aorta is opened and continuous perfusion of the interior of the left ventricle started.

20

The descending aorta is now divided. A preclotted graft is inverted within itself and inserted into the aortic lumen. It is anastomosed to the aorta as previously described, and the inverted portion is withdrawn. This simplifies one of the more difficult parts of the operation. After completion of the anastomosis to the head vessels the flow rate is increased to 500 ml/min, to fill the graft and remove air. The proximal end of the graft is clamped and full flow restored for rewarming while the proximal anastomosis is made. The remaining steps of the operation are as already described.

Haemorrhage is a particular hazard with this technique and fresh blood and platelet-rich plasma must be available in liberal quantities for transfusion after termination of the bypass.

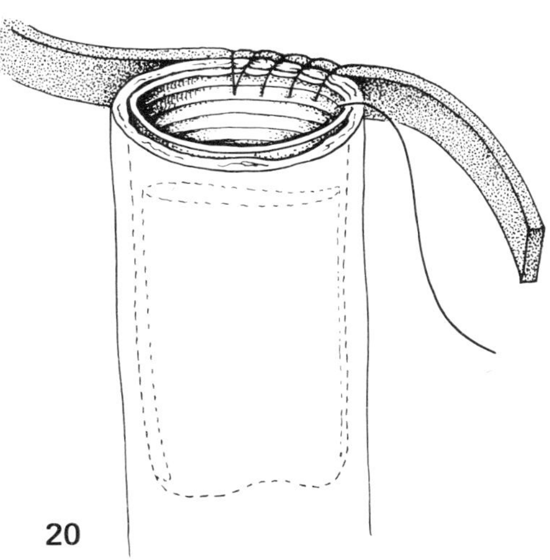

20

ANEURYSMS OF DESCENDING THORACIC AORTA

These are best approached by a left posterolateral thoracotomy. Aneurysms, such as those resulting from deceleration accidents, which are situated near the origin of the descending aorta and the left subclavian artery, can be dealt with through a third, fourth or fifth intercostal space incision. With more extensive aneurysms involving most of the length of the descending thoracic aorta it is often better to make use of two separate intercostal incisions, one high and the other at about the level of the ninth space. Some of these aneurysms are saccular and can be dealt with by lateral aortorrhaphy, if necessary with a Dacron patch repair. The suturing can be made easier by clamping the aorta above and below the region of the neck of the sac for a few minutes. When one is dealing with a fusiform aneurysm, or when it is necessary for any other reason to clamp the aorta for a longer period, a different method must be used in order to protect the spinal cord and the kidneys from the effects of ischaemia. This can be done by means of a left atriofemoral artery bypass (*see* Chapter on 'Methods of Providing Facilities for Open Heart Surgery', pages 22–25) or a left atrial-descending aorta bypass if a short length of normal aorta is available for cannulation just above the diaphragm.

The patient is placed in the left lateral position with the pelvis rotated backwards a little and the left leg fully extended at the hip joint.

The left common femoral artery is exposed. A left thoracotomy is made and with the lung retracted backwards the pericardium is incised over the left atrial appendage just anterior to the left phrenic nerve. After heparinization a 3/8 inch catheter with multiple side holes is inserted into the left atrium through a small incision controlled by a purse-string suture. The system is filled with blood and connected via a reservoir to a cannula inserted into the left femoral artery. A pump on the arterial side of the reservoir is now started up slowly and the flow rate is gradually increased. The aorta can now be clamped above and below the aneurysm and the flow rate through the pump adjusted to maintain an arm blood pressure 10 or 20 mmHg above the normal level. This requires a flow of 1–3 l/min. A heat exchanger can be incorporated in this circuit, allowing the use of moderate hypothermia in addition. This arrangement certainly provides an adequate blood flow to protect the kidneys. Protection of the spinal cord is usually adequate but because of the variation in the anatomical distribution of the intercostal arteries which supply the spinal cord, absolute protection cannot be guaranteed. Indeed, complete resection of the aneurysm may involve tying the one or two intercostal arteries which carry the main blood supply to the cord.

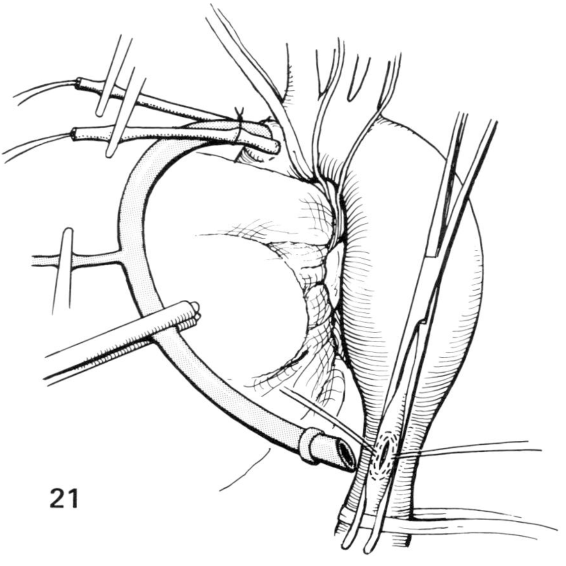
21

21

These partial bypasses involve whole body heparinization, with its attendant problems of control of haemorrhage both during and after the actual bypass. Bleeding can be minimized by utilizing as a bypass a heparin-bonded shunt from the ascending to the descending aorta. The shunt is inserted through small incisions in the aortic walls and fixed in place by tightening controlling purse-string sutures. The ascending aortic end is inserted first, the shunt is filled with blood and clamped, and the distal end then inserted into the descending aorta with slight release of the clamp so as to prevent the entry of air. On removal of the shunt the purse-string sutures are tied and the incisions oversewn with 4/0 Prolene.

22, 23 & 24

Once the bypass has been shown to function satisfactorily, the aorta is dissected and encircled with tapes above and below the aneurysm. Clamps are applied at these sites, the sac entered, and the contained clot rapidly removed. Bleeding from intercostal arteries is controlled by suture-ligating these vessels from within the lumen. Blood loss may be heavy from these branches, and therefore the blood is collected by a low pressure sucker placed inside the aorta, and returned to the patient using one of the techniques of autotransfusion (*see* Chapter on 'Methods of Providing Facilities for Open Heart Surgery', pages 22–25). The proximal and distai ends of the aorta are dissected free and anastomosed to a preclotted woven Dacron graft with a continuous suture of 3/0 polypropylene, incorporating a wide margin of aortic cuff. The distal clamp is removed so as to fill the graft with blood just before the suture line is completed. The proximal clamp is removed, the bypass stopped, and protamine given if the patient was heparinized.

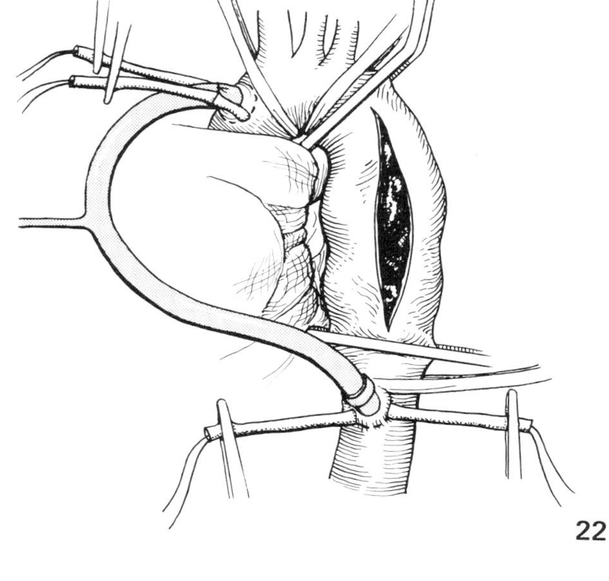

22

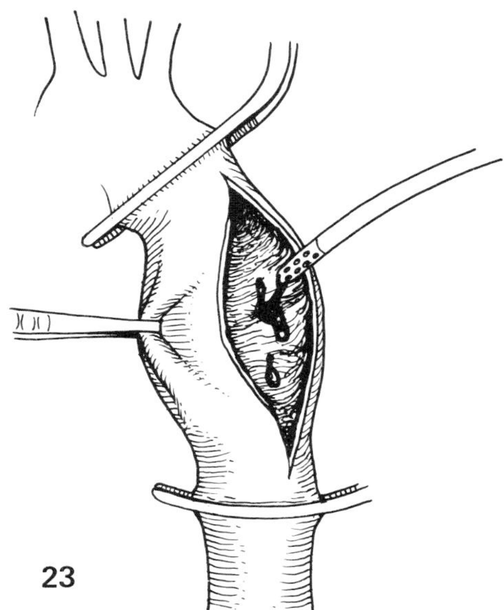

23

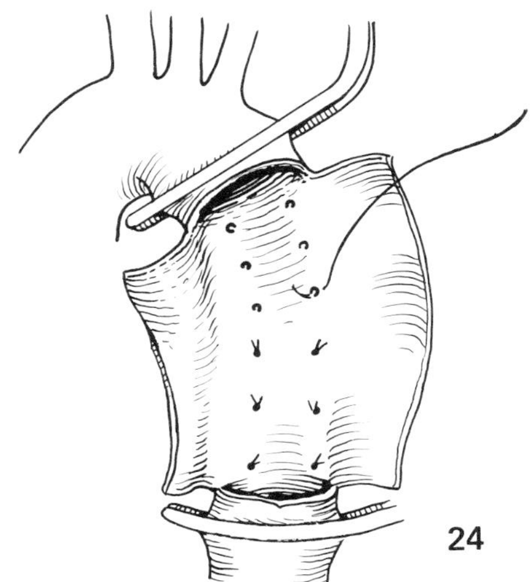

24

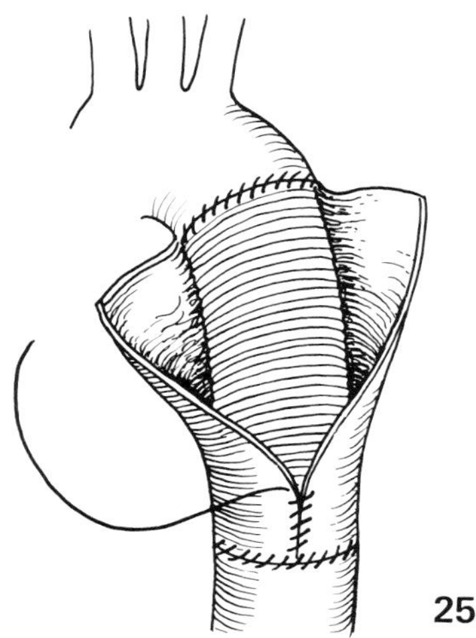

25

25

The excess of aneurysmal wall is excised, and the remainder sutured over the graft, so as to prevent a subsequent communication of the suture lines with the lung or bronchus. Meticulous haemostasis is secured, two pleural drains inserted, the left lung re-inflated and the wound closed in layers.

Recently evidence has been accumulating that the incidence of paraplegia following occlusion of the descending thoracic aorta is no greater when a shunt is not used, provided that the time of occlusion does not exceed 45 min, and that hypotension is avoided. This technique, however, can be recommended only for experienced surgeons who can guarantee to complete the procedure within the time limit.

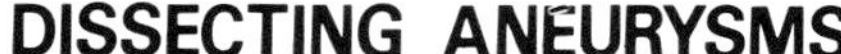

DISSECTING ANEURYSMS

PRE-OPERATIVE

Dissecting aneurysms resulting from an intimal tear or intramural haemorrhage are usually due to cystic medial necrosis. The condition occurs in Marfan's disease, and it has also been described in association with the Ehlers-Danlos syndrome, Turner's syndrome, coarctation of the aorta, and pregnancy. Hypertension is present in more than 80 per cent of cases. The intimal tear is found in the proximal ascending aorta in more than half of the patients, and then with diminishing frequency along the arch. The mortality in untreated patients is very high, 25 per cent dying within 24 hr and 75 per cent within 4 weeks. Extension of the dissection retrogradely may result in intrapericardial rupture, coronary artery occlusion, or aortic regurgitation from distortion of the aortic valve ring. In about one-third of the cases the dissection extends from the ascending aorta to or past the bifurcation, and it may occlude any of the major aortic branches, causing cerebral, renal, mesenteric or limb or spinal cord ischaemia. Rupture may occur into the pleural, mediastinal or retroperitoneal spaces.

Clinical features

Nearly all patients present with excruciating chest pain, often going through to the back and down the legs. There may be absent peripheral pulses, or neurological signs due to interference with the cerebral or spinal cord blood supply. Murmurs of aortic regurgitation or pericardial friction are often found. About half the patients are found to have a raised blood pressure, but in many others the hypertension is masked by the effects of haemorrhage or impaired left ventricular function.

Diagnosis

The typical history of intense pain in the chest going through to the back is obtained in nearly all cases. Clinical examination may reveal absent pulses, and the signs of aortic regurgitation or of pericarditis. Chest radiographs may reveal enlargement of the aortic shadow, or a pericardial or pleural effusion. The E.C.G. may show evidence of myocardial ischaemia. Aortography from the aortic valve to the bifurcation is necessary in all cases to establish the diagnosis and to determine the site of origin and extent of the dissection.

26

Principles of treatment

Dissecting aneurysms are classified into three types depending on the site of the initial intimal tear and the extent of spread of the dissection. As a result of trials of medical and surgical treatment, it is now generally agreed that immediate surgical treatment is the method of choice for type I and type II dissections, whereas type III dissections respond satisfactorily to medical treatment, operation being reserved for certain late complications.

Surgical treatment involves resection and graft replacement, although occasionally repair with end-to-end anastomosis of the aorta is possible. The fenestration operation is no longer used on the aorta, although it may be useful to relieve obstruction in its branches. The regurgitant aortic valve is re-suspended or replaced. Local procedures may be required to restore the flow in the major aortic branches.

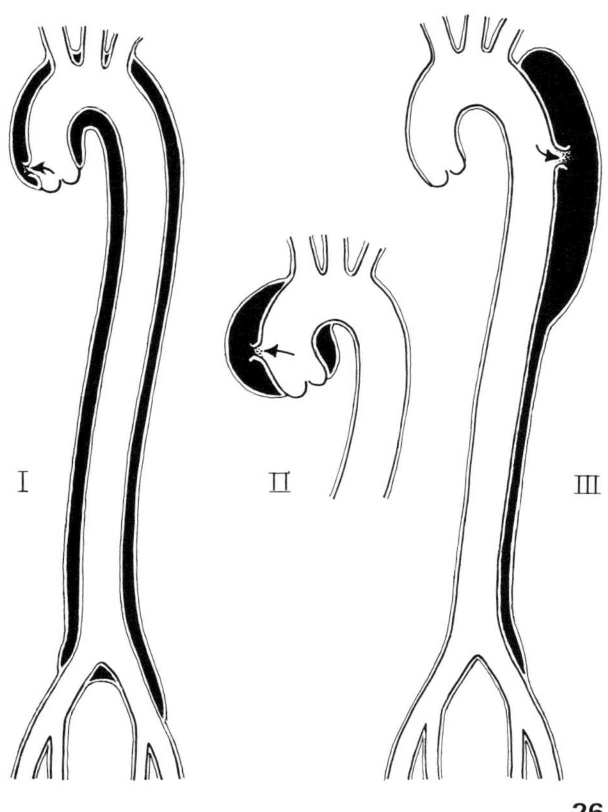

26

Medical treatment

The patient must be closely observed in an intensive care unit with standard monitoring methods under the management of a cardiothoracic surgeon. Treatment involves lowering the blood pressure and diminishing the force of cardiac contraction. This is used as a temporary measure in types I and II while preparations for aortography and operation proceed, and definitively in type III dissections.

The systolic blood pressure is reduced to around 100 mmHg by means of an intravenous drip of trimetaphan 1–2 mg/ml which is used for up to 48 hr. The head of the bed is elevated and reserpine 1–2 mg or propranolol 1 mg is given intramuscularly every 4–6 hr. The last two drugs may be given in combination, e.g. reserpine 0·25 mg twice daily and oral propranolol 20 mg four times daily. Guanethidine 25–50 mg is given by mouth twice a day. Chlorpromazine may be added to the regime if control of the blood pressure is inadequate.

Aortography is performed as soon as possible. If the site of the intimal tear cannot be identified, medical treatment is continued. Type I or II dissections are treated by immediate operation. Drug treatment is continued for type III dissections, but operation is carried out if evidence of extension of the dissection appears. This evidence is manifest by an increase in the size of the aortic haematoma, changing aortic murmurs, occlusion of major aortic branches, oliguria or anuria, electrocardiographic evidence of myocardial ischaemia or right bundle branch block, or the development of a pleural or pericardial effusion. A decision in favour of surgical treatment is also made if the treatment fails to control the patient's pain or hypertension.

Operation for type I and type II dissections

The ascending aorta is approached through a median sternotomy and cardiopulmonary bypass instituted with arterial return via a femoral artery cannula. The patient is cooled to 30°C. A left ventricular vent is inserted. The aorta is cross-clamped just proximal to the innominate artery, and the aortic root perfused with 500 ml of Hartmann's solution at 4°C. Pericardial cooling is then started. (Coronary perfusion may be used as an alternative.)

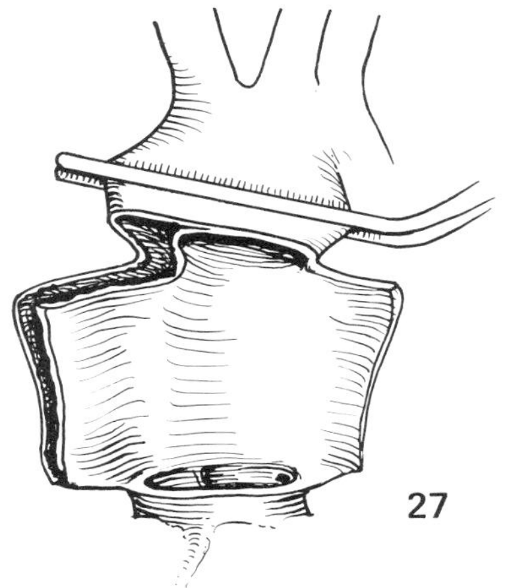

27

27&28

The aorta is incised longitudinally and divided proximal to the innominate artery. In a type I dissection, the two layers of the distal ascending aorta are sutured together with a continuous 3/0 polypropylene suture to obliterate the false lumen. The tissues may be very friable and thinned, and if the sutures tend to cut out the suture line is reinforced with strips of Teflon felt which may be applied both to the internal and external surfaces.

The aorta is now transected just above the upper limit of the commissures of the aortic valve cusps. The aortic valve is inspected to determine whether resuspension is possible or whether replacement is required. Replacement of the valve is necessary only when the ring is grossly dilated or the cusps cannot be made to co-apt.

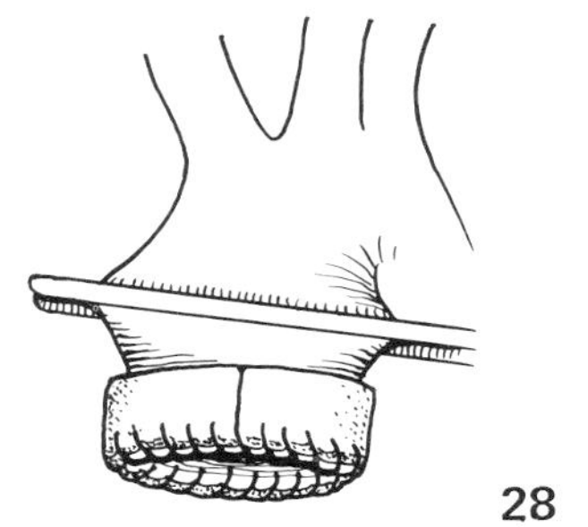

28

29

Resuspension is carried out by the placement of one or two mattress sutures at or above each commissure. These sutures are buttressed with pledgets of Teflon felt, passed through the full thickness of the aortic wall across the aortic haematoma, and tied over Teflon pledgets on the outside.

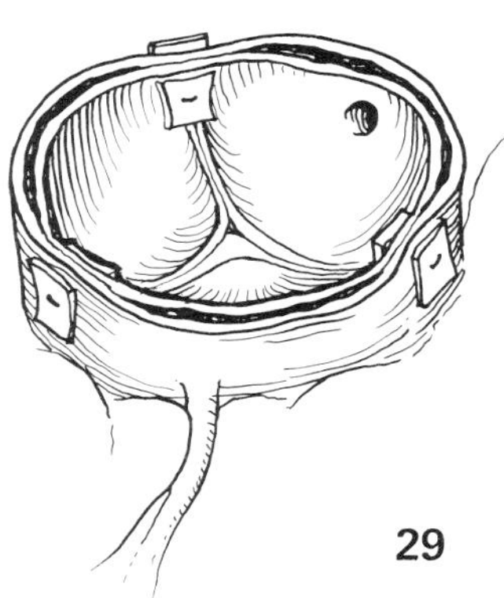

29

A suitable sized graft, which should be smaller than the diameter of the aortic annulus, is now anastomosed to the proximal dissected layers after these have been sutured together with a continuous 4/0 polypropylene suture. A continuous suture of 3/0 polypropylene is used, and the aortic side of the suture line is buttressed with a strip of Teflon felt. The distal anastomosis is made in a similar manner. The heart is filled with blood to evacuate air from the left ventricle and aorta just before the suture line is completed. The aortic clamp is removed, and the suture lines inspected carefully for leaks. These are controlled by mattress sutures tied over Teflon pledgets. Within 2–3 min the heart can be defibrillated. The outer layers of the aortic wall are sutured over the graft to assist in haemostasis. Bypass is discontinued, decannulation performed and protamine given.

Operation for type III dissection

When this procedure is indicated, approach is via a left posterolateral thoracotomy, and one of the methods already described for maintenance of the blood flow to the kidneys and spinal cord is used. Blood loss is liable to be heavy, and therefore a heparin-bonded shunt, which avoids systemic heparinization, is recommended. The technique to be used is that described for aneurysms of the descending thoracic aorta.

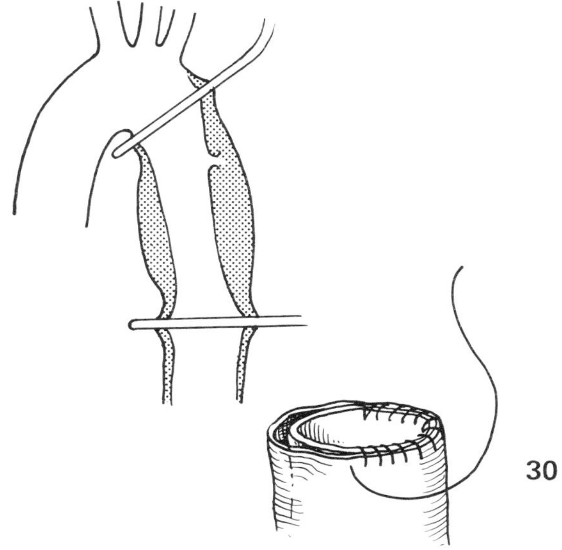

30

30&31

After the aorta has been clamped, it is transected just beyond the left subclavian artery, which is usually just proximal to, or at the level of, the intimal tear. A second transection is made just proximal to the distal clamp, and if the dissection is seen to proceed beyond this point, the two layers are sutured together before carrying out the anastomosis to the graft. If the layers are soft and attenuated, the suture line is re-inforced with a Teflon felt strip on the outside and inside. A preclotted woven Dacron graft is then attached to the two ends of the aorta in the manner already described.

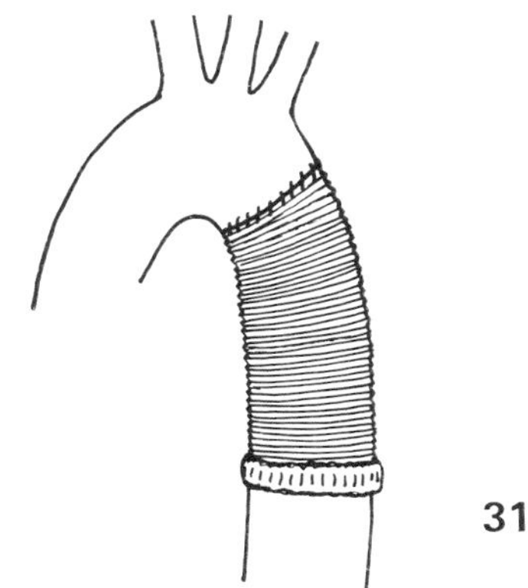

31

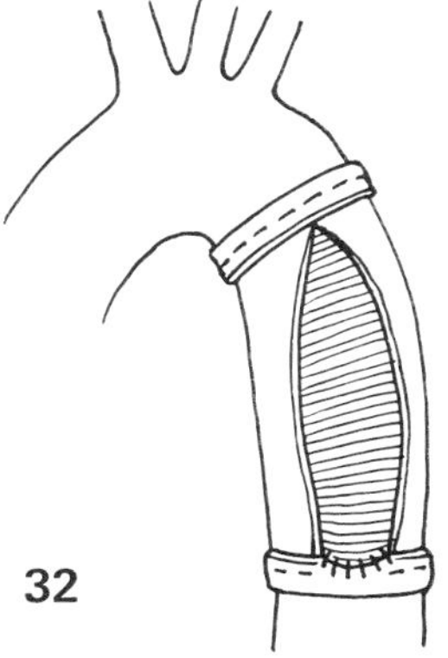

32

32

In some cases it is possible to attach the graft entirely within the aorta, using a continuous horizontal mattress suture which passes through the full thickness of the aorta and through a Teflon felt strip on the outer surface. This technique should be used whenever possible as it involves far less dissection and therefore a considerable reduction in operative blood loss.

POSTOPERATIVE CARE

The patient should be nursed in an intensive care unit specializing in cardiovascular cases. The pericardium is drained by at least two tubes, and each pleural cavity, if it has been opened, by one or two tubes. The tubes are all connected to a single measuring cylinder in which a negative pressure of 50 mmHg is maintained. The blood loss is recorded every 15 min, and an amount equal to this is transfused.

A nasogastric tube is inserted to prevent gastric distension, and a urinary catheter to allow accurate measurement of urine flow, which should be maintained at a minimum of 20 ml/hr.

Artificial ventilation is continued for 12–24 hr after the operation, that is, until the patient's cardiovascular condition has stabilized. Spontaneous respiration is suppressed by the use of a muscle relaxant, or by frequent injections of papaveretum or Diazepam. The endotracheal tube facilitates frequent and regular tracheobronchial suction. If an inspired oxygen concentration of 50 per cent fails to provide an arterial pO_2 of 12–15 kPa, positive end-expiratory pressure of 10 cm of water should be added.

The blood pressure and central venous pressure are measured every 15 min, and kept within prescribed limits by transfusion or the administration of vasopressor or vasodilator drugs. Hypertension is not uncommon after these operations, and may lead to excessive bleeding. Diazoxide 150–300 mg will give an immediate reduction in blood pressure. A more sustained effect can be obtained with chlorpromazine, the dose of which may vary from 2·5–25 mg.

Frequent measurements of the blood gases and electrolytes permit early detection of hypo- and hyperkalaemia, and metabolic or respiratory acidosis which must be corrected by appropriate respirator adjustment or administration. A central venous catheter for measuring pressure and for drug administration, and a radial artery cannula for arterial blood gas measurement are essential.

Haemorrhage is the most important complication following these operations. If the rate of blood loss appears to be increasing, attention should first be directed to controlling the blood pressure. At the same time a sample of blood should be examined for deficiency of clotting factors, and platelet-rich plasma, fibrinogen or epsilonaminocaproic acid given as indicated. The blood volume must of course be maintained, and this may necessitate transfusion of larger quantities of blood. Although a certain latitude must be allowed in these cases, if the bleeding persists the wound must be explored to seek a remediable surgical cause for the haemorrhage. Anticoagulants are not used after these operations; they are not only unnecessary but actually dangerous.

Prophylactic antibiotics are discontinued after 3 days. The drainage tubes are removed when the hourly drainage remains below 25 ml which is usually 24–48 hr after operation.

A chest radiograph is obtained within a few hours of the operation, mainly to detect the presence of a pneumothorax or haemothorax, and daily films are taken until the tubes have been removed.

If the lungs are functioning normally, artificial ventilation can be discontinued the day after operation, and the endotracheal tube removed.

References

Appelbaum, A., Karp, R. B. and Kirklin, J. W. (1976). 'Surgical treatment for closed thoracic aortic injuries.' *J. thorac. cardiovasc. Surg.* **71**, 458

Cooley, D. A., DeBakey, M. E. and Morris, G. C., Jr. (1957). 'Controlled extracorporeal circulation in surgical treatment of aortic aneurysm.' *Ann. Surg.* **146**, 473

Crawford, E. S. and Rubio, P. A. (1973). 'Reappraisal of adjuncts to avoid ischaemia in the treatment of aneurysms of descending thoracic aorta.' *J. thorac. cardiovasc. Surg.* **66**, 693

Daily, P. O., Trueblood, H. W., Stinson, E. B., Wuerflein, R. D. and Shumway, N. E. (1970). 'Management of acute aortic dissections.' *Ann. thorac. Surg.* **10**, 237

Gott, V. L. (1972). 'Heparinized shunts for thoracic vascular operations.' *Ann. thorac. Surg.* **14**, 219

Krause, A. H., Ferguson, R. B. and Weldon, C. S. (1972). 'Thoracic aneurysmectomy utilising the TDMAC – Heparin shunt.' *Ann. thorac. Surg.* **14**, 123

Wheat, M. W., Jr. (1973). 'Treatment of dissecting aneurysms of the aorta : current status.' *Prog. cardiovasc. Dis.* **16**, 87

Treatment of Left Atrial Tumours

H. H. Bentall, F.R.C.S.
Professor of Cardiac Surgery, Royal Postgraduate Medical School, London;
Consultant Thoracic Surgeon, Hammersmith Hospital, London

PRE - OPERATIVE

By far the most common tumour of either atrium is the myxoma. This lesion, which accounts for 50 per cent of all cardiac tumours, is to be regarded as a true tumour for local recurrence is possible, as also is distal seeding. Tumours of the left atrium outnumber those of the right atrium by at least 5:1. Description is therefore given of the myxoma of the left atrium. Similar principles may be applied for removal of tumours from the right atrium.

Indications

Tumours of the left atrium may manifest themselves in a number of different ways. (*1*) General symptoms, suggesting a diagnosis of subacute bacterial endocarditis. (*2*) Embolic phenomena. (*3*) Symptoms and signs suggestive of mitral valve disease associated with rapidly developing pulmonary hypertension. (*4*) Physical signs which may vary with posture, very rarely accompanied by postural syncope.

If these types of presentation are kept in mind the diagnosis is likely to be made clinically. Confirmation is usually possible by echocardiography. Opacification of the left atrium by contrast delivered into the pulmonary artery reveals the tumour by the presence of a radiolucent area. The tumour may be seen descending partly into the left ventricle during diastole returning wholly or partly into the left atrium in systole. The operation for removal of a tumour is indicated as soon as the diagnosis is made, and no patient is considered too ill for operation.

Pre-operative preparation

A brief period of pre-operative preparation by medical management may be required but, in general, operation is proceeded with even in the presence of pulmonary oedema, for removal of the tumour produces an immediate relief of left atrial pressure.

Anaesthesia

Endotracheal positive pressure anaesthesia is used according to the routine of the unit. Most patients will receive intermittent positive pressure ventilation for the first few hours after operation; very sick patients in pulmonary oedema may need a longer period of ventilation.

Choice of approach

Median sternotomy is now the route of choice to the left atrium. Approach to the tumour may be through the atrial septum starting in the fossa ovalis. This permits a direct examination and excision of the base of the tumour and closure of the atrial septum is usually straightforward. Some surgeons prefer the approach through the inter-atrial groove as is used for mitral valve replacement; this is less convenient for excision of the base of the tumour. Catheterization of both venae cavae should be used to permit the opening of the right atrium even if the posterior approach to the left atrium through the inter-atrial groove is used. Caval snares are required.

In view of the fact that the pedicle of left atrial tumours almost invariably arises from the atrial septum at the rim of the fossa ovalis, the author prefers deliberate excision of the base of the tumour from the atrial septum.

Position of patient

The recumbent posture is used for the median sternotomy.

Perfusion technique

Total cardiopulmonary bypass is used according to the practice of the unit and it is the author's preference to use hypothermia to a temperature of 32°C with electrical fibrillation of the heart. The use of this degree of hypothermia affords extra protection for the short period of aortic clamping which is required to prevent tumour embolism during manipulation.

THE OPERATION

1

Insertion of catheters

The great vessels are taped in the routine manner and venous-drainage catheters inserted through separate incisions in the right atrium into the superior and inferior vena cava.

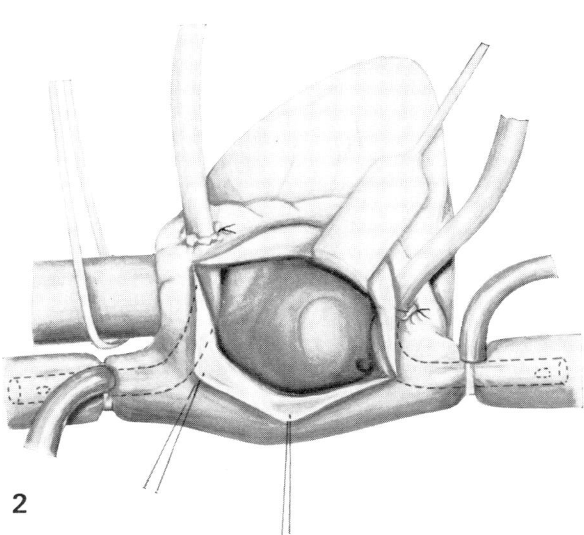

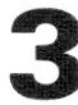

2

Opening of right atrium

The cavae are snared. The right atrium is opened by an oblique incision and a Kelly retractor inserted. The fossa ovalis is exposed.

3

The incision

The temperature having been lowered to 32°C, the heart is fibrillated electrically and the aorta cross-clamped. A short incision is made in the atrial septum in its upper portion close to the rim of the fossa ovalis. The pedicle of the tumour will usually readily be displayed and is excised from the atrial wall. A stay suture inserted into the pedicle may be useful. The incision in the atrial septum is then extended in front and behind and the tumour begins to extrude itself.

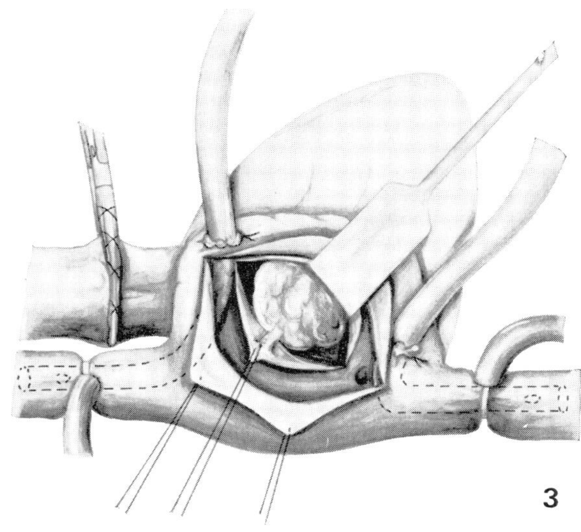

3

4

Withdrawal of tumour

Ovum forceps are gently applied to the tumour and, with the greatest care, the tumour is withdrawn. During withdrawal the tumour is often gripped by the mitral valve ring and disimpaction by finger and retractor may be necessary. The utmost gentleness should be used to minimize damage to the very friable tumour. After removing the main bulk of the tumour, the left atrium, the orifices of the pulmonary veins and the interior of the left ventricle are carefully inspected for detached remnants.

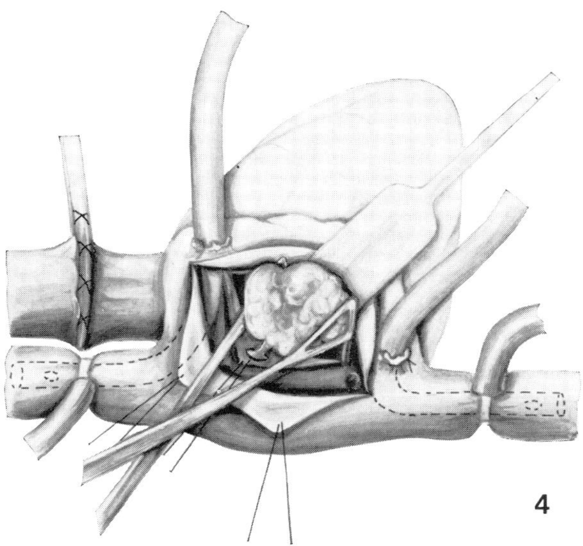

4

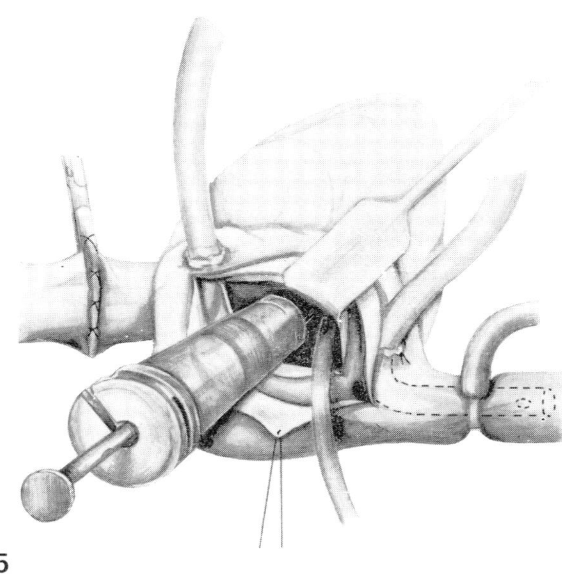

5

5

Flushing of atrium and ventricle

A syringe of saline is used to flush the interior of the left atrium and left ventricle and the discard sucker is used to remove the washings. Careful attention is given to the pulmonary veins into which tumour may have fallen.

6

Closure of septum

The aortic clamp is removed, the left side of the heart refilled with blood and the atrial septum closed, special care being given to the removal of all trapped air from the left atrial appendage, left atrium and left ventricle by catheter or wide-bore needle. A small air needle is inserted into the root of the aorta and the heart is defibrillated electrically by d.c. counter-shock.

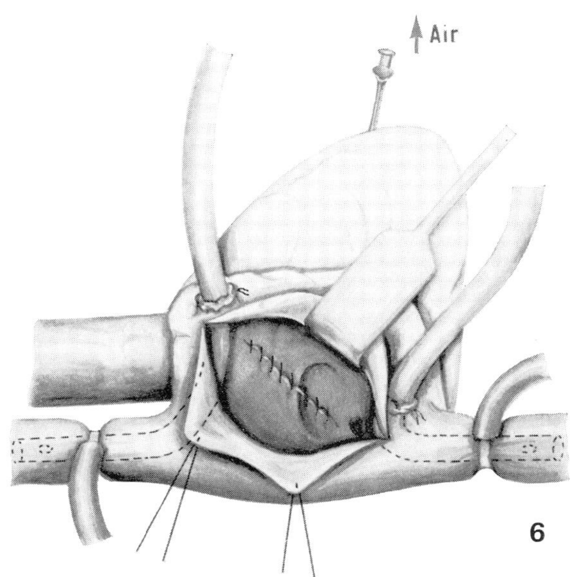

6

7

Closure of right atrium

The right atrium is closed, the caval snares released and the cardiopulmonary bypass stopped.

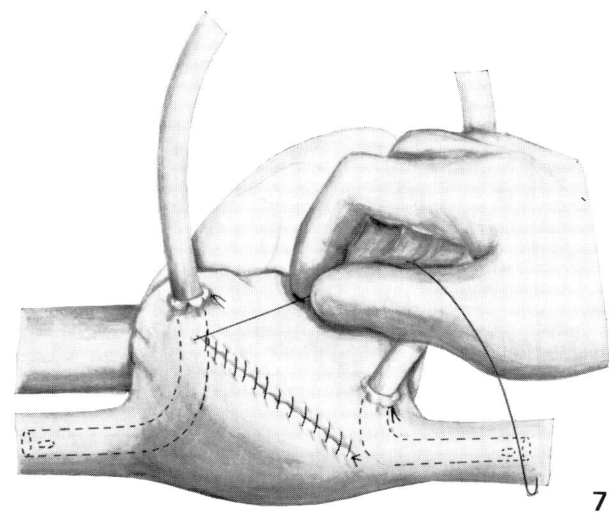

7

POSTOPERATIVE CARE

In the great majority of patients, no special treatment is required, the benefits of this operation being so considerable. Those patients who had pulmonary oedema, however, may require intermittent positive pressure respiration for a few days.

FOLLOW-UP

Long-term results of operation in these patients is most encouraging. Recurrence of tumour has not been noted in the author's series of 17 patients followed for up to 15 years, although occasional reports of local recurrence and distant seeding have appeared in the literature.

References

d'Allaines, Cl., Marchand, M., Gay, J., Leduc, G., Farge, Cl. and Dubost, Ch. (1976). 'Myxome récidivé de l'oreillete gauche; A propos d'un cas opéré avec succès.' *Annls Chir. thorac. cardiovasc.* **15**, 99

Bigelow, N. H., Klinger, S. and Wright, A. W. (1954). 'Primary tumours of the heart in infancy and early childhood.' *Cancer* **7**, 549

Blondeau, Ph. and Dubost, Ch. (1973). 'Discussion de la technique d'exérèse des myxomes auriculaires gauches.' *Annls Chir. thorac. cardiovasc.* **12**, 751

Croxon, R. S., Jewitt, D., Bentall, H. H., Cleland, W. P., Kristinsson, A. and Goodwin, J. F. (1972). 'Long term follow-up of atrial myxoma.' *Br. Heart J.* **34**, 1018

Goodwin, J. F., Stanfield, C. A., Steiner, R. E., Bentall, H. H., Sayed, H. M., Bloom, V. R. and Bishop, M. B. (1962). 'Clinical features of left atrial myxoma.' *Thorax* **17**, 91

Read, R. C., White, H. J., Murthy, M. L., Williams, D., Chao, N. S. and Flanagan, W. H. (1974). 'The malignant potentiality of left atrial myxoma.' *J. thorac. cardiovasc. Surg.* **68**, 6

Spencer, W. H., Peter, R. H. and Orgain, E. S. (1971). 'Detection of a left atrial myxoma by echocardiography.' *Archs intern. Med.* **128**, 787

Wise, J. R. (1970). 'Atrial myxoma and angiocardiography.' *Ann. intern. Med.* **72**, 756

Zachai, A. H., Weber, D. J., Ramsby, G. and Wong, B. (1974). 'Recurrence of left atrial myxoma.' *J. cardiovasc. Surg.* **15**, 467

[*The illustrations for this Chapter on Treatment of Left Atrial Tumours were drawn by Miss S. Barker.*]

Bronchoscopy. Rigid Instrument

PRE-OPERATIVE

Indications

Diagnostic bronchoscopy is one of the most common methods of investigation used in the study of chest disease. The mobility of the vocal cords, the patency and mobility of the tracheobronchial tree, the state of the mucosa, the presence of tumours and secretion must all be noted. Biopsy of tissue and aspiration of secretions for laboratory examination can be carried out. Lobar sampling of inspired gases and the study of the respiratory movements of the bronchial tree in the assessment of pulmonary function are further applications of the technique. Therapeutic bronchoscopy permits the aspiration of tracheobronchial secretion and inhaled vomit and the removal of intrabronchial foreign bodies.

Contra-indications

There are no absolute contra-indications to bronchoscopy *per se*, but the passage of the instrument may be rendered impossible by severe deformities and rigidity of the neck and by oedema of the larynx. Bronchoscopy, if possible, should be postponed until dental sepsis is cleared. It is unwise to bronchoscope patients suffering from florid superior vena caval obstruction–since laryngeal oedema may be precipitated.

Anaesthesia

In experienced hands the procedure can almost always be carried out under general anaesthesia, provided that no relaxants are given until the surgeon is assured that the lights and suction are in working order, and that spare sucker tubes are available. For most diagnostic bronchoscopies in adults succinylcholine and thiopentone are adequate. Oxygen is given by the Sanders technique in which an intermittent jet of oxygen entrains air by the Venturi effect, and the entrained air inflates the lungs. In the anoxic patient requiring tracheobronchial aspiration for retained secretions relaxants should be avoided; the bronchoscope should be passed under general anaesthesia with the patient breathing spontaneously, or under local anaesthesia.

Position of patient

The distressed patient with the bronchial tree filled with secretion is best bronchoscoped while sitting upright in bed; otherwise it is usual for the patient to be lying supine on an operating table without pillows, and with the head moderately extended.

To prevent injury, the eyes (but not the nose) are covered with a sterile towel. The upper teeth and gum are protected by a gauze swab.

THE OPERATION

1

Introduction into oropharynx

The operator stands behind the patient and holds the proximal end of the bronchoscope between the finger and thumb of the right hand like a pen. The instrument is lubricated and then introduced in the mid-line gently past the uvula into the back of the pharynx.

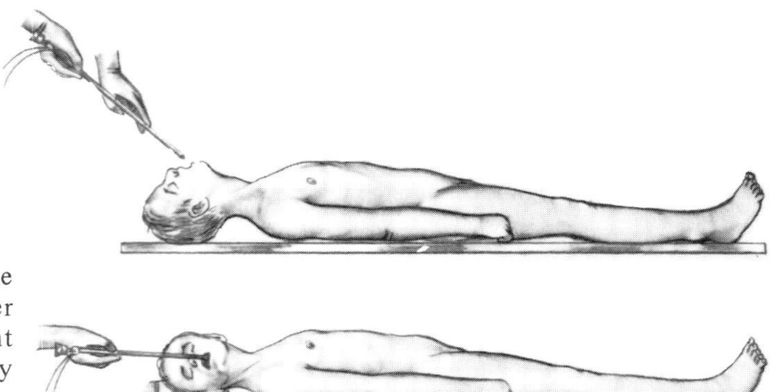

1

2

Identification of epiglottis

At this stage the anterior end of the instrument, lifted forward by the operator's left hand, is used to displace the root of the tongue anteriorly and bring the epiglottis into view. Throughout the procedure the utmost gentleness should be used, and any tendency to use the patient's upper jaw as a fulcrum must be avoided.

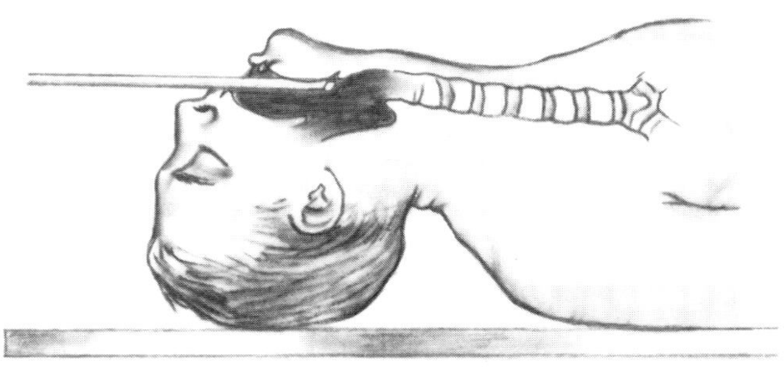

2

3

Visualization of cords

The epiglottis is then in turn lifted forwards by slipping the tip of the bronchoscope beneath it; the vocal cords will then be seen. The bronchoscope, rotated so that its beak lies in the same axis as the laryngeal inlet, is then passed gently onwards into the trachea.

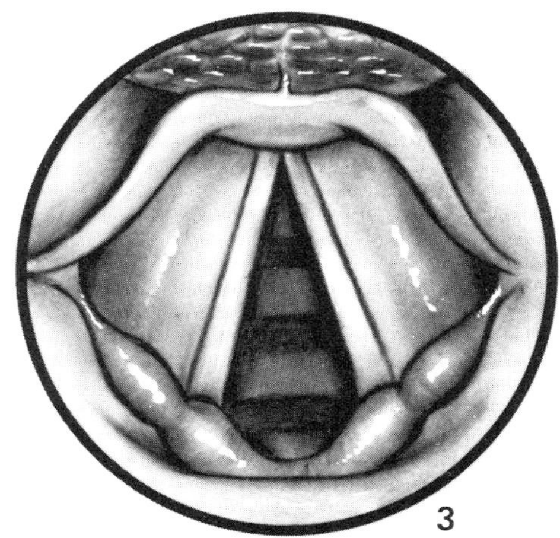

3

4

Advancing to the carina

Once in the trachea, the instrument is advanced to the carina, and any variation in the normal mobility and sharp edge of this structure should be noted.

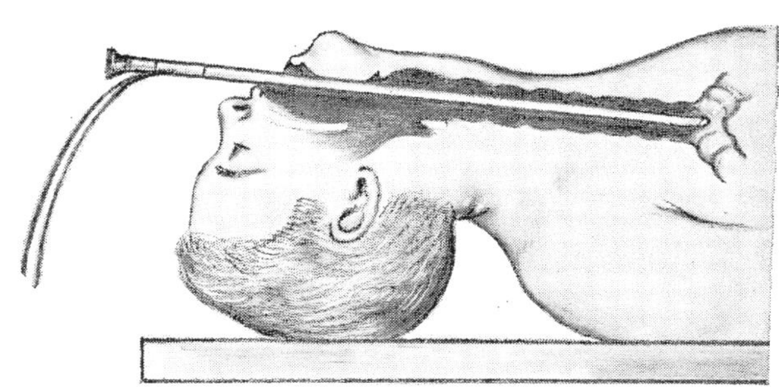

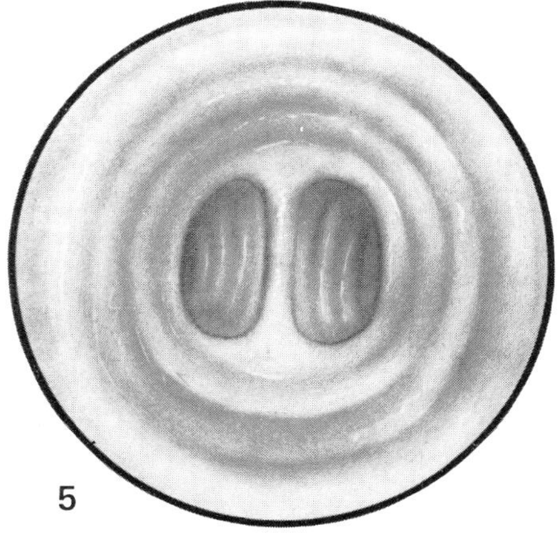

5

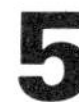

5

Inspection of bronchial tree

It is usual to examine the bronchial tree on both sides, starting with the presumed normal side first. To enter the left or right main bronchus, the head is slightly extended and deviated to the opposite side while the bronchoscope is advanced.

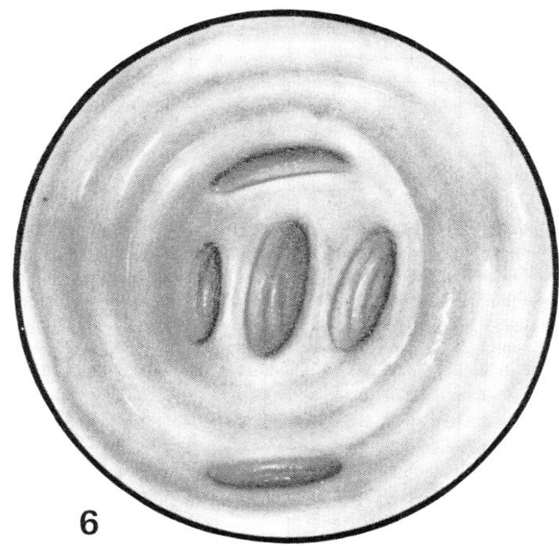

6

6

Upper lobe bronchi

The bronchi to the upper lobes can be examined either by direct view or with the aid of angled, illuminated telescopes. To get a good direct view into the upper lobes the head should be deviated and rotated well to the opposite side. The right upper lobe and its segmental divisions can usually be seen in this way without a telescope; the left side is less accessible and an angled telescope is often useful.

7

The bronchi

The basal segments of both lower lobes and the segmental divisions of the middle lobe and lingula can be inspected by direct vision, the view being magnified by a straight telescope if necessary.

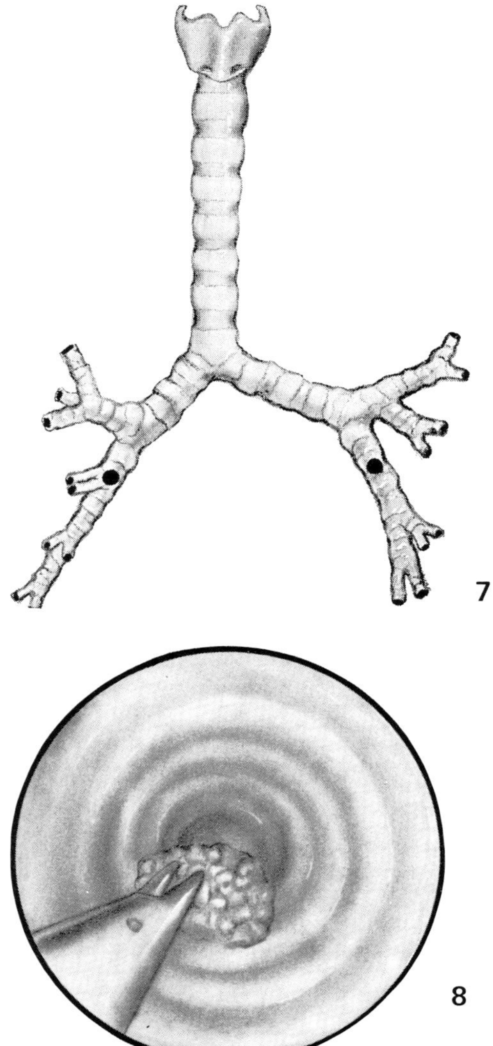

8

Biopsy of tumours

In about two out of three cases of carcinoma a tumour will be seen and biopsy can be readily carried out with the use of Brock's bronchoscopic biopsy forceps. Occasionally a 'blind' biopsy obtained from the depths of a bronchus may be helpful but such a procedure can cause severe haemorrhage and is rarely justified. Biopsy should be left as the final step of the investigation, it must never be done until the patient is able to cough and breathe spontaneously and should always be followed by careful aspiration of any blood or secretion.

Removal of foreign bodies

Prior to carrying out bronchoscopy for this purpose, the operator should be sure that there are available a good selection of suitable grasping forceps. The foreign body is usually to be found on the right side but may be obscured by secretions and mucosal swelling. If the foreign body is large it may not be possible to remove it through the instrument, and therefore the forceps and bronchoscope must be withdrawn together. The bronchial tree should be carefully inspected at the end of the procedure to ensure that no fragments have been missed and that all infected material is aspirated.

Difficulties

Difficulty is sometimes experienced in visualizing the larynx in patients with prominent teeth. In these circumstances the bronchoscope should be introduced between the molars rather than the incisors—choosing the side of the mouth opposite to that where the bronchial pathology is presumed to lie. The bronchoscope will then be in the line of the appropriate main bronchus.

Some operators prefer to expose the cords with a Negus operating laryngoscope to facilitate the passage of the bronchoscope.

POSTOPERATIVE COMPLICATIONS

Anoxia

Prolonged examination in the apnoeic patient will give rise to anoxia and may lead to cardiac arrest. When bronchoscopy is carried out under a relaxant the anaesthetist's duty to maintain the patient's oxygen saturation must take priority over the needs of the surgeon.

Bleeding

Some bleeding is almost inevitable after bronchial biopsy and usually causes no trouble if the patient is coughing and breathing well at the time the biopsy is taken. More serious haemorrhage can follow the biopsy of vascular tumours such as the adenoma. In these circumstances the patient should immediately be turned on the affected side and tilted head down to prevent obstruction of the good lung by blood. The bronchoscope should be removed gently when it is clear that the patient is breathing well and, even then, the instrument should be kept readily available lest respiratory obstruction by blood clot occur.

Oedema of larynx

Laryngeal oedema may follow the passage of too large an instrument in children. Nursing in a steam tent will usually be sufficient in the way of treatment, but steroids may be necessary.

Reference

Sanders, R. D. (1967). 'A ventilating attachment for bronchoscopy.' *Delaware med. J.* **39**, 170

[*The illustrations for this Chapter on Rigid Bronchoscopy were drawn by Mr. G. Lyth.*]

[*This Chapter has been taken from the Second Edition of Operative Surgery and amended by Mr. S. F. Stephenson.*]

Bronchoscopy. Flexible Instrument

S. F. Stephenson, F.R.C.S.
Thoracic Surgeon, East Birmingham Hospital, Birmingham

PRE - OPERATIVE

General

The bronchial fibrescope, being slender and flexible, penetrates further into the bronchial tree and gives a greater range of vision than the rigid instrument, especially within the upper lobes. But the fibrescope does not supercede the rigid bronchoscope which is still essential for the assessment of bronchial rigidity, the aspiration of copious secretions and the removal of foreign bodies.

Choice of technique

The easiest method is to pass the fibrescope through a rigid bronchoscope provided that the operator is experienced in the use of the rigid instrument and preferably under general anaesthesia. The second method, which causes less postoperative discomfort for the patient, is to pass the fibrescope through an endotracheal tube. This is very suitable for peripheral lesions, but for this technique general anaesthesia and oxygen inflation are essential since the fibrescope partially obstructs the airway. The third technique is to pass the instrument through the nose, with or without a short nasal tube, under local anaesthesia. This is usually well tolerated by the patient and it can be performed as a diagnostic procedure in the theatre, out-patient room or at the bedside. It is also a useful method for aspirating secretions in the ill patient at the bedside or in the intensive therapy unit.

THE OPERATIONS

1

USING A RIGID BRONCHOSCOPE

The rigid bronchoscope is passed as described in the previous section. The patient's head is adjusted so that the rigid instrument lies in the trachea directed at the carina and remains in position without being held. This frees both the operator's hands, one of which firmly holds the proximal end of the fibrescope and the other guides the warmed instrument into and through the bronchoscope, and is then free to take brushings or biopsies, to inject saline for bronchial washings or to clear the suction/biopsy channel of secretions, or to attach the camera and take photographs.

2

USING AN ENDOTRACHEAL TUBE

The anaesthetist passes the tube under general anaesthesia and gives oxygen intermittently through the side arm of a Nosworthy connection. The operator passes the fibrescope through a perforated cap on the end of the connection. The shaft of the instrument should be lubricated so that it slides easily.

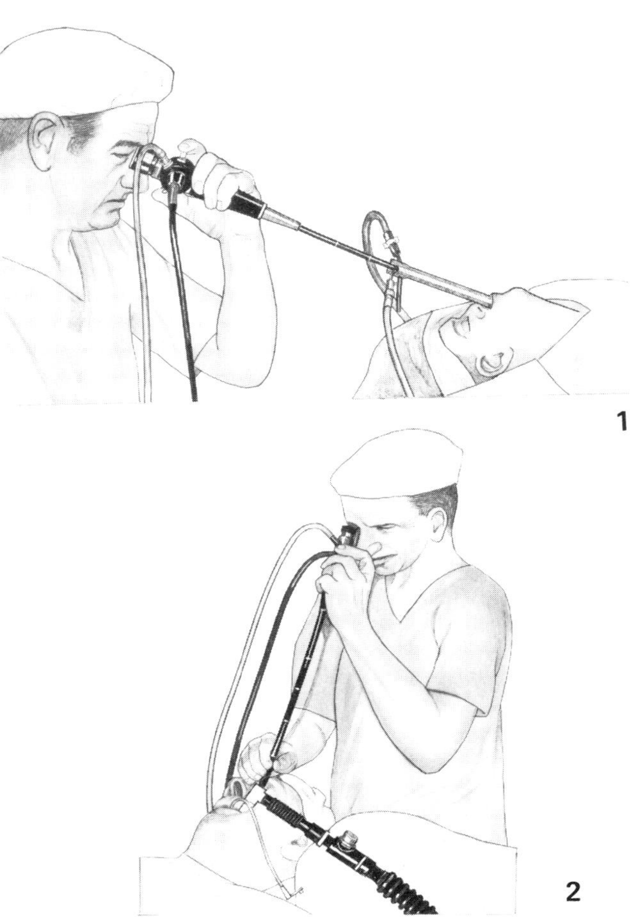

1

2

THE TRANSNASAL METHOD

Position of patient

The patient may be lying down or propped up on pillows or seated in a dental chair. The operator sits or stands facing the patient.

3

Passage of the fibrescope

Under local anaesthesia to the nose and pharynx a short nasal tube may be passed in either nostril. The lubricated fibrescope is passed through the tube and emerges above the larynx. Local anaesthetic is now injected onto and between the vocal cords. Practice is needed to manipulate the tip of the fibrescope behind the epiglottis and between the cords, and more local anaesthesia may be needed as the instrument advances to the carina and main bronchi.

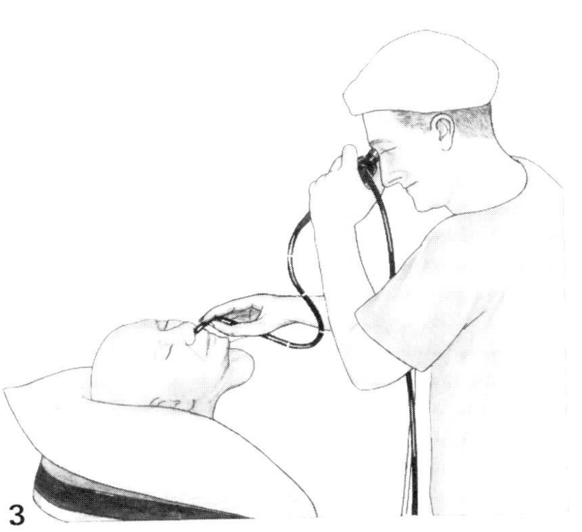

3

Difficulties

Considerable practice is needed before consistent results can be obtained with the bronchial fibrescope. Bronchial secretions or blood may obscure vision and are removed by suction, with irrigation if necessary. Biopsy instruments may cause further obscuration by pushing secretions out of the suction channel. Patience and experience enable the operator to get round these difficulties.

Complications

Complications are unusual. Haemorrhage may arise from biopsy sites or from using strong suction in small bronchi, but it is rarely if ever severe. Anoxia due to airway obstruction by the instrument may occur and is avoided by using general anaesthesia and oxygen inflation. Patients on mechanical ventilators need especial care. Passage of a fibrescope through an endotracheal tube under local anaesthesia should be avoided.

Care of instruments

Fibrescopes are delicate and expensive instruments. They should only be handled by staff trained in their use, and should be serviced regularly.

[*The illustrations for this Chapter on Flexible Bronchoscopy were drawn by Mr. F. Price.*]

Bronchography

L. L. Bromley, M.Chir., F.R.C.S.
Consultant Thoracic Surgeon, St. Mary's Hospital, London

PRE - OPERATIVE

Indications

Outlining the bronchial tree with contrast material can be valuable in the diagnosis of certain pulmonary conditions, notably bronchiectasis. It can be helpful in distinguishing bronchial carcinoma from subacute or chronic inflammatory conditions of the lung.

Choice of method

For children a general anaesthetic is necessary, the radio-opaque contrast being injected through a catheter passed down an endotracheal tube. For adults two methods are available under local anaesthesia. Injection down a catheter introduced into the trachea via the nose and pharynx, or direct introduction of a fine plastic tube into the trachea by puncture through the skin of the neck. The choice of method is largely individual and arrived at through the operator's familiarity with each technique.

Pre-operative preparation

Full explanation to adults of the nature of the procedure is necessary to achieve confidence and co-operation. Mild sedation given orally 1 hr beforehand with 10 mg Diazepam is helpful. If the patient is habitually coughing large amounts of sputum as in bronchiectasis a spell of tipping just before the examination is important.

Contrast material

Dionosil (propyliodone) is an organic iodide compound which is hydrolysed and absorbed from the bronchial tree within 2 or 3 days. It is excreted in the urine; iodides and iodine are not produced during degradation, thus sensitivity reactions should not be a problem. Aqueous and oil suspensions are available; rather less surface anaesthesia is needed if the oily suspension is used.

Bilateral examination

As a rule the side most under suspicion should be done first but where both sides are under review it is best to do the right first. In all cases the procedure is carried out in the radiological department.

THE OPERATION

1

NASOTRACHEAL CATHETER

One or other nasal passage and the oropharynx are sprayed with 2 per cent lignocaine. A few minutes later the laryngopharynx is sprayed and again a few minutes later the larynx is visualized by direct laryngoscopy and the cords themselves sprayed whilst the patient is inhaling deeply. If direct laryngoscopy is not possible the larynx and major bronchi may be surface anaesthetized by injection of 2 ml of 2 per cent lignocaine directly into the trachea through the skin in the mid-line of the neck. This injection is made rapidly at the moment of full expiration, the fluid being inhaled and sprayed upwards and downwards by the short coughing bout that follows. Not more than 8 ml of lignocaine should be used altogether. A fine plastic catheter is then passed through the nose and during deep breathing is passed on into the trachea–its arrival in the trachea being heralded by breath sounds in the tube itself. Previous measurement of the catheter length in relation to the patient's size and nasopharyngeal curve allows for placement of the tip about 2 cm above the carina. The catheter is fixed to the nose by adhesive strapping. The patient is then positioned leaning at 45° towards the side to be examined and the contrast material is injected. For an average adult 10 ml is adequate and it is injected over about 20 sec whilst the patient is told to breathe evenly and slightly more deeply than normal. He is asked to avoid coughing.

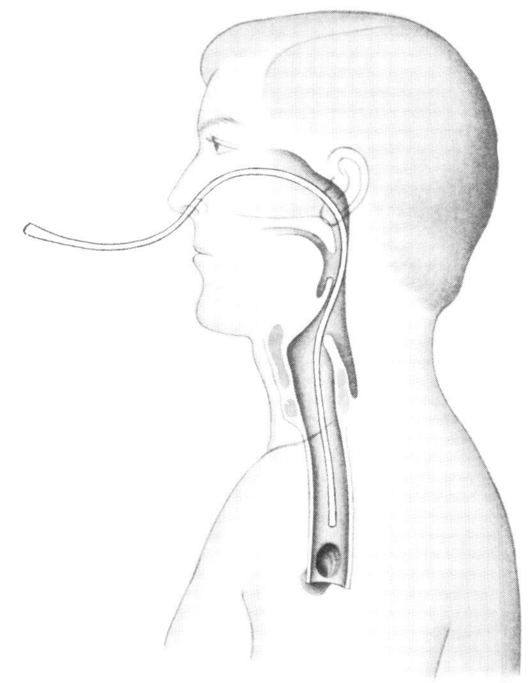

1

Positioning the patient

2

Position 1

For either side the positioning drill is the same. The basal segments will fill during injection of the contrast. Immediately the injection is finished the patient lies on his side, the head supported by one pillow. This position is held for 10 sec and should effect upper lobe filling.

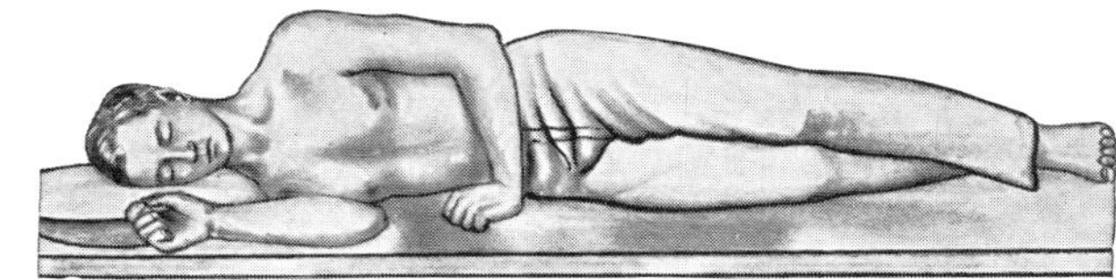

2

3

Position 2

The patient is then turned fully on to his face and kept in this position for 10 sec; this should effect filling of the middle lobe or lingula, and of the anterior segments of the upper and lower lobes.

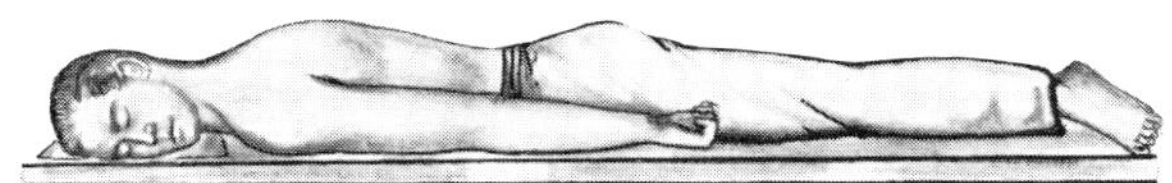

3

4

Position 3

He is now turned on to his back, the x-ray table is angled to give 15° Trendelenburg tilt; this should effect filling of the apical segments of the upper and lower lobes.

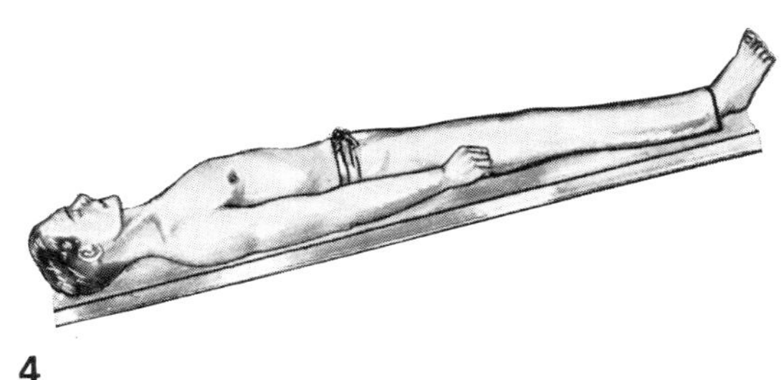

4

5

Position 4

The patient is now turned on to his side and the table is given a 10° reverse Trendelenburg tilt. It is important that these changes in position should be carried out smoothly and without delays. From the moment of starting to introduce the medium into the mouth to completion of the x-rays need not take more than 3 min. Radiographs are taken–lateral, oblique and anteroposterior views during held inspiration.

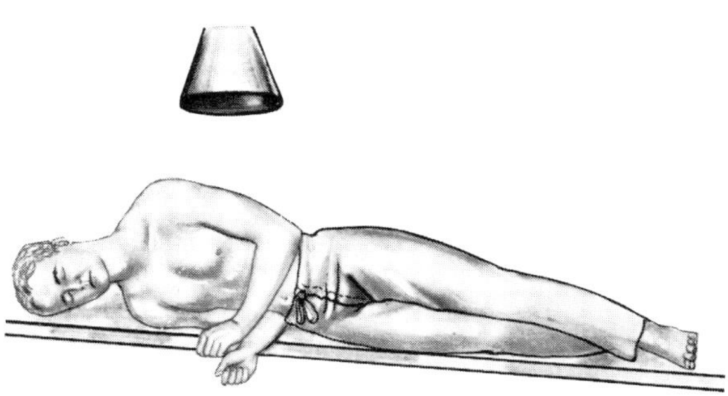

5

TRACHEAL PUNCTURE

Several suitable plastic intravenous cannulae are presently available. One of these, introduced via the lumen of a needle, is quite satisfactory for the purpose of tracheal puncture provided it has an internal diameter of about 1·5 mm (e.g. Bard 1-catheter).

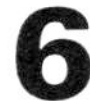

6

The skin and subcuticular tissues overlying the crico-thyroid membrane or upper 2 cm of the trachea are anaesthetized with 2 per cent lignocaine and the needle advanced into the trachea. Three millilitres of local anaesthetic are then injected as previously described and the needle withdrawn. The needle catheter unit is then introduced along the same track. When the trachea is entered the catheter is advanced and the needle withdrawn and secured if required in a plastic lock to avoid any risk of movement and subsequent cutting at the catheter/needle point junction. The injection of contrast material is then made as previously described.

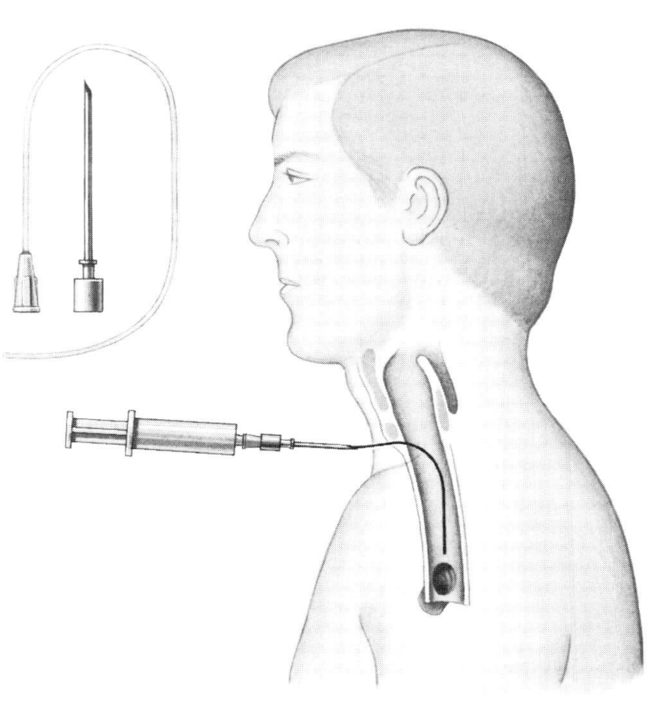

6

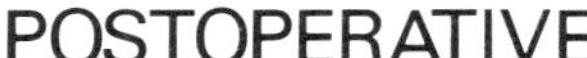

POSTOPERATIVE

After the radiographs are developed and judged satisfactory, the patient is tilted 20° head down and encouraged to cough up as much of the contrast material as he can. Because of the local anaesthetic of the laryngopharynx he is not allowed to drink or eat for 4 hr after the procedure.

[*The illustrations for this Chapter on Bronchography were drawn by Mr. G. Lyth and Mr. M. J. Courtney.*]

Aspiration of the Chest, Pleural Biopsy and Needle Biopsy of the Lung

L. L. Bromley, M.Chir., F.R.C.S.
Consultant Thoracic Surgeon, St. Mary's Hospital, London

ASPIRATION OF THE CHEST

PRE-OPERATIVE

Indications

Aspiration of the pleural cavity is indicated for diagnostic and therapeutic reasons. When fluid is present it may be serous, serosanguinous, purulent, pure blood or chyle. Thus aspiration of the chest may be required in a variety of acute and chronic clinical situations where laboratory examination of a specimen of the fluid is required to aid diagnosis. For therapy it may be necessary to remove fluid (often a large volume) to allow expansion of a compressed lung and thus improve respiration.

Biopsy of the parietal pleura is a useful adjunct to the procedure especially to help in the diagnosis of tuberculous and malignant effusions. There are no special contra-indications to the procedures except for those patients who may have a coagulation defect (e.g. already on an anticoagulant or with severe liver disease).

Anaesthesia

The procedure is done under local anaesthesia of the chest wall using lignocaine hydrochloride 1 per cent solution. This is 10 mg/ml. The maximum dose is 200 mg; thus up to 20 ml can be used. Usually, however, only 5–10 ml are needed.

A small intradermal wheal is raised with a fine needle at the chosen site. The needle is then changed to a long fine one and this is advanced through the muscles of the chest wall and into the intercostal space. Local anaesthetic is introduced.

It is important to keep the needle towards the lower part of the space away from the neurovascular bundle which lies in the subcostal groove. When the parietal pleura is reached the patient may experience a sharp pain; the slow advance of the needle is then stopped and 2 ml local anaesthetic are introduced. The needle is then withdrawn.

TECHNIQUE

1

Equipment

Special equipment is illustrated. The success and comfort of an aspiration is largely dependent on the use of a good two-way stopcock, which must possess an adequate lumen, have a tap that can be moved without the application of force and which does not leak.

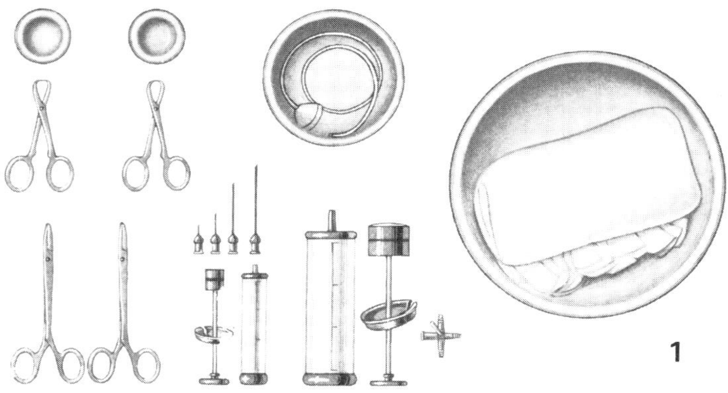

1

Pleural aspiration

2

Site of puncture and introduction of aspirating needle

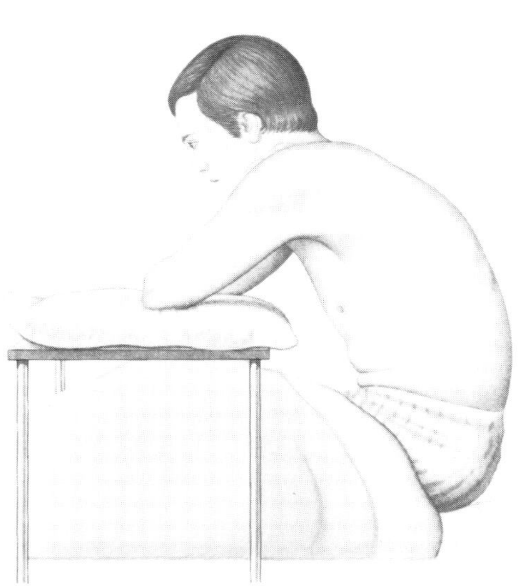

2

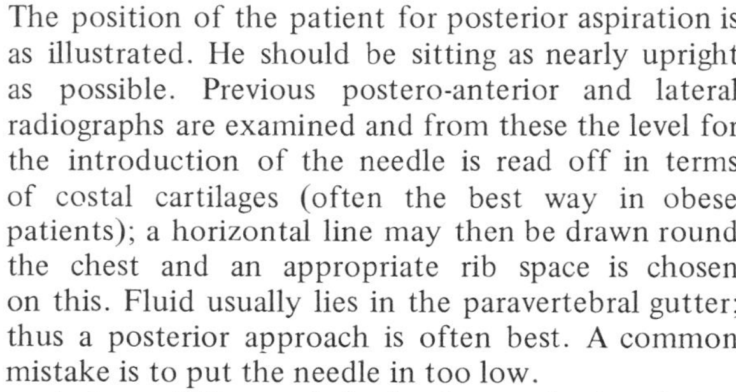

The position of the patient for posterior aspiration is as illustrated. He should be sitting as nearly upright as possible. Previous postero-anterior and lateral radiographs are examined and from these the level for the introduction of the needle is read off in terms of costal cartilages (often the best way in obese patients); a horizontal line may then be drawn round the chest and an appropriate rib space is chosen on this. Fluid usually lies in the paravertebral gutter; thus a posterior approach is often best. A common mistake is to put the needle in too low.

A few millilitres of the local anaesthetic solution are drawn up into a 20 or 50 ml syringe, the two-way tap fitted, and then a suitable wide-bore aspirating needle is fixed to the distal end of the tap. The discharge tubing is connected to the other outlet of the tap. The needle is then introduced along the track previously infiltrated with local anaesthetic and as the parietal pleura is approached very slight suction is applied to the plunger of the syringe. Arrival in the pleural cavity is indicated when more fluid appears in the syringe. With some fluid already in the syringe, it is easier to see and feel when the intrapleural collection is reached than if a dry empty syringe is used.

3

Withdrawal of fluid

This should be conducted steadily and slowly. A Spencer-Wells forceps will, if clamped on the needle at skin level, hold the needle at the desired depth. As a general rule in aspirations other than for diagnosis, as much fluid as possible should be removed; in the case of a loculated effusion more than one puncture will be necessary. Towards the end of the procedure it is often found that fluid enters the syringe in a jerky fashion, coming most easily on expiration—a sign that the amount of fluid remaining is small. It is important that air should not be sucked into the chest by leakage at the joints in and around the tap.

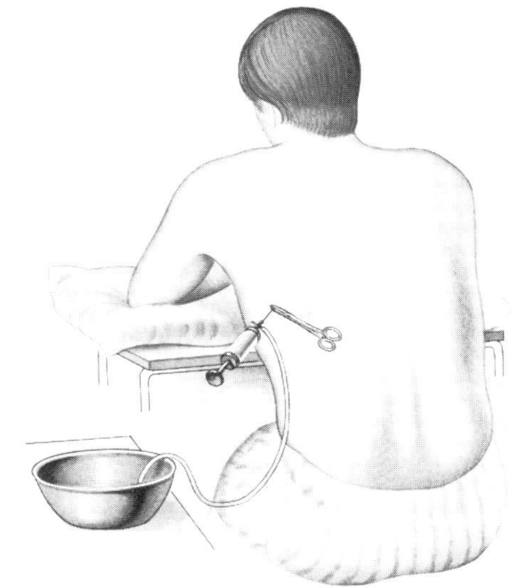

3

PLEURAL BIOPSY

4

Pleural aspiration and pleural biopsy can be satisfactorily combined by the use of the Abrams needle. Having established the position of the intrapleural collection of fluid by aspiration of a small amount as already described, a 5 mm skin incision is made at the site of the original intradermal wheal and the Abrams needle introduced into the chest wall. A three-way tap and syringe are then connected, the needle advanced further and the pleural cavity entered. The inner trocar of the needle is then rotated anticlockwise fully into a locked position and free withdrawal of the fluid is now possible. When sufficient has been removed the whole needle is slightly angulated and slowly pulled back until the side window is felt to catch on the parietal pleura. The inner trocar of the assembly is then rotated sharply clockwise and as it advances it will cut off a small specimen. The whole needle is then withdrawn and the specimen for histology retrieved from within the needle tip.

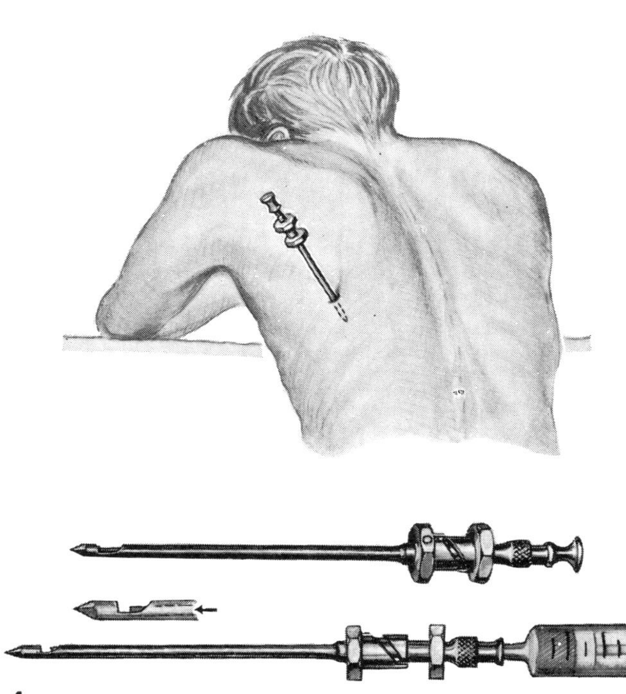

4

NEEDLE BIOPSY OF THE LUNG

Indications

Obtaining a small sample of lung for microscopy is very useful in the diagnosis of many general diseases of the lung, e.g. fibrosing alveolitis and selective biopsy of a localized peripherally situated lung lesion is possible with x-ray image intensifier guidance.

Anaesthesia

Local infiltration of the chest wall and parietal pleura overlying the segment of the lung to be biopsied is made with 1 per cent lignocaine.

5

Drill biopsy

After making a 3 mm nick in the skin a specially designed needle (Steel pattern) is introduced as far as the parietal pleura and its trocar withdrawn. The needle is then connected to a high-speed compressed air drill and the patient asked to hold his breath in full inspiration. The air flow button is then pressed down and the needle rapidly and fully advanced. The drill is then replaced by a syringe containing 5 ml of saline and suction applied as the needle is withdrawn. The specimen is then ejected into a container for examination.

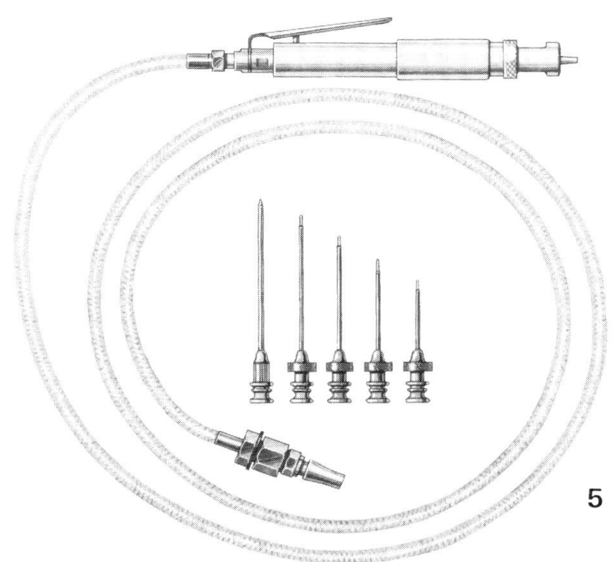

5

6

Needle biopsy

A 'Trucut' needle may be used with similar local anaesthesia.

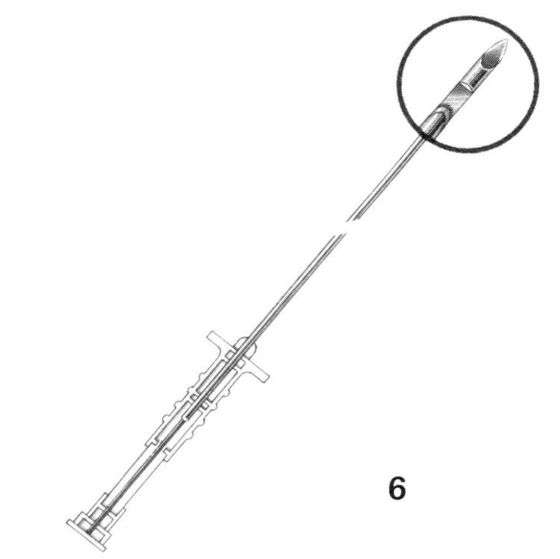

6

POSTOPERATIVE CARE

The development of a small pneumothorax is not uncommon but it is rare to be large enough to require tube drainage. A chest x-ray should be taken 1 hr after the procedure or sooner if there is any respiratory distress.

Occasionally there develops some staining of the patient's sputum but significant haemoptysis is unlikely unless the biopsy needle is introduced too deeply towards the hilum of the lung.

[*The illustrations for this Chapter on Aspiration of the Chest, Pleural Biopsy and Needle Biopsy of the Lung were drawn by Mr. M. J. Courtney and Mr. R. N. Lane.*]

Mediastinoscopy and Anterior Mediastinotomy

H. C. Nohl-Oser, D.M., F.R.C.S.
Consultant Thoracic Surgeon, Harefield, Hillingdon and West Middlesex Hospitals

MEDIASTINOSCOPY

PRE-OPERATIVE

Indications and contra-indications

This procedure is of value in the diagnosis of any case of hilar or mediastinal lymphadenopathy and can also be used to assess the operability of cases of bronchial carcinoma. Mediastinoscopy will often establish the diagnosis of intrathoracic disease—especially when all other diagnostic methods have failed to yield results—such as bronchial carcinoma, Hodgkin's disease, sarcoidosis, mediastinal glandular tuberculosis, pneumoconiosis and other conditions.

Thymic growths and other anterior mediastinal tumours cannot be approached safely by this method as these tumours lie in front of the great vessels. Superior vena caval obstruction is not a contra-indication *per se.* Once the bleeding from the skin incision has been stopped and the distended veins in the neck retracted laterally, there are no engorged veins in the pretracheal area and it is safe to take a biopsy.

Complications

Serious haemorrhage can occur while taking a biopsy, through injury to the superior vena cava, vena azygos, arch of the aorta, pulmonary arteries or even the left atrium in front of the left main bronchus. In such an event the mediastinum must be packed tightly with swabs through the mediastinoscope and a postero-lateral thoracotomy performed on the side from which the biopsy was taken. It is a mistake to try the anterior approach through a median sternotomy.

Other complications known to occur are injury to the left recurrent laryngeal nerve and pneumothorax.

Special equipment and apparatus

Diathermy for coagulation of small vessels, Langenbeck retractors, Carlen's mediastinoscope or a Negus laryngoscope, Brock's short (28 cm) cupped broncho-scopy biopsy forceps, crocodile forceps for carrying small swabs and blunt dissection, a sucker and a long aspirating needle with attached syringe, are essential instruments.

Anaesthesia

Mediastinoscopy is frequently combined with a bronchoscopy. Under those circumstances, the mediastinoscopy should always precede the broncho-scopy as this avoids anaesthetic difficulties due to intrabronchial bleeding following bronchial biopsy.

Induction is with thiopentone and succinylcholine. A cuffed endotracheal tube is passed after spraying the vocal cords and trachea with 4 per cent lignocaine. If the mediastinoscopy is to be followed by broncho-scopy, anaesthesia is maintained by nitrous oxide, oxygen and halothane and intermittent positive-pressure ventilation. This technique induces a certain degree of hypotension, which is useful in minimizing bleeding during the procedure; on the other hand, frequent monitoring of the blood pressure is essential and a vein must be kept open for transfusion.

For the bronchoscopy which follows, further succinylcholine is given, preceded, however, by atropine which will give protection against the common bradycardia.

Should mediastinoscopy be the only procedure, then the standard nitrous oxide, oxygen-relaxant technique is satisfactory, although it will not produce the advantageous hypotensive effect.

THE OPERATION

1

Position of patient

The neck is extended by placing a sandbag under the shoulders, while excessive extension and movement of the head are avoided by a U-shaped bolster under the occiput. The table is tilted slightly feet downwards to lessen venous congestion.

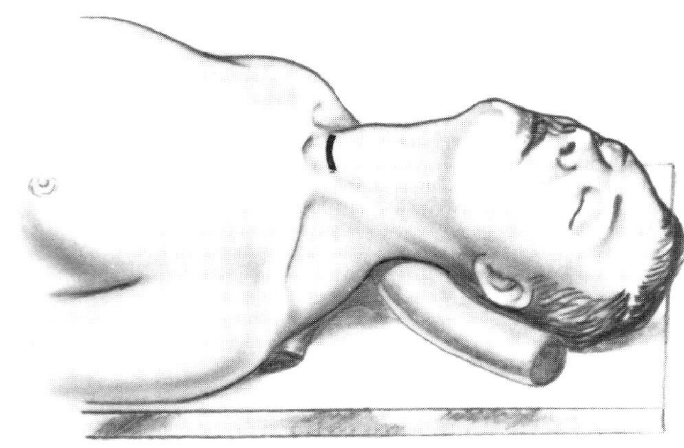

1

2

The incision

A transverse 2 inch (5 cm) incision, in line with the skin folds, is made just above the suprasternal notch. The pretracheal muscles are separated vertically in the mid-line, coagulating small vessels.

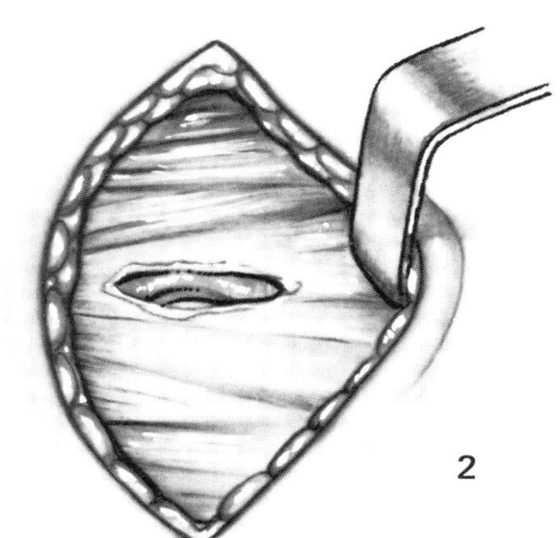

2

3

3

Exposure of trachea

The pretracheal muscles, together with the inferior thyroid veins, are retracted to either side. This exposes the pretracheal fascia, which is incised transversely.

4

Dissection into mediastinum

The lower flap of the pretracheal fascia is lifted up with dissecting forceps and a tunnel is made, downwards into the mediastinum, by blunt finger dissection, keeping the dorsum of the finger all the time in contact with the anterior surface of the trachea.

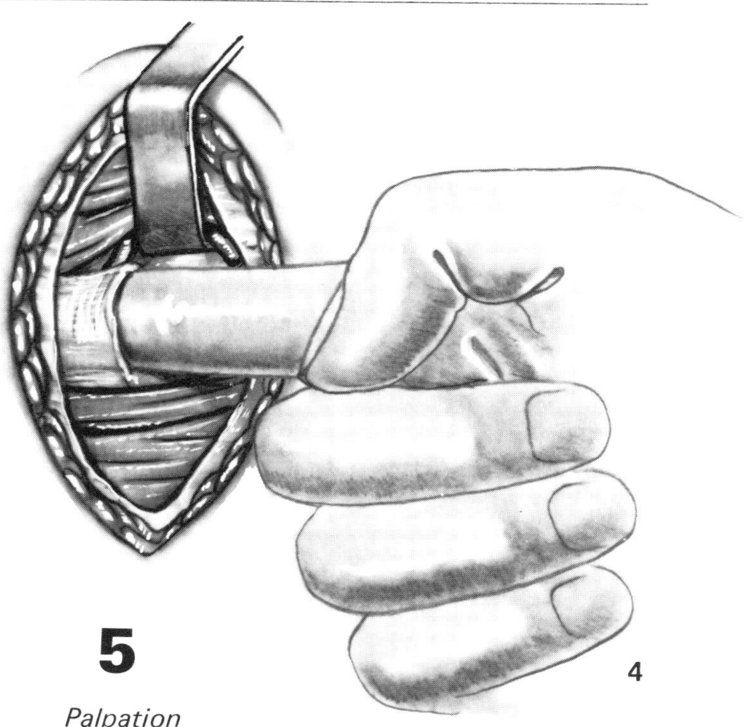

4

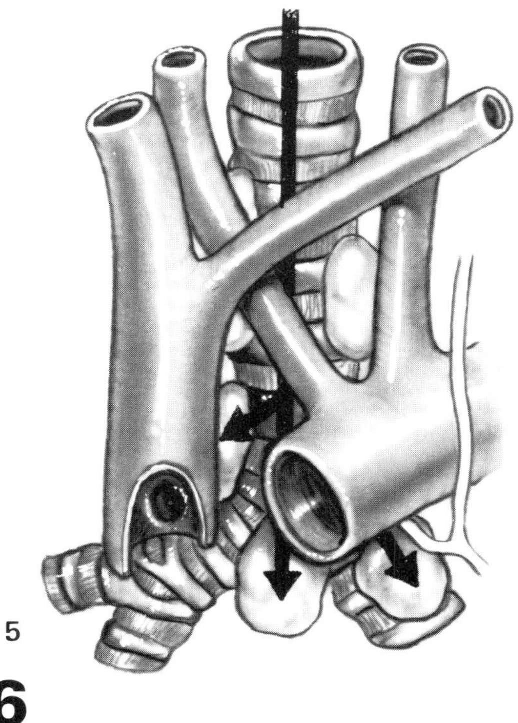

5

5

Palpation

Much information can be obtained by palpation alone. The plane of the dissection (arrowed) lies behind the great vessels, the pulsation of the innominate artery in front and to the right and the arch of the aorta to the left can be felt distinctly. In the majority of cases the origin of each main bronchus can be palpated lower down by feeling for the superior tracheobronchial angle. At this point the finger breaks gently through the pretracheal fascia, as the superior tracheobronchial and paratracheal lymph nodes lie outside this fascial envelope.

6

Biopsy

Carlens' mediastinoscope or the Negus laryngoscope is next introduced into the prepared tunnel. Further dissection is carried out with the crocodile forceps. The paratracheal lymph nodes, the superior tracheobronchial nodes and those in the subcarinal (inferior tracheobronchial) region are accessible. Before a biopsy is taken aspiration of the tissue is advisable for the inexperienced operator, as these nodes lie in proximity to the large vessels. The biopsy itself is best achieved with Brock's bronchoscopy biopsy forceps.

Closure

The pretracheal muscles are approximated with a catgut suture and a subcutaneous interrupted catgut suture will obliterate the dead space.

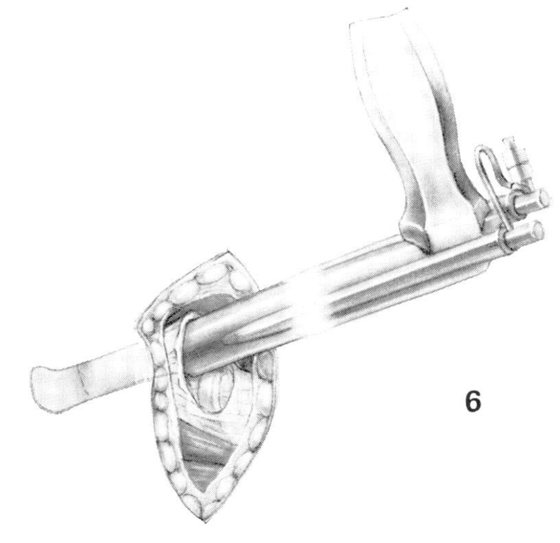

6

ANTERIOR MEDIASTINOTOMY

Indications

This procedure gives access to any structures lying in the anterior mediastinum, i.e. in front of the great vessels, which cannot be approached by mediastinoscopy. Some surgeons advocate anterior mediastinotomy in addition to mediastinoscopy in the pre-operative assessment of bronchogenic carcinoma of the left upper lobe, as there is evidence that the lymphatic spread from that lobe is frequently to the anterior mediastinal group of nodes. Other surgeons maintain that the field of vision during mediastinoscopy is too restricted and therefore prefer mediastinotomy. It is also recommended by some authors, because the wider exposure makes it possible, by opening the pleura, to inspect the hilum of the lung and even take lung biopsies, if necessary. This in fact, amounts to a limited thoracotomy.

It is only possible to explore one or the other side of the mediastinum with this technique, so that careful operative radiological assessment is necessary.

THE OPERATION

7

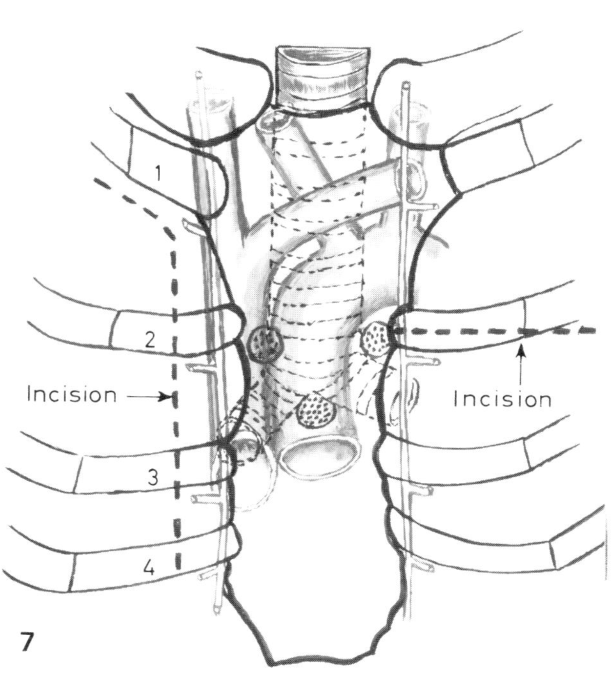

7

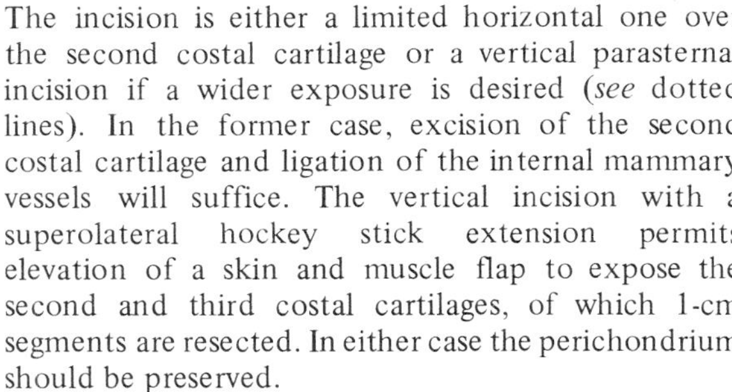

The incision is either a limited horizontal one over the second costal cartilage or a vertical parasternal incision if a wider exposure is desired (*see* dotted lines). In the former case, excision of the second costal cartilage and ligation of the internal mammary vessels will suffice. The vertical incision with a superolateral hockey stick extension permits elevation of a skin and muscle flap to expose the second and third costal cartilages, of which 1-cm segments are resected. In either case the perichondrium should be preserved.

By blunt dissection behind the sternum, pushing the pleura and phrenic nerve laterally, the anterior mediastinal space is entered. With the vertical parasternal incision it is possible, on the right, to expose the right paratracheal and subcarinal nodes by developing a plane of dissection between the superior vena cava and the ascending aorta; on the left side, the anterior hilar area at the pulmonary artery root and the subaortic area can be examined. Should no pathology be found in the lymph node areas, then entrance into the pleural space allows further evaluation of the extent of any tumour present or permits a lung biopsy to be taken.

A drainage tube is inserted down to the operation site before the incision is closed and connected to an under-water seal.

References

Mediastinoscopy, Proceedings of an International Symposium, Edited by Otto Jepson and H. Rahbek Sorensen, Odense University Press, Denmark, 1971.

Stemmer, E. A., Calvin, J. W., Chandor, S. B. and Connolly, J. E. (1965). 'Mediastinal biopsy for indeterminate pulmonary and mediastinal lesions.' *J. thorac. cardiovasc. Surg.* 49, 405

[*Illustrations 1–6 for this Chapter on Mediastinoscopy and Anterior Mediastinotomy were drawn by Mr. G. Lyth. Illustration 7 was drawn by the Author.*]

Surgical Access in Pulmonary Operations

R. H. F. Brain, F.R.C.S.
Consultant Thoracic Surgeon, Guy's Hospital, London

PRE-OPERATIVE

General

Although chest surgery has become standardized in many ways it is still difficult to systematize the thoracic approach even in pure pulmonary surgery, because of the many individual preferences that persist for the same operation.

The surgeon is concerned both with obtaining adequate access to particular parts of the thoracic cavity, and with the provision of sufficient room for manoeuvre inside. In this latter connection — bearing in mind that a lung is a space-occupying and mobile organ — it is not surprising to find, for example, that competition with the anaesthetist was common until the introduction of the double-lumen intratracheal tube made single-lung anaesthesia possible. The use of this tube or the adoption of a similar procedure enables the surgeon to operate at will in a clear field with a quiet, completely collapsed lung.

Importance of the patient's position on the table

Since the position of the patient on the table largely governs the approach, a suitable table, with chest attachments capable of fixing the patient firmly, is very necessary. In addition it should be possible to move the patient easily during the operation by rotation and tilting of the table.

Special positions, such as the 'head up' or 'sitting', the 'head down' or even the 'prone' position, were often used in the past when operating on 'wet' patients liable to produce large quantities of purulent sputum during the operation, with the risk of its aspiration elsewhere in the bronchial tree. Bronchus 'blockers' in the first instance and nowadays double-lumen intratracheal tubes allow, in addition to single-lung anaesthesia, the frequent aspiration of either side without interfering with ventilation.

Pre-operative preparation

Pulmonary operations, other than 'emergencies', should never be hurried. After admission a proper period of acclimatization of the patient to the ward and to the staff is necessary. Not only does this allow all-round confidence to be established but it also gives time for adequate physiotherapy. The latter, in addition to helping respiratory function, also reduces the risks of infection by promoting bronchial drainage and consequently sputum reduction. At the same time it enables general exercises to improve the general health of the patient and builds up 'solid' nitrogen nutritional reserve. During this time stress should be placed on activity; no patient able to get up should be allowed to rest in bed more than is strictly necessary. In this way a tendency to pre- and postoperative venous thrombosis is kept to a minimum.

A complete ban on smoking for only a few days will reduce the amount of postoperative sputum and infection.

Other investigations at this time normally include, in addition to the usual blood studies, ventilation and blood gas measurements. The latter in particular provides a useful baseline for possible respiratory failure problems after surgery.

Chemotherapy is occasionally indicated for serious specific infections by organisms such as the tubercle bacillus or the *Staphylococcus pyogenes*; but the 'routine' use, with its tendency to promote resistant strains, is deplored.

Bronchoscopy performed as an immediate pre-operative measure allows for a final appraisal of the situation and toilet of the bronchial tree.

Anaesthesia

Since the almost total decline of thoracoplasty, local anaesthesia is never used, apart from minor procedures on the chest wall and occasionally in the drainage of empyema. General anaesthesia, using non-toxic drugs, non-inflammable gases, muscle relaxants and mechanically controlled ventilation of the lungs, is now the rule.

1

Double-lumen intratracheobronchial tube (Carlens' or Robertshaw)

After induction, a suitable size of one or other of the double-lumen bronchial catheters available is introduced in the supine position before the patient is placed in position on the table.

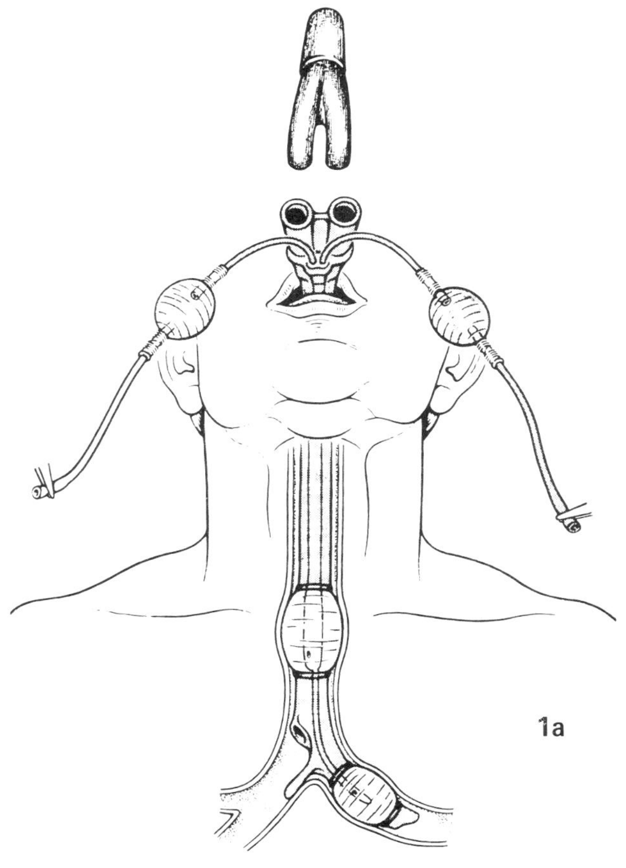

1a

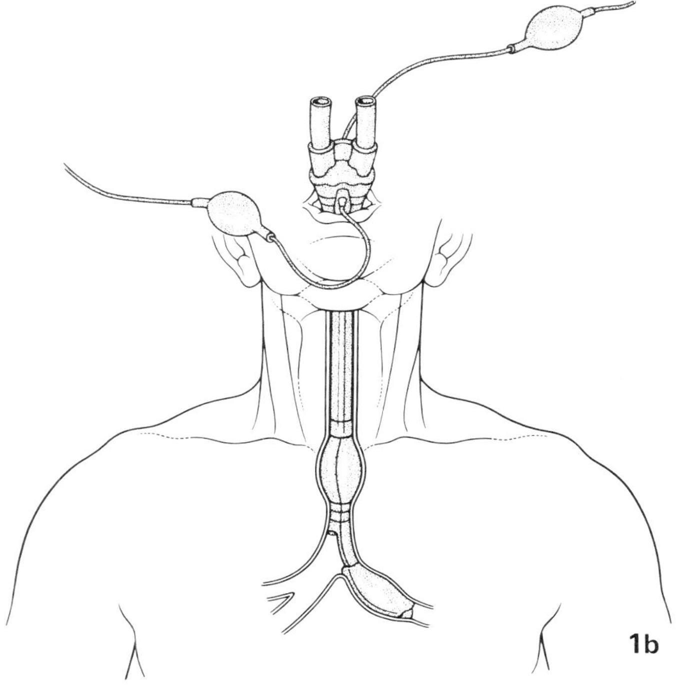

1b

THE OPERATION

Thoracotomy (posterolatero-anterior types)

In the past it has been customary to subdivide the standard lateral approach into posterolateral and anterolateral, depending upon the exact siting of the operative field. This may still apply for the mediastinum, but for lung surgery the incision beginning posteriorly is carried forwards varying distances depending upon the size of the chest opening required. On the whole an easy access makes for safer surgery and a full anterolateral incision is preferred to the division of the back end of the ribs above and/or below the incision, when perhaps later access is found to be inadequate.

For pulmonary surgery it is usual to enter the chest through the bed of the fifth rib for upper lobe operations and whole lung resection, and through the bed of the sixth rib for lower and middle lobe operations.

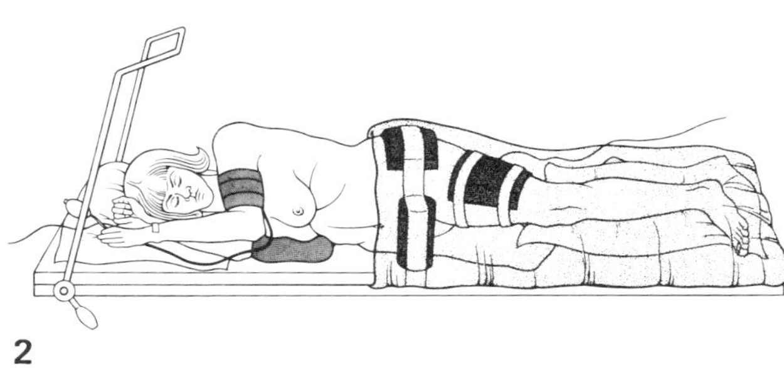

2

2

Position of patient

Attention is drawn, first, to the methods of firm fixation of the patient – movement during the operation is undesirable; secondly, to the intravenous drip position and to the underlying axillary pillow which serves to facilitate thoracotomy by widening the intercostal spaces on the operation side. The diathermy pad is strapped to the uppermost thigh, and its terminal and leads kept well away from the skin of the patient, avoiding the risk of burns.

Excessive heat loss during the operation is avoided by the covering of the lower half of the patient by a heat-reflecting 'space' blanket.

Four towels are arranged, two parallel to the prepared skin incision, with one anterior and one posterior forming a rectangle. A large abdominal sheet over the head of the table covers the anaesthetic screen and the intravenous drip apparatus, while a second large sheet covers a Mayo tray or similar table and the remainder of the patient below the operation area.

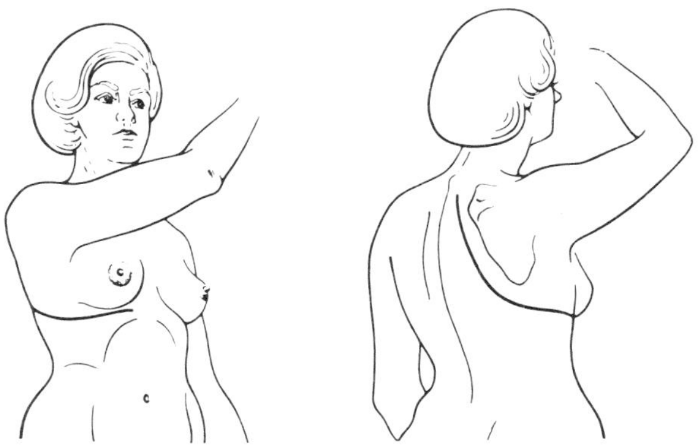

3

3

The skin incision

After towelling it is now customary to cover the exposed wound area with a sterile adhesive plastic sheet that serves both as an additional fixative for the surrounding towels and as a 'guard' against infection for the edges of the wound.

The posterolatero-anterior incision begins in front just lateral to the sternocostal junction and running backwards immediately below the angle of the scapula, then turns upwards running in the line midway between its vertebral border and the mid-line posteriorly to a level nearing the upper border of the scapula, depending upon the chest wall entry level selected.

4

Diathermy

The wound is opened progressively, beginning in front with a 2 – 3 inch (5 – 7·5 cm) incision, all bleeding points are then secured and diathermied before the wound is extended further, thus keeping the blood loss to an absolute minimum.

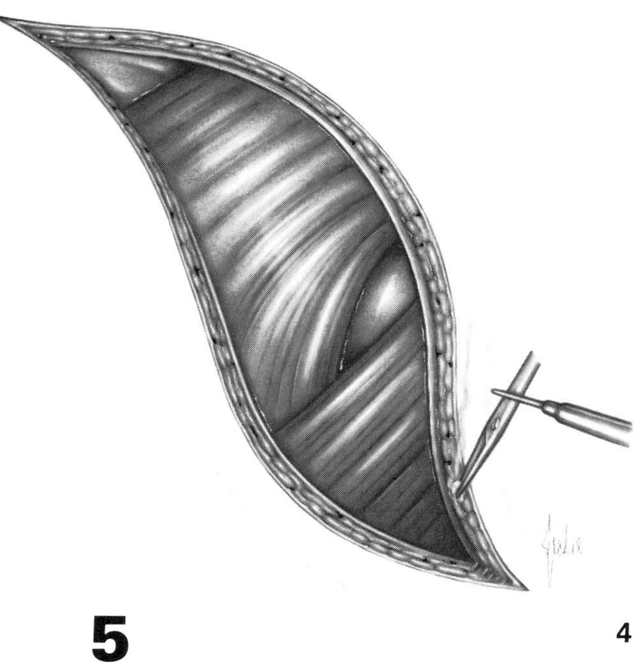

4

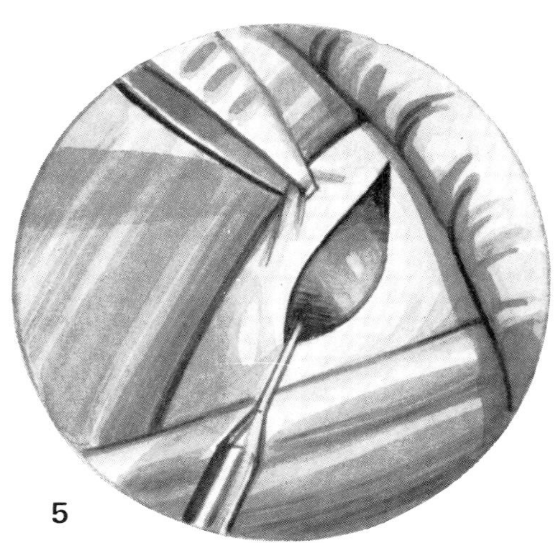

5

5

Exposure of chest wall

Entrance to muscle planes is made easier by first defining the small fascial triangle behind the latissimus dorsi muscle between it and the lateral border of the trapezius muscle, incising through it and the underlying rhomboid muscle until the chest wall is reached.

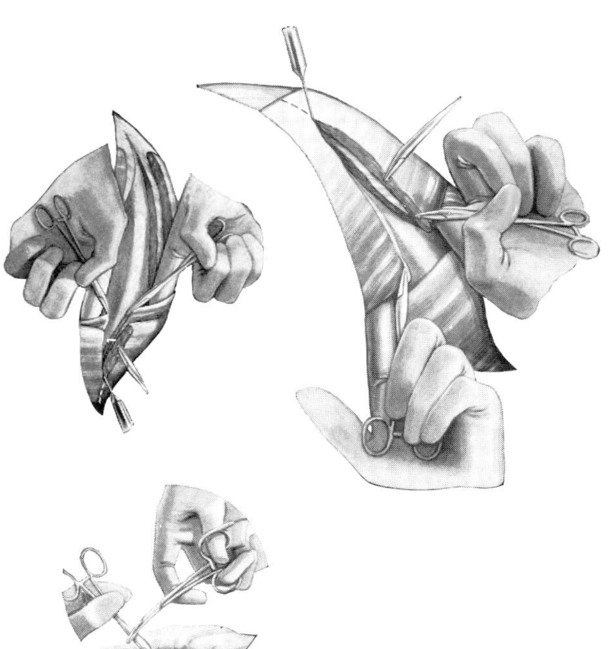

6

6

Incision of muscles

The assistant's and the surgeon's index fingers are used to elevate the muscles, and they are then incised parallel to the wound with a diathermy coagulating current, meticulously picking up and coagulating bleeding points as they are met.

7

Entry through thoracic cage

Selection of rib. The exact rib required is defined by counting from above down under the elevated scapula, beginning at the second; the first is usually impalpable unless the posterior scalene has been divided. The rib chosen will depend on the projected operative procedure; the fifth and the sixth are the more usual ones.

On special occasions a 'double' thoracotomy may be helpful. For example when, through the standard approach, extreme difficulty is encountered in mobilizing a lung from the diaphragm or costophrenic angles; a second incision through the eighth and ninth rib bed performed through the same skin/muscle incision will provide a solution.

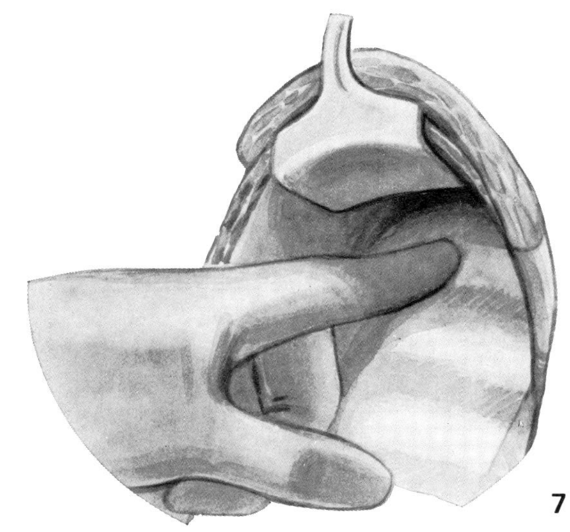
7

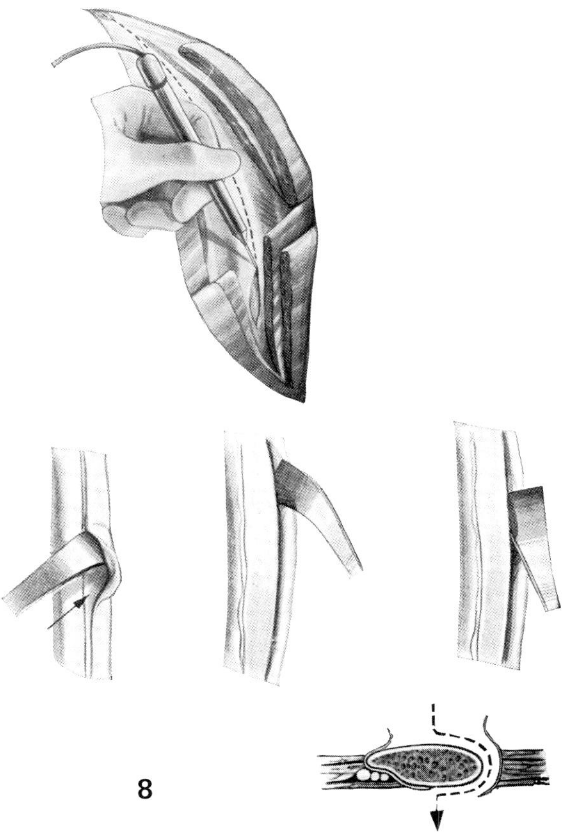
8

8

Incision and eversion of periosteum

The periosteum is incised with diathermy in the mid-rib plane. The periosteum of the upper half of the rib is raised. In this way interference with the intercostal neurovascular bundle below the rib is avoided. Ribs never need to be resected in straightforward thoracotomy.

9

Entry into pleural cavity

Entry into the pleural cavity is made by incising through the rib bed.

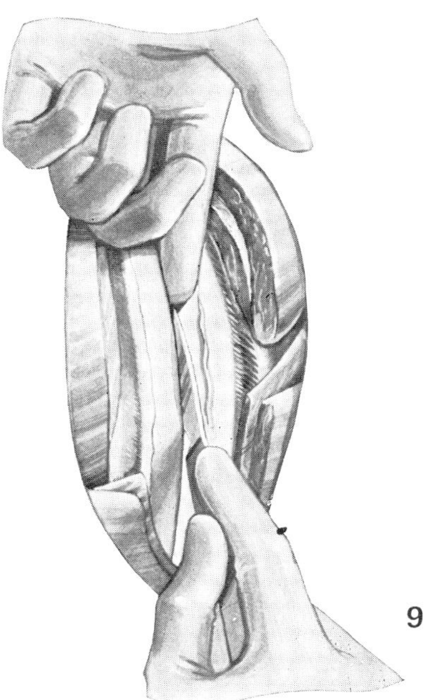

9

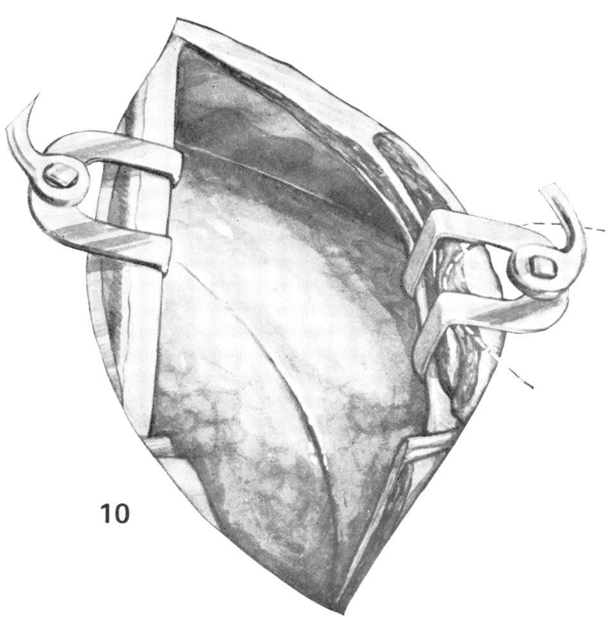

10

10

Introduction of retractor

Adhesions in the neighbourhood of the incision between the chest wall and lung are first divided so that a large self-retaining retractor of the Tudor-Edwards or Price-Thomas type may be introduced, spreading the wound widely without tearing the lung or damaging the ribs.

11 & 12

Drainage of chest

Depending upon the exact operative procedure, it may be necessary temporarily to drain the pleural cavity, usually for the first 48 hr after the operation. An intercostal tube is introduced anterior to the mid-axillary line below the incision immediately prior to closure of the periosteum and later attached to an underwater seal drainage bottle. The tube runs obliquely through the chest wall into the pleural cavity and then laterally around the outer side of the lobe or lung, posteriorly to the apex of the pleural space. In this way the tube will not be angulated and obstructed in the normal supine position in bed, and drainage will be facilitated by gravity. When the tube is removed a simple firm adhesive dressing will be all that is necessary to prevent air entry from the exterior. Suture of the tube drainage site is not recommended because of the risk of infection.

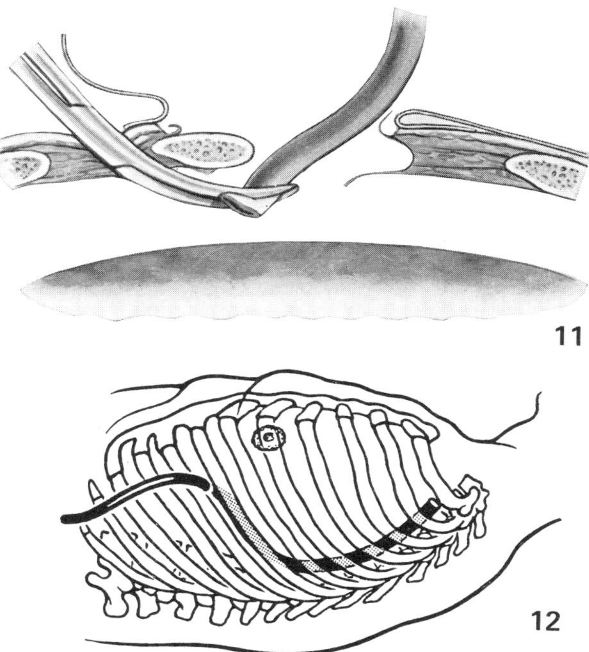

11

12

Closure of wound

13

Approximation of chest wall

At the conclusion of the intrathoracic portion of the operation with the removal of the retractor, manual approximation of the chest wall is usually an easy matter. However, in elderly subjects it may sometimes be necessary to use instrumental approximation.

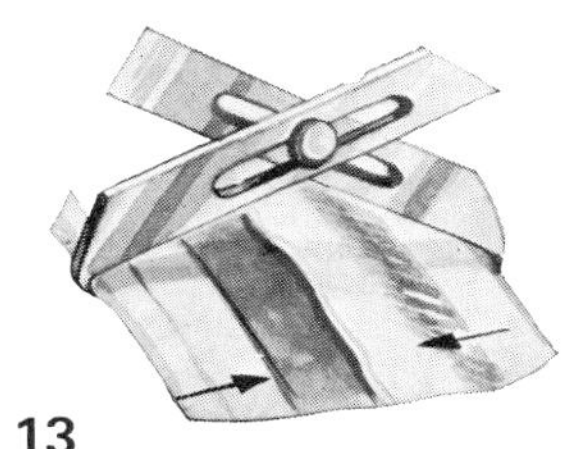

13

Suture of periosteum

The periosteum is sutured with interrupted nylon or catgut stitches at approximately 1 cm intervals.

14

Re-inforced rib approximation

This is recommended, using wire or strong monofilamentous non-absorbable suture material introduced in the transcostal position. A strong airtight closure able to withstand the explosive force of coughing is important; it will prevent dehiscence and the collection of air and fluid from the pleura within the layers of the wound later. The chronic bronchitic, the obese and the elderly are especially prone to this complication.

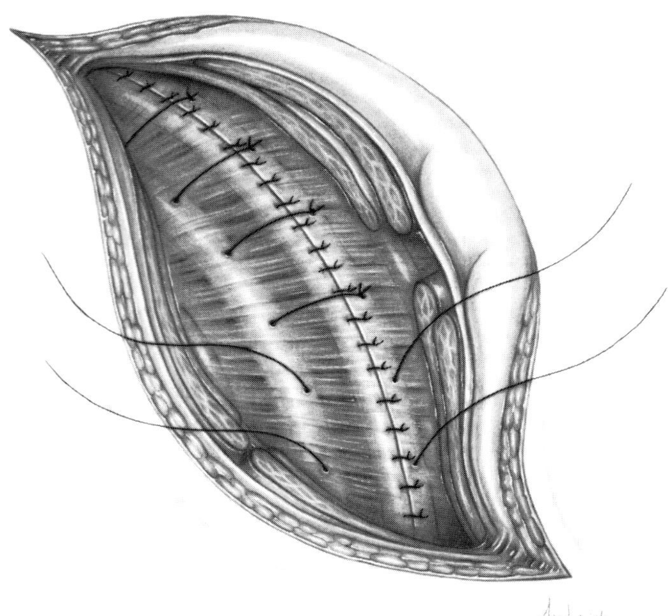

14

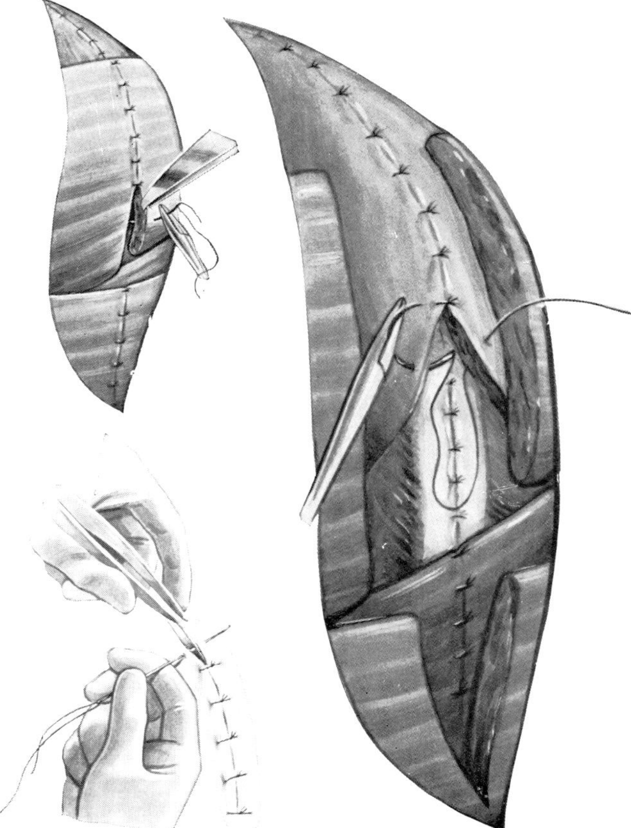

15

15

Closure of muscles and skin

The muscles are closed in layers. Interrupted catgut sutures are preferred but nylon or even stainless steel wire (often continuous) are used.

The skin is sutured with interrupted silk.

The tension of all sutures should be such as to approximate only the wound edges, allowing for swelling in the postoperative period and thus avoiding the risk of necrosis around the stitches with secondary infection.

POSTOPERATIVE CARE

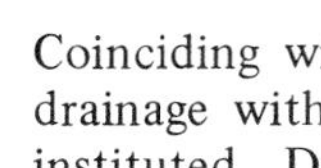

Concern for adequate pulmonary ventilation begins before the patient leaves the operating theatre, and is judged at first by the rate and depth of ventilation and by the general appearance and colour, providing the ventilating gas is air. Auscultation should reveal a full range of dry breath sounds. A radiograph at this stage is helpful.

Bronchoscopy, after removal of the anaesthetic tubes, with careful toilet of the bronchial tree is recommended.

Drainage

Coinciding with closure of the pleural cavity pleural drainage with a water-seal valve mechanism bottle is instituted. Dual tubes are rarely indicated but are preferred by some when a large volume of drainage is expected, for example following decortication operations when both air and fluid losses may be excessive. Dual drainage using two bottles with suction poses a special problem; both tubes must be coupled to the same negative pressure source otherwise fluid is likely to be transferred via the chest from one bottle to the other.

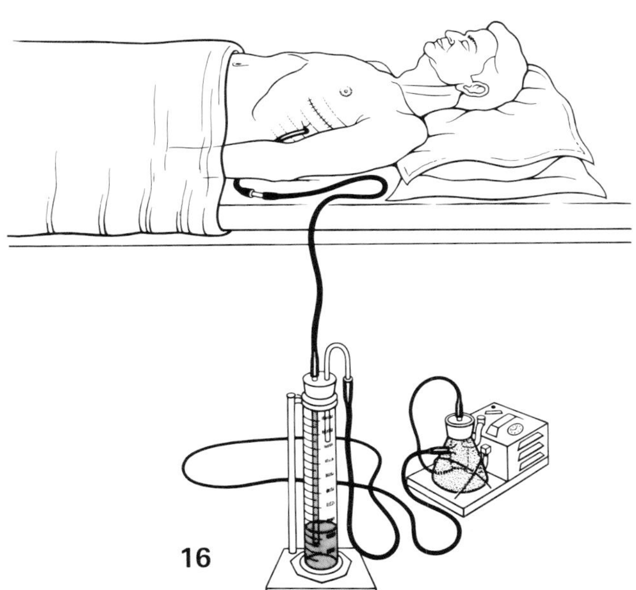

16

Motor suction

Negative pressures of 5 – 10 mmHg may be needed at this stage and should be continued in the ward later.

When transportation from the theatre to the ward means the temporary disconnection of the chest drainage tube from the bottle, care must be taken to see that the intercostal tube or tubes are clamped off beforehand. The pleural tube is removed usually after 24 – 48 hr unless contra-indicated by the persistent leakage of air, blood or chyle. Prolonged leakage of air may pose a special problem.

Physiology

Concern for ventilation coincides with that for the cardiac output. The prompt replacement of all fluid losses during the operation means that the patient leaves the theatre with a near normal blood volume as judged by the usual parameters, aided by swab and sometimes even patient weighing. Return of the patient to the ward poses the following problems.

Pain control

Control of pain is usually obtained by analgesics in small repeated doses, although long-acting local anaesthetics to the chest wall and the extradural space have been used successfully. Special care with the elderly, the very young and patients with poor respiratory function must be taken – over-sedation suggested by a low respiratory rate and/or an inadequate tidal volume may precipitate sputum retention and respiratory failure.

Restlessness

This may be due to many factors but the most important is anoxia. Its realization avoids the possible fatal use of sedatives in its management.

Physiotherapy

Physiotherapy by specially trained personnel or the nursing staff is invaluable in maintaining a clear airway. Short but frequent periods (5 min hourly) of deep breathing and cough promotion is preferable to prolonged, often agonizing and tiring sessions twice per day. In the presence of obstruction from intrabronchial viscid mucopurulent exudate these measures are augmented by the inhalation of steam, 'wetting' and/or mucolytic agents, postural drainage and, as a final resort, bronchoscopy.

Bed posture

In the thoracic patient this is important. Generally, it should be flat but changing, and with 10 – 15° elevation of the lower limbs above the right heart. Such a position aids bronchial drainage, venous return from the legs and, at the same time, facilitates diaphragmatic movements by allowing full unrestricted movements of the abdominal wall. Further benefits from this position are the equal distribution of weight over the posterior aspect of the patient, avoiding the notorious 'pressure points' with their tendency to ulceration; the more even intrapulmonary blood distribution avoids plethoric lung bases with their tendency to promote too easy gas absorption and consequent atelectasis at a time when ventilation may be poor. The head raised or the sitting positions are reserved for patients with left heart obstruction, those with an incompetent oesophageal cardia, and in the very obese where the excess of intra-abdominal fat displaces the diaphragm upwards.

Ambulation

Following pulmonary operations it is usual to mobilize patients after 48 hr; this does not mean sitting at rest in a chair. At first, short frequent periods of walking with a return to the horizontal position in bed should be the rule.

COMPLICATIONS

Acute respiratory failure

Sputum retention is, without doubt, the commonest complication following thoracotomy and is potentially fatal from the rapid onset of acute respiratory failure. This complication may arise very early, either in the theatre or during transit to the ward due to inadequate ventilation. Its early signs may be easily 'missed' and all too often an anoxic failing heart is attributed to 'surgical shock' from a variety of reasons and the urgency for immediate proper ventilation is not appreciated. Routine recovery 'wards' or 'areas' near the theatre with proper supervision until patients are fully recovered from anaesthesia and with facilities for their immediate transfer to intensive care help to eliminate this complication.

Sputum retention

Freedom from this complication will depend largely upon the preservation of good respiratory movements and an effective cough reflex which together will keep the tracheobronchial tree clear. Regular observations of the blood gases and their correlation with the clinical features may be essential. If physiotherapy, the careful control of pain and the use of mucolytics, such as steam and alevaire, are insufficient then an early bronchoscopy, if necessary repeated, will be needed. When these simpler measures fail, often due to fatigue from the effort of over-ventilation, then complete control must be assumed with full sedation, intubation and mechanical ventilation. Frequent aseptic aspiration and toilet of the air passages with specific chemotherapy, when appropriate, will assist recovery. Tracheostomy is a last resort because of its own special morbidity.

The ventilating gases will require humidification and oxygen enrichment up to 40 per cent. Over this figure for more than a few hours runs the risk of permanent alveolar capillary damage with impairment of gas transfer.

Wound infection

Unfortunately, in minor forms, this is all too common and follows an imperfect aseptic theatre technique. Secondary infection from the surface in a well sutured wound is impossible. A wound haematoma adds to the extent and the severity of the infection. Although a wound rarely secondarily infects the pleural space, nevertheless the converse of a deep infection presenting through the wound is not uncommon.

Careful appraisal of the situation will dictate proper treatment.

Rib fractures

Fractures of the rib usually arise as the result of the forcible mechanical retraction of the wound and are avoidable. Nevertheless, when created they are no great handicap to the patient, providing that sharp edges of the rib are trimmed before closing so that they do not produce wounds in the lung.

Injury to an intercostal vessel

This is one of the common causes of a haemothorax—an avoidable complication.

Injury to the intercostal nerve

This may be responsible for the exaggeration of postoperative wound pain and sometimes for a persistent late neuralgia, often with skin anaesthesia. The use of the supracostal technique when entering the chest minimizes the incidence of this complication.

Dehiscence of the wound

Major wound dehiscence in the absence of infection is uncommon, although small intercostal openings allowing the leakage of pleural fluids and air into the wound are not unusual. Extensive rib separations must be resutured as soon as possible using transcostal sutures (*see Illustration 14*).

Surgical emphysema

This is common in its minor form but rarely is it of importance unless the pleural cavity is inadequately drained so that a large persistent air leakage is allowed to accumulate within the pleura to be coughed out at intervals around the tube into the tissues of the chest wall and beyond. Skin drainage incisions are never required.

Traction and compression nerve injuries to the brachial plexus

Such injuries are very uncommon and usually arise as a result of bad positioning or rough handling of the patient on the table or during transit back to the ward while the patient is unconscious. Children in particular are prone to this complication.

Haemothorax

Haemothorax from bleeding chest wall or bronchial vessels within the mediastinum may need re-exploration. X-ray control is essential when managing this complication, as the pleural space may 'hide' litres of clotted blood which must be replaced in the circulation and later removed from the pleura restoring the vital capacity and possibly avoiding a late fibrothorax deformity. Pulmonary bleeding is almost never important except in the rare and usually fatal event of a slipped ligature from an artery or vein.

Pneumothorax

The leakage of air from the lung surface is rarely uncontrollable by drainage and suction. Persistence of a small air leak after 10 – 14 days calls for a careful check of the tubes, the apparatus and the surface drainage wound. If the leakage is confirmed as pulmonary, drainage continues, probably with its conversion to the open method. At this stage the natural pleurodesis renders open drainage of small spaces safe and can be compared with the similar procedure used in empyema.

Bronchopleural fistulae (see also pages 340–346)

On the whole these are re-explored at the outset before infection becomes established. Drainage in the late cases, with or without resuture of the bronchus, is practised. The dangers of this complication in association with the use of a further general anaesthetic must be emphasized. Preliminary pleural drainage, bronchoscopy before or during induction, and the use of either a one-lung anaesthetic tube or the double-lumen intratracheal catheter, will eliminate the risk to the patient of drowning in his own pleural fluid.

[*The illustrations for this Chapter on Surgical Access in Pulmonary Operations were drawn by Miss P. Archer.*]

Intercostal Drainage

John W. Jackson, M.Ch., F.R.C.S.
Consultant Thoracic Surgeon, Harefield Hospital, Middlesex

The insertion of an intercostal tube may be a life-saving measure. The technique is simple and, if correctly carried out, safe and relatively painless. The method should be understood by the most junior members of the thoracic surgical team and every casualty officer. The necessary equipment should be available in every casualty department.

PRE-OPERATIVE

Indications

Whenever a lung is collapsed by a volume of air or fluid sufficient to interfere with or embarrass respiration, consideration must be given to the insertion of an intercostal tube. This is particularly so if the trouble is bilateral, in recurrent and tension pneumothorax and the pneumothorax following chest injury especially when this is associated with a bloodstained pleural effusion. Most cases of traumatic haemothorax respond to intercostal drainage, two tubes may be necessary particularly if artificial ventilation is likely to be required. Bleeding from a torn lung usually ceases once the lung is re-expanded. Persistent drainage of blood through the chest tubes, in cases of penetrating injury, may be an indication of injury to a major blood vessel and call for thoracotomy. Chylothorax resulting from interruption of the thoracic duct by accident or at operation should be relieved by aspiration; if it persists and tube drainage is deemed necessary then open operation and ligation of the duct should also be considered before nutrition and metabolism are disturbed.

Intercostal tube drainage should be avoided in malignant pleural effusion unless it is associated with tension pneumothorax and respiratory distress. There is a risk of tumour implant in the tube track and a bronchopleural fistula may be present and perpetuate the air leak.

A shallow pneumothorax without respiratory symptoms is probably best left alone, the use of needles and intravenous-type cannulae should be avoided—they are likely to cause surgical emphysema and confuse the issue. Small pleural effusions should be aspirated initially with a needle and syringe so that their nature can be determined and treatment initiated.

Empyema is now an uncommon complication of pulmonary infection but may still occur when initial treatment had been delayed or was inadequate. It should be controlled by daily aspiration and the instillation of the appropriate antibiotic while systemic antibiotics are maintained.

Tube drainage may be required:

(*1*) in children;

(*2*) where there is virulent infection that cannot be controlled by antibiotics;

(*3*) where a lung abscess has ruptured into the pleura causing a positive pressure pyopneumothorax;

(*4*) where an empyema ruptures into the lung and threatens to drown the patient;

(*5*) where there is a postoperative bronchopleural fistula for which immediate surgery is not feasible.

Apical and basal tubes may be required.

Following operation it may be necessary to insert an intercostal tube because the tubes placed at operation were not in the correct position or have become displaced or removed prematurely.

Equipment

1

The Tudor-Edwards empyema trocar and cannula is still preferred because it is sharp, has a flange and allows the catheter to run freely into the chest as it is introduced. Three sizes are available:

Small 1/4 inch (6 mm) accepts a 16 Ch catheter
Medium 5/6 inch (8 mm) accepts a 22 Ch catheter
Large 3/8 inch (9·5 mm) accepts a 28 Ch catheter.

The small size should be used in infants only, the medium size may be used in children and to release air, as an apical tube, in adults. A plastic or rubber urethral catheter may be used.

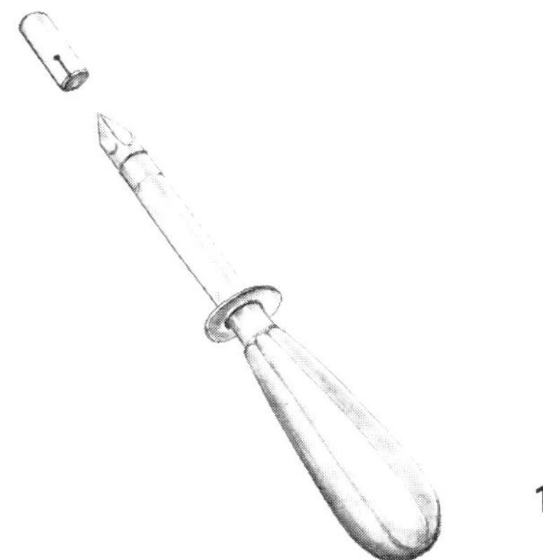

1

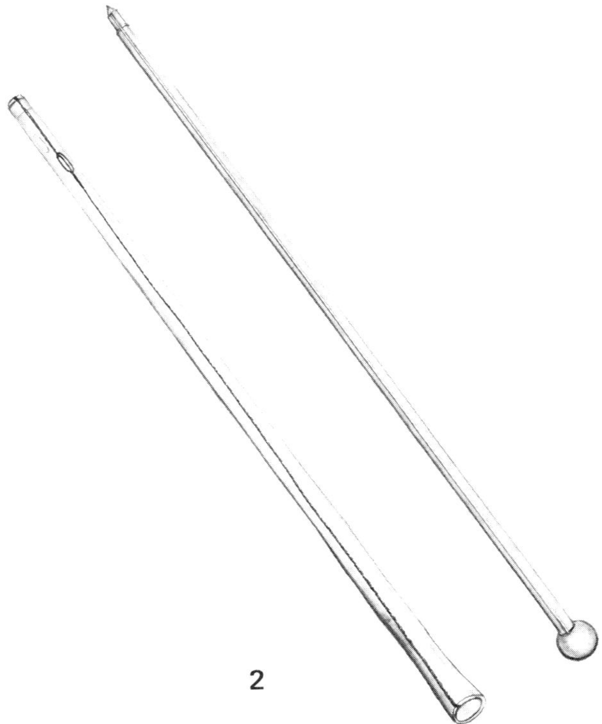

2

2

The 'Argyle' type thoracic catheter is conveniently packaged and contains a radio-opaque marker line which is interrupted at the most proximal side-eye so that its position can be easily identified on x-ray. It also comes with a central metal introducer so that it can be inserted on its own. The tip is not so sharp as a trocar and more force is required to push it through the chest making it not so easy to feel one's way between the ribs; it may plunge, even if a clip is applied to its side, and in its unchecked passage it may penetrate lung or other vital structures. This tube may be used without its introducer in association with a trocar and cannula.

3

The Malecot or De Pezzer catheter on an introducer has advantages in that the mushroom head can be located near the chest wall.

A Foley-type catheter with an inflatable balloon is not suitable as its walls are too soft and the outer end will not pass through the cannula.

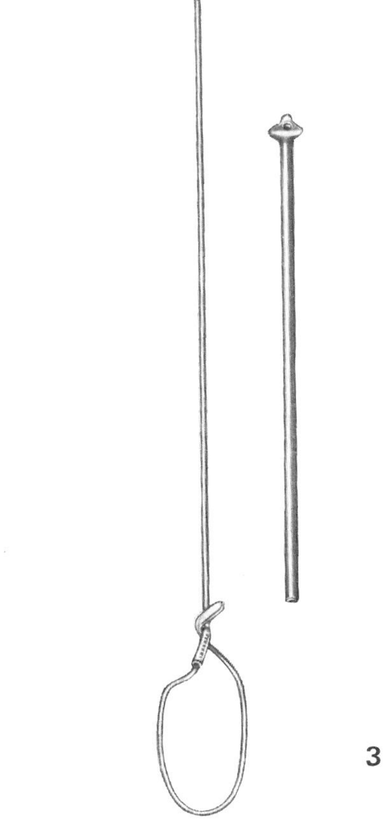

3

Position of patient

4

If the patient is shocked or unconscious the tube should be inserted with the patient in the recumbent position with the affected side uppermost. This position ensures that the lung and diaphragm are out of the way and is thus suitable for the insertion of apical or basal tubes.

To relieve a tension pneumothorax a tube may be inserted through the second intercostal space anteriorly 5 cm from the sternal edge. For this the patient may be sitting up or lying down.

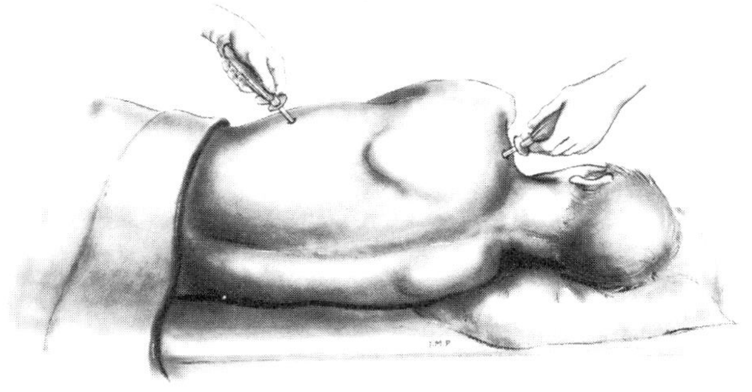

4

5

If the patient is confined to bed or has a broncho-pleural fistula and is coughing up an empyema, he should be upright leaning forward over a bedtable and pillows. If he can get out of bed he should be seated comfortably astride a chair by the bedside resting his head on pillows on the bed. This is a more stable position and ideal for dealing with empyema and pneumothorax. While inserting a basal tube the forearm on the side affected should rest on the bed in front of the patient, but for an apical tube the arm should be by the side and the patient asked to grip the seat or a leg of the chair with his hand. This ensures that the scapula is out of the way.

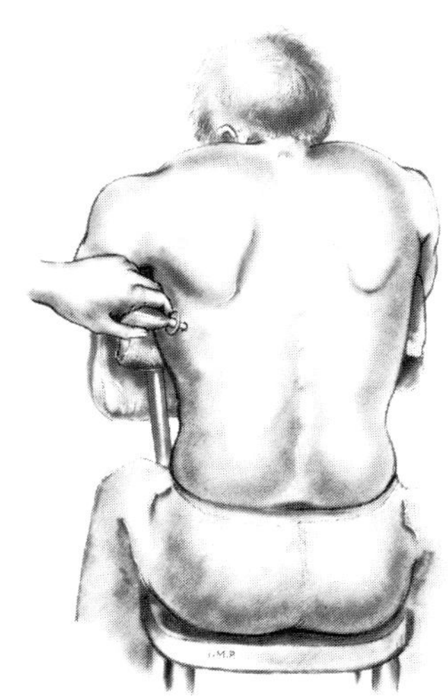

5

Site of drainage

First check the *side* with reference to the clinical signs and x-ray appearances. For empyema and effusion select a site posteriorly in the paravertebral gutter one space above the lowest level of the fluid. If necessary hold the x-ray film against the patient's chest.

Anaesthesia

Lignocaine 0·5 per cent in a 20 ml syringe should be used. A subcutaneous swelling at the selected site is raised using 5–10 ml of solution, the intercostal muscles are infiltrated with 5 ml and injecting is continued advancing the needle so as to get a good infiltration of the extrapleural tissues. The tip of the needle is advanced until the pleura is entered and air or fluid obtained. A sample of fluid must be preserved for laboratory examination. If the pleural space is not entered an alternative site is selected.

A few minutes are allowed for the anaesthetic to achieve its full effect and the interval is used to prepare the instruments and sutures and to check that the tubing fits the cannula, connections and underwater seal drainage bottle.

THE OPERATION

6

A vertical incision long enough to accept the trocar and cannula is made.

A mattress suture, to be tied at a later date when the tube is removed, is inserted.

The trocar and cannula are held firmly and advanced between the ribs until the pleura is entered.

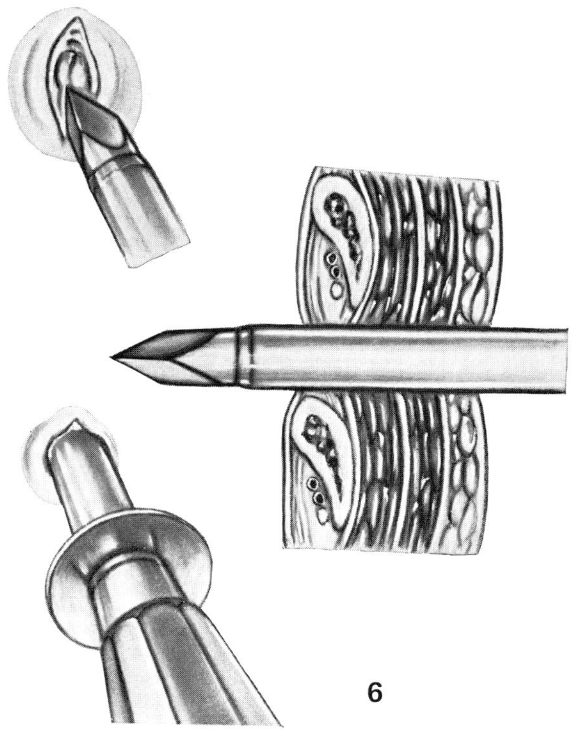

6

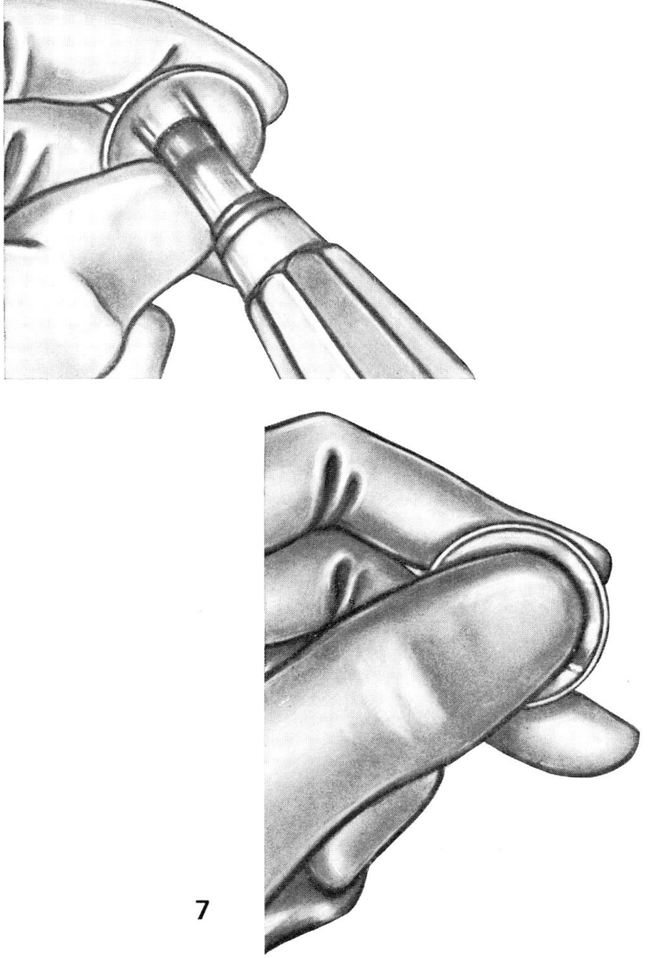

7

7

The cannula is supported between the fingers and thumb and the trocar is removed.

The opening in the cannula is sealed with the thumb to prevent air entering or fluid spilling from the chest.

8

The expanded end of the catheter is occluded with a forceps.

The thumb is removed from the cannula and the tip of the catheter is introduced until it is well inside the chest. No force should be required.

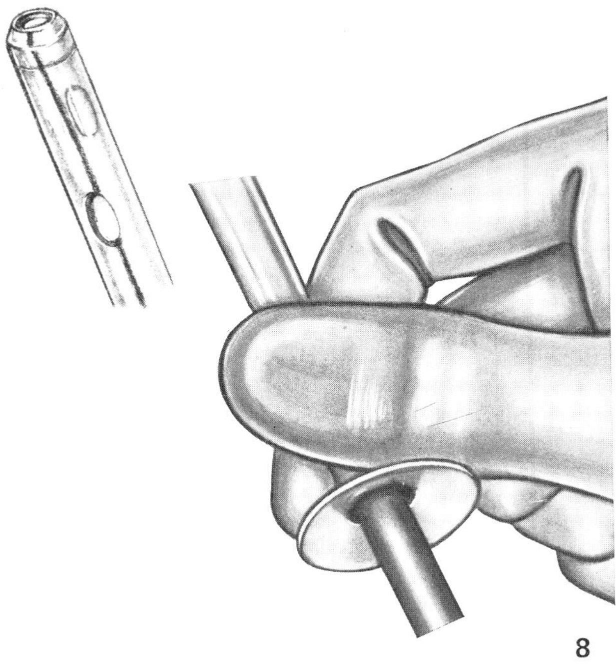

8

9

The catheter is held and the cannula removed from the chest.

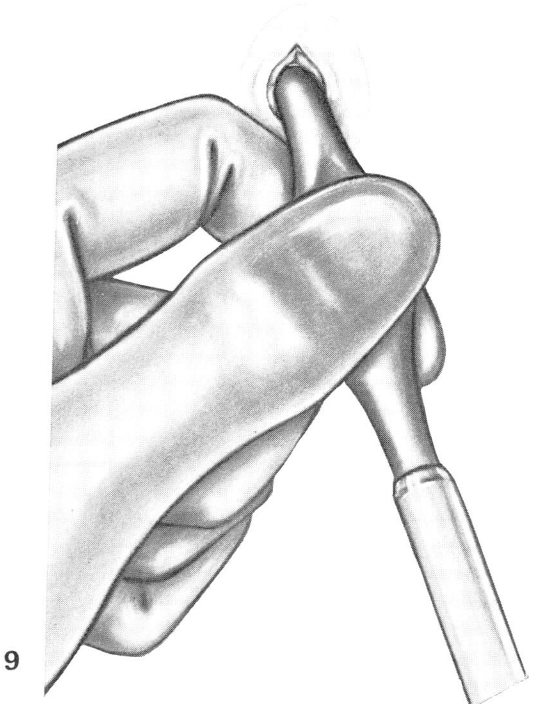

9

10

The catheter is clamped between the cannula and the chest. The first clamp is released and the cannula is drawn over the end of the tube.

The position of the tip of the catheter in the pleura is adjusted.

The catheter is secured to the skin with a second nylon stitch.

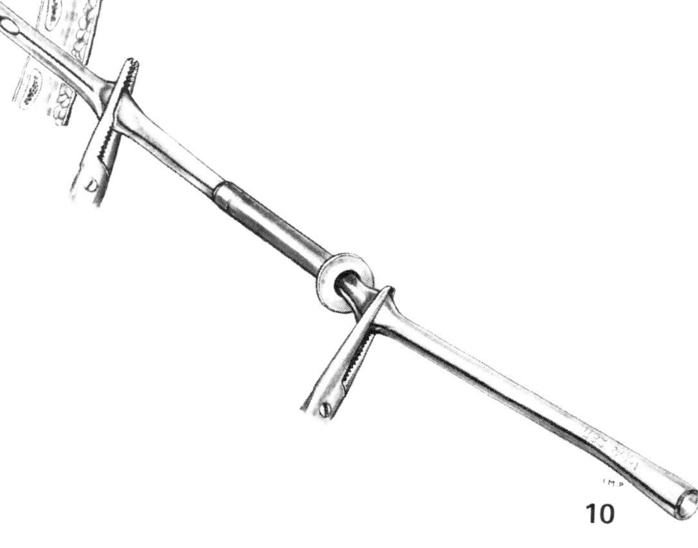

10

11

The catheter is connected to the underwater tube of the underwater seal bottle.

The clamp is released and the catheter allowed to drain.

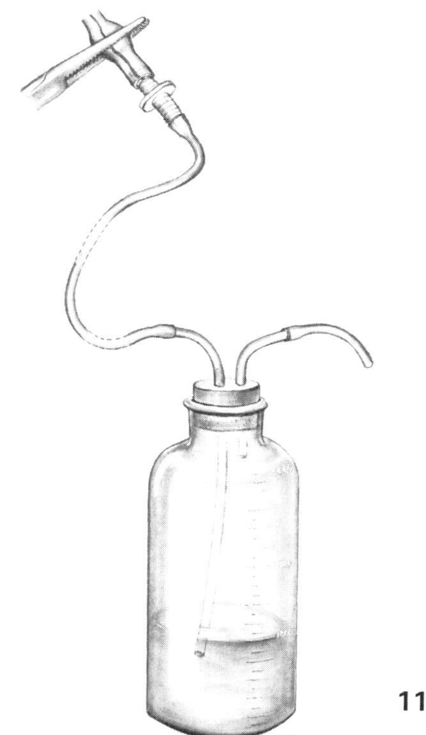

11

POSTOPERATIVE CARE

The drainage system

Each underwater seal bottle must be kept at floor level. All tube connections and the bung of the bottle must be secured with tape. Large clamps are kept at hand and must be applied immediately to the chest drain, as it leaves the patient, should accidental disconnection occur, also when a bottle is being changed or lifted across a bed or trolley.

Suction apparatus, at 35 cm of water (1 inch of mercury), may be applied to the short tube of the underwater seal bottle. If there are two or more sets of tubes and bottles they must all be connected to the same suction apparatus using branched connections. The volume of drainage is measured and recorded hourly, or more frequently until a stable state is established. Clean bottles are applied each day and a specimen of the drainage fluid sent to the laboratory.

The patient

If infection is present antibiotics are continued.

An x-ray is taken next day or sooner. It will show: (*a*) how much air and fluid has been removed; (*b*) how much the lung has re-expanded; (*c*) the position of the tubes.

If there is lobar collapse or mediastinal displacement bronchoscopy may be necessary to exclude tumour or to remove a foreign body or retained secretions.

Physiotherapy is started as soon as possible to encourage chest wall movements, to promote re-expansion of the lung, to clear the airways of accumulated secretion and to assist in pleural drainage. Once the patient is well enough to sit upright in bed he may be moved to a chair and later allowed to stand up and move about the room while still attached to his drainage system.

12

Soon it may be possible to replace the underwater seal system by a one-way valve (Heimlich) connected to a Uribag. This can be pinned to the patient's clothing and will allow him to walk about freely inside and outside the hospital.

The single valve allows drainage by gravity, in the double valve the proximal chamber is compressible and by squeezing it intermittently a negative pressure is developed and is an efficient and convenient way of continuing suction.

Tubes are removed only when there is satisfactory clinical and radiological re-expansion of lung, leakage of air should have ceased for 24–48 hr and drainage become minimal. The opening in the skin is closed by tying the suture placed at the time of tube insertion.

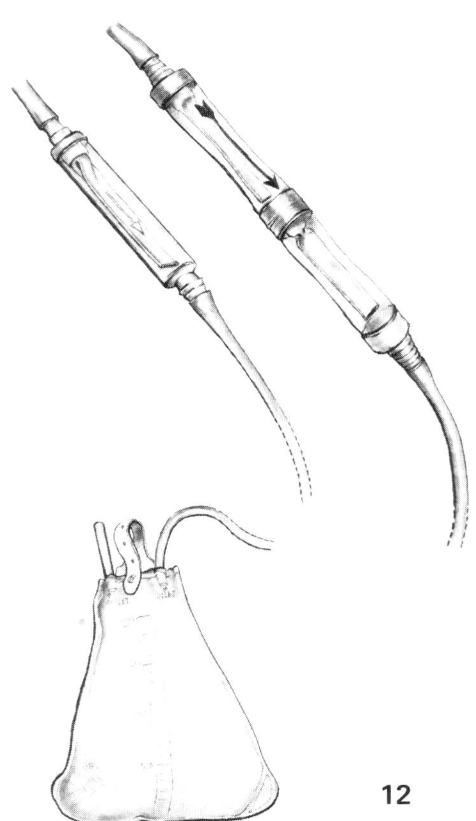

12

COMPLICATIONS

Pain is not a problem unless the tube is a tight fit or the ribs crowded.

Surgical emphysema indicates that it is easier for air to pass round the tube than through it and suggests that the tube is too small, blocked or misplaced, or that suction is inadequate. If a tube is blocked it should be cleared by milking.

After 10 days the tube track is likely to be infected and there is a risk of haemorrhage from pressure erosion of an intercostal vessel. If there is evidence of a residual pleural pocket or bronchopleural fistula, a sinogram should be carried out.

At this stage a decision must be taken whether to continue with drainage or proceed to decortication. If there is pleural thickening and the patient is otherwise fit and infection is under control, decortication gives the best chance of restoring normal function and minimizing deformity. If the patient is frail or elderly or if there is persistent infection in the underlying lung, drainage of the pleura should be continued by re-inserting the intercostal tube at a fresh site or doing a rib resection (*see* Chapter on 'Rib Resection for Empyema', pages 273–278).

[*The illustrations for this Chapter on Intercostal Drainage were drawn by Miss P. A. Archer and Mrs. I. M. Prentice.*]

Rib Resection for Empyema

Vernon C. Thompson, F.R.C.S.
Consulting Thoracic Surgeon to The London Hospital
and London Chest Hospital

[*This Chapter should be studied in conjunction with the preceding Chapter on Intercostal Drainage.*]

PRE - OPERATIVE

Indications and contra-indications

Rib resection for empyema should only be employed when more conservative methods have failed. It should never be employed as the primary treatment. Rib resection is essentially an open method of drainage and the size of the empyema cavity must be reduced to the smallest possible dimensions by aspiration and possibly intercostal drainage beforehand.

The primary treatment of empyema is by aspiration and the instillation of suitable antibiotics. A sterile empyema of a persistent nature is best treated by resection. A pure tuberculous empyema should never be treated by open drainage.

It is only when conservative measures fail or are doomed to fail that rib resection should be employed. The causes of failure of conservative measures are: (*1*) infection with an organism resistant to all antibiotics; (*2*) loculation of the empyema by massive deposits of fibrin or blood clot; (*3*) persistent re-infection by a bronchopleural fistula or by an oesophageal fistula; (*4*) postoperative infections of the pleural cavity by bronchial fistula after lung resection or by oesophageal fistula after oesophago-gastric resections; (*5*) underlying lung disease, such as bronchiectasis or tumour.

Anaesthesia

If there is no bronchial fistula the patient may be given a general anaesthetic, but if a fistula is present local anaesthesia should be employed. The technique is a little more elaborate than that for intercostal drainage. The line of incision should be infiltrated together with the subcutaneous and deep fascial planes. The intercostal spaces above and below the rib to be resected can be infiltrated after they have been exposed.

Site of drainage

It is essential that drainage should be at the lowest point; but this requires some qualification. The lowest point should be in relation to the patient's normal position in bed, which is semirecumbent. The site for gravitational drainage should therefore almost invariably be posterior. Another consideration which must be borne in mind is that the diaphragm always rises in the obliteration of an empyema space. Allowance must be made for this, and the tube should be introduced one rib space above the diaphragm, otherwise the rising of the diaphragm may seal off the end of the tube.

The site of drainage must be determined after a study of postero-anterior and lateral x-rays and a careful rib count. The lowest point of the empyema can be most clearly demarcated by preliminary injection of Dionosil into the empyema space.

Finally the site is confirmed by aspiration above and below the rib selected for resection, after exposure by a vertical incision.

THE OPERATION

Position of patient

1

If there is no bronchopleural fistula and if the patient is able to lie on the contralateral side without distress the operation can be carried out in the lateral position under a general anaesthetic.

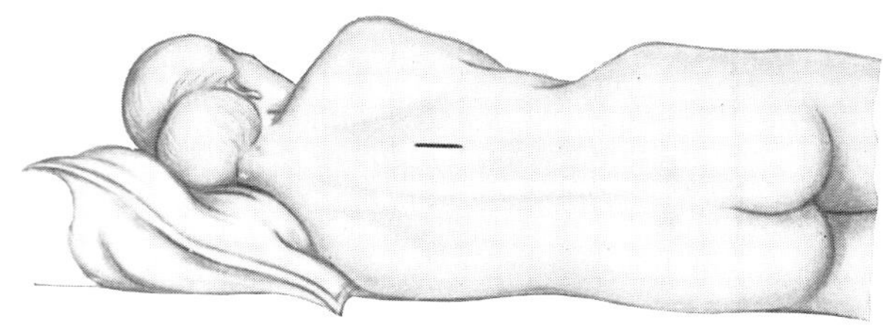

1

2

In bronchopleural fistula

If there is a bronchopleural fistula and the patient is unable to lie on the contralateral side, the operation should be carried out under local anaesthesia with the patient sitting on a stool leaning forward with the arms supported over the operating table.

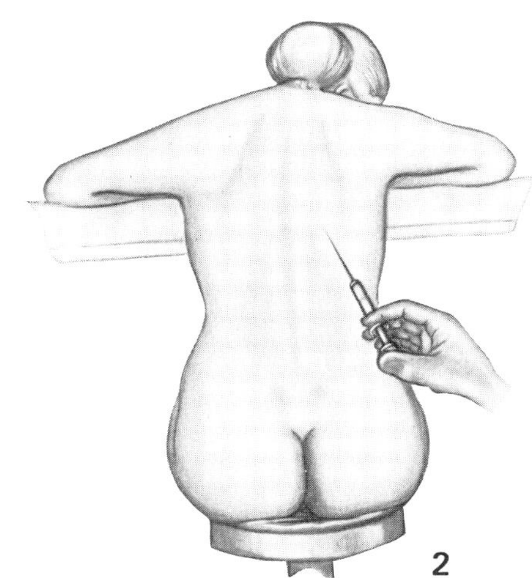

2

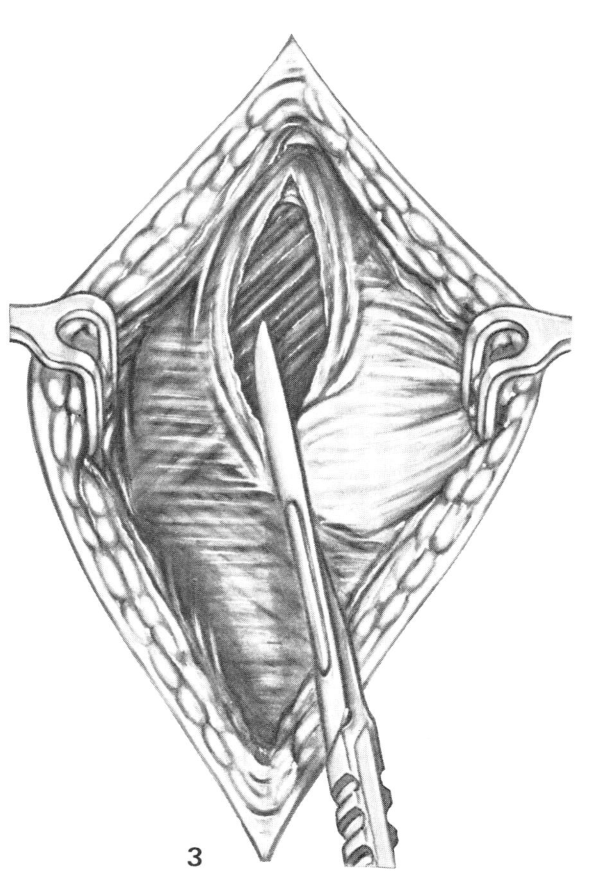

3

3

The incision

The incision should be a vertical one 3 inches (8 cm) in length. This allows extension upwards or downwards if it is not quite correct as shown by aspiration above and below the rib previously selected for resection. The incision is carried through skin, subcutaneous tissues, deep fascia and muscle to the ribs and intercostal muscles.

4

Incision in periosteum

When the rib has been exposed and selected for resection, the edges of the wound are retracted along the line of the rib and the periosteum is incised for 2–3 inches (5–7·5 cm) with the diathermy knife.

Before resecting the rib aspiration should be performed above and below the rib to confirm that the site is well chosen.

A specimen of pus should be sent to the laboratory to identify the organisms present and to determine their sensitivities to antibiotics.

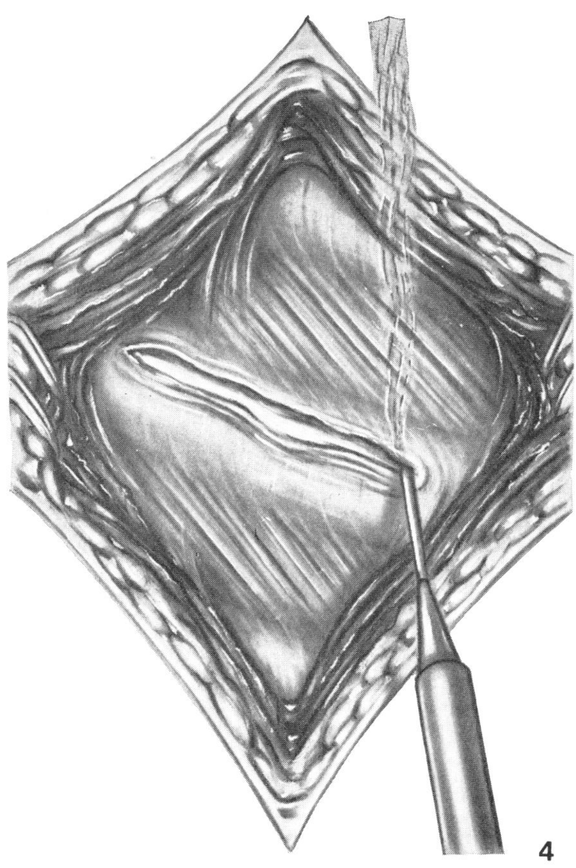

4

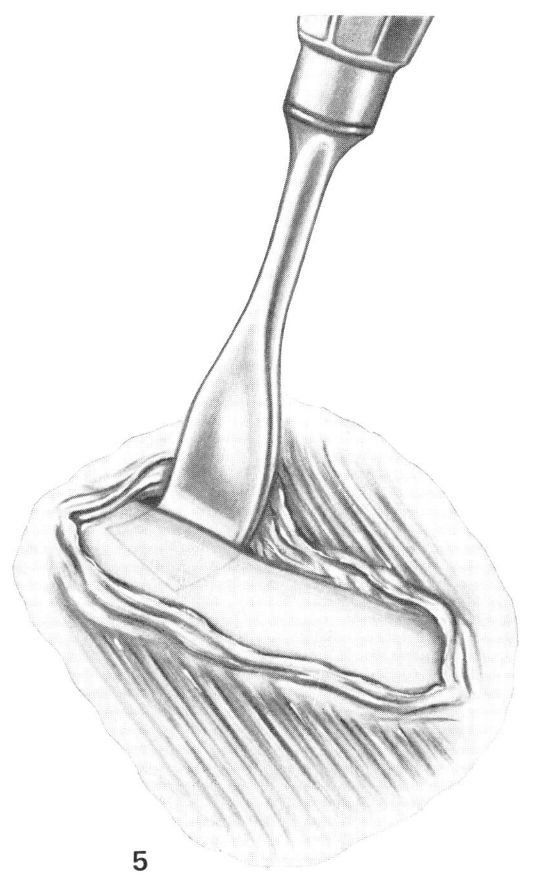

5

5

Elevation of the periosteum

With a rugine the periosteum is separated from the rib. On the upper surface of the rib the rugine should be carried forwards in the direction of the intercostal muscle fibres and on the lower surface it should be carried backwards. In this way the part of the rib to be resected should be completely freed from its periosteum.

Care should be taken to keep close to the rib and not to tear the periosteum which should be left intact. If this procedure is not carried out carefully there is a risk of tearing the intercostal vessels with troublesome haemorrhage which will require ligation of the vessels after the segment of rib is removed.

If the vessels are ligated care must be taken to preserve the intercostal nerve as it has an important motor and sensory supply to the anterior abdominal wall.

6

Resection of a segment of the rib

With a costotome, of which there are many varieties, and almost any can be employed providing it cuts the rib cleanly, a portion of the rib 2–3 inches (5–7·5 cm) in length should be resected.

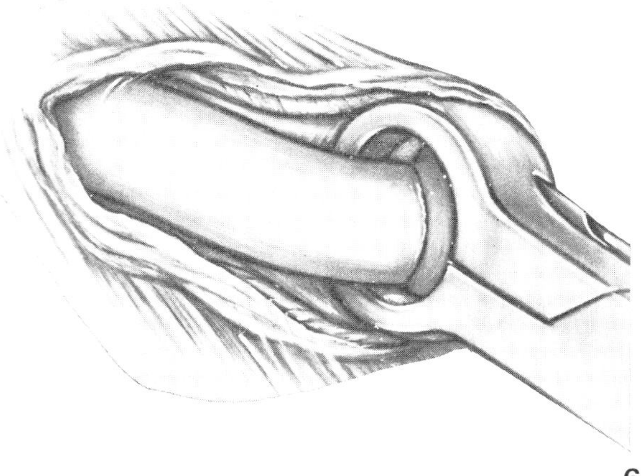

6

7

Opening of the pleura and cleaning of the empyema space

The periosteum and pleura deep to the rib should be incised keeping well above the leash of intercostal vessels and nerve. The contents of the empyema are removed with a sucker. The empyema cavity is inspected with a Nelson light and great care should be taken to remove all fibrinous deposits from the surface of the pleura with the sucker, leaving the space quite clean. A portion of parietal pleura is excised and sent for histological examination.

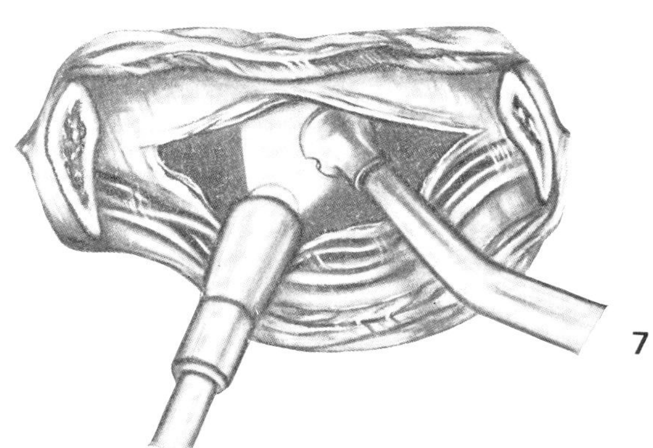

7

8

8

Inserting tube into pleural cavity

A wide bore rubber or plastic tube is then inserted into the pleural cavity; its external diameter should be about 2 cm, and it should project into the cavity about the same distance. The pleura and deep periosteal layer should then be sutured round the tube as closely as possible.

9

Suture of the wound

The muscles, deep fascia, subcutaneous tissue and skin are then loosely sutured round the tube, using catgut for the muscles and unabsorbable sutures for the skin.

No attempt should be made to suture the tissues tightly as some drainage to the wound itself must be allowed. Tight suture will cause oedema of the wound and possibly cellulitis; this may tend to withdraw the tube from the empyema space.

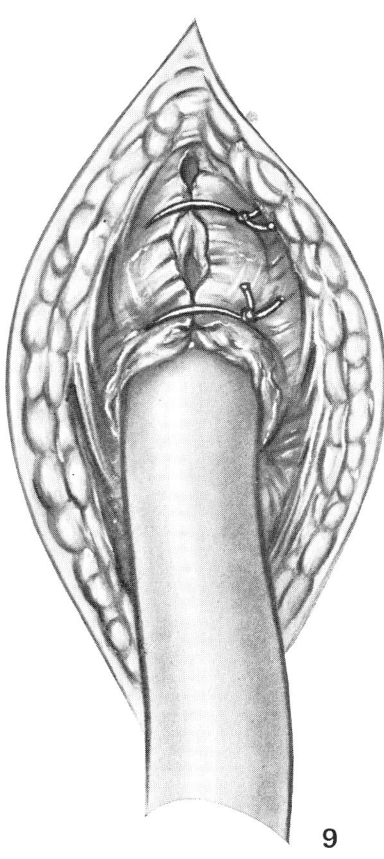

9

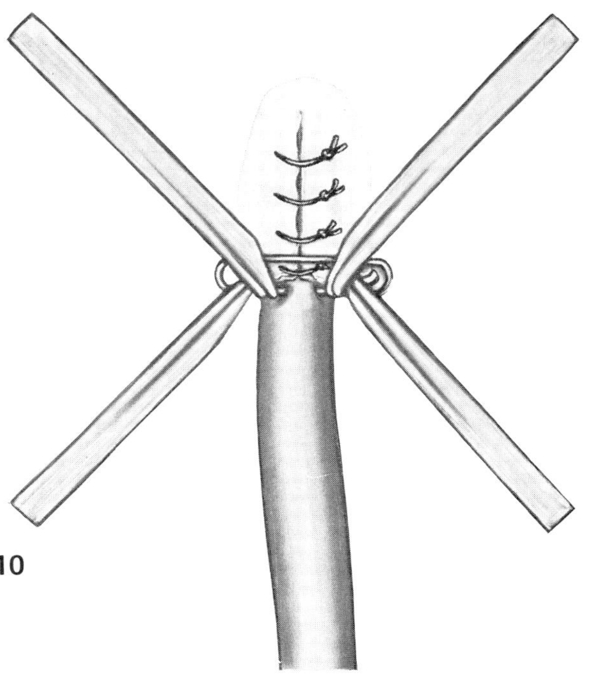

10

10

Fixation of the tube

The tube should be anchored by the insertion of a safety pin through the upper wall of the tube (not through the middle of the lumen, as this may cause obstruction by clots) and the safety pin should be fixed to the skin by adhesive strapping taken round the arm of the safety pin that pierces the tube as illustrated. The length of each piece of strapping should be 8 inches (20 cm), the width 0·5 inches (1 cm), and the angles between the arms of the strapping should be 90°.

The tube should be connected to an underwater seal bottle and the patient should be nursed as detailed in the previous chapter.

POSTOPERATIVE CARE

Breathing exercises of the inspiratory type should be instituted from the day after operation. Suction at about 30 cm of water should be applied to the exit tube from the bottle. The patient should be allowed out of bed and encouraged to take exercise as soon as possible; on such occasions the tube can be disconnected from the suction apparatus, but this should be applied whenever the patient is in bed.

X-ray examination should be made weekly at first to show the diminution in the size of the pleural space. When this is no longer visible on direct radiography the space can be outlined by filling it with a radio-opaque material such as Dionosil.

The technique is to remove the tube, to lie the patient so that the wound in the chest wall is uppermost and to fill the space with Dionosil with a syringe and catheter until it overflows. The sinus is then packed with gauze, all Dionosil on the skin is cleaned off, a metal marker is placed on the sinus at skin level which is then sealed off with adhesive strapping and radiographs are taken in the erect lateral and postero-anterior positions.

The fundamental points in the management of the tube are that the end of the tube should be at the bottom of a cavity, but when a long track exists the end of the tube should be about 1 inch (2·5 cm) from the end of the track. If the end of the tube is kept at the bottom of a long track it is highly probable that a bottle-neck will seal off the top of the track.

Once an empyema has reduced itself to a long track, it may be necessary to lengthen the tube. A good rule is to remove the tube once a week, to measure the length of the track with a gum elastic bougie and to adjust the tube so that it is 1 inch (2·5cm) shorter than the track.

The tube should not be finally removed until the pleural space has become completely obliterated and only the tube track in the chest wall remains.

Causes of chronic empyema

The commonest causes of chronic empyema are mismanagement of acute empyema:

Drainage has been too soon or too late.

Drainage has been in the wrong place.

The drainage tube has been too small.

The tube has been removed too soon.

Foreign bodies (for example, tubes) have been lost in the pleural cavity.

A bottle-neck has developed in the empyema cavity leaving a persistent undrained space.

Other causes of chronic empyema are:

Serious underlying disease in the lung such as tuberculosis.

Unrecognized foreign body, adenoma or carcinoma.

Specific infections of the pleura such as tuberculosis or actinomycosis.

Persistent bronchopleural or oesophageal fistula.

Osteomyelitis of rib or spine.

[*The illustrations for this Chapter on Rib Resection for Empyema were drawn by Miss P. Archer.*]

Decortication

Pleurectomy: Excision of Empyema

W. P. Cleland, F.R.C.P., F.R.C.S.
Surgeon, The Brompton Hospital; Consulting Thoracic Surgeon, King's College Hospital;
Senior Lecturer in Thoracic Surgery, Royal Postgraduate Medical School;
Civilian Consultant in Thoracic Surgery to the Royal Navy

PRE-OPERATIVE

Aim of operation

The object of the operation is the removal of the fibrous wall of the empyema cavity both from the lung surface and from the chest wall and diaphragm leaving the lung free and unhampered to fill the space formerly occupied by the empyema.

Decortication can be combined with resection of lung (pleurolobectomy; pleuropneumonectomy) if the latter is diseased.

Indications

The operation is used in the treatment of subacute or chronic empyema where simpler measures (repeated aspirations, drainage) have failed to eliminate the empyema cavity.

Contra-indications

The operation is a severe one and patients who are frail or elderly or whose general condition is poor should not be submitted to it.

The operation should not be performed in a postpneumonic empyema until the signs of pneumonia have disappeared.

Pre-operative investigations

An empyema is never a primary condition and every attempt should be made to determine its cause before embarking on surgical treatment. In addition, a precise knowledge of the state and condition of the underlying lung is essential before pleurectomy is undertaken.

Investigations which will be required are: (*1*) cytological and bacteriological examination of the pleural fluid and sputum; (*2*) bronchoscopy; and (*3*) bronchography.

Pre-operative preparations

(*1*) The empyema should be aspirated repeatedly before operation and sterilized by intrapleural antibiotics.

(*2*) Full ambulation and vigorous breathing exercises are essential for as long as is practicable before operation.

(*3*) Systemic chemotherapy is advisable for 2–3 days before operation or longer if much sputum is present.

Anaesthesia

General anaesthesia with intratracheal intubation is employed. (Intrabronchial occlusion or one lung anaesthesia is not usually necessary.)

Hypotensive agents (Arfonad) may be useful in reducing the oozing from the chest wall and lung during mobilization.

THE OPERATION

1

The incision

The approach is through a standard posterolateral thoracotomy with the patient lying on the unaffected side and the arm pulled well forwards. This incision will give reasonable access to both the apex of the thoracic cavity and the diaphragmatic aspect (the two most difficult regions to mobilize). The trapezius and rhomboideus major behind and the latissimus dorsi and serratus anterior in front are divided in the line of the skin incision.

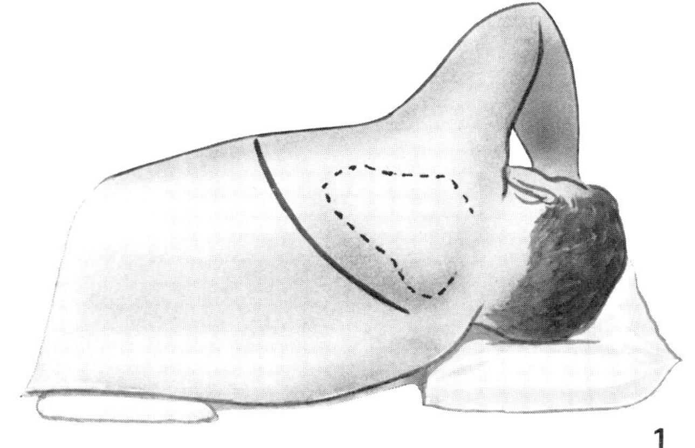

1

2

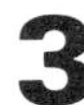

2

Entry into extrapleural layer

The fifth or sixth rib is resected subperiosteally from the neck to the mid-axillary line and the posterior layer of periosteum is incised longitudinally. The extrapleural layer is entered by blunt dissection with the finger and the outer wall of the empyema is stripped from the chest wall in all directions by a combination of blunt and sharp dissection. Considerable force is often required to complete the mobilization.

3

Mobilization of empyema

Due care must be exercised when stripping the outer wall from the apex of the thorax and from the diaphragm to ensure that the underlying structures are not injured. Mobilization should be carried out under direct vision if possible.

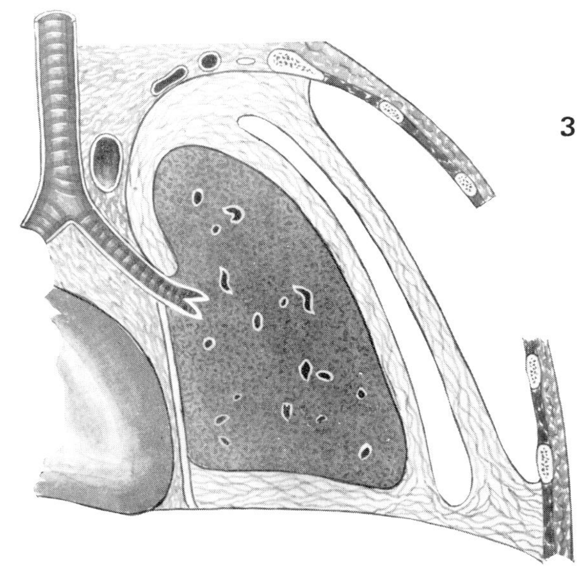

3

4

Stripping of outer wall

Mobilization from the mediastinum is usually easier than from the parietes as the fibrous tissue is less dense. Care must be taken not to injure the innominate vein on the left side or the superior vena cava and azygos vein on the right side as well as the vagus and phrenic nerves.

Mobilization from the diaphragm may be particularly tedious. It is easy to detach the diaphragm from the chest wall during mobilization but it should be re-attached at the end of the procedure.

On completing the mobilization, the empyema will have been completely detached from all its parietal attachments but still remains adherent to the lung.

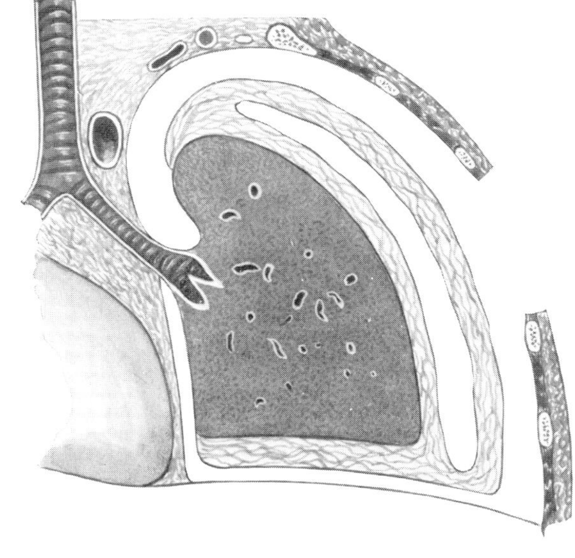

4

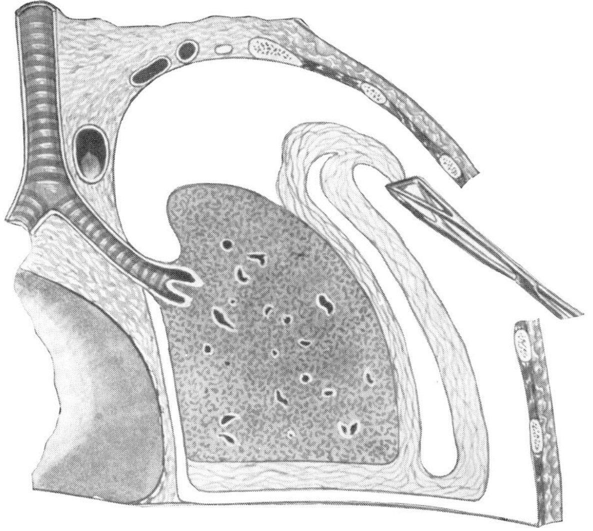

5

5

Stripping of inner wall

The inner wall of the empyema is now 'peeled off' the lung surface. An area of minimal adherence is selected initially to provide the right plane for dissection and the mobilization is carried out gently by a combination of blunt and sharp dissection, taking care to injure the lung as little as possible.

6

Freeing of fibrous attachments

Having removed the empyema sac, any remnants of fibrous tissue left attached to the lung surface which are deforming the lung are removed either by blunt dissection with a swab on a holder or by sharp dissection.

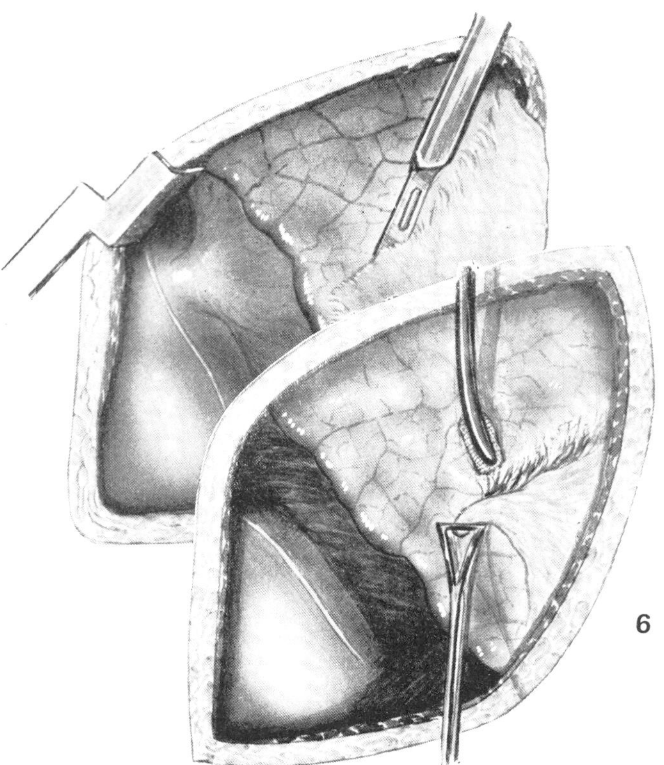

6

7

Opening of lung fissures

Finally the fissures between the lobes are opened up and any puckerings or bucklings of the lung are undone. The lung is completely separated from all parietal and mediastinal attachments so that it is left free to expand fully.

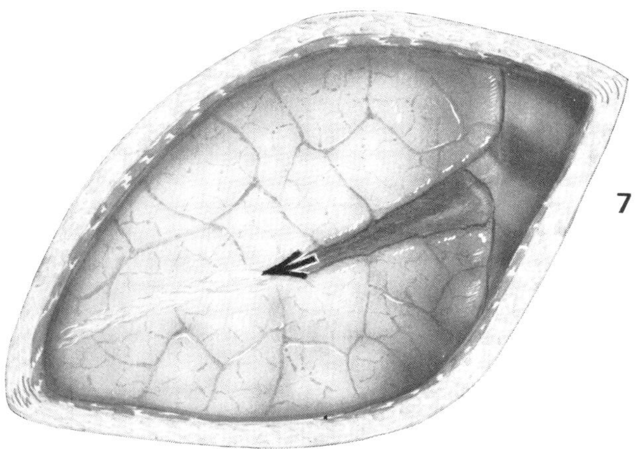

7

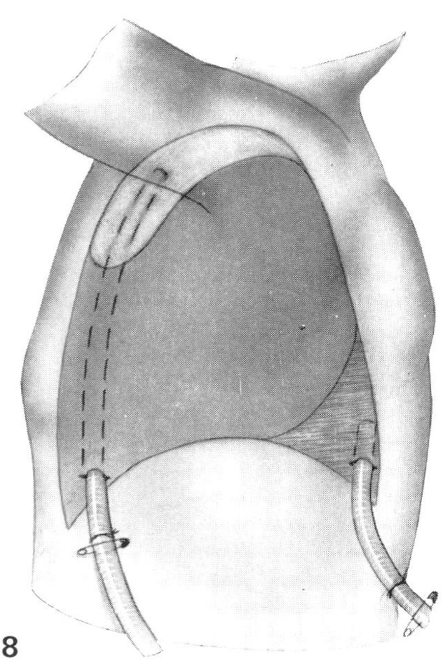

8

8

Drainage

At least two tubes are required for drainage purposes. One lies at the apex of the chest and is designed to remove any air which leaks from the lung surface, whilst the other removes fluid which accumulates at the base. Both are inserted through separate stab wounds. They should never be brought out through the thoracotomy incision.

The wound is closed carefully in layers.

POSTOPERATIVE CARE AND COMPLICATIONS

Management

The success of the operation depends on obtaining early and complete expansion of the decorticated lung so that the space occupied by the empyema is completely obliterated and no dead space persists to encourage fresh infection or result in pleural thickening. Rapid expansion of the lung is achieved by: (*1*) applying strong suction to both drainage tubes (negative pressures of several inches of mercury are often required); (*2*) nursing the patient lying on his unaffected side (in this position the upper thoracic cavity is enlarged and increased lung expansion encouraged); (*3*) the employment of vigorous breathing exercises and early ambulation.

The tubes are removed when leakage of air and fluid have ceased but in any case should not be retained for longer than 1 week. Any subsequent accumulation of air or fluid should be aspirated.

Complications

Bronchopulmonary secretions may give rise to serious complications of atelectasis, pneumonitis or suppurative bronchitis. Coughing exercises and postural drainage are usually sufficient to keep the bronchial tree clear but if they do not suffice, catheter suction or bronchoscopic aspiration is required.

Air leakage is often considerable for several days and occasionally for longer periods preventing full lung expansion. Temporary phrenic paralysis and the induction of a pneumoperitoneum may be employed in order to reduce the space and decrease the leakage. Additional drainage tubes connected to suction will often encourage expansion of unexpanded lungs.

Re-infection of the pleural space is likely to occur if the lung does not expand to fill the pleural cavity completely. Infected pockets should be treated by repeated aspirations and the instillation of antibiotics; further drainage may be required if aspirations fail to control the infection.

References

Eggers, C. (1923). *Ann. Surg.* 77, 327
Price Thomas, C. and Cleland, W. P. (1945). *Lancet* **1**, 327
Sarot, I. A. (1949). *Thorax* **4**, 173
Sellors, T. H. and Cruickshank, G. (1951). *Br. J. Surg.* **38**, 411

[*The illustrations for this Chapter on Decortication were drawn by Mr. F. Price.*]

Thoracoplasty with Apicolysis

W. P. Cleland, F.R.C.P., F.R.C.S.
Surgeon, The Brompton Hospital; Consulting Thoracic Surgeon, King's College Hospital;
Senior Lecturer in Thoracic Surgery, Royal Postgraduate Medical School;
Civilian Consultant in Thoracic Surgery to the Royal Navy

PRE-OPERATIVE

Aim of operation

The operation is designed to produce concentric relaxation of the tuberculous upper lobe by apical mobilization; the relaxation is obtained by subperiosteal resection of the ribs overlying the mobilized area.

Lateral thoracoplasty is used occasionally in place of thoracoplasty with apical mobilization for apical disease. It was used extensively in the treatment of tuberculous empyema but has now largely been superseded by pleurectomy and decortication. It consists of excision of the ribs as described above without apicolysis.

Indications

Thoracoplasty is only employed for the occasional patient with chronic fibrocaseous or cavernous lesions in the upper lobe which cannot be controlled by chemotherapy and which are considered unsuitable for resection. It is of particular value for patients whose organisms are resistant to all or most antibiotics.

Contra-indications

Children, and adults over the age of 50 years, are generally regarded as unsuitable for thoracoplasty. Operation should be delayed in the presence of active, progressive disease or when toxicity is marked.

Patients whose general condition is poor or whose respiratory reserve is low should not be submitted for operation.

Associated conditions (asthma, chronic bronchitis, emphysema and ischaemic heart disease), if severe, add to the hazards of the operation.

Pre-operative preparation

Every patient should have an adequate period of antituberculous chemotherapy before operation.

Diaphragmatic breathing exercises, coughing exercises and arm and shoulder movements should all be given beforehand.

Patients with excessive amounts of sputum should be treated with the appropriate antibiotics.

Anaesthesia

Either general or local anaesthesia can be employed.

(*1*) General anaesthesia is effected by thiopentone, a relaxant, nitrous oxide and oxygen using an intratracheal cuffed tube.

(*2*) Adequate premedication is essential with local anaesthesia. Omnopon 20 mg and scopolamine 0·4 mg together with a barbiturate are usually effective. Supplementary intravenous doses of Omnopon can be given during the operation if required.

The skin and muscles in the line of the incision are infiltrated extensively with 0·2 per cent lignocaine (Xylocaine) with 0·5 ml 1:1000 adrenaline using a total volume of about 400 ml.

A paravertebral block of the upper 7 thoracic nerves is carried out using 0·4 per cent lignocaine and a lower brachial plexus block is sometimes performed in addition.

THE OPERATION

1

The incision

The skin incision is 'J' shaped, curving two fingers' breadth below the angle of the scapula with the arm hanging well forward. The vertical limb is placed 2–3 cm from the vertebral spines. It extends from the level of the first thoracic spine to the posterior axillary line.

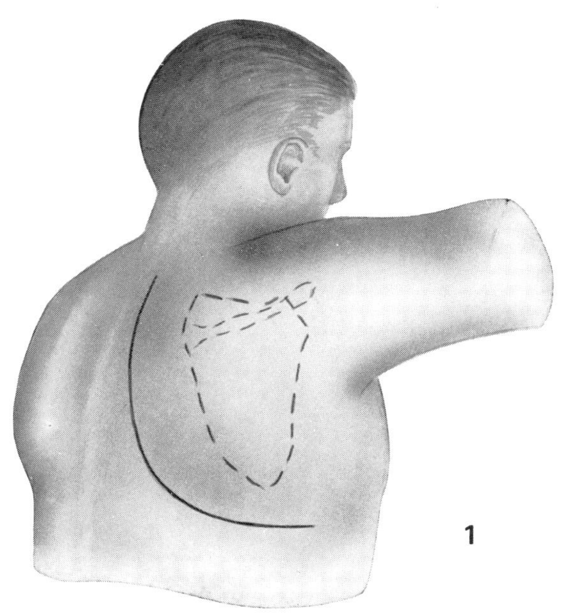

1

2

Division of muscles

The superficial (trapezius and latissimus dorsi) and deeper (rhomboids and serratus anterior) layers of muscle are divided in the line of the incision.

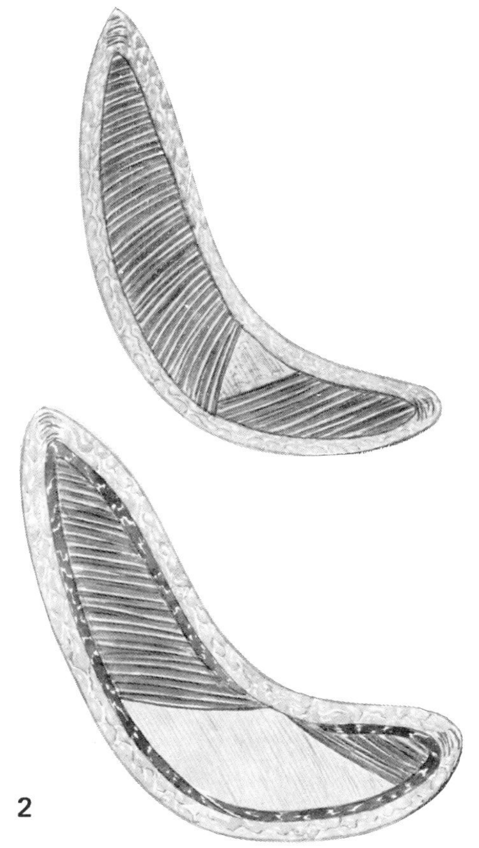

2

3

Exposure of ribs

The scapula is elevated vertically to expose the layer of areolar tissue between it and the chest wall. This layer is incised and the scapula displaced forwards and elevated further to expose the posterior aspect of upper digitations of the serratus anterior muscle. The narrow gap between the scalenus medius and the uppermost digitation of the serratus is opened and developed by blunt dissection in the areolar plane on the anterior surface of the serratus (that is, in the axilla). In this way the digitations of the serratus arising from the upper ribs are isolated and can now be cut with scalpel or diathermy close to their origin from the ribs and intercostal spaces to the level of the fourth rib.

The serratus posterior superior is excised and the upper ribs are now completely exposed. The insertions of the scalenus medius and posterior are then detached from the first and second ribs.

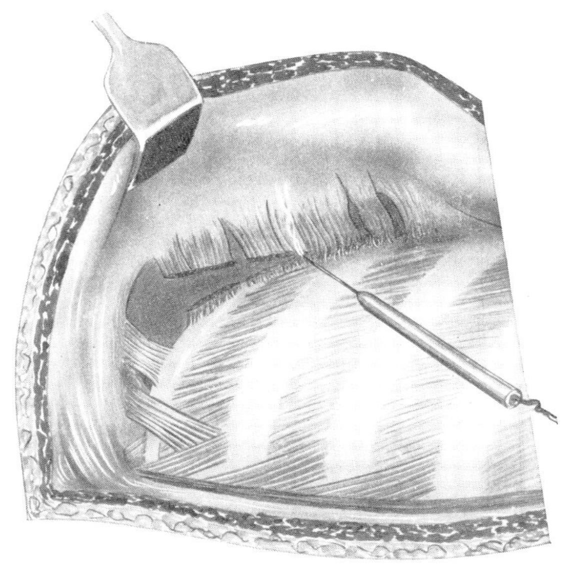

3

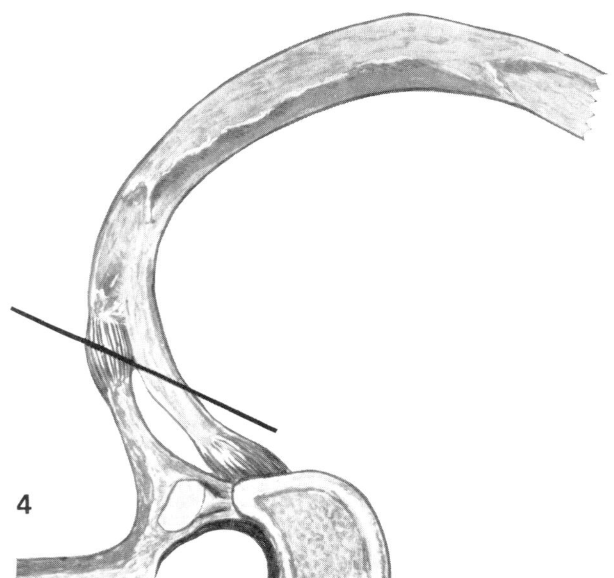

4

4

Removal of second and third ribs

The periosteum of the third rib is incised with diathermy from its costotransverse joint to the anterior axillary line and is then stripped from the rib. The erector spinae muscle is then retracted to expose the costotransverse ligament; this is divided with right-angled bone shears and the blades of the latter are then advanced obliquely downwards and inwards to divide the neck of the rib obliquely. The rib is then divided transversely at its anterior end. The second rib is treated similarly.

Removal of first rib

5

Posterior portion

The first rib is denuded of periosteum throughout its entire length. Care is then taken not to injure the axillary vessels and brachial plexus which lie closely applied to its inner border. The rib is divided near its centre and removed in two portions. The posterior portion is mobilized by dividing the costotransverse ligament and with the fragment pulled forwards it is removed by dividing through the neck.

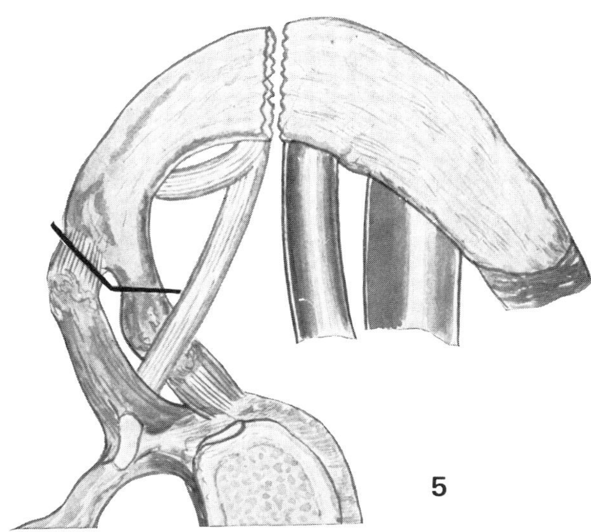

5

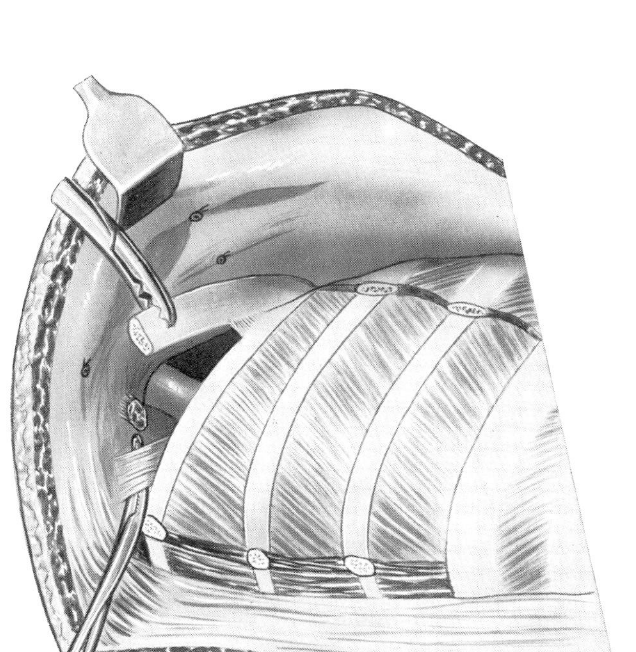

6

6

Anterior portion

The anterior fragment is firmly grasped in bone-holding forceps and pulled downwards to expose the costoclavicular ligament. This is divided with scissors or rugine and the rib removed by cutting through the costochondral junction.

The first intercostal muscle is then excised in order to give an unhampered view of the apex.

7

Apical mobilization; division of Sibson's fascia

Apical mobilization is best achieved by deliberately and cleanly exposing the first dorsal nerve, the subclavian artery and the innominate vein. The exposure of these structures involves division of Sibson's fascia and its three thickenings (bands of Sibelau). The first band lies superficial to the nerve, the second between the artery and the nerve and the third in front of the artery. These bands are isolated and divided and the intervening, less dense, fibrous fascia also divided.

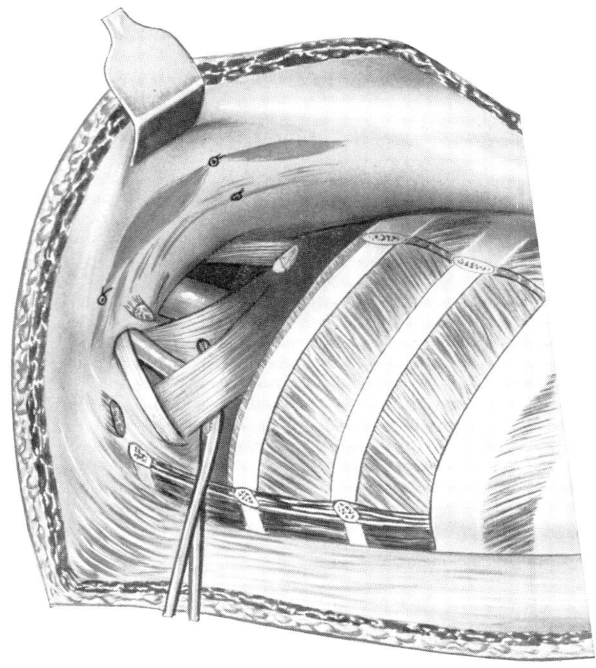

7

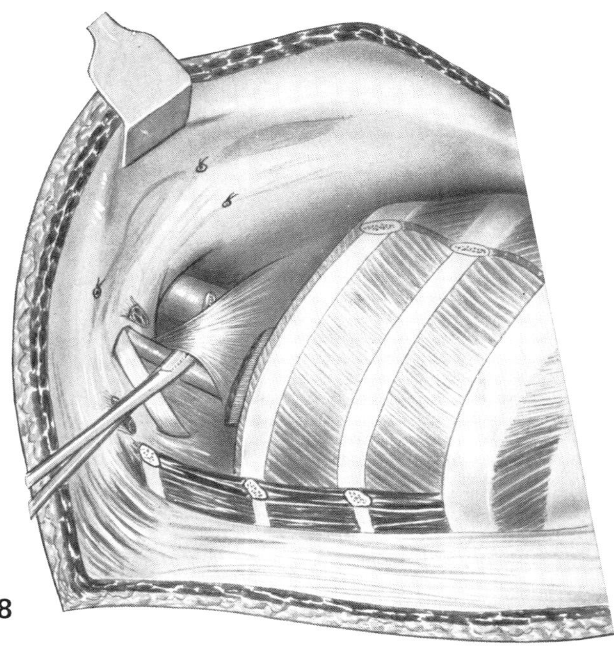

8

8

Exposure of the innominate vein

Some fibres of the scalenus anterior which insert into the pleura (scalenus pleuralis) require division in order to expose the innominate vein with the internal mammary artery running across it.

9

Further mobilization

The mobilization is carried downwards separating the lung from the mediastinal structures by a process of sharp and blunt dissection until the azygos vein is reached on the right side and the aortic arch exposed on the left side.

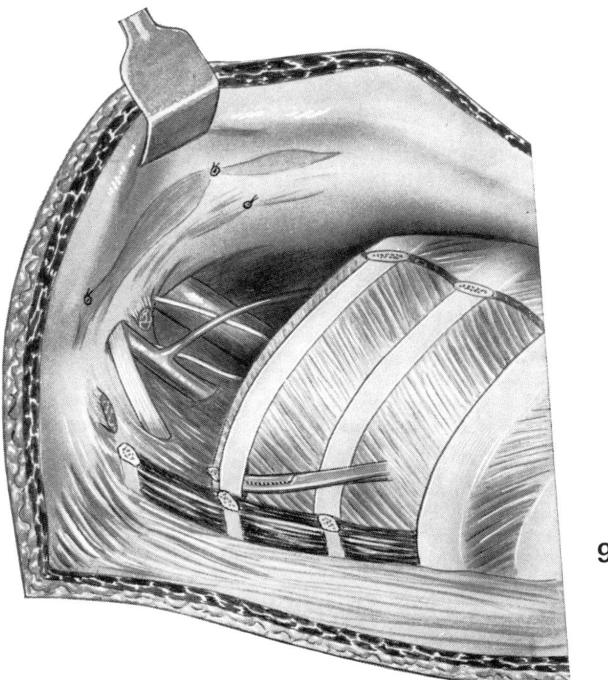

9

10

Division of the intercostal bundles

The upper three intercostal bundles and muscles will require division between ligatures during the later stages of the mobilization. Streptomycin powder is sprinkled over the mobilized apex.

The wound is closed carefully in layers without drainage of the space.

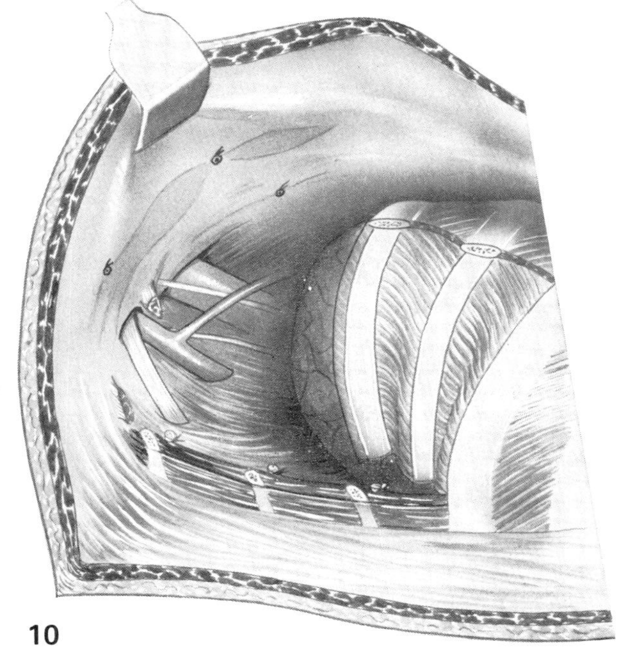

10

11

SECOND STAGE

This is performed 2 weeks after the first stage. The original wound is re-opened and the scapula mobilized. Blood and clot are removed from the extra-fascial space.

Two or more ribs are resected subperiosteally and removed as already described. The bundles and muscles are divided posteriorly and further apical and posterior mobilization of the lung is carried out especially in the paravertebral gutter. Third and subsequent stages are performed at intervals of 2 weeks until the necessary number of ribs has been removed to relax the diseased area. It is unusual to require more than two stages.

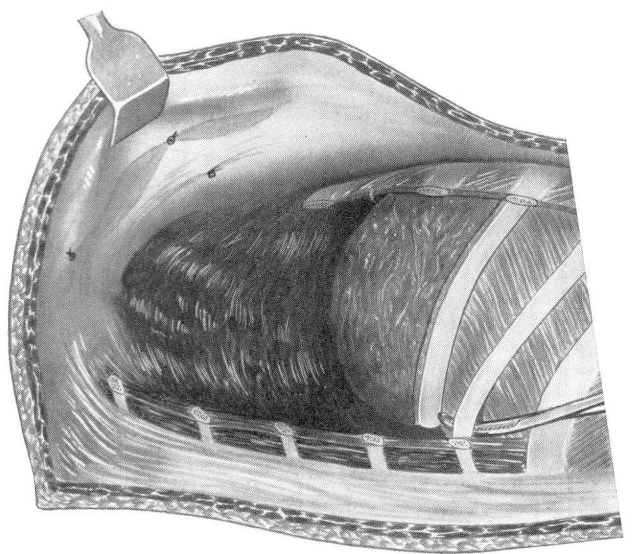

11

References

Björk, V. O. (1954). *J. thorac. Surg.* **28,** 14
Brock, R. C. (1955). *Thorax* **10,** 1
Price Thomas, C. and Cleland, W. P. (1942). *Br. J. Tuberc.* **36,** 109
Sellors, T. H., Jackson, J. W. and Callanan, J. G. (1955). *Thorax* **10,** 191
Semb, C. (1935). *Acta chir. scand.,* Suppl. 37

[*The illustrations for this Chapter on Thoracoplasty with Apicolysis were drawn by Mr. F. Price.*]

Management of Spontaneous Pneumothorax

L. L. Bromley, M.Chir., F.R.C.S.
Consultant Thoracic Surgeon, St. Mary's Hospital, London

INTRODUCTION

Spontaneous pneumothorax results from the rupture of an air vesicle, bulla or cyst on the surface of the lung. The patient presents with a varying degree of collapse of the lung. When this is less than 50 per cent as assessed by chest radiography and, if the patient is not dyspnoeic, conservative management can be adopted. With lung collapse of more than 50 per cent and with moderate dyspnoea on exertion, hospital admission is necessary; the situation being managed by temporary tube drainage of the pleural cavity. For recurrent or chronic pneumothorax the situation may be treated by iodized talc poudrage and tube drainage or by thoracotomy with oversewing of the air leak and parietal pleurectomy.

INSERTION OF AN INTERCOSTAL TUBE

Position of patient

The patient lies supine or semisupine in bed or on the operating table. A convenient site for introduction of the tube is through the second intercostal space in the mid-clavicular line.

Anaesthesia

One per cent lignocaine is infiltrated into the skin and intercostal space at the chosen site.

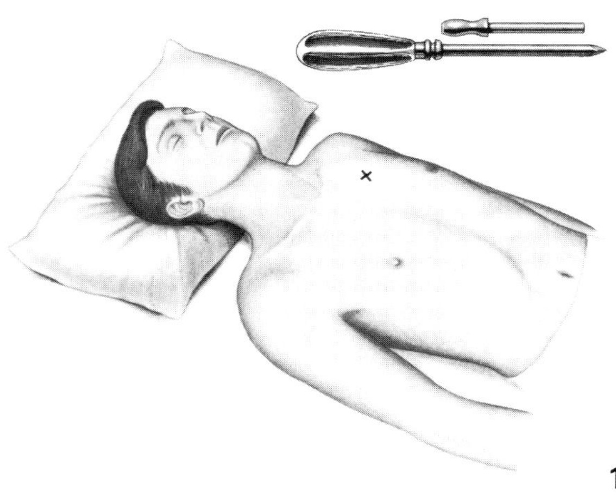

1

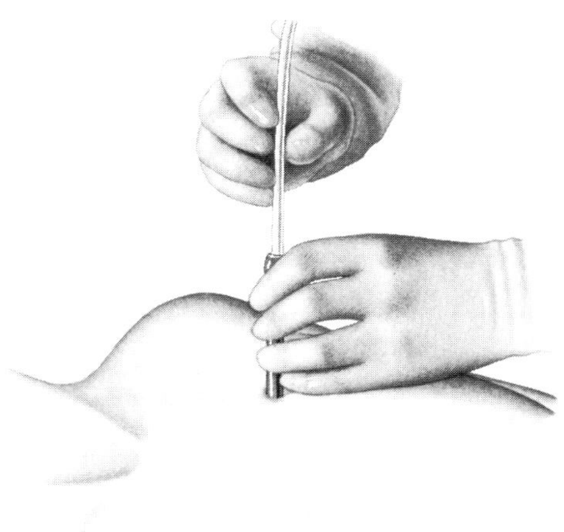

2

2 & 3

Insertion of trocar and cannula

A 1·5 cm incision is made through the skin. At this stage it is most convenient to insert a vertical mattress suture of silk through the centre of the incision and to tie the ends in a loop. This stitch is to be tied when the tube is ultimately removed. A second suture is placed at the edge of the skin incision. The trocar and cannula are then advanced into the pleural cavity and the trocar is withdrawn. A suitable plastic catheter is then threaded down the cannula and the cannula withdrawn. The tube is then anchored in position by tying down the second silk suture around the tube.

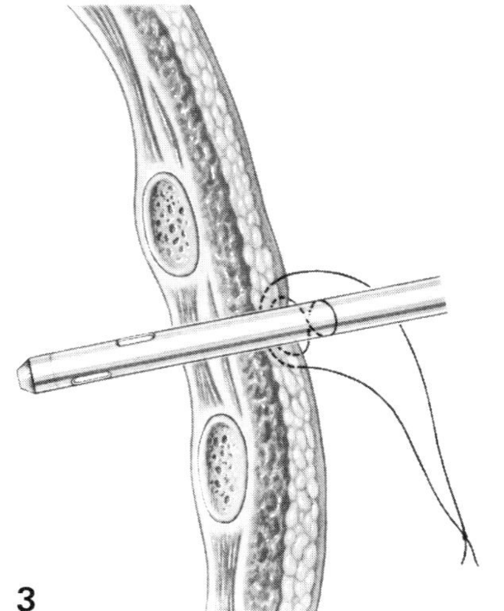

3

4

A combined trocar and tube (Argyle) can be used but great care is necessary with its introduction to avoid pushing it in too far.

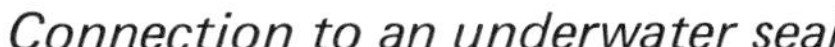

4

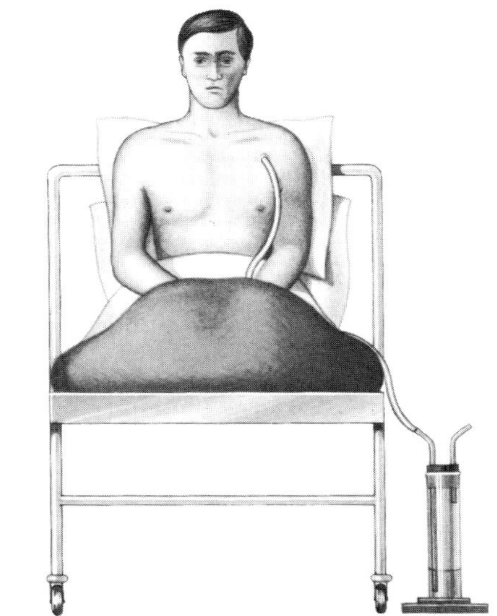

5

Connection to an underwater seal

5

The catheter is connected via a length of plastic or rubber tubing to a chest drainage bottle which provides an underwater seal. If the pneumothorax is large and with a continuing air leak the outlet from the bottle can be connected to a low-pressure suction apparatus (Roberts pump) which assists air removal and expansion of the lung.

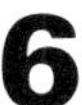

6

An alternative to the waterseal system is to connect the catheter directly to a simple rubber flutter valve contained in a plastic unit (Heimlich valve). With this system the patient can be ambulant.

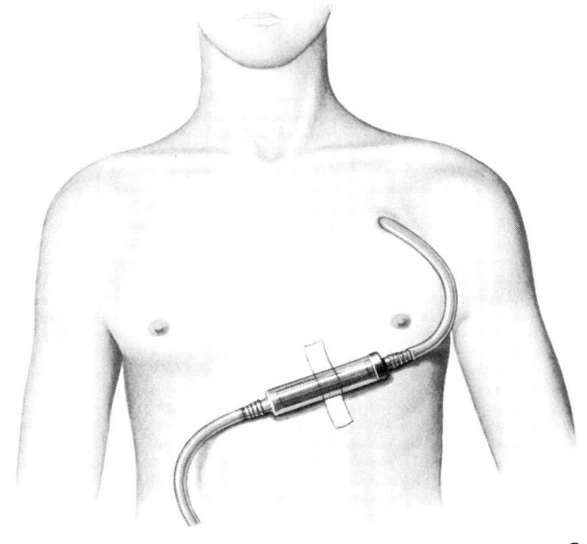

6

Postoperative care

Dressings are applied and the tube further anchored by adhesive strapping. The tube is removed and the original mattress suture tied when the air leak has stopped and the lung has fully expanded.

7

TALC POUDRAGE

A chronic or recurrent pneumothorax being present a trocar is inserted through the second intercostal space as described. Through the trocar 2–3 g of iodized talc are puffed into the pleural cavity via an insufflator. A catheter is then inserted, the trocar withdrawn and the catheter connected to an underwater seal. Iodized talc produces pleural irritation and adhesion formation.

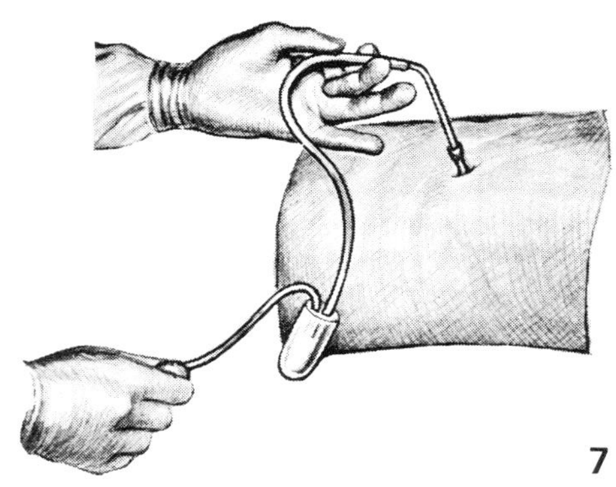

7

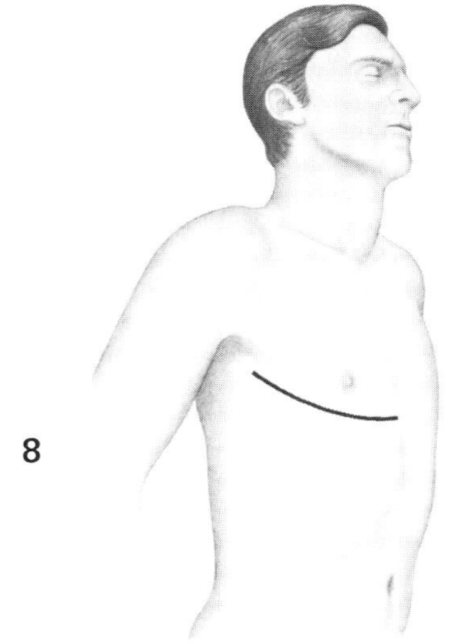

8

THORACOTOMY, OVERSEWING OF BULLAE AND PLEURECTOMY

8

Position of patient

Supine but with the affected side of the chest slightly elevated.

Anaesthesia

Full general. A double lumen tube can be most helpful as ventilation of the affected side can be controlled. In all cases, however, high inflation pressures must be avoided.

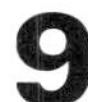

Incision

The skin incision is slightly curved below the nipple or in the inframammary fold. The inferior part of the pectoralis major is divided and the anterior end of the fourth intercostal space exposed. With diathermy the periosteum on the upper border of the fifth rib is divided and the pleural cavity entered immediately above this rib. A retractor is inserted.

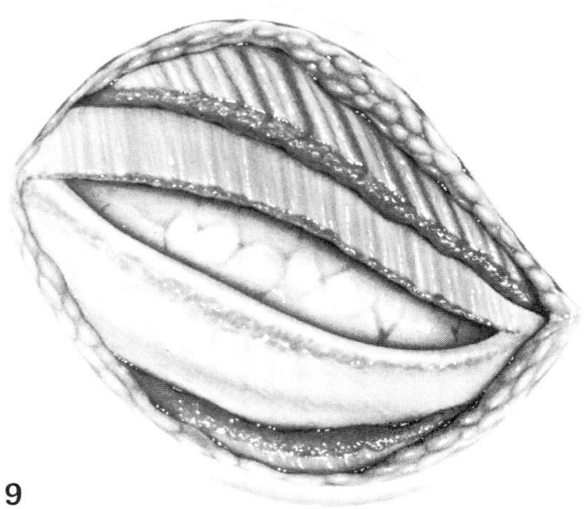

9

10

Oversewing bullae

All parts of the lung are examined. It is most common to find small bullae at the apex of the upper lobe but they may be present at several sites. They are oversewn using fine suture material on an atraumatic needle.

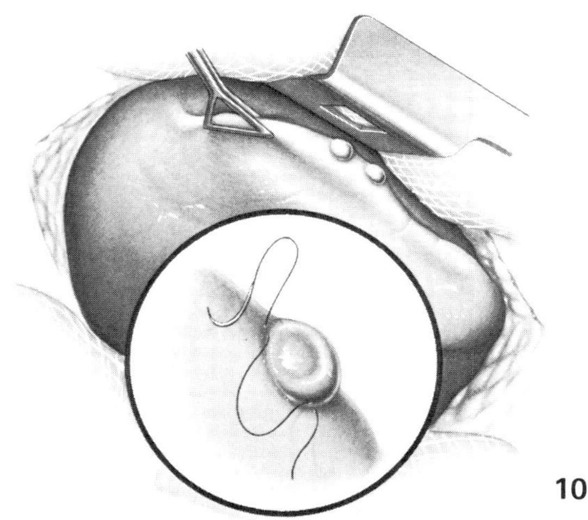

10

11

Parietal pleurectomy

Starting at the margins of the incision a plane of cleavage is established between the parietal pleura and the inner chest wall. The pleura is then stripped off and excised from all areas except the mediastinum and diaphragm.

Apical and basal drains are inserted and connected to underwater seals.

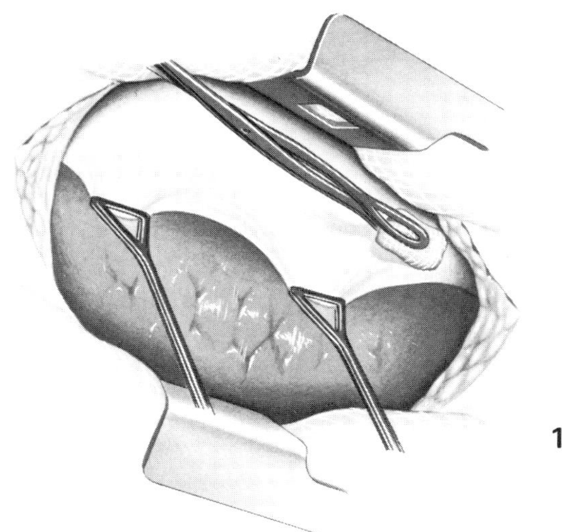

11

Closure

As for routine thoracotomy.

Postoperative care

Some degree of air leak and a moderate serosanguinous exudate is to be expected. It is normal, however, to be able to remove the chest drains 36–48 hr postoperatively.

[*The illustrations for this Chapter on Management of Spontaneous Pneumothorax were drawn by Mr. M. J. Courtney.*]

Pulmonary Cysts

J. R. Belcher, M.S., F.R.C.S.
Surgeon, London Chest Hospital; Thoracic Surgeon, The Middlesex Hospital; Consulting Thoracic Surgeon, North West Thames Regional Health Authority

PRE-OPERATIVE

Indications and contra-indications

There are two different groups of air-containing cysts of the lung: emphysematous and anepithelial cysts.

Air-containing cysts should only be removed when they are causing dyspnoea. No patient can be too gravely dyspnoeic to be recommended surgery if the cyst occupies more than one-third of one lung field. The bigger the cyst the better the result is likely to be. Bilateral cysts should be treated separately on their merits, the larger one being dealt with first and the other one only when the residual symptoms justify it.

The operative mortality in patients with respiratory failure is about 10 per cent.

As the operation does nothing to improve the disease in the rest of the lung, it should not be advised if less than one-third of a lung field is involved.

Pre-operative preparation

This is the same as that for any thoracotomy, with the proviso that more care than usual must be taken to be certain that infection has been eliminated from the lung as far as possible. Figures of blood gas analyses (pCO_2, pO_2, pH) should be available to act as a base line in assessment after the operation.

Anaesthesia

The technique is of paramount importance, as the normal method of paralysis and manual ventilation is very hazardous until the chest wall is open. (There is a risk of causing a tension pneumothorax which may be lethal.) Intubation under local anaesthesia followed by inhalation anaesthesia is the method of choice.

THE OPERATION

The incision

A standard posterolateral thoracotomy is used.

1

Removal of cysts

The purpose of the operation is to remove the mechanical interference with respiration caused by large cysts—not to remove them all.

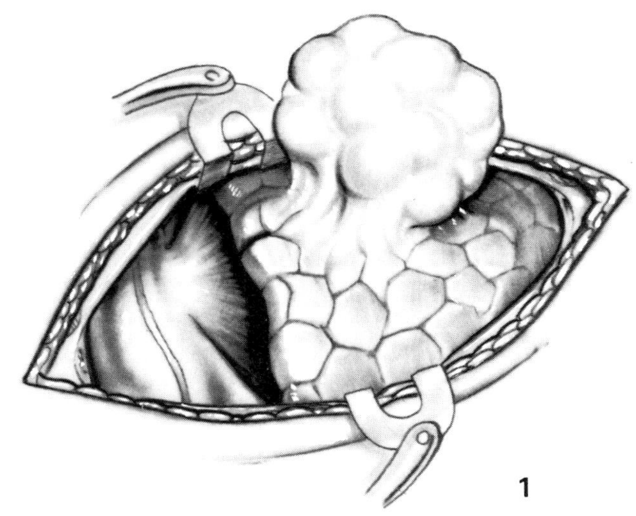

1

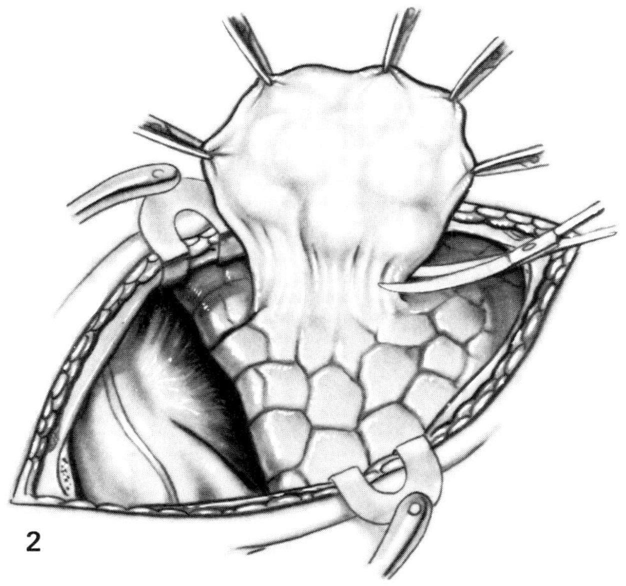

2

2

Opening of cysts

The cysts to be removed are opened near the point where they merge with normal lung, and the incision is carried right round the base of the cyst. (Trans-illumination is valuable in delineating the boundary.)

3

Division of trabeculae

Trabeculae are divided near the normal lung, and the cyst wall which consists of visceral pleura is removed. Where the cyst arises from a narrow pedicle, simple ligature and excision is all that is required.

If it is apparent that the whole lobe is destroyed by the emphysematous process, and there are virtually no functional alveoli in it, a lobectomy is done.

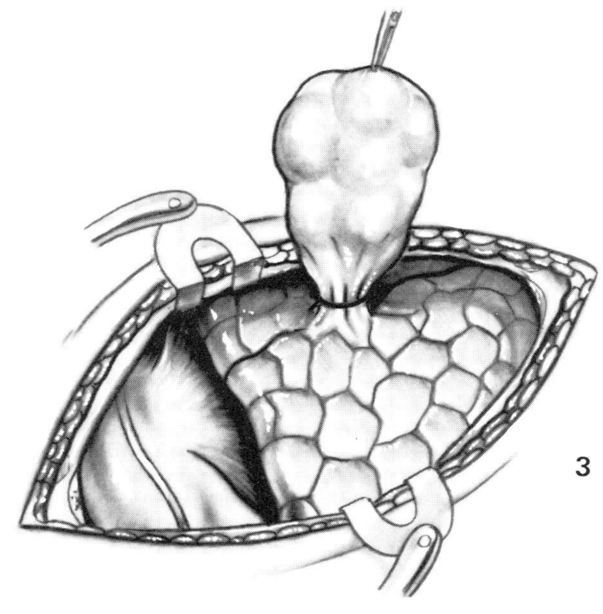

3

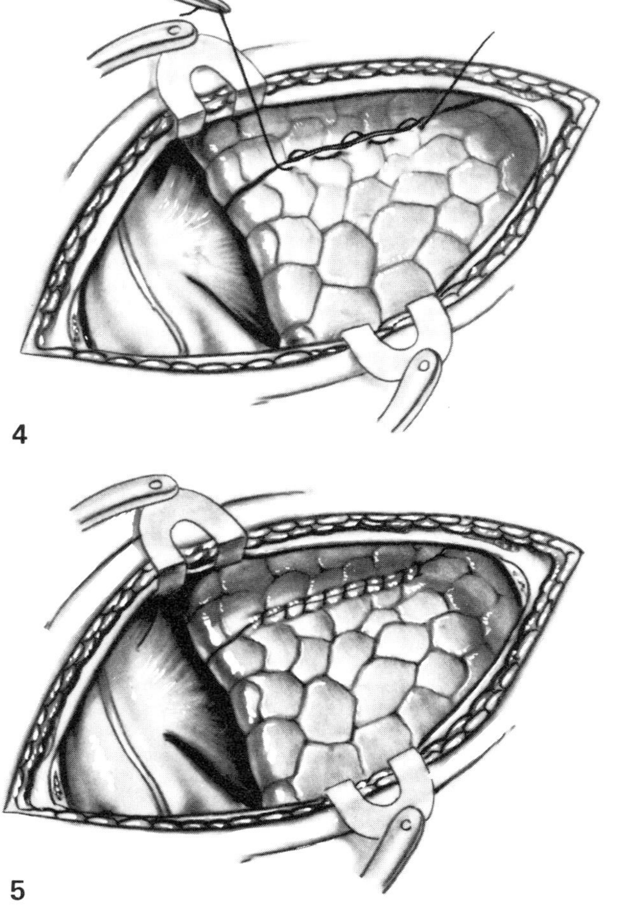

4

5

4 & 5

Oversewing the raw area

A running purse-string suture is used to co-apt the raw surfaces left behind after the removal of the cyst. Particular attention must be paid to haemostasis before this is done.

Drainage

At least two drains (one at the base and the other at the apex) are used, as severe leakage of air is often a problem immediately after operation.

The lung is inflated by the anaesthetist, and the chest is closed in the usual way.

POSTOPERATIVE CARE

The two major problems are leakage of air and abnormalities of the blood gases.

Maintenance of tube patency

It is essential that both tubes remain patent until the leakage stops, and that suction is applied to them, for if a large volume of air accumulates in the pleura, the patient may succumb with respiratory insufficiency. Also, if the lung is not kept in a fully expanded state, it may never become as efficient as it should do.

The tubes are only removed when the leakage of air has ceased.

Biochemical changes

Many patients operated on for this condition have had a high pCO_2 for some time and adjustment of the respiratory centre to the normal after operation may take some time. Thus, hypoxia has to be watched for and treated should it occur. Excessive air leak from the lungs may cause a dramatic reduction of the pCO_2 to levels well below normal, and repeated gas analyses may be required before the situation becomes stable.

Complications

Subcutaneous emphysema may occur rapidly if the patency of the tubes is jeopardized, but it can be readily treated by adjustment or replacement of them.

Atelectasis is uncommon, but must be treated with more than usual promptitude should it occur.

Where the residual lung is too small to fill the pleura, empyema is liable to occur and has to be treated on its merits.

[*The illustrations for this Chapter on Pulmonary Cysts were drawn by Mr. G. Lyth.*]

Pulmonary Hydatid Cysts

N. R. Barrett, M.Chir., F.R.C.S.
Consulting Surgeon, St. Thomas's Hospital, London

INTRODUCTION

Hydatid cysts are a phase in the life cycle of the tapeworm, *Taenia ecchinococcus.* This disease remains an important scourge in many parts of the world where it is endemic; and since the time that elapses between infestation and the diagnosis of a hydatid cyst is usually measured in years, travellers can carry it to places where experience in its diagnosis and management is limited.

Hydatid cysts are most commonly found in the liver and the lungs. They may be solitary or multiple, 'simple' or 'complicated' by rupture and infection. A solitary lung cyst may be the only abnormality in the patient; equally, a solitary lung cyst may be only a part of a diffuse infestation.

Whenever it is technically feasible hydatid cysts should be removed, and this is especially true in the lung. The reason is that 'simple cysts' not only occupy space that should be filled with lung, but they are liable to rupture and this is followed by daughter cyst formation, sepsis, and sometimes by anaphylaxis. If a lung cyst has already ruptured it is almost certain that a hydatid abscess will have formed in the lung, and in this sepsis is perpetuated by unabsorbable fragments of chitinous endocyst.

There are several techniques that deal efficiently with solitary simple lung hydatid cysts. In all, the object is to get the cyst out of the body without tearing its membrane or spilling its contents. If hydatid fluid is spilled into the lung cavity, the pleural cavity, or into the incised structures of the chest wall, it is possible that hydatid elements will be implanted in one or all of these sites and that secondary cysts will form. To avoid this some surgeons inject 10 per cent formalin into the hydatid before taking it out. This kills the germinal membrane; but this technique is dangerous in the management of a lung cyst, because if the cyst ruptures during the operation the bronchial tree may be flooded with dilute formalin.

The following techniques are advised for treating lung cysts.

'Simple cysts'

(*1*) Cysts up to 1 inch (2·5 cm) in diameter are best removed by segmental or wedge resection of the part of the lung that contains the cyst.

(*2*) Cysts up to 5 inches (12·5 cm) in diameter can be taken out by enucleation (as described below) or by excising the cyst together with its adventitia intact. The adventitia is the compressed zone of normal lung that surrounds, and is closely applied to, the chitinous membrane of the cyst.

(*3*) Very large cysts are most safely treated by lobectomy.

'Complicated cysts'

Lobectomy is essential. If, during the course of removal of a pulmonary hydatid cyst, the membrane is ruptured and the liquid contents are spilled, the wound and the pleural cavity should be liberally flushed out with warm normal saline.

ENUCLEATION OF 'SIMPLE' PULMONARY HYDATID CYST

These patients are clinically well, unless the cyst is so large that it causes dyspnoea. Do nothing that might rupture the cyst before operation, and *never aspirate* to verify the diagnosis. A few drops of hydatid fluid implanted into the tissues of the host can cause dangerous anaphylaxis.

No special anaesthesia is required beyond that used for a routine thoracotomy. But if the cyst is large the bronchus leading to the invaded lobe may with advantage be blocked off with a balloon. This is a safeguard against flooding the bronchial tree by untimely rupture.

If the cyst ruptures spontaneously during induction, immediate bronchoscopic aspiration of liquid and membranes may be necessary. Anaphylaxis under general anaesthesia is said not to occur.

The usual approach is by lateral thoracotomy. The pleural cavity is usually free in these cases and the cyst can be seen or palpated. Before proceeding to enucleation cover the wound edges with polythene towels.

THE OPERATION

1

Typical 'simple' cyst

A typical 'simple' hydatid cyst is approaching the surface of the lung. The pale discoloured tissue is the adventitia of the host: it is never the parasite itself. If a cyst impinges so much upon the surface of the lung that the laminated membrane itself has become exposed, the cyst herniates spontaneously out of the lung into the pleural cavity, and in so doing it generally ruptures and disseminates the disease.

1

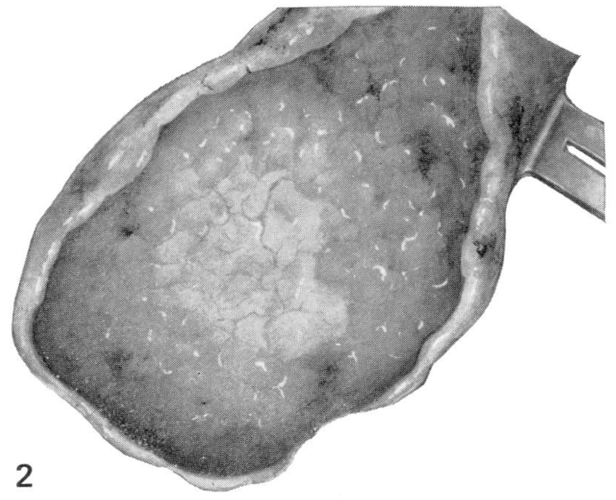

2

2

Elevation of lobe into wound

Protective polythene towels have been placed over the exposed tissues of the wound, and the lobe containing the parasite has been elevated into the wound by placing a large swab behind the lobe.

3

Exposure of laminated membrane

The adventitia is being incised to expose the laminated membrane and the latter is prevented from herniating immediately out of the lung by placing a finger along the incision. This is important because, if the cyst herniates through too small an incision in the adventitia, the neck of the herniated part is constricted, and this favours rupture. The cyst is kept inside its pulmonary cavity until the incision in the adventitia is large enough to allow the parasite to fall out. The laminated membrane is pure white in colour.

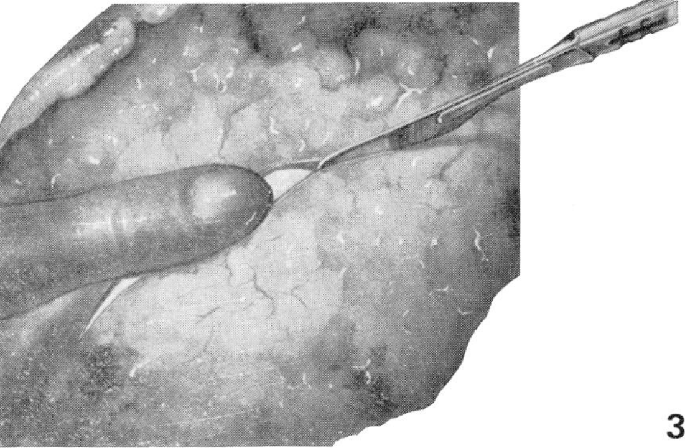

3

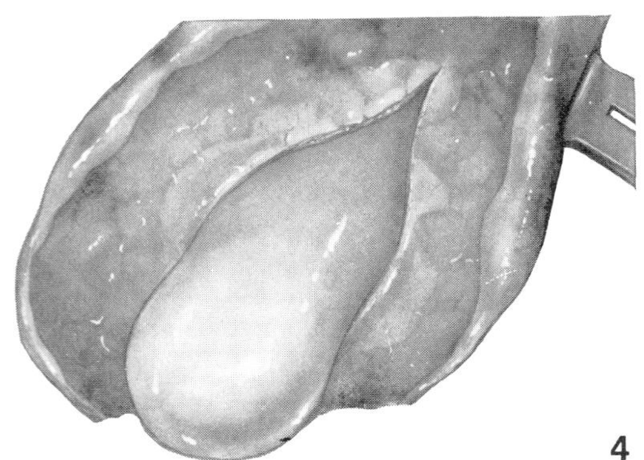

4

4&5

Herniating of parasite from lung

The surgeon must, at this point, have patience. Enucleation can be helped by the anaesthetist increasing the intrabronchial pressure, by an assistant placing his hand behind the lobe and elevating it, and by tilting the operating table towards the side of the surgeon. Immediately after the cyst has rolled out of the lung one or more bronchial fistulae often become apparent in the adventitia of the host. These should be closed by sutures; and the efficacy of the sutures should be tested by filling the cavity in the lung with saline and noting the presence or absence of air leaks. Haemorrhage from delicate veins in the unsupported adventitia may occur after enucleation but this is seldom serious.

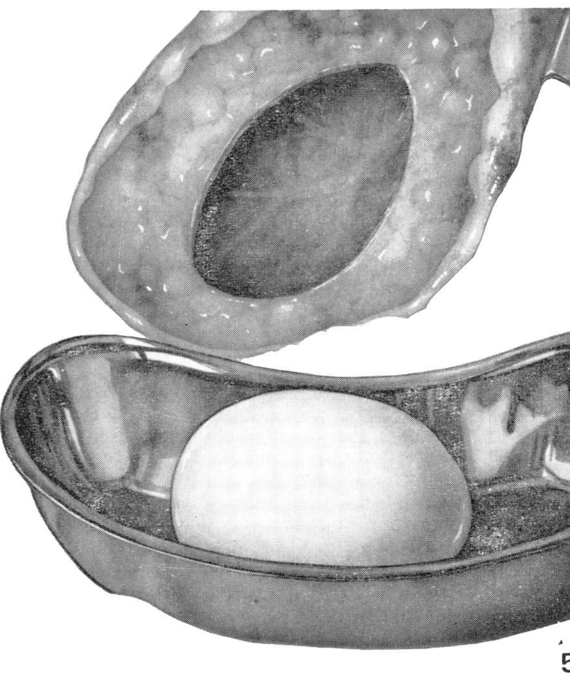

5

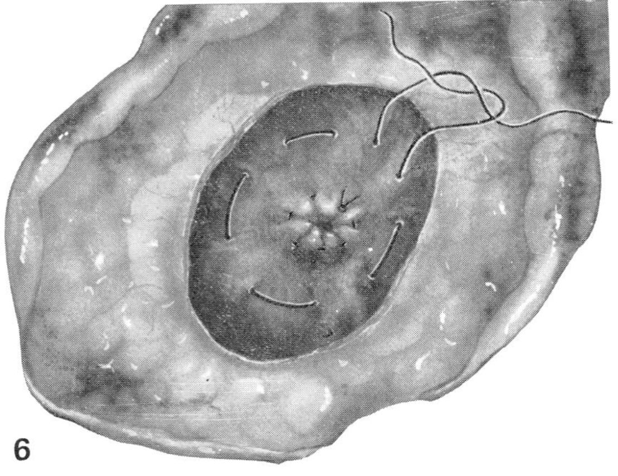

6

6

Closure

The parasite has herniated out of the lung and the space it occupied is being obliterated by concentric rows of stitches. If this is not done the cavity in the lung may persist for a long time and a bronchopleural fistula is inevitable.

After obliterating the empty sac the visceral pleura is sewn over the incision in the lobe. The chest is closed with temporary pleural drainage.

[*The illustrations for this Chapter on Pulmonary Hydatid Cysts were drawn by Miss J. Dewe.*]

Flail Chest and Non-penetrating Injuries

Bryan P. Moore, F.R.C.S.
Consultant Thoracic Surgeon, Brook General Hospital, London

PRE-OPERATIVE

The objectives of management of flail chest, due to blunt injury, which may be unilateral or bilateral are as follows: (*1*) to restore or maintain adequate spontaneous ventilation and voluntary expectoration of secretions; (*2*) to prevent or correct deformity of the chest wall; (*3*) to avoid the need for mechanical positive-pressure ventilation or tracheostomy whenever possible. Operative stabilization is essential in the more severe cases. In unconscious patients (e.g. from concomitant brain injury) the use of an oro- or naso-tracheal tube or tracheostomy may be required for the aspiration of bronchial secretions.

The bronchoscope provides the most efficient means of aspirating secretions, blood or foreign material from the lower respiratory passages and also of locating haemorrhage or a torn bronchus. Care must be taken to ensure against hypoxia and a venturi system attached to the bronchoscope is of great assistance.

Initial treatment includes attention to blood volume and fluid and electrolyte balance, unilateral or bilateral pleural drainage for the removal of air and blood by intercostal tube (normally inserted with local anaesthesia) with under-water seal and clearance of airways of blood, debris and secretions. If significant hypoxaemia or hypercarbia exists, ventilation as a resuscitative measure may be needed. The stomach should be kept empty and urine excretion monitored.

Appreciation of the severity of flail chest is frequently incorrect. Paradoxical movement may be obvious with respiration but will be exaggerated with coughing. Palpation of the chest wall, particularly of the costal cartilages and anterior and wall ribs is very helpful and may reveal many fractures which are invisible in the straight and lateral chest x-rays.

Multiple rib and costal cartilage fractures tend to loosen and displace progressively during the first few days following a blunt injury. Deterioration from progressive accumulation of bronchial secretions and pulmonary atelectasis must be anticipated.

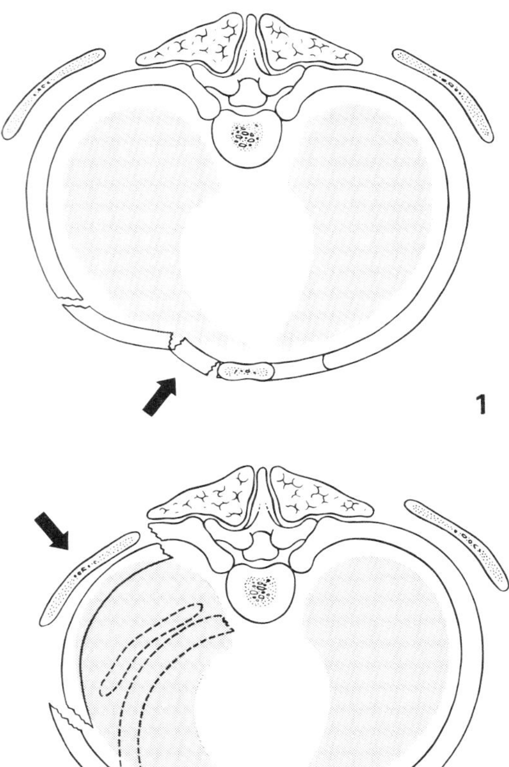

1 & 2

The injuries may be divided into anterolateral (typical of the motor car driver trapped behind the steering wheel in a head-on collision) and posterolateral (typical of the victim who has time to turn away and present the back of the shoulder to the on-coming force).

OPERATIVE STABILIZATION OF THE FLAIL CHEST WALL

The most effective method is individual medullary pinning of the multiple fractures with wires or fine nails.

The best exposure depends upon the part of the chest, anterolateral or posterolateral, more affected.

3

Anterolateral injuries

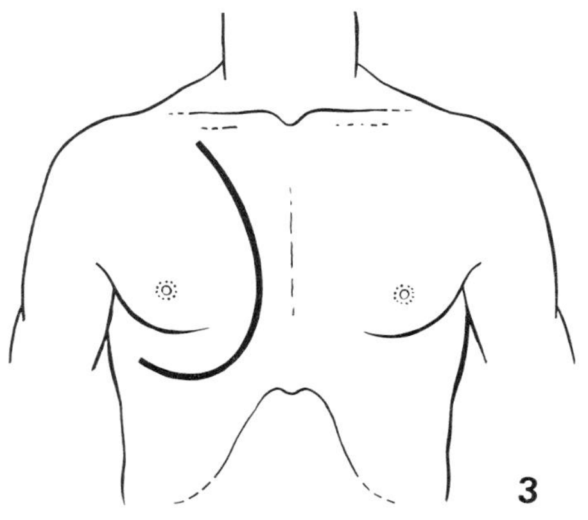

Anterolateral injuries with fractures of the costal cartilages and anterior ends of the ribs, particularly of the second to fifth ribs, which are most liable to produce paradoxical movement, may be exposed by a curved incision lying vertically over the costo-chondral junctions beside the sternum which is extended upwards and outwards to below the mid-point of the clavicle and downwards and outwards below the breast in the line of the fifth or sixth rib.

A broad flap of skin and subcutaneous tissue should be reflected outwards. The fractures can be exposed individually by separating the fibres of pectoralis major. As many fractures are pinned as are reasonably accessible through the approach. The pleura will almost always be found to be torn and pleural drainage will be necessary. The pleural cavity can be explored adequately if the incision is extended laterally and deepened through all layers, but this is not usually indicated.

Perfect stability with multiple or comminuted fractures may be unobtainable but even a single firm bridge across a flail segment may prove of great value and will avoid or diminish the need for mechanical ventilatory support.

Posterolateral injuries

Posterolateral injuries of the upper part of the chest wall are frequently effected by the scapula or shoulder joint being momentarily forced into the chest with disruption of the shoulder girdle. Two series of fractures are likely to occur, in successive ribs, one at the outer border of the erector spinae muscles and a second in the posterior axilla. The lower ribs are unprotected by the scapula.

4

In severe cases of this nature, and in those in which visceral damage is suspected, thoracotomy is advised through a standard or modified posterolateral approach and accompanied by stabilization with medullary pinning of all accessible rib fractures. For better exposure of the highest three ribs, the standard incision can be extended upwards midway between the spine and the medial border of the scapula. For the lowest four ribs, a T-shaped incision may be made downwards and toward the mid-line.

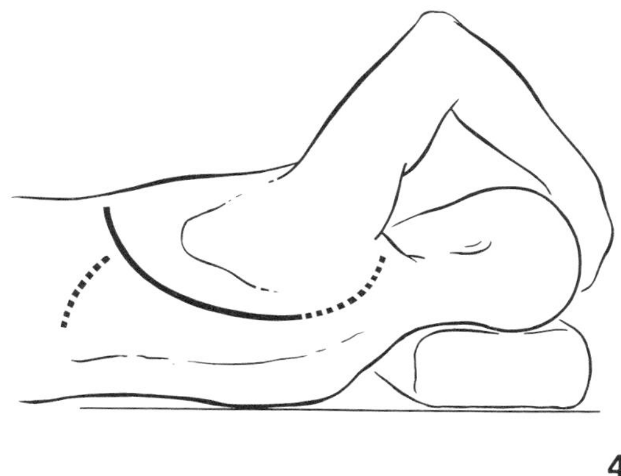

4

5 & 6

Technique of intramedullary rib and costal cartilage fracture stabilization

The fracture is located and, in the case of the ribs, the periosteum should be bared over a small area about 3 cm away. The rib or cartilage is grasped with bone-forceps (not the fingers for fear of injury) and a small perforation of the cortex made with a bone awl or a drill. A Kirschner wire, held in the appropriate holder, is suitable and should be manipulated into the medulla and across the fracture into the medulla of the opposing fragment until it impacts in the curving cortex. A short length of the redundant wire may be angled down towards the rib to discourage displacement.

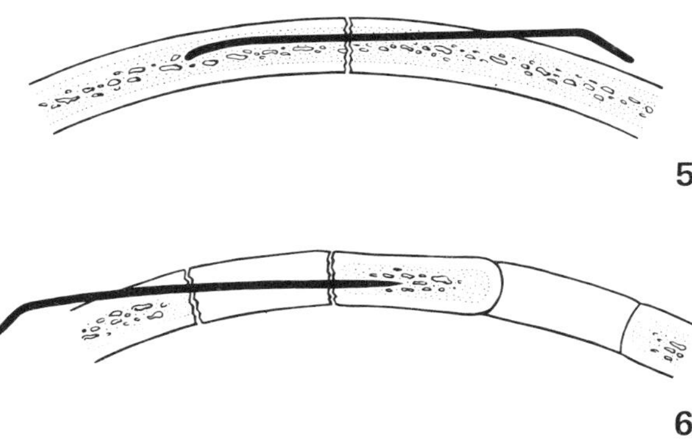

5

6

Fractures of the sternum

Fractures of the sternum contribute towards instability of the chest wall and paradoxical movement. They may be caused by direct or indirect violence. In either case, if unstable or displaced but not impacted, the fractures should be reduced or fixed by a medullary nail (Kirschner, Rush or Steinmann). The approach is through a vertical mid-line incision centred upon the fracture site and deepened down to the periosteum.

Compression injuries of the chest in children, adolescents and young adults are likely to be accompanied by visceral injury in the absence of obvious flail chest wall or even rib, cartilage or sternal fracture. Laceration and disruption or extensive contusion of a lobe (particularly a lower lobe) may be present without prominent haemoptysis or air leak. If this condition is suspected, exploratory thoracotomy, preferably early, is mandatory so that a severely damaged lobe can be removed before irreversible infection supervenes.

POSTOPERATIVE CARE

Homeostasis in respect of fluid and electrolyte balance, blood volume and arterial blood gases and pH must be maintained. The importance of physiotherapy cannot be over-stressed together with early mobilization. In multiple injuries and particularly if mobilization is impossible, prophylactic anticoagulation against deep vein thrombosis may be advisable. Infection should be treated prophylactically and definitively with antibiotic therapy.

[*The illustrations for this Chapter on Flail Chest and Non-penetrating Injuries were drawn by Mr. M. J. Courtney.*]

Penetrating Wounds of the Chest

Bryan P. Moore, F.R.C.S.
Consultant Thoracic Surgeon, Brook General Hospital, London

WOUNDS OF THE CHEST WALL

Superficial wounds should be explored, devitalized tissue excised and sutured or left open for delayed suture according to general principles.

Penetrating wounds of all layers of the chest wall, including the parietal pleura will breach the vacuum of the pleural space and may allow the development of a pneumothorax from without in the absence of a wound of the underlying lung. This condition of 'sucking chest wound' demands urgent effective closure by pressure, pack or suture and early drainage of the pleural space by intercostal tube with underwater seal. In projectile wounds, revision, debridement and delayed suture must be modified to include closure of the pleura.

Wounds of the chest wall including the parietal pleura are likely to divide major branches of the intercostal or internal mammary arteries or veins. Haemorrhage into the pleural space may be profuse or gradual but is always augmented by the negative pleural pressure and respiratory movement. Reactionary haemorrhage is common and must be anticipated.

When evidence of intrapleural haemorrhage exists, an intercostal pleural drainage tube of not less than 6·5 mm internal diameter (28 Ch) should be inserted under local anaesthesia and attached to a drainage bottle with underwater seal. Blood lost must be replaced.

Many penetrating wounds of the chest wall have been safely treated by intercostal drainage alone but if the least doubt exists concerning continued haemorrhage or visceral damage, it is far safer to explore the chest by thoracotomy.

1

By far the most useful exposure is a full postero-lateral thoracotomy through the bed of the fifth rib (fourth intercostal space).

The rib should be stripped of periosteum along the superior border and the posterior end may be divided just distal to the vertebral transverse process after retraction of the erector spinae muscles medially. If the wound is low in the chest, a lower rib bed should be substituted but it is seldom necessary to open below the seventh rib bed (sixth intercostal space) which allows reasonable access to the diaphragm also. The ribs should be counted by palpation from above downwards with the hand beneath the scapula.

Penetrating wounds through or close to the sternum which are judged to involve the heart or mediastinal structures may require an alternative exposure.

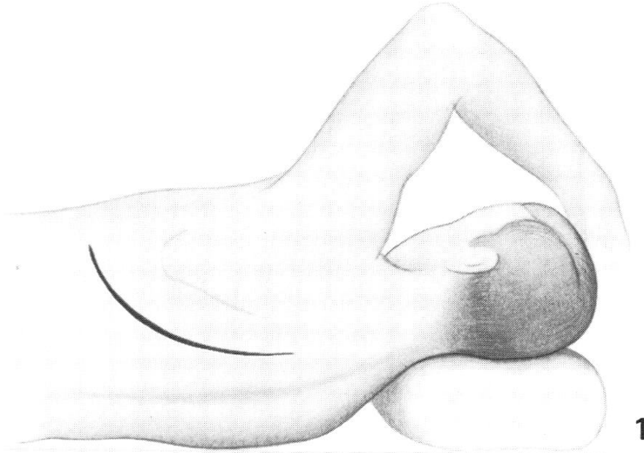

1

2

The best general approach to the heart and anterior mediastinum is through a complete median (vertical) sternal split. The median incision extends from the upper border of the manubrium to 3 cm below the tip of the xiphoid process.

Division of the sternum is normally made with an oscillating saw but can also be made with a Gigli saw (passed behind with a very long forceps) or with a Lebsche chisel. These instruments may not be available in some emergency situations. This approach is not satisfactory for dealing with any wound of either lung.

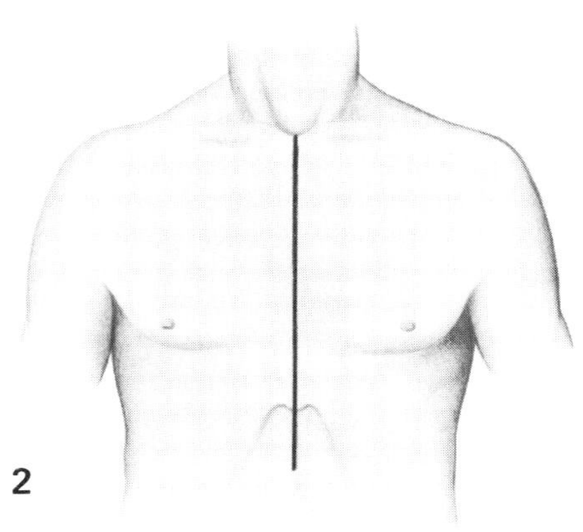

2

3&4

In the emergency situation, and in selected cases, the heart may be approached through a left anterior sub-mammary, fourth intercostal space incision extending from the left border of the sternum to the mid-axilla. The exposure will be very limited unless a self-retaining chest retractor is available. It may be improved either by dividing costal cartilages above and below the incision or by extending the incision medially across the sternum after control of the internal mammary vessels. The division of the sternum is normally performed with the Gigli saw or Lebsche chisel but other osteotomes are effective.

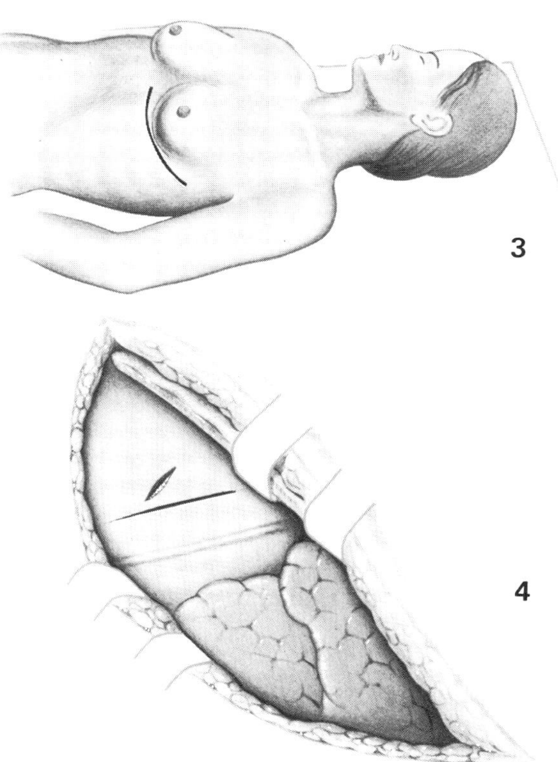

3

4

WOUNDS OF THE LUNG

Stab wounds

5

The visceral pleura should never be closed over a deep incised wound of the lung because anaesthetic gases may be forced out of lacerated bronchi into open pulmonary vein tributaries producing coronary and other air embolus.

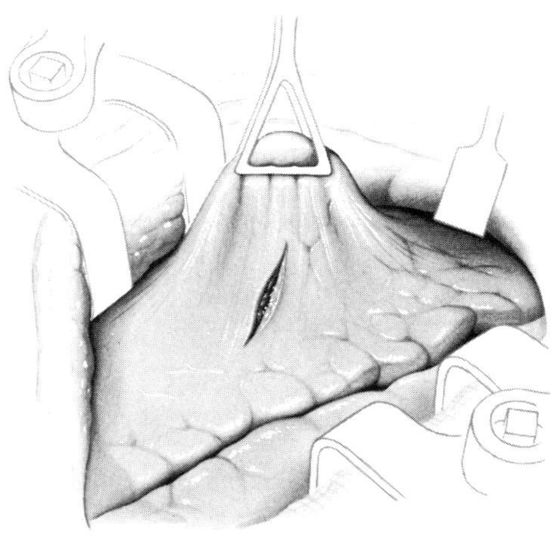

5

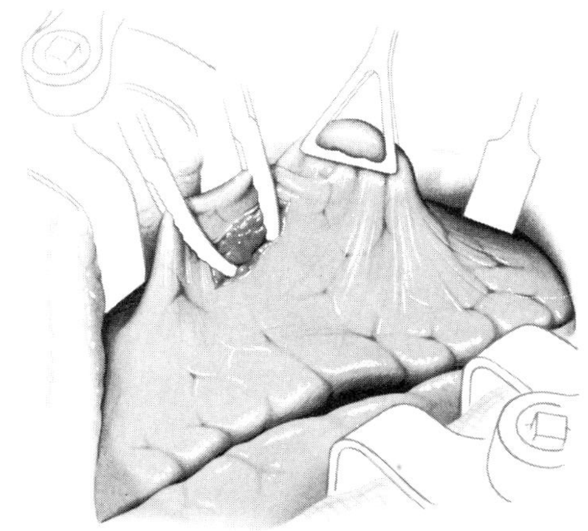

6

6,7&8

A deep incised wound which is bleeding or leaking air may be explored by extending the limits in the lines of the intersegmental planes of the bronchopulmonary segments. The deflated lung can be divided between (Roberts) lung clamps and this tissue oversewn with catgut to control air-leak and haemorrhage. Individual bronchi and vessels can be sutured but drainage to the pleura must be permitted. The pleural space should be drained by two intercostal tubes with underwater seal before closure of the wound.

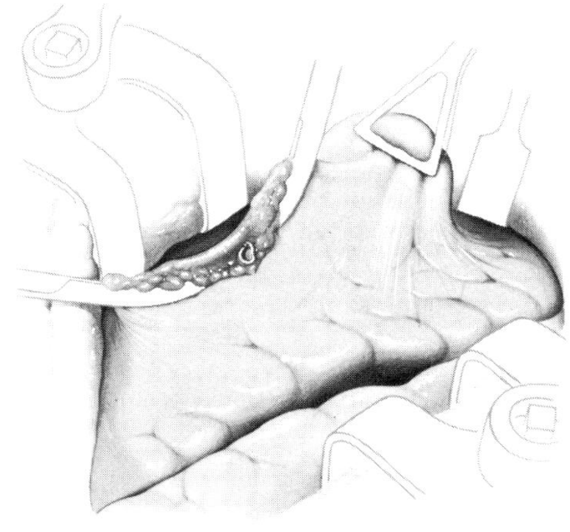

7

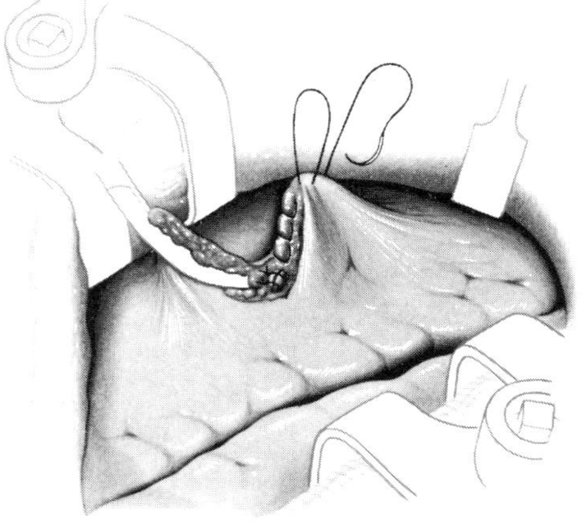

8

Projectile wounds

These vary very widely according to the nature and velocity of the projectile. Relatively low-velocity revolver bullets may perforate one or more lobes of the lung with little damage and after inspection, only drainage of the pleural space may be required. High-velocity perforating wounds are accompanied by more damage to tissue adjacent to the track. If the degree of damage is extensive, lobectomy or pneumonectomy may be necessary.

Bomb fragments, because of irregular shape, commonly carry with them pieces of rib and are associated not only with severe haemorrhage and air-leak from torn pulmonary vessels and bronchi but also with haemorrhage from irregular entry and exit chest-wall wounds. Control of haemorrhage by thoracotomy may need to precede the desirable degree of resuscitation.

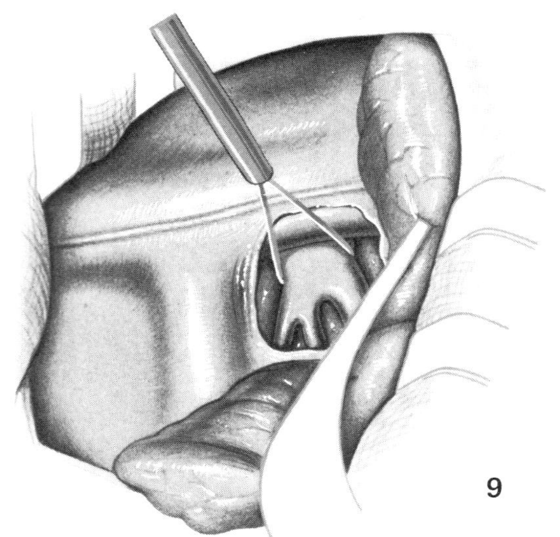

9

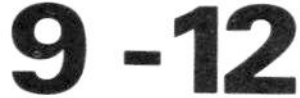

Severe bleeding from the lung should be temporarily controlled at right or left thoracotomy by first isolating the main pulmonary artery in the hilum and passing a tape or stout ligature round as a snare and secondly treating the superior and inferior pulmonary veins in the same way. This procedure is much facilitated if the lung is deflated (by the use of a double-lumen anaesthetic tube).

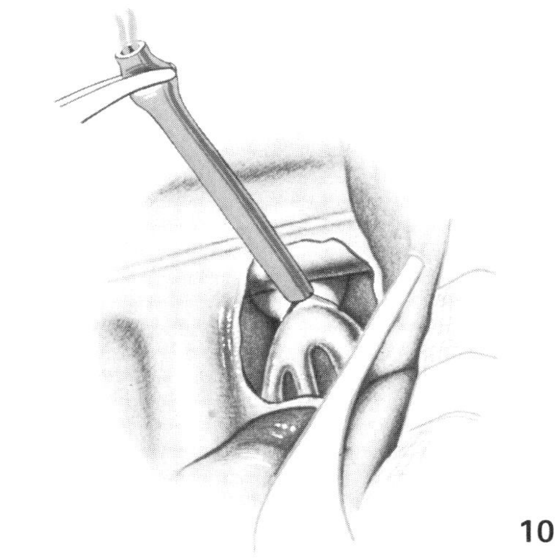

10

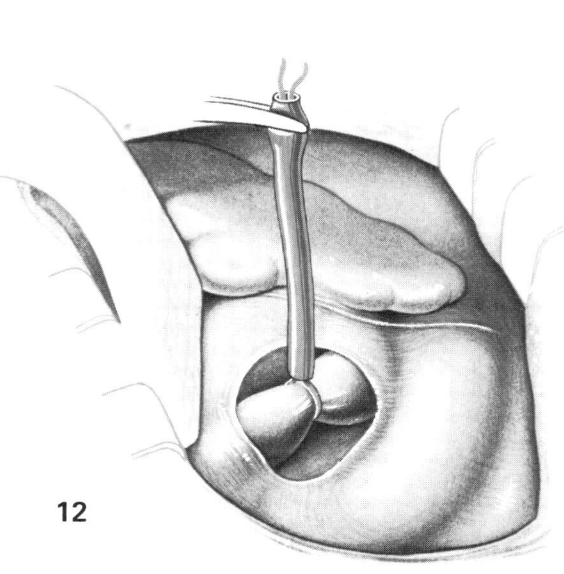

12

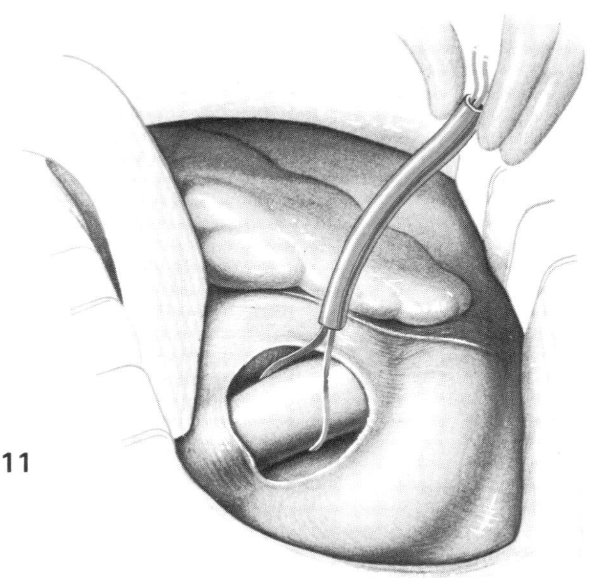

11

WOUNDS OF THE HEART

The immediate cause of circulatory arrest by any wound of the heart is tamponade. Relief is by widely opening the pericardium and this is possible through any one of the approaches mentioned above.

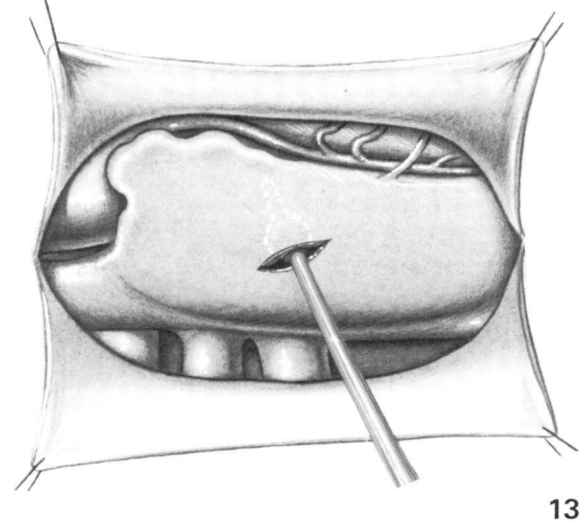

13

13-16

Clots and fluid blood gush out of the pericardium and are likely to be followed by bleeding from the original heart wound. Control of this is usually possible with one finger because larger wounds are unlikely to allow survival. Firm traction on the incised margins of the pericardium with forceps or stitches will be helpful. Should resuscitation be required before closure of a heart wound a Foley catheter may be useful, inserted and inflated and then drawn back as a tampon.

To aid suture of a wound of the right or left atrial wall, an atrial or large vascular clamp may be applied and a continuous suture inserted. No attempt should be made to apply a clamp to either ventricle. The wound, which will be small, should be closed with interrupted sutures placed carefully to avoid any obvious coronary artery.

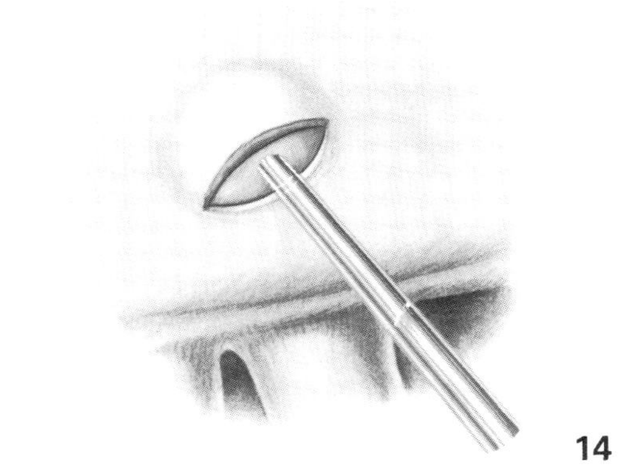

14

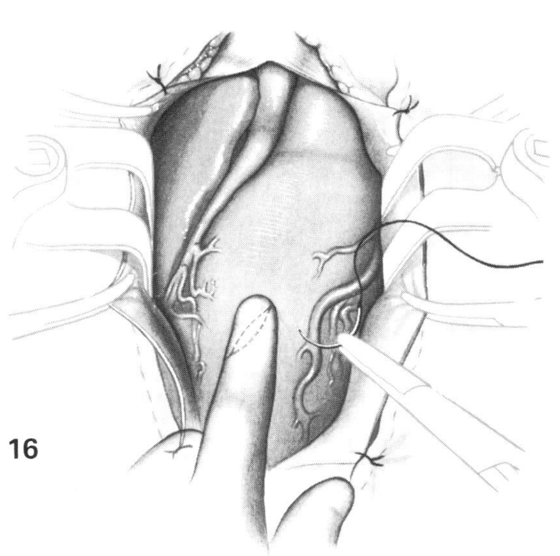

16

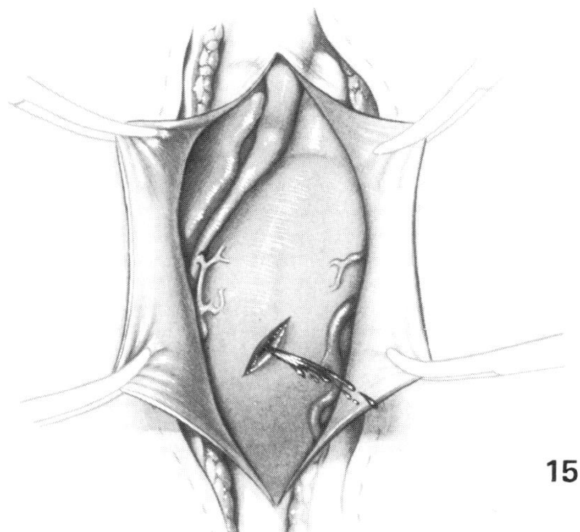

15

17

If the heart muscle is friable or the stitch holes bleed, horizontal mattress sutures supported on either side by small patches of Teflon felt may have to be added.

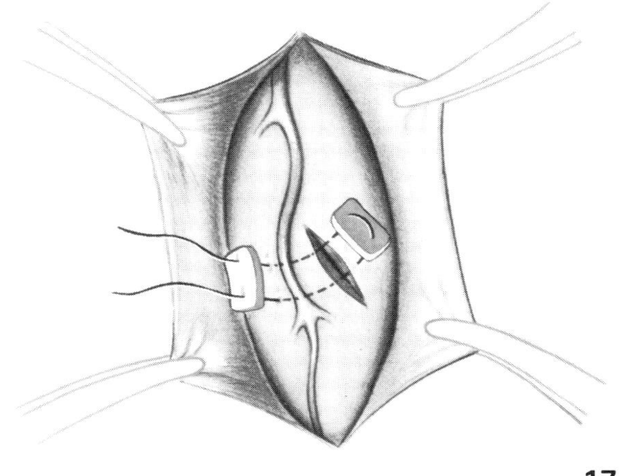

17

The pericardium must be able to drain freely so that the tamponade will not recur.

Following right or left thoracotomy the pericardium should be resutured only enough to prevent prolapse of the ventricles through the opening. After median sternotomy, the pericardium need not be resutured and two drains (minimum size 6·5 mm internal diameter, 28 Ch should be inserted through dependent stab wounds into the anterior mediastinum and unsutured pericardium.

[*The illustrations for this Chapter on Penetrating Wounds of the Chest were drawn by Mr. M. J. Courtney.*]

Resection of Lung

R. Abbey Smith, Ch.M., F.R.C.S.
Thoracic Surgeon, Walsgrave Hospital, Coventry

PRE - OPERATIVE

Indications

In Britain about 90 per cent of lung resections are carried out for carcinoma of the lung. Four methods of resection are routinely used: pneumonectomy, lobectomy, sleeve resection and segmental resection. The methods may be used in combination; for instance, right upper lobectomy with resection of the apical segment of the right lower lobe for carcinoma involving the upper end of the main fissure, or left lower lobectomy with segmental resection of the lingular segment of the left upper lobe for bronchiectasis.

Pneumonectomy

Few indications exist for this operation except where a diagnosis of lung carcinoma is firmly established before operation, or by frozen section examination during operation. Occasionally it is impracticable to do any operation less than the removal of an entire lung for such conditions as unilateral bronchiectasis affecting all segments, or tuberculosis with complete lung destruction on one side. Following long-standing main bronchus obstruction from a carcinoid tumour or stricture of the bronchus resulting in pulmonary suppuration, the only satisfactory surgical treatment may be pneumonectomy.

In the case of carcinoma the pneumonectomy will include removal of as much of the lymphatic drainage as is practicable; clearance of the lymphatics in the mediastinum cannot be complete. It is not proven that removal of involved lymph nodes improves the long-term prognosis. Areas of parietal pleura where the lung has become adherent should also be excised if the carcinoma is palpable in the lung beneath. When there is extension of growth into the chest wall, ribs or diaphragm, the involved portion should also be removed and the defects repaired (le Roux, 1964).

The value of extending pneumonectomy so as to ligate the pulmonary artery and veins within the pericardium is debatable when the growth is situated at some distance from the points of entry of these vessels into the pericardial cavity. When the growth can be felt close to and possibly invading the pericardium, there can be no doubt that it is both wiser and easier to open the pericardium. Portions of pericardium may be resected and the main pulmonary artery and veins more safely secured (Allison, 1946). When the growth extends along the pulmonary veins a portion of the left atrium can be excised if this is necessary to ensure complete removal of the tumour.

Surgeons use different descriptive terms for resection of a carcinoma which has extended beyond the lung. The terms used—intrapericardial, radical, extended, palliative and non-curative pneumonectomy have, however, no generally accepted meaning.

Lobectomy

If all macroscopic carcinoma can be removed by lobectomy this operation is preferred to pneumonectomy in the treatment of carcinoma. Other indications for lobectomy include bronchiectasis, tuberculosis, aspergilloma, lung abscess which has not responded to prolonged chemotherapy and some cases of metastatic carcinoma and sarcoma if the primary is controlled.

The extent of bronchiectasis requires accurate anatomical pre-operative assessment by bronchograms which show all the segmental and subsegmental divisions of both lungs. Once the anatomical extent of the disease is known it is possible to decide whether the patient's symptoms justify resection. Resection is contra-indicated in bilateral cases if a total of seven or more lung segments are involved. Bronchiectatic changes in the bronchi cannot be felt or seen at operation; therefore the extent of the operation must be planned beforehand by careful scrutiny of the bronchograms. Generally, all bronchi showing dilatation on the bronchograms should be removed, although dilatation is occasionally reversible. Ideally, no normal segmental bronchus should be resected, but this is not always possible.

In tuberculosis, residual lung abscess and aspergilloma, the extent of the disease in the lobe may make lobectomy necessary, although satisfactory eradication of the disease may be achieved by segmental resection. Operation should be postponed until the maximum benefit from the appropriate antibiotic has been achieved. Compared with lobectomy for carcinoma, technical problems during lobectomy for these three diseases are greater. The presence of sputum, the possibility of early spread of the disease to other parts of the lungs, the frequency of adhesions between the two layers of the pleura, the need for an extrapleural dissection, particularly in peripheral aspergilloma or tuberculous cavitation, obliteration of the fissure or of the normal spaces between vessels and bronchi and the generalized distortion of the hilar anatomy are all recognized difficulties. An increased incidence of intra- and postoperative bleeding and of bronchopleural fistula exists. Lobectomy in these circumstances can be amongst the most difficult operations in surgery. A history of an empyema or of a previous operation on the side to be operated upon, gross flattening of the chest wall and radiological evidence of thickened pleura or calcification in hilar lymph nodes warn the surgeon of difficulty.

Sleeve resection

The commonest indication for this operation is carcinoma seen at bronchoscopy to involve the origin of either upper lobe bronchus. Standard upper lobectomy will not remove the portion of the carcinoma present in the main bronchus. Upper lobectomy is combined with resection of a sleeve of the main bronchus and resuture of the two ends. It is this operation which is referred to as 'sleeve resection'. It removes bronchial tissue involved, conserves normally functioning lobes and allows a wide clearance of the lymphatic drainage. If the carcinoma involves the pulmonary artery (the left pulmonary artery is a close posterior relation of the left upper lobe bronchus) a sleeve of the pulmonary artery may also be resected and the ends re-united by a continuous arterial suture. Sleeve resection of the main bronchus may be indicated in a tuberculous stricture or a stricture following a neglected traumatic rupture of the bronchus. If the lobe is irreparably damaged this also is resected.

Segmental resection

Segmental resection is the removal of a segment or segments of a lobe by isolation of the bronchus to the segment; the segmental bronchus is isolated in the hilum of the lung, divided and gentle traction applied to the distal end. The associated segmental artery and vein are also divided. If a small (under 2·5 cm in diameter), peripheral lesion in the lung is resected between clamps, the operation is referred to as 'wedge resection'. Segmental resection requires a knowledge of the detailed anatomy of the lung hilum. The operation is used for selected patients with tuberculosis (especially the tuberculoma), bronchiectasis, small peripheral carcinomata, chronic lung abscess when only one segment is involved and a variety of uncommon conditions such as benign tumours, arteriovenous aneurysms and the post-inflammatory 'tumours' (histiocytomata). A hamartoma in the lung is removed by local enucleation.

Before embarking on segmental resection it is necessary to have an exact knowledge of the segmental distribution of the disease. A study of the postero-anterior and lateral chest radiographs, two-plane tomography, adequate bilateral bronchograms and the findings at bronchoscopy using the fibre-optic bronchoscope as well as the rigid instrument, usually provide the required information. Palpation of the lung at operation will help to confirm the extent of the disease, although a bronchiectatic segment cannot be palpated. Facilities for immediate frozen section examination are essential.

Segmental resection of one segment of a lobe is usually a straightforward operation. When more than one segment is resected the operation may have to be abandoned in favour of lobectomy. An isolated normal segment should not be left if it is very small, if there is much air leak from its raw surface, if it does not readily remain inflated or if its blood supply has been damaged.

Pre-operative preparation

Pre-operative preparation has these important aims: to improve the patient's general health, to reduce the quantity of sputum and render it sterile if possible and to give the patient insight into and an explanation of the contribution he can make towards a rapid postoperative recovery. Instruction in breathing exercises and clearing of sputum is given by the physiotherapist. Much will depend on the patient's ability to clear sputum from the bronchial tree after operation. About 2 weeks may be spent in pre-operative preparation.

Full pre-operative clinical assessment of lung function combined with respiratory function studies allow a patient to be placed in one of three groups: those fit for lung resection, those unfit and those whose postoperative lung function can only be guessed. This group cannot be rejected for surgery by any rule of thumb method. A history of increasing winter bronchitis with morning sputum and diminishing exercise tolerance over the preceding few months, the signs of emphysema, excessive obesity, an inability to improve cardiorespiratory function by supervised exercise, evidence of airways obstruction, abnormalities in the electrocardiogram after exertion and abnormalities in blood gas analysis may be decisive.

Position of patient on operating table

Most surgeons perform lung resection with the patient in the lateral position on the operating table. To control sputum and to be able to deal with any complication arising during the resection (haemorrhage, opening of an incipient bronchopleural fistula, sudden release of pus distal to a bronchial obstruction or displacement of tumour fragments) a double-lumen endobronchial tube (Robertshaw, 1971) is used.

There are surgeons and anaesthetists who prefer to use an endotracheal tube with the patient in the prone position. This position allows secretions from the lung during operation to run by gravity into the trachea, from which they may be aspirated. There are advantages and disadvantages in both positions. The writer prefers the patient in the prone position and the use of an endotracheal tube for all lung resections, for the reasons stated by Parry Brown (1973). Because the majority of surgeons use the lateral position, the steps of the operations will be depicted with the patient in this position.

Sequence of dissection

There is much variation in the ease of lung resection. Some steps in the operation may prove difficult in one case and easy in another. It is wise to start the dissection in the easiest area. In the illustrations that follow the sequence adopted is: arteries, veins and finally bronchi. Various circumstances such as the position of the main mass of the carcinoma, fusion of a fissure, deviations from the normal anatomy and loss of the normal landmarks in the lung hilum from malignant or inflammatory infiltration may require this sequence to be altered. Recognition of a vessel as an artery or vein may not always be easy unless the vessel can be traced to its parent trunk. Individual vessels are dissected free by picking up the sheath of a vessel with non-toothed dissecting forceps and cutting the sheath with scissors. A hilar dissection clamp completes the isolation of the vessel preliminary to its ligation. In malignant disease the veins should when possible be ligated as the first step, to prevent embolization of tumour fragments. Whenever a clamp is placed on a bronchus the lungs should be inflated to confirm that only the bronchus to the lung or lobe that is being removed is occluded. In a difficult dissection excessive ventilatory movement of the lung may be reduced by the anaesthetist changing from machine ventilation to hand ventilation for short periods.

PNEUMONECTOMY

LEFT PNEUMONECTOMY

1

Exposure

The pleural cavity has been opened by the removal of a length of the sixth left rib. The Price-Thomas rib-spreader separates the ribs. A free pleural cavity is exposed in the lower half. In the upper part of the pleural cavity anteriorly there are multiple pleural adhesions which can be divided with scissors. Posteriorly the adhesions are so dense that it is necessary to strip the lung from the chest wall in the extrapleural plane. An incision has been made into this plane and finger dissection will separate the lung from the chest wall. Care must be taken in doing this not to damage the vessels from the aortic arch or intercostal vessels. When an anterior extrapleural strip is necessary the phrenic nerve and the internal mammary vessels are endangered. Dissection in this plane may result in considerable blood loss.

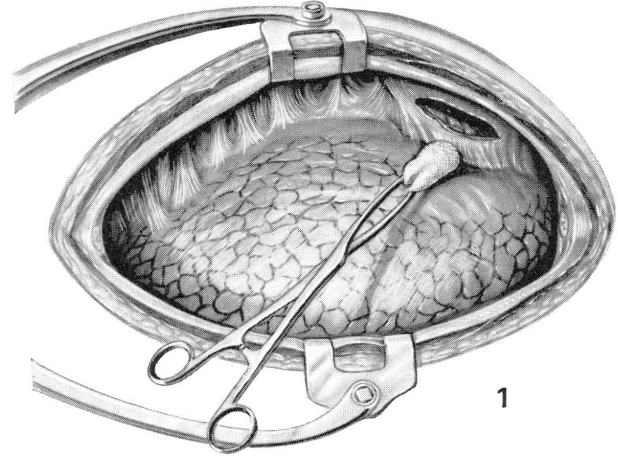

1

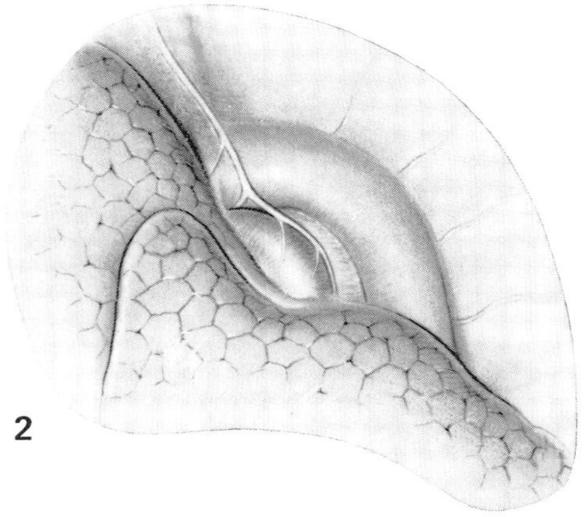

2

2

Commencement of dissection

Having examined and palpated both lobes, the hilum and the mediastinum, the lung is retracted downwards and forwards. The pleura is incised at the line of its reflection on to the lung. The dissection starts at the upper part of the hilum by picking up the sheath of the left main pulmonary artery over its posterolateral surface and between the ligamentum arteriosum and the first branch. This tissue is cut with scissors.

3

Exposure of the pulmonary artery

The vagus nerve has been cut distal to its recurrent laryngeal branch, which hooks around the ligamentum arteriosum. The space between the pulmonary artery and the left main bronchus has been defined. Dissection is continued round the pulmonary artery in that portion of the vessel between the ligamentum arteriosum and the first branch of the pulmonary artery to the upper lobe. A clamp has been placed beneath the vessel; gentle opening of this clamp clears the tissue from the medial aspect of the pulmonary artery preliminary to its ligation.

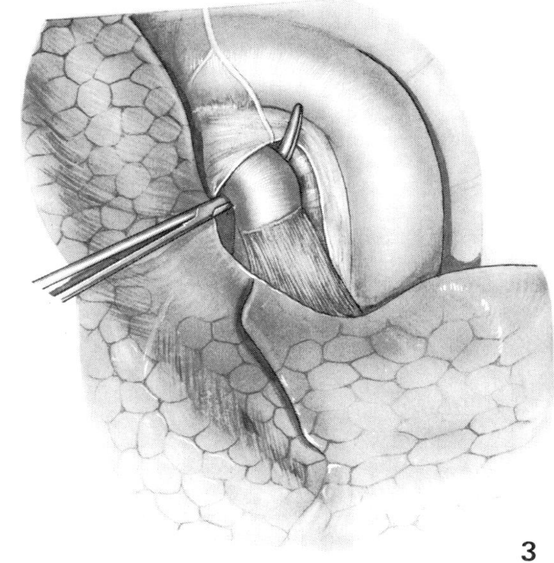

3

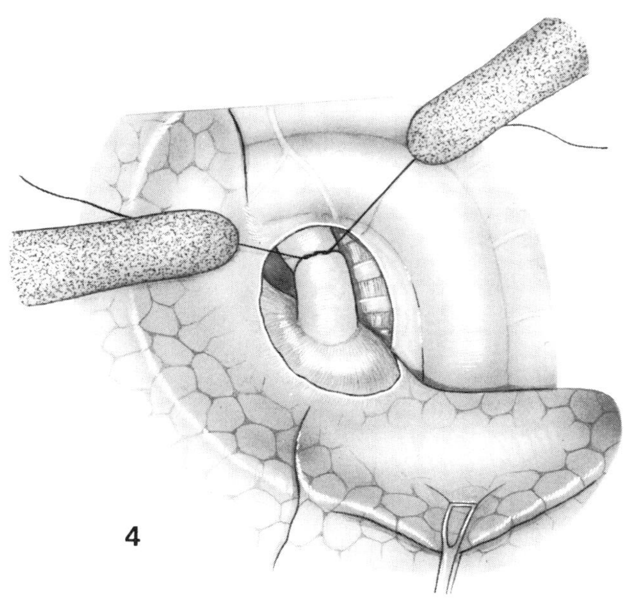

4

4

Ligation of the pulmonary artery

A strong ligature (No. 20 Barbour's linen thread) has been passed round the vessel and is being tied with a surgeon's knot in the position in which the vessel lies. Pulling or shearing of the vessel may tear its wall. Some surgeons use a second ligature or a transfixion stitch. A ligature or clamp is placed on the distal end. The vessel is divided, leaving a symmetrical cuff at least 1 cm long distal to the ligature. If a cuff of this length is not obtainable the vessel should be clamped and sutured (*see Illustration 10*).

5

Exposure of superior pulmonary vein

Having divided the pulmonary artery, the lung has been retracted backwards to expose the anterior aspect of the hilum. The superior pulmonary vein has been dissected out between the point of union of the branches within the lung and the entry of the vessel into the pericardial cavity. The vessel may be secured in a similar way to the pulmonary artery, depending upon the surgeon's preference.

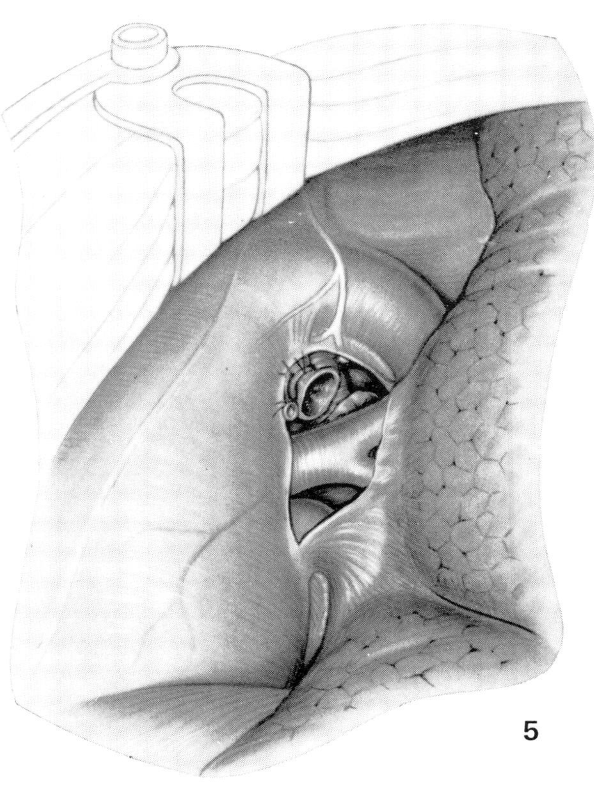

5

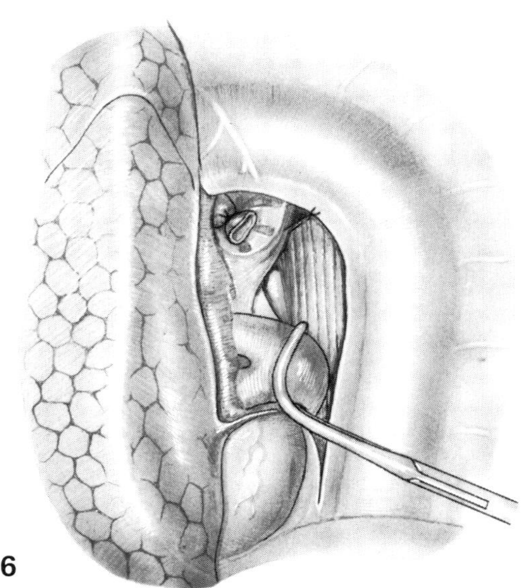

6

6

Exposure of inferior pulmonary vein

The lung is retracted forwards and the pulmonary ligament divided. One or more vessels in the pulmonary ligament may require ligation. The pericardium shows through the divided pulmonary ligament. The tissues covering the posterior surface of the vein have been divided by sharp dissection and an instrument has been passed around the vessel.

7

Clamping of the bronchus

The lung is now attached only by the bronchus. Before applying clamps any bronchial vessel should be controlled by diathermy. A subcarinal lymph node has been removed, exposing the carina. A Thompson non-crushing bronchus clamp has been applied just distal to the carina and the Price-Thomas toothed bronchus clamp distally. The bronchus is held in the clamps and is being divided; a long stump is to be avoided.

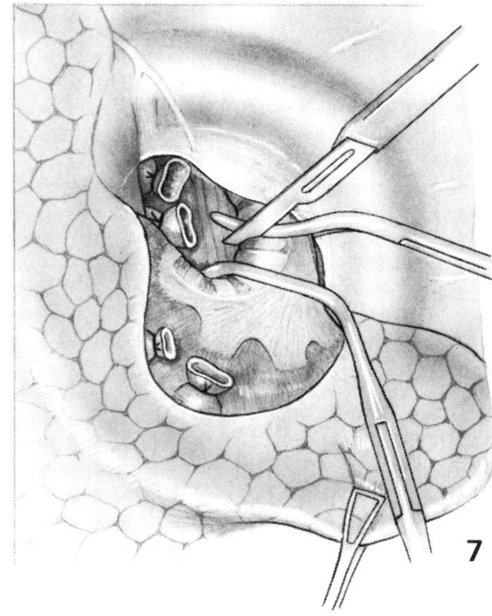

8

Closure of the bronchus

The lung has been removed and the Thompson bronchus clamp taken off the bronchial stump before insertion of any sutures. If an endotracheal cuffed tube is used instead of an endobronchial blocker in the right main bronchus, removal of the Thompson clamp will cause loss of anaesthetic gas pressure and the clamp should not be removed until the anaesthetist confirms that the time is opportune. Secretions are sucked out from within the bronchial stump by a gum elastic catheter. Any small residual bleeding point is diathermied. The bronchial stump is being closed with interrupted Ethiflex eyeless sutures on 25 mm half-circle needles. The sutures are placed about 0·4 cm apart; some six or seven sutures are sufficient for a stump of average dimensions. The posterior bronchial wall is friable material and liable to be torn if the suture is pulled on as it is tied. The stump should be pushed under the aortic arch and not pulled toward the operator as the suture is tightened. The left main stump is more difficult to close than the right because of the presence of the aortic arch and the tendency of the left main bronchus stump to retract beneath it.

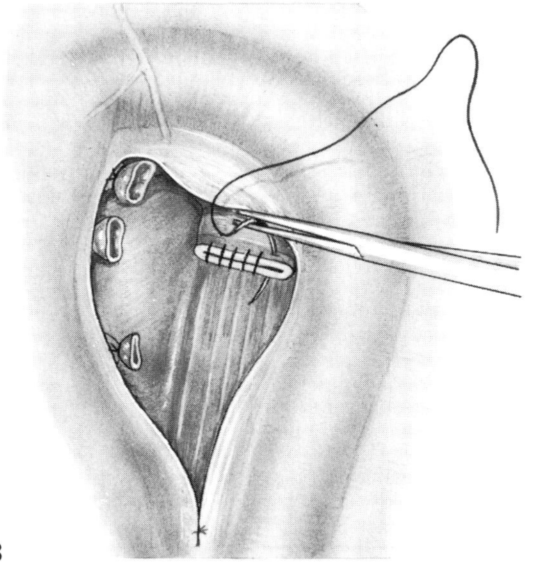

9

Alternative method of bronchial closure

A continuous monofilament wire has the advantage of great strength (provided it is not kinked whilst being inserted) and it is inert in the tissues. It is used as a continuous suture, starting at one end, across the bronchial stump and back to the point of commencement, where it is knotted. This end must be kept away from the aorta. It is desirable to cover the bronchial stump to support the suture line. In pneumonectomy for lung carcinoma, when all adventitious tissue has been removed with the lymphatic drainage, the oesophageal muscle may be used to cover the bronchial stump. This method is illustrated. The bronchial suture is of continuous monofilament wire and the covering sutures are of linen thread.

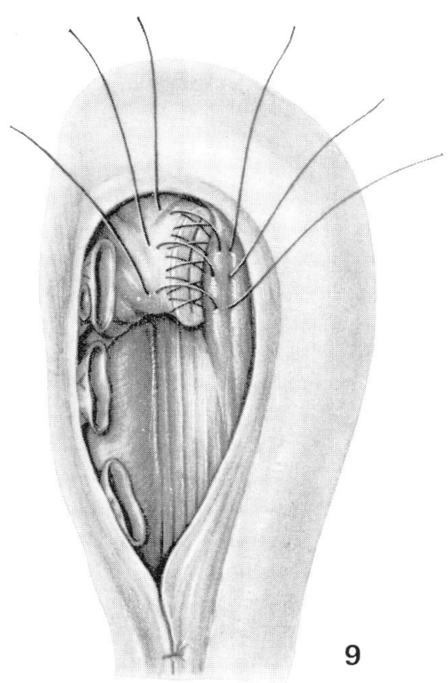

9

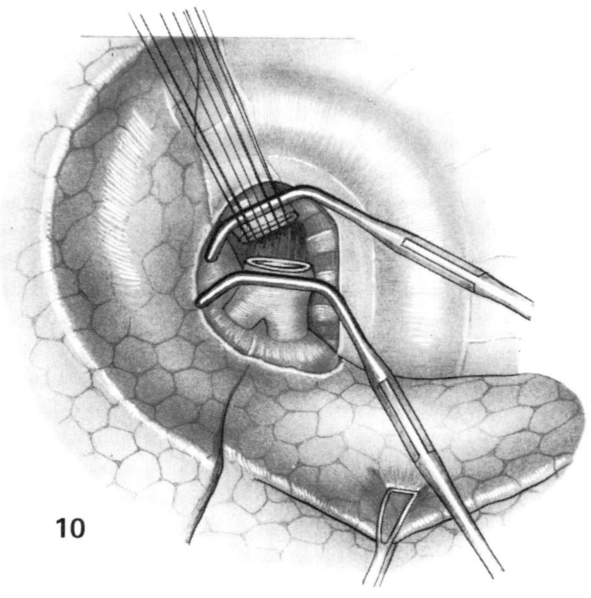

10

10

Alternative method of securing the artery

When the length of the exposed pulmonary artery is short because of the proximity of a tumour to the pulmonary artery, ligation and division of the artery may be judged unsafe. In these circumstances a right-angled Satinsky vascular clamp is placed just distal to the ligamentum arteriosum and the artery divided between clamps. The proximal end is sutured with atraumatic linen sutures and the ends left long until haemostasis is confirmed, when the clamp is removed. Additional sutures may be necessary. Bleeding from a needle hole may be controlled by tying adjacent sutures together or the insertion of another suture. The clamp may have to be re-applied.

LEFT RADICAL INTRAPERICARDIAL PNEUMONECTOMY

When mediastinal lymph nodes are extensively involved by carcinoma it is possible that the prognosis may be improved by radical clearance of the lymphatics at the time of pneumonectomy. In addition, the pulmonary artery and veins may be so involved in their extrapericardial course that intrapericardial control is necessary.

11

Preliminary dissection

The pleural incision extends from the apex of the pleura to the diaphragm. The dissection includes the lymph nodes in the front of the hilum and those in the pulmonary ligament; the dissection is carried up behind the inferior pulmonary vein. The muscle of the oesophageal wall is exposed and the subcarinal nodes removed.

The vagus nerve is usually divided immediately distal to the origin of the recurrent laryngeal branch, which should be carefully preserved whenever possible. Sometimes the nerve must be divided when the nodes in front of the trachea and beneath the aortic arch are removed. The phrenic nerve also may have to be divided. Paralysis of the left side of the diaphragm results in a much greater rise of the dome post-operatively than occurs if the nerve can be left intact. The pericardial cavity is opened at a point furthest away from the carcinoma and a finger inserted to palpate the vessels intrapericardially.

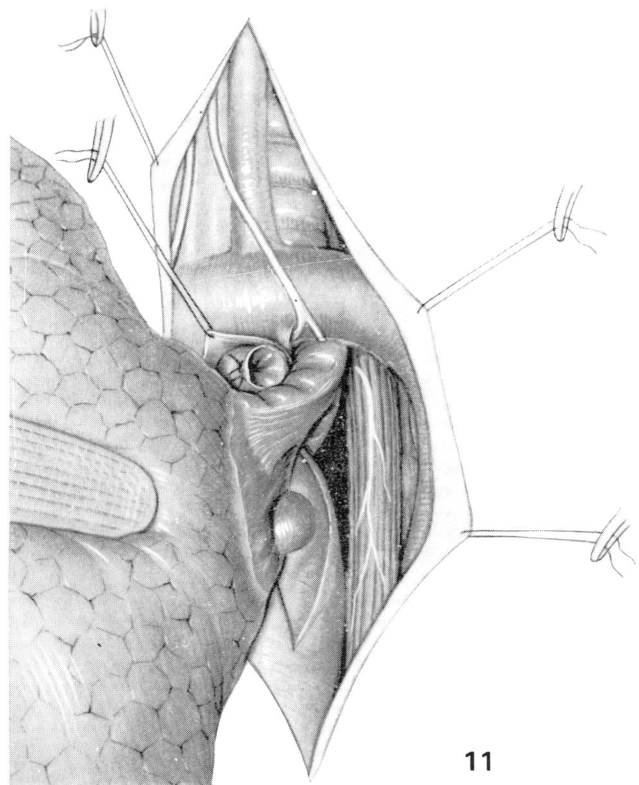
11

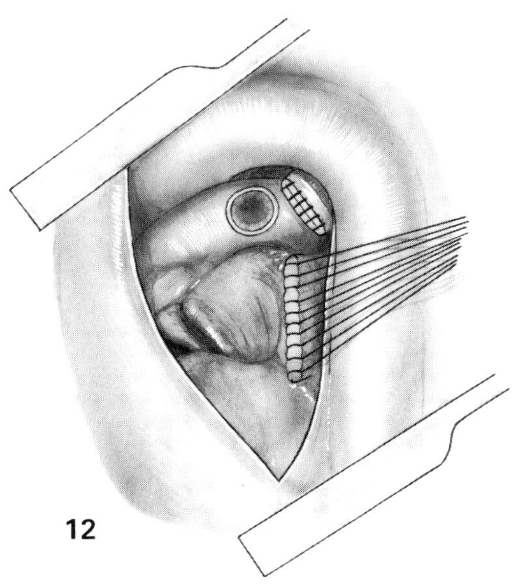
12

12

Intrapericardial control of the vessels

Generally it is not necessary to secure both the pulmonary artery and the veins intrapericardially. Occasionally this is necessary and wide excision of the pericardium is required. The pericardium is picked up in forceps as far away from the tumour edge as possible and cut with scissors.

On the left side a clamp may readily be passed round both pulmonary veins as they enter the atrium. The atrial wall has been sutured and the Satinsky clamp removed. The left pulmonary artery has been ligated intrapericardially and the right trunk can be seen. This vessel may be damaged when a tumour grows close to the bifurcation of the main pulmonary artery.

13

Closure of the pericardium

The pericardial defect must be closed to prevent the serious complication of herniation of the heart. The pericardium must not be tightly closed or tamponade may result. The large defect shown has been repaired by 1 cm wide Teflon strips sutured to the pericardial edges. For smaller defects (of 4 cm or so in diameter) a lattice of catgut sutures is a satisfactory method.

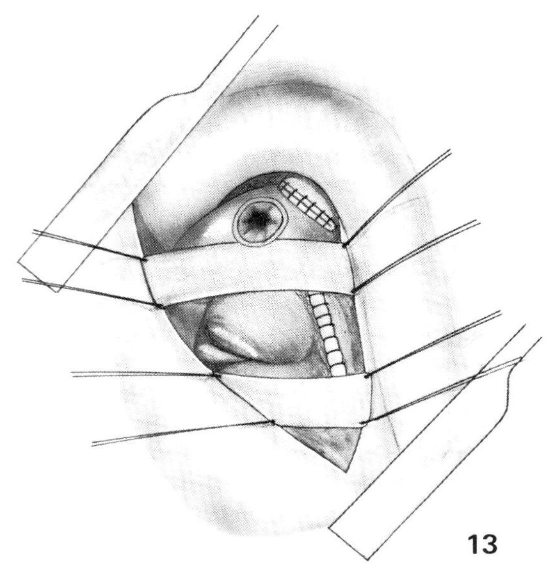

13

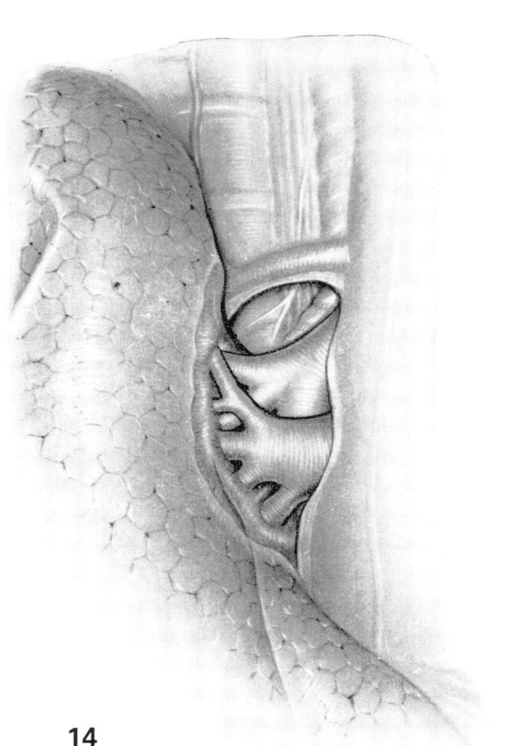

14

RIGHT PNEUMONECTOMY

14

Dissection

In simple pneumonectomy the azygos vein need not be divided. The anterior aspect of the hilum is usually dissected first. The most anteriorly-placed structure is the superior pulmonary vein and between it and the bronchus, which lies posteriorly, is the pulmonary artery. The artery and vein are demonstrated by a combination of sharp and blunt dissection. The vein draining the apical segment of the upper lobe is seen crossing the arterial branches to the upper lobe.

15

Division of main vessels

The view is the same as in the previous illustration after division of all the main vessels. The superior vena cava may need retracting forward to simplify ligation of the artery. The vessels are secured in a similar way to left pneumonectomy. The inferior pulmonary vein is more easily approached from the posterior aspect. After dividing it, the bronchus is approached from in front, as shown. The clamp is placed so that when the bronchus is divided there is a short bronchial stump.

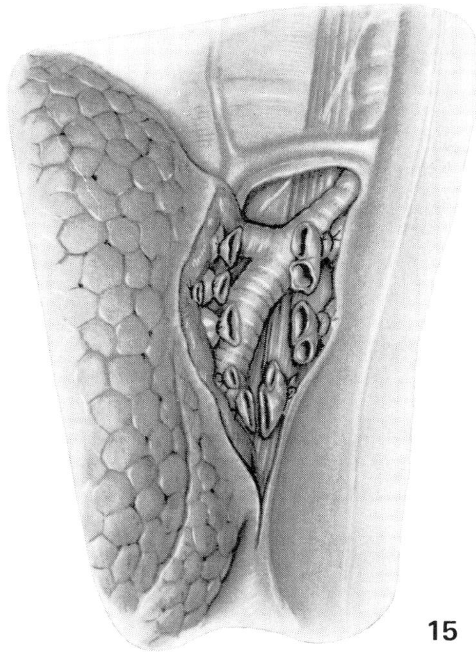

15

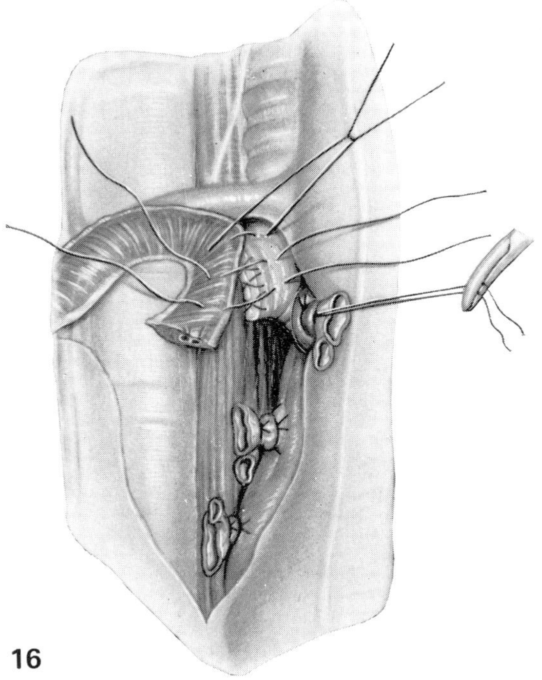

16

16

Bronchial closure

When the lung has been removed and the bronchus closed the bronchial stump seems to protrude into the pneumonectomy space, unlike the left side, where the stump retracts under the aortic arch. It is thus more difficult on the right side to cover the stump with living tissue. In an attempt to reduce the incidence of bronchopleural fistula, some surgeons (especially when operating for the rare inflammatory conditions which require pneumonectomy) use a pedicled graft of intercostal artery and muscle to suture firmly over the closed stump. This step, which is illustrated, may assist bronchial stump healing and separate the stump from the pneumonectomy space.

RIGHT RADICAL INTRAPERICARDIAL PNEUMONECTOMY

17

Preliminary dissection

The pleural incision is similar to that on the left side, extending from the apex to the diaphragm. On the right side an *en bloc* dissection of pleura, lymph nodes and any adventitious fatty tissue over the oesophagus, trachea and superior vena cava may more easily be achieved than on the left side. The vagus and the phrenic nerve may also be resected. The azygos vein has not been divided, but in the usual radical operation it should be. The only reason for not dividing the azygos vein is its function as a means of collateral circulation when the development of superior vena caval obstruction later is anticipated.

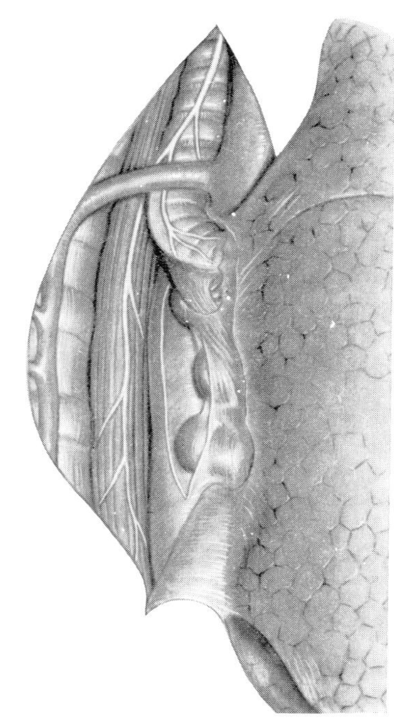

17

18

Intrapericardial control of the vessels

The azygos vein has now been divided and the bronchial stump sutured. The lung has not yet been removed. The pericardial cavity has been entered posteriorly by cutting the pericardial reflection off the posterior wall of the pulmonary artery, lifting this reflection up, cutting it and entering the cavity posterior to the superior pulmonary vein. The pericardial cavity may be opened at any other convenient spot. A Satinsky clamp has been placed proximally on the divided pulmonary artery which lies posterior to the intrapericardial course of the superior vena cava. When the pulmonary artery has been sutured, the pulmonary veins, united to form a single trunk at the veno-atrial junction, will be clamped and sutured. On the right side it is not possible to pass a clamp around the common venous trunk inside the pericardial cavity until the reflection of the pericardium on to the inferior vena cava has been divided.

A further incision of the pericardium (along the dotted line) may be necessary. Injury to the left atrium may occur if the clamp is forced bluntly through this reflection.

Teflon closure of the pericardial defect is seldom required after right intrapericardial pneumonectomy.

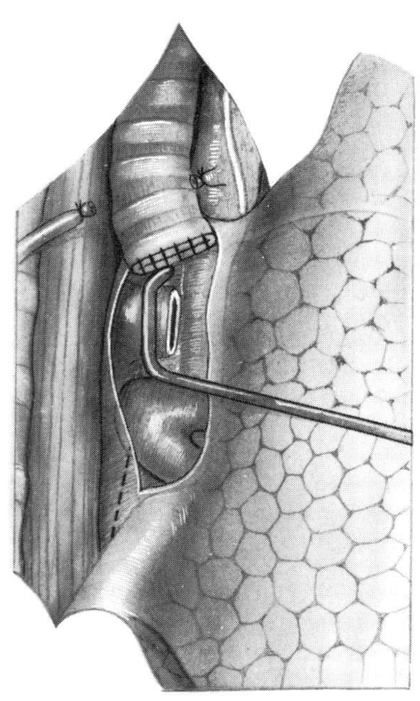

18

Drainage after pneumonectomy

In most cases drainage can be omitted. It is essential, however, if there is oozing from the chest wall following an extrapleural operation. This oozing may be difficult to control by coagulation with the diathermy button or by any other means. The tube should be placed dependently through an intercostal space and connected to an under-water seal. Some prefer to clamp the tube and release the clamp every 3 hr. Drainage is painful and provides a potential route for infection to reach the pneumonectomy space.

LOBECTOMY

There are many variations in the bronchovascular patterns in the lungs (Boyden, 1955). The illustrations depict the anatomy of the vessels commonly found. It is essential, when resecting a lobe or segment of lung, to expose the hilar structures and make sure which vessels and bronchus lead to and from the pathological segment, lobe or lobes to be removed.

LEFT LOWER LOBECTOMY

19

Lobar artery and vein

By opening the fissure, which in this case was almost complete, a little dissection only was required to reveal the pulmonary artery and its branches. The artery to the apical segment of the lower lobe is divided separately; it is never possible to ligate the artery to the lower lobe as a single trunk without also occluding the lingular artery. The inferior pulmonary vein is approached from the posterior aspect as described under Pneumonectomy, page 323. Ligatures of a smaller gauge linen thread are used for the lobar arteries than for main arterial ligation in pneumonectomy.

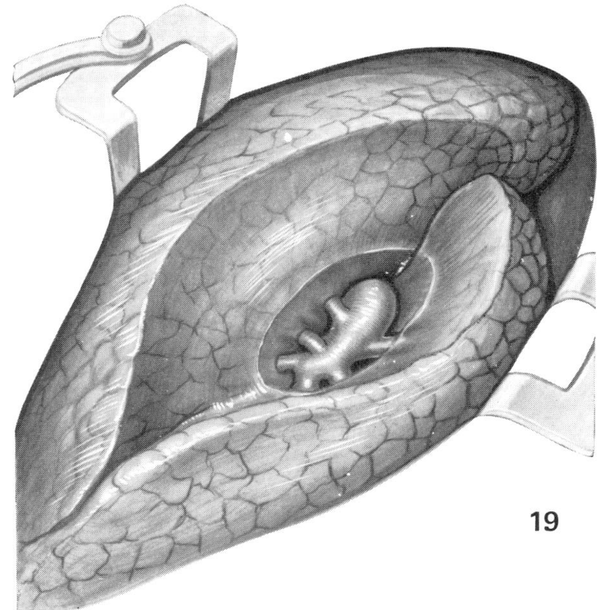

19

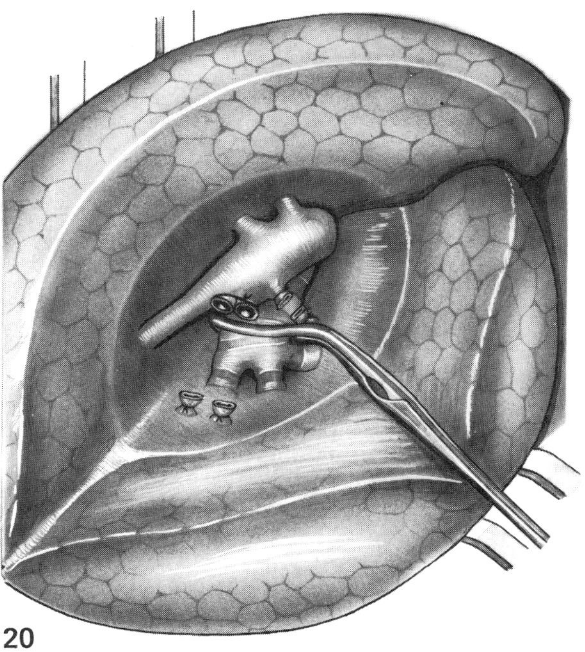

20

20

The bronchi

The apical segment artery and the arteries to the basal segments have been divided separately. The large branch to the lingula can be seen. A Thompson non-crushing bronchus clamp has been applied to the whole of the lower lobe bronchus. It is seldom necessary to clamp the apical segment bronchus separately. A second clamp, sometimes more easily placed in the reverse direction, is applied and the bronchus divided between the clamps. The proximal clamp is removed, the lumen of the bronchus sucked out and the open bronchus sutured, leaving a short stump. When there is an excessive amount of pus in the lower lobe (which cannot be reduced by pre-operative preparation) the bronchus may be clamped as the first step of the operation. Occasionally this is difficult to do.

LEFT UPPER LOBECTOMY

21

Arterial branches to upper lobe

The left pulmonary artery runs posteriorly to the left upper lobe bronchus. The upper part of the fissure has been developed to display the arterial branches to the upper lobe. The first branch which may or may not immediately divide into two is usually large and awkwardly placed. It may have to be clamped and sutured rather than ligated. It has the apical branch of the superior pulmonary vein as a close anterior relation.

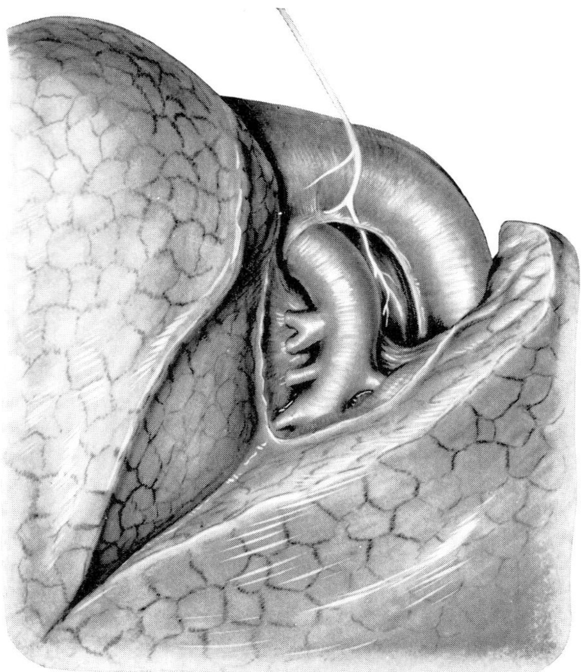

21

22

Exposure of upper lobe bronchus

The pulmonary artery is retracted medially and the upper lobe gently pulled on to show the upper lobe bronchus and its segmental branches to the apico-posterior and the lingular segments. The vein draining the apical segment of the lobe is just visible running to join the superior pulmonary vein, which lies immediately anterior to the bronchus.

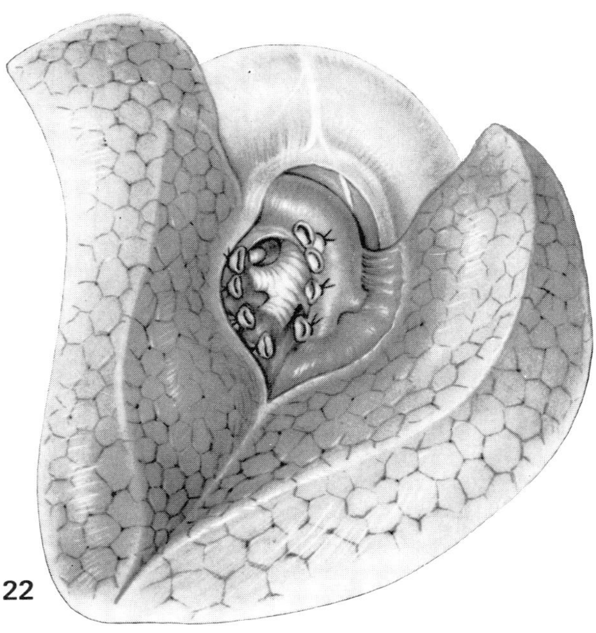

22

23

Closure of bronchus and division of superior pulmonary vein

A hilar dissecting clamp has been passed gently anterior to the bronchus to separate the superior pulmonary vein from it. The bronchus is divided, the stump closed and a toothed bronchus clamp placed on the distal portion. The pulmonary vein is seen between the two ends of the divided upper lobe bronchus. The vein is dissected free, ligated and divided. Gentle traction on the bronchus clamp will expose any adventitious tissue holding the upper lobe to the lower lobe and this tissue is divided with scissors, or the diathermy needle.

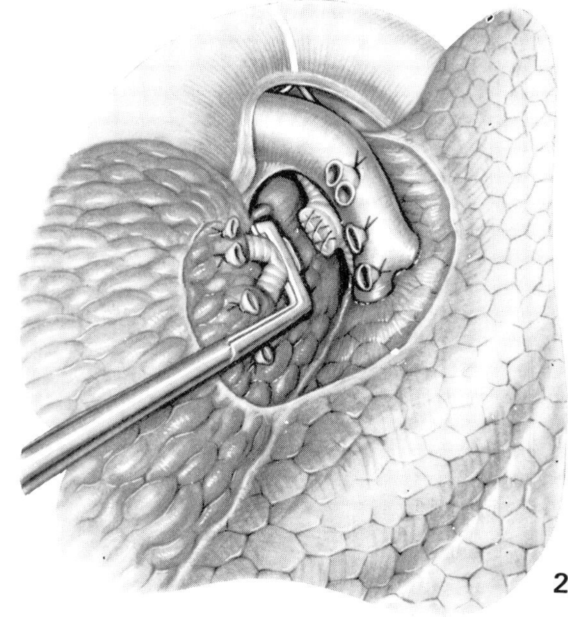

23

RIGHT LOWER LOBECTOMY

24

Exposure of the artery

The fissures have been dissected and the middle lobe retracted anteriorly. The artery to the apical segment and three basal segment arteries are shown. The middle lobe artery, seen running anteriorly, is always closely related to the lower margin of the superior pulmonary vein; this vein is visible. The artery to the apical segment of the right lower lobe must be ligated separately, to prevent damage to the middle lobe artery. This artery would be obstructed if an attempt was made to ligate the lower lobe artery as a single trunk.

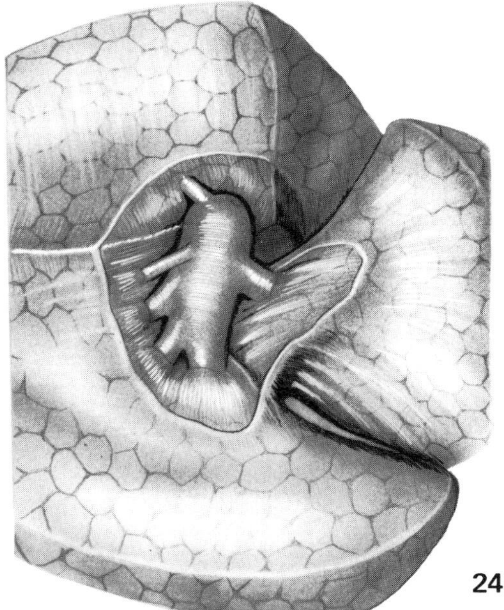

24

25

Division and closure of bronchi

Division of the right lower lobe bronchus should always be carried out in two steps. First, division of the apical segment bronchus followed by division of the bronchi to the basal segments. Attempts to divide the whole bronchus to the lower lobe as a single trunk will damage the bronchus to the middle lobe. In the illustration the arteries to the basal segments have been divided and the bronchus to the apical segment divided and sutured. The apical segment artery will be ligated and divided and a clamp placed across the bronchi to the basal segments.

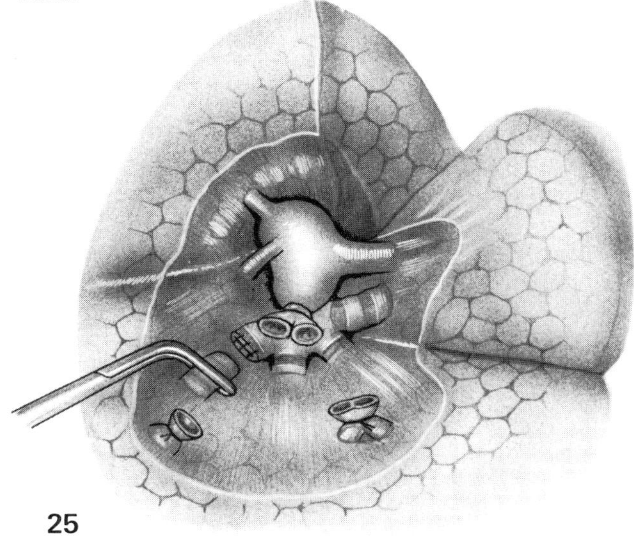

25

26

After removal of lobe

The lobe has been removed and the ligated inferior pulmonary vein, the basal segments and the apical segment artery are shown. The suture line in the bronchi of the basal segment is shown. The separate suture line in the apical segments bronchus is hidden by the ligated basal segment artery. The middle lobe bronchus and the middle lobe artery are preserved. The only other artery visible is the artery to the posterior segment of the right upper lobe.

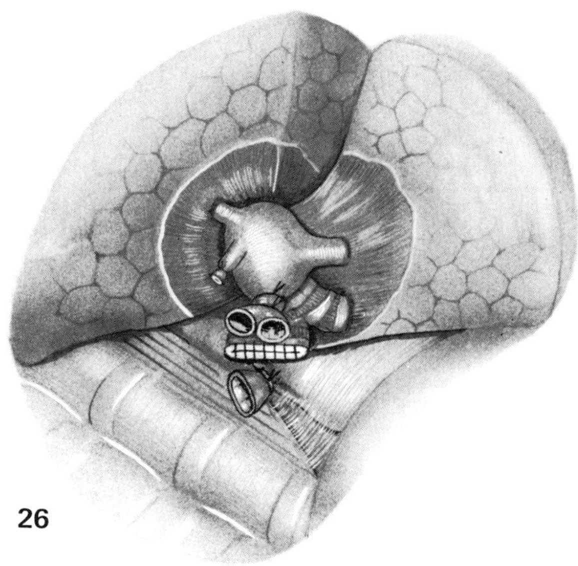

26

RIGHT UPPER LOBECTOMY

27

Ligation of artery to upper lobe and dissection of superior vein

The hilum is approached anteriorly. The main pulmonary artery lies anterior to the bronchus and posterior to the superior pulmonary vein. The upper lobe is usually supplied by a large branch of the main pulmonary artery, which has been dissected and looped with a ligature. This main branch divides into a branch to the apical segment and a branch to the anterior segment, both also looped with ligatures. Preliminary dissection and division of the superior pulmonary vein may facilitate this step. The middle lobe vein draining into the superior pulmonary vein must be preserved. The artery to the posterior segment of the upper lobe is not visible in this view but may be found by dissection in the greater fissure.

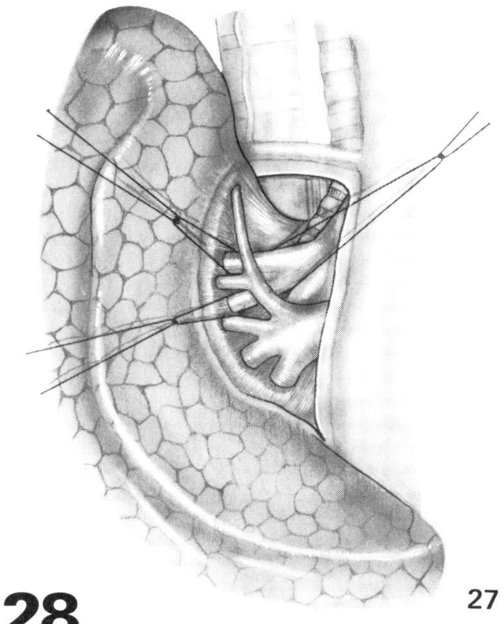

27

28

Exposure of upper lobe bronchus

The upper lobe has been retracted forwards to expose the upper lobe bronchus from behind. Only two of the segmental divisions are visible. The anterior segmental bronchus is not visible from this view. The bronchus has been cleared of adventitious tissue by gauze dissection and a hilar dissection clamp has been passed around it. Two bronchus clamps are then applied.

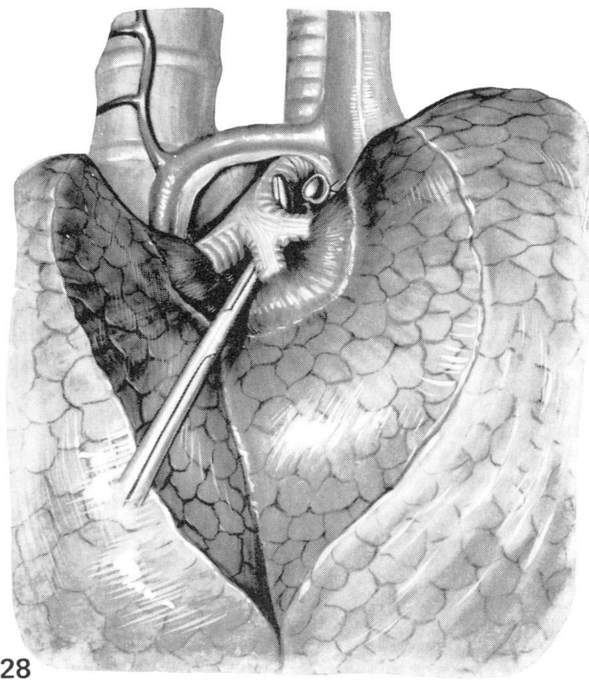

28

29

Division of the bronchus

The bronchus has been divided, the proximal clamp removed and the stump sutured flush with the main bronchus. The arterial branch to the posterior segment of the upper lobe is seen. Of the arteries to the upper lobe this branch arises most distally from the main arterial trunk. This artery to the upper lobe is also seen in *Illustration 25*. The resection is completed by ligation and division of this branch.

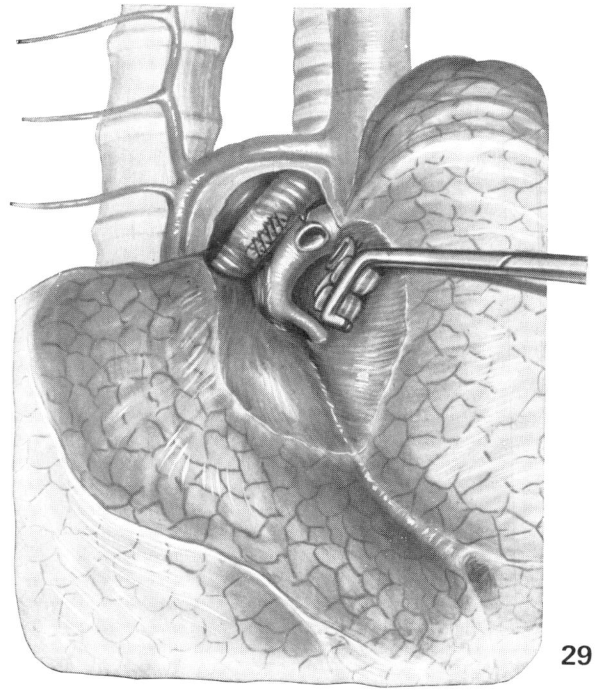

29

SEGMENTAL RESECTION OF LUNG

REMOVAL OF THE APICAL AND POSTERIOR SEGMENTS OF THE LEFT UPPER LOBE

30

Arterial dissection

The hilum is approached from above and behind as for left upper lobectomy. The pulmonary artery has been dissected into the fissure, so that its branches to the upper lobe are displayed. The most proximal artery is usually a branch to the anterior segment of the upper lobe and this is shown left intact. The next two branches (one dividing immediately) have been identified as those supplying the segments to be removed and have been divided between ligatures. The fourth branch shown is the lingular artery and can be seen to run posterior and caudally to its segmental bronchus.

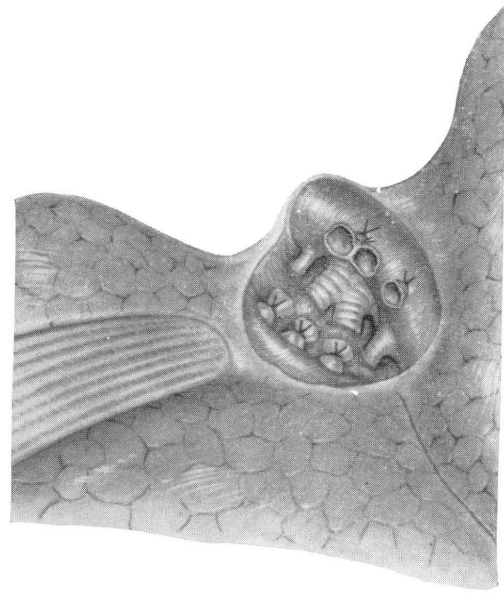

30

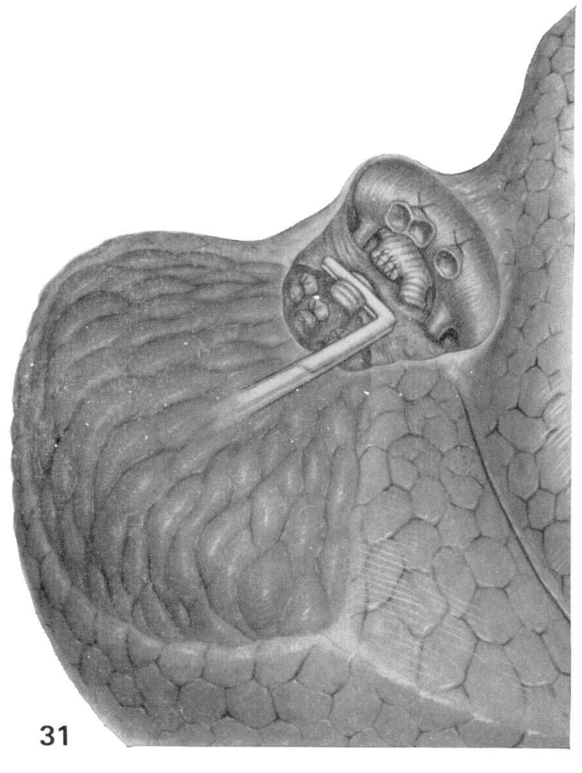

31

31

Division of bronchus

After dividing the arteries, the bronchus to the upper lobe is seen beneath and can be dissected free to identify the two divisions visible from the posterior approach. The apicoposterior bronchus has been clamped distally and divided. The suture line is seen. The lingular bronchus and artery are preserved.

32

Separation of segments

After dividing the arteries and veins, gentle traction on the bronchus clamp, division of visceral pleural bands with the diathermy needle and the use of the index finger begin the separation of the segments in the intersegmental plane. It is an advantage to have the lung fairly well inflated; the collapsed segments being removed will then be more easily distinguishable. Should the intersegmental plane be crossed an air leak will result.

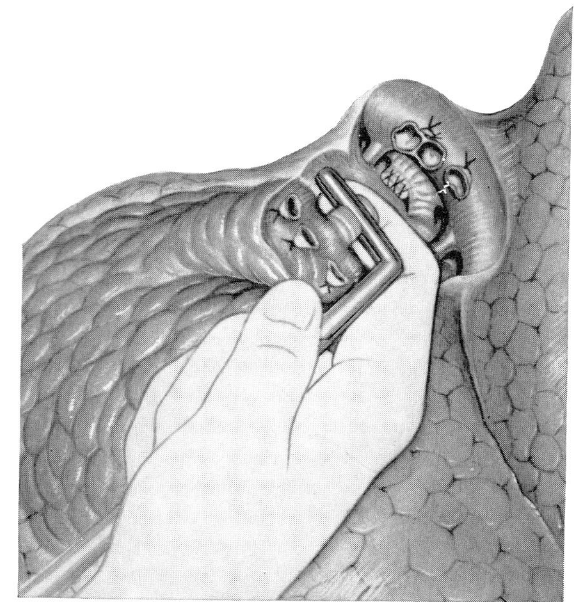

32

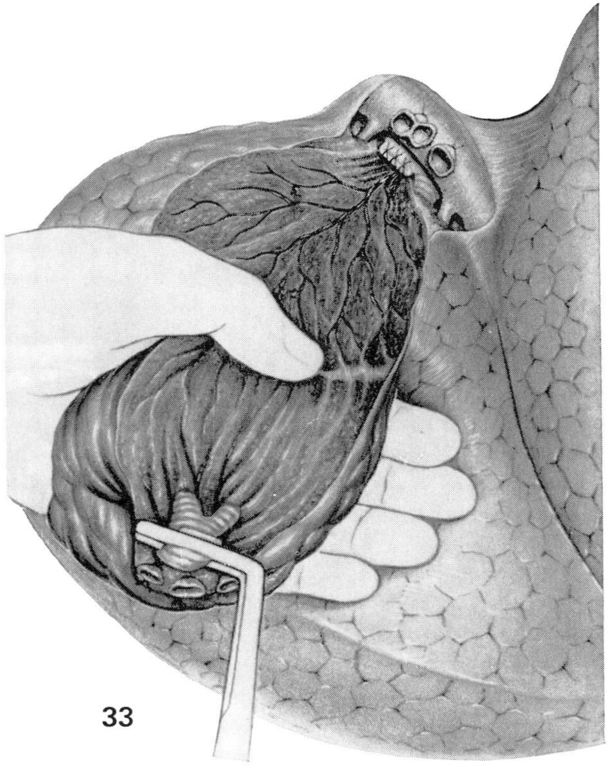

33

33

Removal of segments

Once the separation has started in the correct plane, the segments are removed by a gentle pulling, invaginating manoeuvre. The intersegmental veins can be seen and confirm that the separation is in the correct plane. Haemorrhage is not gross; tributaries of the vein may require to be ligated.

34

Division of visceral pleura

The segments being removed are now held only by the visceral pleura, which is cut with scissors. Bubbles show the site of a small air leak from the remainder of the upper lobe. A swab is then applied to the raw surface for a minute or so and haemostasis confirmed.

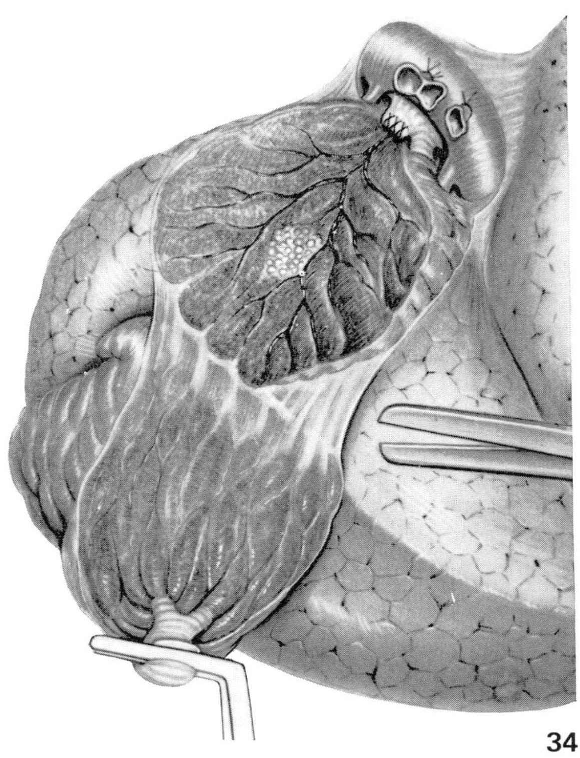

34

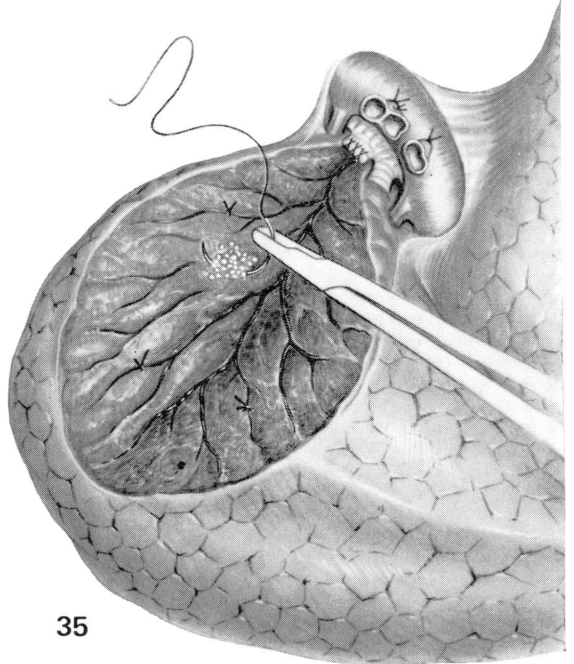

35

35

Closure of air leak

An air leak from a bronchiole is being closed with an atraumatic suture. The anaesthetist should inflate the lung fully to test for other air leaks and to make sure that the remaining bronchi have not been obstructed. It is inadvisable to suture the raw surfaces of the lung together. Such sutures inevitably create further air leaks. On full inflation the remainder of the lung will take up its natural position, obliteration of the space being completed in the early postoperative period by the raw surface adhering to the parietal pleura or adjacent lung. Two drainage tubes are placed (*see* page 259).

LINGULECTOMY WITH LEFT LOWER LOBECTOMY

36

Identification of lingular bronchus

This shows the appearance after left lower lobectomy in a case without adhesions between the lingula and lower lobe. The lingular segment has also been shown by bronchography to be bronchiectatic and is to be removed. When the ligated artery is lifted up the lingular bronchus can be identified.

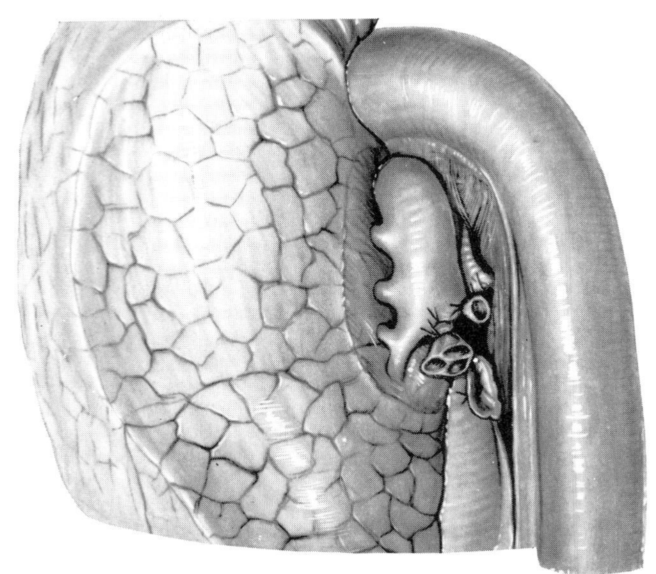

36

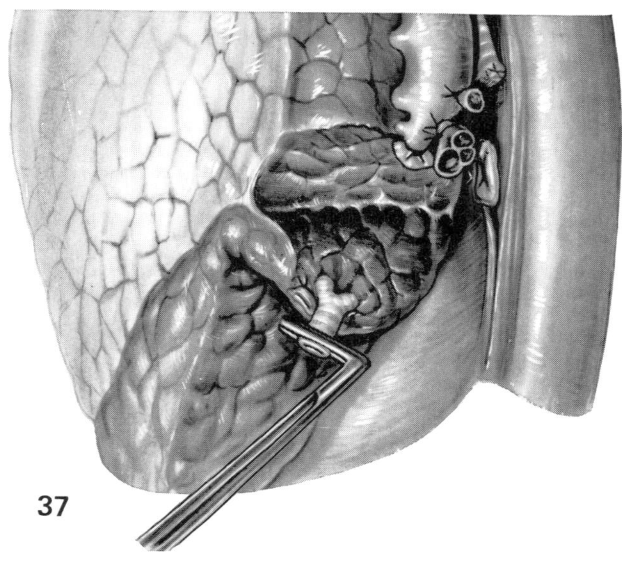

37

37

Separation of lingula

The lingular bronchus has been divided and sutured proximally. The stump is hidden by the ligated lingular artery. The ligated apical segmental branch and the basal segmental branches of the pulmonary artery to the resected lower lobe are seen. The vein, lying anteriorly, is not yet visible. Gentle traction on the bronchus clamp is separating the airless lingula from the rest of the upper lobe.

38

REMOVAL OF THE APICAL SEGMENT OF THE LEFT LOWER LOBE

The pulmonary artery is seen lying in the fissure; its branch to the apical segment of the lower lobe has been ligated and divided, just proximal to its division into two branches. Beneath the divided artery the bronchus is visible. The vein will be approached from the posterior aspect of the segment. It usually lies posterior to the bronchus and drains into the inferior pulmonary vein. It may run between the apical and the basal segmental bronchi.

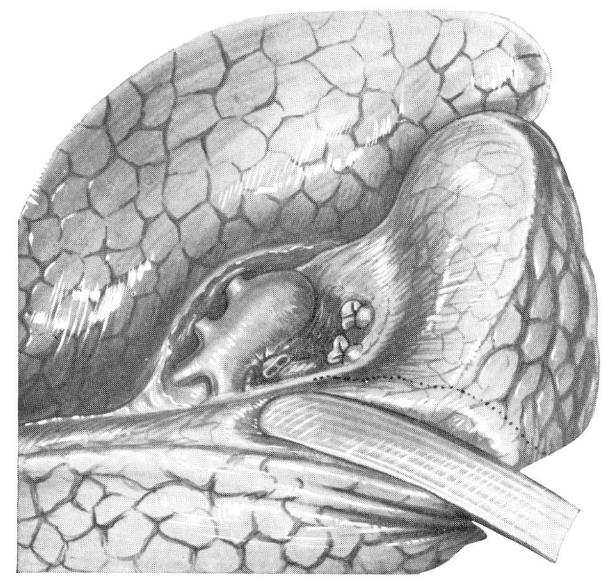

38

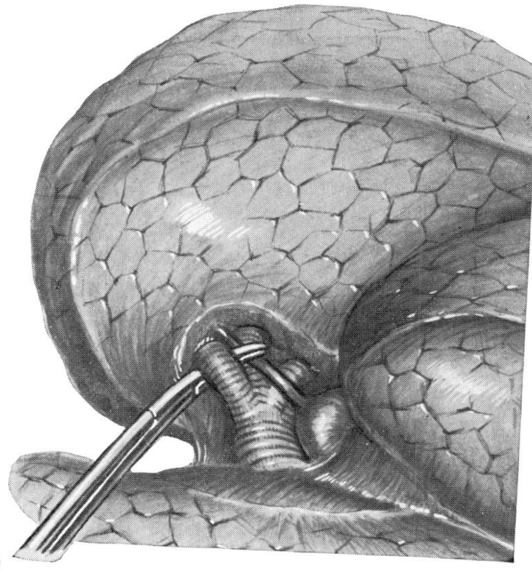

39

39

REMOVAL OF THE POSTERIOR SEGMENT OF THE RIGHT UPPER LOBE

The upper lobe bronchus has been approached from behind after separating the upper and lower lobes and is seen to divide into its three main divisions. A clamp has been passed around the bronchus to the posterior segment. The artery to this segment is clearly seen; it arises as the most distal of the upper lobe branches from the main pulmonary artery. The segmental vein is anterior.

SLEEVE RESECTION

Excellent exposure of both main bronchi is provided with the patient in the prone position on the operating table. One-lung anaesthesia with an endobronchial tube in the contralateral main bronchus is preferred. This allows an unhurried suturing of the two ends of the divided bronchus. The knots on the tied interrupted bronchus sutures should be outside the lumen of the bronchus whenever possible. Similar suture material is used for this operation as for bronchial closure in other lung resections. Suture material with a needle on both ends of the suture allows it to be passed outwards from within, in a forehand direction through each end of the divided bronchus. The needle must not pierce or pick up the sheath of the adjacent pulmonary artery. On completion of the bronchial resuture a flap of pleura must be inserted to separate the bronchial suture line from the pulmonary artery, which helps in preventing secondary haemorrhage into the bronchus. The pulmonary ligament should be divided and the lower lobe freed completely from the diaphragm, to prevent pull on the suture line from diaphragmatic movement.

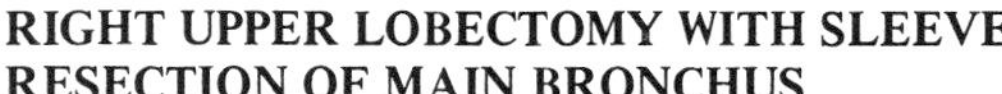

RIGHT UPPER LOBECTOMY WITH SLEEVE RESECTION OF MAIN BRONCHUS

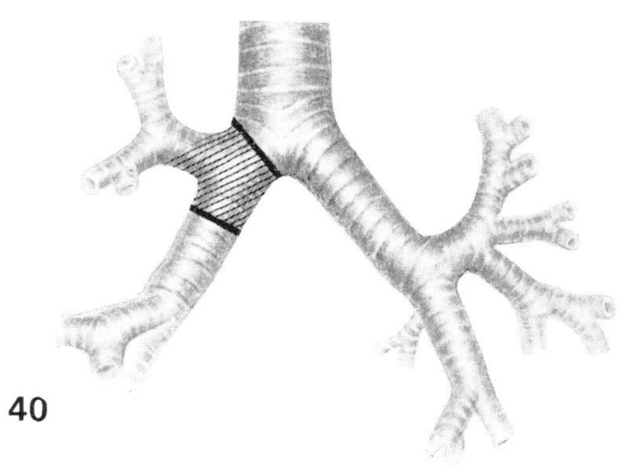

40

40

The shaded area marks the extent of resection of the main bronchus required for a carcinoma growing from the lower lip of the right upper lobe bronchus with involvement of the main bronchus. A standard right upper lobectomy could not achieve total removal of the tumour. Although it appears from this anatomical diagram that the right middle lobe bronchus (and the apical segment bronchus to the right lower lobe, which cannot be seen) are some distance away, this is not so when the bronchial branches are exposed at operation. The incision across the distal main bronchus must never compromise the orifice of the middle lobe or the apical segment of the lower lobe bronchus.

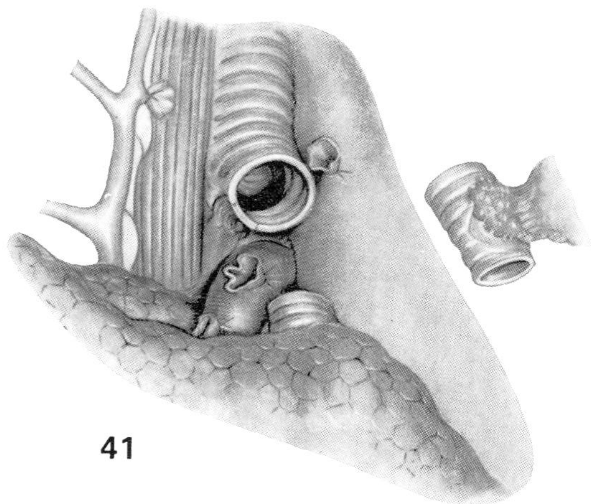

41

41

Exposure and removal of segment of main bronchus

The azygos vein has been divided. The pleura over the medial wall of the right main bronchus has been incised and a finger inserted in front of the bronchus. By gentle finger dissection the main bronchus is lifted off the pulmonary artery. The upper lobe vein is tied. The resected cylinder of main bronchus containing the upper lobe bronchus is shown. A clean division of the bronchus can best be made with a pair of sharp long-bladed straight scissors, with the finger protecting the pulmonary artery.

42

End-to-end anastomosis of bronchus

The two ends of the bronchus are of unequal size and re-anastomosis requires a careful technique. Different surgeons use different methods of overcoming the inequality in size. The distal end may be cut obliquely to increase its width. Two interrupted sutures may be placed in the lateral wall of the main bronchus to reduce its width, or, as in the case illustrated, a wedge of main bronchus may be resected and a repair carried out as shown. Before the final sutures in the bronchus are placed the patency of the middle lobe and the apical segment of the lower lobe bronchus must be confirmed and any blood removed from the lumen of the upper and lower portions of the main bronchus by suction with a soft rubber catheter. There need be no fear of damage to the suture line by vigorous coughing in the early postoperative period.

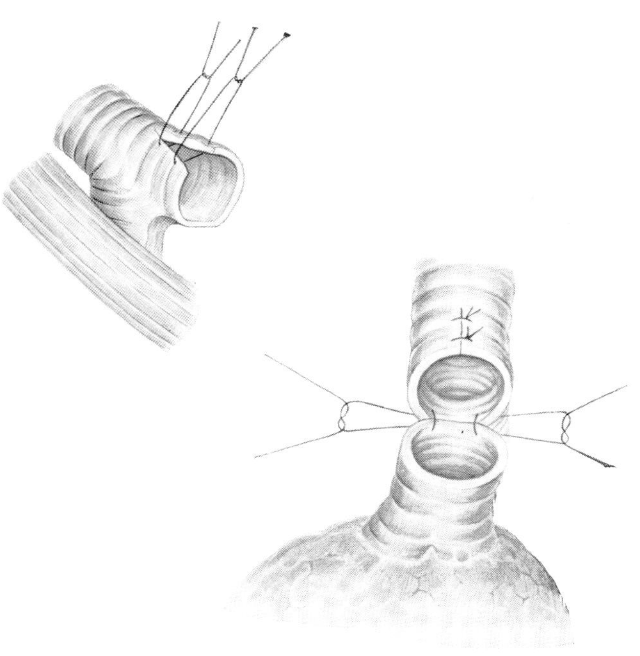

42

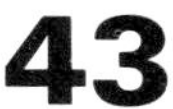

LEFT UPPER LOBECTOMY WITH SLEEVE RESECTION OF MAIN BRONCHUS

The shaded area represents the resection necessary for a carcinoma of the upper lip of the left upper lobe orifice growing into the lumen of the main bronchus. The re-attachment of the lower lobe bronchus to the trachea or divided main bronchus is technically more difficult on the left side owing to the position of the aorta. Cummings' aortic retractor (G. U. Manufacturing Co. Ltd.) improves the exposure. Because of the close relationship of the pulmonary artery to the posterior wall of the left upper lobe bronchus a carcinoma in the situation described sometimes involves the pulmonary artery. As well as a cylinder of bronchus, a segment of the main pulmonary artery may also have to be removed and the artery anastomosed end to end. Anticoagulants should be given because of the frequency of thrombosis at the arterial suture line. For lesser degrees of involvement of the pulmonary artery, particularly if one or more of the segmental branches are involved and ligation is difficult, the involved arterial wall may be cut away after temporary occlusion of both ends of the pulmonary artery. The defect in the wall of the artery can be repaired by a continuous longitudinal suture of the arterial wall. The lumen is narrowed but the blood flow is adequate.

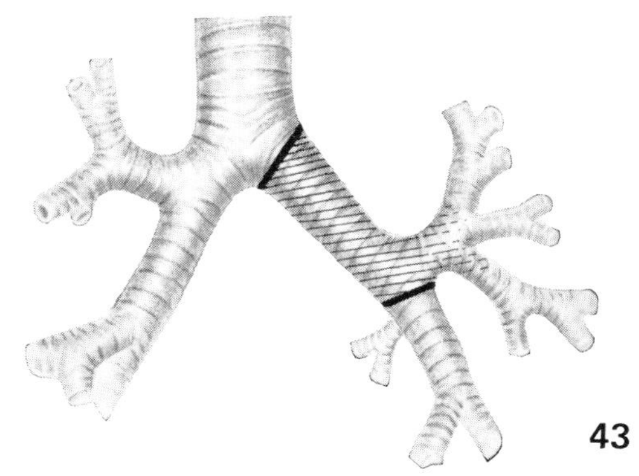

43

Drainage after lobectomy, segmental and sleeve resection

After any partial resection it is necessary to place at least one intrapleural tube before the chest wall is closed. For the details *see* page 259.

References

Allison, P. R. (1946). 'Intrapericardial approach to lung root in the treatment of bronchial carcinoma by dissection pneumonectomy.' *J. thorac. Surg.* **15**, 99

Belcher, J. R. and Grant, I. W. B. (1955). *Thoracic Surgical Management*, 2nd Edition. London: Bailliere, Tindall and Cox

Boyden, E. A. (1955). *Segmental Anatomy of the Lungs.* London: Blackiston

Brock, Sir Russell and Whytehead, L. L. (1955). 'Radical pneumonectomy for bronchial carcinoma.' *Br. J. Surg.* **43**, 8

Holmes Sellors, T. (1952). 'Posture and approach in thoracic surgery.' *J. int. Chir.* **12**, 1

Johnston, J. B. and Jones, P. H. (1959). 'The treatment of bronchial carcinoma by lobectomy and sleeve resection of the main bronchus.' *Thorax* **14**, 49

le Roux, B. T. (1964). 'Maintenance of chest wall stability.' *Thorax* **17**, 397

Parry Brown, A. I. (1973). 'Posture in anaesthesia.' *Proc. R. Soc. Med.* **66**, 339

Robertshaw, F. L. (1971). 'Control of secretions and haemorrhage in the lungs during operation.' *General Anaesthesia*, Third Edition, Vol. II, p. 217. Edited by Gray, T. C. and Nunn, J. F. London: Butterworths

Thompson, V. C. (1965). *Clinical Surgery*, Vol. 5, p. 173, Edited by C. Rob and R. Smith. London: Butterworths

[*The illustrations for this Chapter on Resection of Lung were drawn by Mr. R. N. Lane and Mr. F. Price.*]

Use of Stapler in Lung Surgery

S. C. Lennox, F.R.C.S.
Consultant Surgeon, The Brompton Hospital, London;
Senior Lecturer, Cardiothoracic Institute, University of London

Instruments

Automatic staplers are being increasingly used in pulmonary surgery. The following texts and illustrations show some of their uses. The instrument used in this series is the Auto Suture, Models TA 30, TA 55 and GIA.

1

Closure of the bronchus

The bronchus is prepared as described in the Chapter on 'Resection of Lung', pages 313–336. The stapler (Model TA 30) is applied to the bronchus in the same way as a proximal clamp would be used, that is flush with carina for a pneumonectomy or as proximal as possible for a lobectomy. For a pneumonectomy 4·8 mm staples are generally used. For a lobectomy either 4·8 or 3·5 mm staples are used according to the thickness of the tissues. After discharging the staples the bronchus is divided flush with the stapler. Bronchial stump closure should then be tested. It is unusual to have to insert any further sutures. The bronchus is seen (*insert*) to be closed with two rows of interdigitating staples.

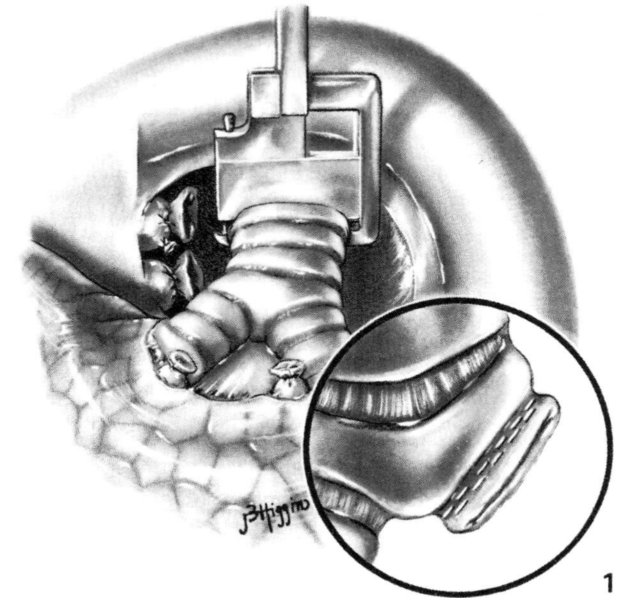

1

2

Closure of the pulmonary artery

The pulmonary artery can be safely closed with the stapler using 3·5 mm staples. The main indication for their use is when there is insufficient length of the artery to allow it to be tied safely. The stapler is used in the same way as for closure of the bronchus.

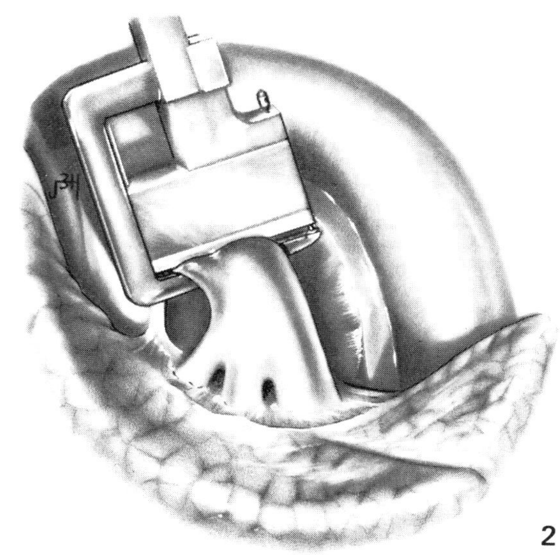

2

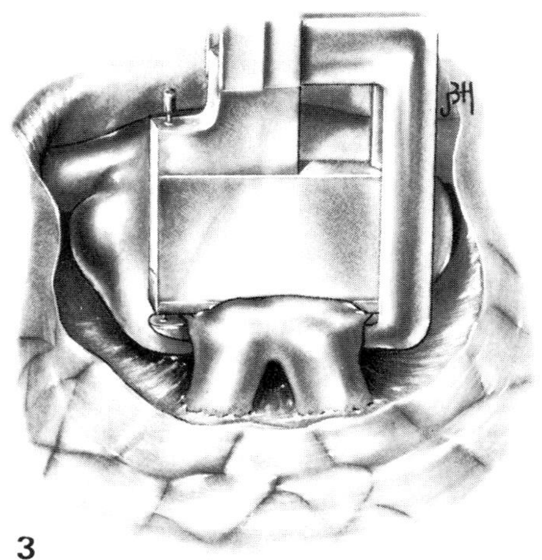

3

3

Closure of the left atrium

The stapler is particularly useful for those patients with involvement of the pulmonary veins. The stapler (Model TA 55) with 3·5 mm staples, is applied to the left atrium, distal to the tumour. After discharging the staples the left atrium is cut flush with the stapler.

4a&b

Open lung biopsy

This can be carried out through a small cosmetic incision either in the axilla or through the auscultatory triangle. The incision (*Illustrations 4a* and *b*) need only be large enough to allow palpation of the lung, thereby enabling the appropriate tissue to be biopsied. Through the small incision a stapler can be introduced and the biopsy performed. If the material to be biopsied is peripheral then the Model TA 30 or TA 55 can be used with 3·5 mm staples as shown in *Illustration 4c*. If, however, the tissue to be biopsied is deeper in the lung, then it is more suitable to use the Model TIA which enables a deep wedge of tissue to be removed.

Incomplete fissures in the lung can be similarly divided during resection of a lobe.

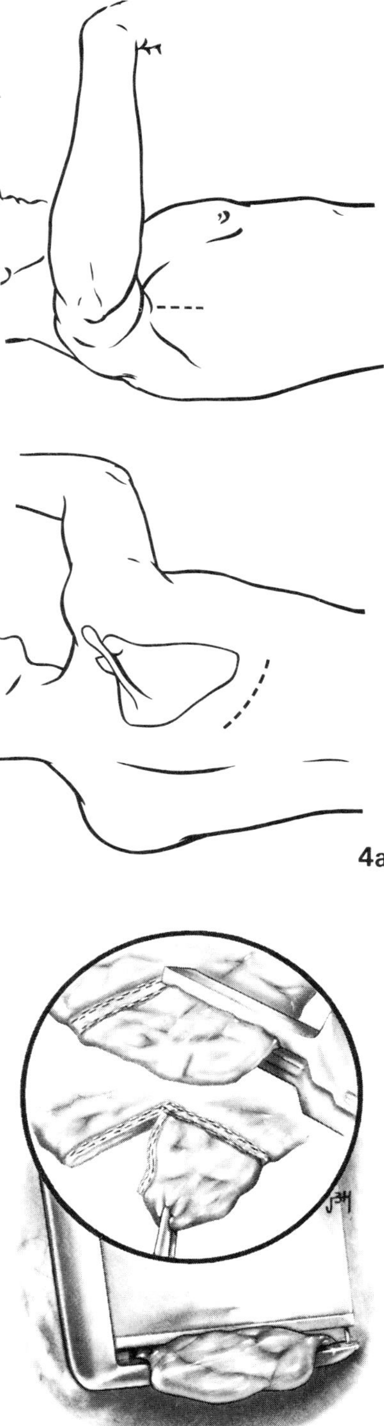

4a

4b

[*The illustrations for this Chapter on Use of Stapler in Lung Surgery were drawn by Mr. B. Higgins.*]

Bronchopleural Fistula after Pneumonectomy

M. F. Sturridge, M.S., F.R.C.S.
Consultant Thoracic Surgeon, The Middlesex Hospital, London;
Consultant Surgeon, London Chest Hospital;
Honorary Consultant Thoracic Surgeon, The National Hospital for Nervous Diseases, London

INTRODUCTION

Bronchopleural fistula is the commonest cause of morbidity and mortality following pneumonectomy. The seriousness of the condition is due to the large volume of fluid that normally accumulates in the pleural space after pneumonectomy, entering the airway rapidly to produce sudden drowning or more gradually to interfere with the function of the remaining lung. In the long term, infection of the pleural space, and of the respiratory tract leads to chronic debilitating illness.

The fistula is caused by an abscess in the suture line. Predisposing factors are infection which is generally present in the lung of patients requiring pneumonectomy and interference with the blood supply of the bronchial stump by mediastinal dissection. Unusually, bronchopleural fistula may result from technical problems, associated with closure of the bronchus.

A bronchopleural fistula may form at any time following pneumonectomy, but most cases present between the seventh and twenty-first days after operation. The mode of presentation and the management of this complication is dependent upon the size of the fistula and is described accordingly.

VERY SMALL BRONCHOPLEURAL FISTULA

The very small fistula produces no clinical manifestation of its presence. The patient, who recovered normally from the operation, is found on routine follow-up x-ray to have increased the amount of air present in the pleura, as assessed on straight postero-anterior chest x-ray. There is no alteration of temperature, pulse or respiratory rate, no cough, haemoptysis or increase in sputum. The patient is completely unaware of the event.

The condition is brought about by the presence of a pin hole leak in the suture line which allows air to pass into the pleura, but does not permit the fluid to pass back into the airway. Alteration of pressure in the pleura towards atmospheric, arrests transudation of fluid into the space and may lead to re-absorption of the fluid across the pleura.

The passage of air into the space is synonymous with the presence of a bronchopleural, oesophago-pleural or pleurocutaneous fistula. The first is most common and the last most easily excluded. The oesophagopleural fistula is usually associated with mucus and saliva in the pleural effusion and the presence of gram negative organisms. If this is suspected, radiographic examination with a barium swallow will confirm or refute the diagnosis in most cases.

Patients with a very small bronchopleural fistula need to be kept under careful observation, although their clinical state causes no alarm. Untreated, the fistula may heal spontaneously and, following re-absorption of air from the pleura, transudation will progressively replace it, with an end result identical to that following uncomplicated pneumonectomy.

In some patients, particularly those in whom the fistula develops late, the fistula may close spontaneously but the pleura loses its ability to transude fluid. The space remains empty with a high negative pressure, and this, plus contraction of fibrous tissue, may lead to progressive, and perhaps, gross mediastinal displacement, with over-distension of the remaining lung. Provided the pleura is sterile, once the fistula has closed and the intrapleural pressure is negative, the space can be filled artificially by instilling normal saline at body temperature through a drip apparatus at the same time allowing any gas within the space to escape through a separate small cannula. This procedure seems to arrest mediastinal displacement.

If infection enters the space while the fistula is present, even though the fistula subsequently closes, a postpneumonectomy empyema may develop. (The management of this is dealt with in the Chapter on 'Postpneumonectomy Empyema', pages 347–348.

SMALL BRONCHOPLEURAL FISTULA

These fistulae measuring 2–3 mm in diameter and often valvular in type are the most difficult to diagnose, and produce the most severe symptoms and rapid deterioration of the patient's condition. The patient becomes distressed, often cyanosed with peripheral vasoconstriction. The pulse rate is elevated and atrial fibrillation often occurs. The patient develops a cough which may be unproductive, or may produce moderate quantities of clear, frothy sputum. A small streak of red blood may precede or accompany the onset of symptoms. The respiratory rate rises and moist sounds can be heard over the lung. The diagnosis is easily confused with a primary cardiac arrhythmia, myocardial infarction, infection of the remaining lung, pulmonary embolism or respiratory insufficiency.

The possibility of a bronchopleural fistula should be foremost in the clinician's mind and must be disproved before accepting any alternative diagnosis. Clinical evidence of development of a fistula can be obtained by listening for vocal resonance over the gas in the pneumonectomy space. Under normal circumstances the pressure in the space is negative and vocal resonance is poor. Immediately the pressure becomes atmospheric or above, vocal resonance is markedly accentuated and the sudden change is almost diagnostic.

1a & 1b

Diagnosis is confirmed by comparison of consecutive chest x-rays; an alteration in the airspace can be appreciated. A normal triangular outline formed at the apex by the chest wall, the mediastinum and the fluid level, becomes 'dome-shaped' with widening of the fluid level, which will progressively fall, as long as the fistula persists.

The positive objective radiological evidence described, is all that is required to make the diagnosis. Neither pleurocutaneous nor oesophagopleural fistulae will produce so profound a systemic disturbance. Other investigations including measurement of intrapleural pressure, injection of indicator fluids into the pleura, bronchoscopy and bronchography for diagnostic purposes are unreliable and serve only to reduce the clinician's confidence and thus the likelihood of the patient receiving the correct treatment.

The patient's condition is explained by the gradual passage of the hypotonic contents of the pleural space into the respiratory tract. Large volumes of this fluid may be absorbed giving rise to hypervolaemia and an inflammatory reaction is produced in the airway causing respiratory embarrassment and anoxia. Cardiac irregularities are probably secondary to these causes. Fluid does not enter rapidly enough to cause postural coughing or the production of recognizable amounts of pleural fluid in the sputum.

The treatment of these patients is a surgical emergency. The patient should be laid on his side with the pneumonectomy space dependent and the chest is aspirated. The patient is then transferred to the operating theatre as soon as possible for closure of the fistula.

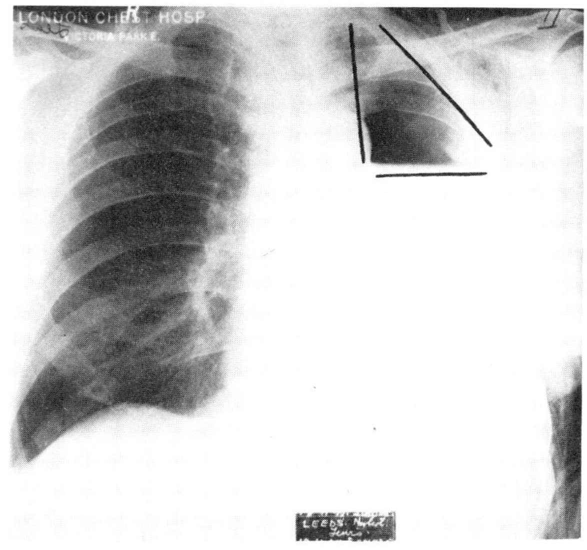

1a

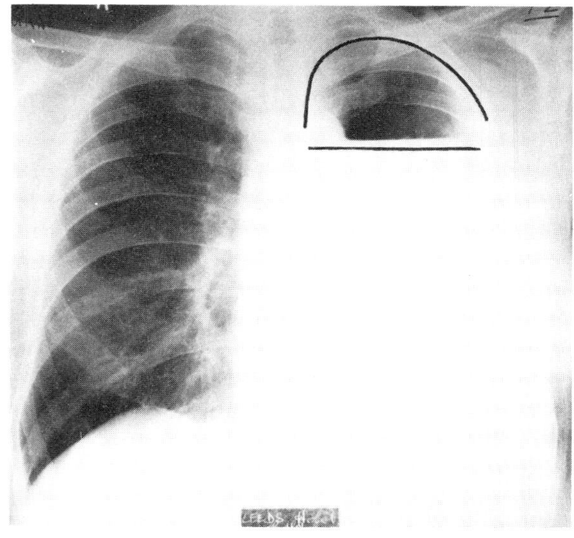

1b

LARGE BRONCHOPLEURAL FISTULA

The development of a large bronchopleural fistula, that is one greater than 3 mm in diameter, is usually heralded by the production of a small amount of fresh blood staining in the sputum. Further events will depend on how much fluid is present in the pneumonectomy space. If the amount is large, the patient may drown from a sudden rush of pleural fluid into the airway. The only hope of saving this patient is to immediately turn him onto the side of his pneumonectomy. Endotracheal intubation and aspiration may be needed to restore the airway provided the heart is still beating but if cardiac arrest has occurred the chances of successful resuscitation are remote. External cardiac massage, which is normally effective only because the lungs support the heart in the mid-line, cannot be relied upon after pneumonectomy, the ventricles easily move aside on compression of the sternum. Immediate thoracotomy will provide the only hope.

If the pneumonectomy space is less full, the patient may cough up a volume of characteristic pleural fluid, so large in amount that it may appear to have been vomited. This alarming occurrence will be repeated at any time that the patient leans away from the pneumonectomy side. As long as the patient remains upright or inclined towards the operated side he is perfectly well, without cough and undistressed. The diagnosis is confirmed by chest x-ray which shows a gross increase of the air in the pneumonectomy space and reduction in the height of the fluid level, but the mediastinum remains central.

The explanation for this event is that fluid only enters the airway when the patient leans over, and then enters at such a rate that it immediately stimulates a cough reflex. As long as the patient is not overwhelmed by the amount of fluid entering, the airway is rapidly cleared. Absorption is minimal and it appears that respiration is only intermittently affected.

The ideal treatment is aspiration of the chest to remove as much fluid as possible followed by early elective operation to close the fistula. These fistulae are rare these days except following unsuccessful attempts to repair a bronchopleural fistula. Such patients and those who are grossly debilitated *before* they develop a fistula or require resuscitation at the time of development can be successfully treated by initial drainage, followed by education in postural drainage via the fistula and then closure of the pleurocutaneous drainage wound. The end result however, is never as good as that following successful operative closure of a fistula.

CLOSURE OF BRONCHOPLEURAL FISTULA

THE OPERATION

The patient is brought to theatre, well propped-up on a trolley, inclined towards the side of pneumonectomy and breathing oxygen from a mask.

Anaesthesia

The principle of anaesthesia is to achieve isolation of the fistula from the airway without further spillage occurring in the process. This is best achieved by the passage of a double-lumen endobronchial tube under local anaesthesia. Once the tube is correctly and securely situated, general anaesthesia can be induced, and the patient is carefully positioned on the operating table in the lateral position, with the pneumonectomy space uppermost, remembering that however successfully the pleural space has been emptied beforehand, there is likely to be at least 500 ml of fluid remaining. If difficulty is encountered, and doubt remains about the correct siting of the tube, it is safer to operate on the patient in the prone position.

The exposure

The pneumonectomy wound is re-opened, removing all suture material layer by layer. The ribs are spread very gradually to avoid breaking them and the pleura is then sucked dry. The parietal pleura below the level of the wound is stripped from the chest wall as far as the diaphragm, and is excised. This serves the dual function of removing any infected granulation tissue and promoting a healthy blood supply to the pleural space from the underlying muscle. The apical and mediastinal pleura are then cleared of any infected material, and granulation tissue, by gently rubbing the surface with a nylon mesh, and the pleura is then washed out with a dilute solution of Flavine in water, which acts as a mild antiseptic and assists clearance of remaining debris. If a muscle graft was applied to the bronchial stump at the first operation, this must be amputated at the chest wall and excised since it will be infected.

Mobilization of the bronchial stump

Patients being treated soon after their original operation present no difficulty in locating the bronchial stump. Fistulae occurring later, when the mediastinum is covered by a layer of fibrous tissue, present more difficulty. Usually there is a tract leading down from the surface of the pleura into the fistula, but in some cases this may be obliterated by granulation tissue. The method of dissection varies on each side.

2

RIGHT-SIDED BRONCHOPLEURAL FISTULA

Dissection is begun posterior to the fistula by making a longitudinal incision in line with the oesophagus. This is carried through the fibrosed pleura with care until the muscle of the oesophagus can be identified. Usually, it is slightly distorted and adherent to the bronchial stump. Great care must be exercised not to perforate the mucosa. The incision is gradually extended until a finger can be insinuated between the oesophagus and the trachea above the level of the bronchial stump. The azygos vein is divided between ligatures to facilitate this procedure. The tissues of the mediastinum are usually relatively normal despite the previous dissection, and the oesophagus can be separated from the bronchial stump by gradually working downwards in this plane until the carina is reached. Starting back above the level of the stump, the pleura is separated from the trachea, until a finger can be passed between the trachea and the superior vena cava, and this plane is developed until it reaches the previous one, below the level of the fistula. Care is necessary when separating the stump from the right pulmonary artery at the lower end of the bronchial suture line.

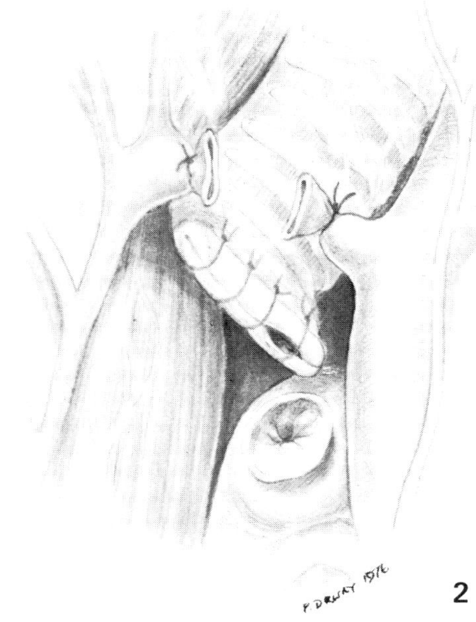

2

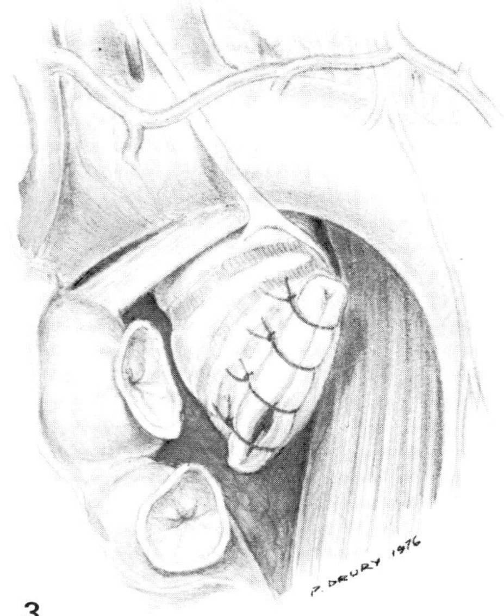

3

3

LEFT-SIDED BRONCHOPLEURAL FISTULA

Because of the important structures closely surrounding the bronchial stump on the left side, including the recurrent laryngeal nerve, the left pulmonary artery and superior pulmonary vein, all of which tend to approximate to the bronchial stump after pneumonectomy, it is safest to approach the bronchus along the fistula tract and to open it completely by removing sutures, incising the overlying fibrous tissue as vision is obtained. Once the stump is fully opened, an incision can be made in the fibrous tissue surrounding it and the stump is mobilized by separating the neighbouring tissues from it. As on the right side, it will be found that once the mediastinal tissues are entered they can be separated quite easily from the bronchus by careful dissection.

Closure of the fistula

No matter how tempting it may appear, the fistula should not be closed by an extra stitch or two as this inevitably, and invariably results in recurrence of the fistula within a remarkably short period of time.

The end of the bronchial stump, including all the tissues that have borne sutures, should be amputated completely to give a clean, fresh bronchus for suture. Usually the tissues are hyperaemic due to the influences of infection and healing. The bronchus is closed in the manner usual to the surgeon, care being taken only to preserve the blood supply and avoid undue tension on the stitches. The bronchial stump can be re-inforced by the application of a pedicle muscle graft, prepared and applied as follows.

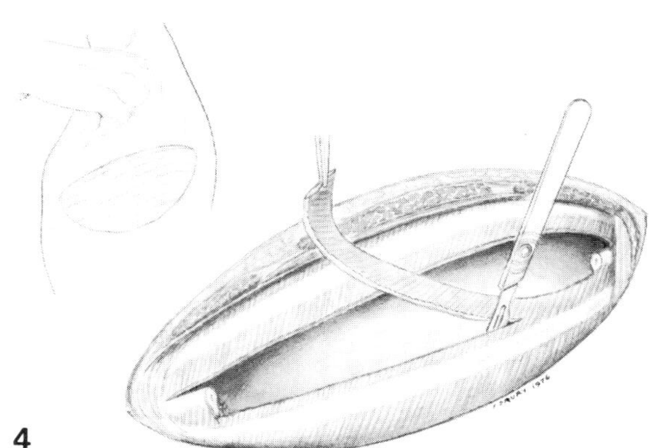

4

4

If the chest has been entered via the upper border of a rib and this rib remains unbroken, the posterior two-thirds of it are carefully resected subperiosteally to expose a sufficient length of intercostal muscle below it to reach from its posterior attachment to the bronchial stump without tension. The intercostal artery is divided anteriorly between ligatures and the muscle is divided with a knife vertically down to the rib below. The graft is then cut from the upper surface of the lower rib leaving a fringe of muscle on the outer aspect and taking great care not to damage the intercostal artery in this process. It is not usually necessary to control bleeding from the graft, but if required it is done by careful suture technique.

If the chest has been entered via the lower border of a rib or if the rib adjacent to the thoracotomy has been broken at any time, it is best to prepare a muscle graft from beneath a nearby intact rib, since only then will the blood supply be known to be intact and the viability of the graft assured.

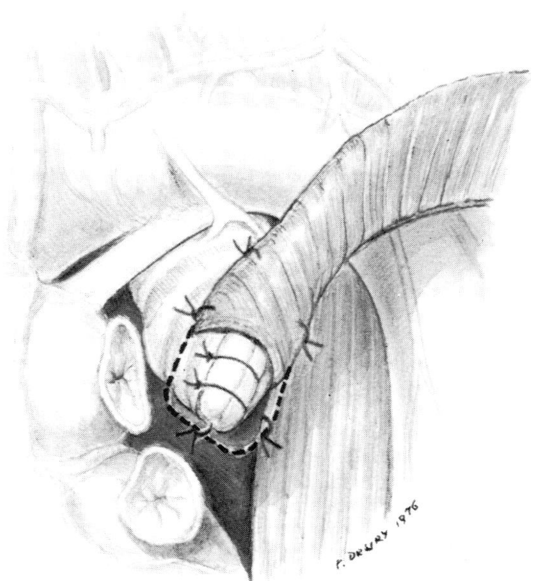

5

5

The graft is brought over the bronchial stump and is fixed by five or six sutures to the bronchial wall proximal to the suture-line, so that it forms a cap over the end of the bronchus. Powdered antibiotics can be placed between the bronchus and the graft. If the graft has a long intrapleural course it is best to support it with an occasional stitch to the mediastinal pleura.

6

Closure of the chest

Now that the fistula has been closed, the pneumonectomy space must be considered as a potential empyema cavity, and will require sterilization by antibiotics in the ensuing days. A plastic nasogastric tube is introduced into the pleura obliquely through a separate incision in the chest wall at a dependent site. (It is convenient to amputate the indwelling end of the tube to enlarge its orifice.) This is firmly fixed to the skin by a surrounding stitch, and the end of the tube is spigotted. If a muscle graft has been prepared, the large defect caused by the absence of the intercostal muscle and the rib, is closed by using three pericostal sutures passed through the lower rib, using a rib-awl and over the upper rib adjacent to the thoracotomy. Tying these from anterior to posterior will usually enable air-tight closure of the chest wall to be achieved by running a second suture to the soft tissues. Careful separation and suture of the muscle layers is important in obtaining a good end result. The skin is closed with interrupted sutures, after careful haemostasis.

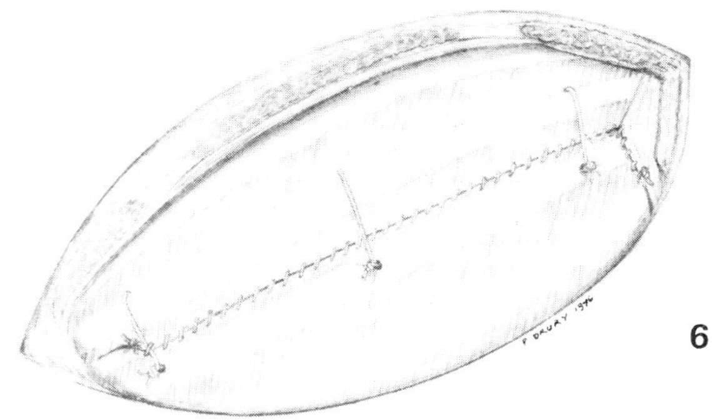

6

POSTOPERATIVE CARE

Care of these patients is essentially that following pneumonectomy, except for the management of the pleura. Every 24 hr after operation the spigot-containing end of the 'nasogastric' tube is amputated. A sample of pleural fluid is aspirated with a syringe for culture. If a specific antibiotic is indicated for a known infection in the pleura, this is injected via the tube and a fresh, sterile spigot applied. If no infecting organism has been identified, 2 mega-units of benzylpenicillin are injected. This process is repeated every 24 hr until three consecutive sterile cultures have been reported. This normally takes 7 days at least. The nasogastric tube is then withdrawn and sterility in the pleural space is checked by aspiration of specimens twice in the following 7 days, and again 7 days later. If sterility is maintained it is safe for the patient to leave hospital. Whatever antibiotic is used in the pleura is also given systemically for 7 days or until the pleura and sputum are sterile.

Persistent infection or re-infection of the space must arouse suspicion of recurrence of the fistula and confirmation of this is sought in the same way as after the initial pneumonectomy. If there is no evidence of recurrence of the fistula the empyema should be treated in the same manner as described in the Chapter on 'Postpneumonectomy Empyema,' pages 347–348.

BRONCHOPLEURAL FISTULA FOLLOWING LOBECTOMY

Bronchopleural fistula is a rare complication of lobectomy perhaps because of the small number of resections for pulmonary tuberculosis and bronchiectasis now performed in this country.

The significance of this complication depends upon the state of the residual lobe. Provided that this is healthy and expanded the patient is usually unaware that a bronchopleural fistula has developed. Occasionally a little blood-stained sputum is produced followed by a small amount of pleural fluid or pus. The diagnosis is made by the appearance in the chest x-ray of a pneumothorax which is usually in the site previously occupied by the resected lobe.

If the pneumothorax is localized and small (less than 5 cm in diameter) it can often be managed conservatively and will become obliterated spontaneously over a period of a few weeks. If a fluid level persists or the pneumothorax is larger, it is best treated by closed drainage followed after a few days by open drainage. The space will then obliterate slowly by expansion of the underlying lung and contraction of the overlying chest wall until only the fistulous track remains. The tube is then withdrawn and the fistula will close spontaneously.

The complication is extremely serious if the residual lobe is infected and atelectatic at the time of fistula formation. There is, in these circumstances, a considerable volume of transudate in the pleura which forms in response to the high negative pleural pressure. The presentation is then identical to that of a bronchopleural fistula after pneumonectomy (q.v.) and the management is the same except that it is nearly always necessary to resect the residual lobe if the patient's life is to be saved.

[*The illustrations for this Chapter on Bronchopleural Fistula after Pneumonectomy were drawn by Mr. P. Drury.*]

Postpneumonectomy Empyema

M. F. Sturridge, M.S., F.R.C.S.
Consultant Thoracic Surgeon, The Middlesex Hospital, London;
Consultant Surgeon, London Chest Hospital;
Honorary Consultant Thoracic Surgeon, The National Hospital for Nervous Diseases, London

Infection of the pleural space following pneumonectomy is an uncommon complication except in association with a bronchopleural fistula (q.v.); it probably results from opportunist bacteria left in the pleura at operation. Empyema usually presents within the first year after operation.

Infection should be suspected in the early postoperative phase if rapid accumulation of fluid in the pneumonectomy space causes mediastinal displacement towards the remaining lung. Such fluid, formed in the presence of positive intrapleural pressure is an exudate and the stimulus to its formation may be infection. Aspiration of the fluid to correct mediastinal displacement allows microscopy and culture. The presence of numerous pus cells and the culture of pyogenic bacteria confirm the diagnosis. Untreated, the empyema will usually track through the recent wound to the surface and discharge.

Cases presenting later after operation usually have general malaise, pyrexia and loss of appetite. The course may start slowly and insidiously but eventually there is a rapid deterioration in health with severe toxaemia and sometimes septicaemia. The pus in the pleura tracks towards the chest wall and presents as a painful tender area with surrounding inflammation. Fluctuation develops and palpation may elicit an expansile cough impulse. This condition is known as empyema necessitans. Aspiration of the chest wall abscess yields an undue volume of pus and rapid refilling of the abscess cavity occurs. The diagnosis is confirmed when the pleural fluid is separately aspirated and pus of the same quality and cultural characteristics is obtained.

TREATMENT

The initial treatment is to reduce the patient's toxicity. Early drainage of the pleura is mandatory. Fluid replacement by intravenous infusion and intravenous administration of a broad-spectrum antibiotic may be indicated before the culture results are ready.

Intercostal drainage of the pleura through either the presenting abscess on the chest wall or at a fresh site if this seems more appropriate, is perfectly adequate in the first stage of treatment. Ideally drainage should be performed in an operating theatre where the pleura can be carefully aspirated as dry as possible. All sloughs and any residual blood clot are removed. Thoracoscopy may be a useful adjunct to this procedure. Great care must be taken to avoid damage to the diaphragm since this may spread the infection to the subphrenic space, a complication which must always be considered iatrogenic in aetiology.

In order to evacuate all the pus it is necessary to introduce air into the pleura but once the fluid has been displaced the drainage tube can be connected to an underwater seal. Pleural washouts may be performed using Flavine 1:5000 in water or Noxyflex (noxytiolin) 1 per cent solution. The fluid is introduced by catheter through the drainage tube with the patient lying on his unaffected side. Air in the pleura can escape around the catheter. After 3–4 hr retention the fluid is allowed to drain out, if necessary letting air into the pleura to displace it.

Samples of pleural fluid should be collected daily for bacterial culture and sensitivity to antibiotics and the subsequent management is dependent upon these results and the patient's progress.

If the fluid cultured is consistently sterile and the patient's condition is good, the drainage tube can be removed when the daily drainage becomes less than 100 ml/24 hr. Fluid should then gradually collect in the space as after pneumonectomy and samples should be aspirated for bacterial culture with intervals of 3, 4 and 7 days between. If all of these are sterile the patient can be discharged.

If bacteria are identified, the patient should be treated with the specific antibiotics orally and by instillation *every 24 hr* into the pleura. As soon as the fluid from the pleura becomes thin and serous a narrow plastic catheter can be introduced into the pleura through the drainage tube which is then withdrawn. Each day a sample is obtained for culture via the catheter and the antibiotics are instilled, until three consecutive daily cultures have been reported sterile. The tube is then removed and continuing sterility checked by aspiration and culture of fluid samples at intervals during the following 2 weeks.

Continuing infection must raise the possibility of a persistent source of infection such as a foreign body, bronchopleural or oesophagopleural fistula. In debilitated patients it may be preferable to perform dependent rib resection and drainage and to leave this for a period until their general condition is improved before re-admitting them to hospital for sterilization of the pleura as described above. It should never be necessary to accept permanent drainage for uncomplicated pleural infection.

Surgical Management of Chylothorax

J. Keith Ross, M.S., F.R.C.S.
Consultant Cardiothoracic Surgeon, Wessex Cardiac and Thoracic Centre, Western Hospital, Southampton

The practical management of chylothorax depends upon an understanding of the surgical anatomy, physiology and pathology of the thoracic duct and its tributaries.

Surgical anatomy of the thoracic duct

The thoracic duct begins at the upper end of the cisterna chyli, near the lower border of the twelfth thoracic vertebra, and throughout its intrathoracic course has a close relationship with the vertebral column. In its lower part, the duct lies to the right of the mid-line between the azygos vein and the aorta, and at about the level of the fifth thoracic vertebra it inclines to the left for the remainder of its intra-thoracic course, ultimately gaining the root of the neck where it ends by emptying into the left jugulo-subclavian junction. This 'normal course' is found in only a little over half of individuals, and two or more main ducts are present at some stage in its course in between 40 and 60 per cent of people.

In addition to the chief ending of the duct, other minor lymphaticovenous anastomoses exist between the thoracic duct system and the azygos, intercostal and lumbar veins. The richness of this collateral circulation is such that the main thoracic duct may be ligated safely at any point in its thoracic or cervical course without harmful effects.

The classically described course of the duct explains why damage to it below the level of the fifth or sixth thoracic vertebra usually results in a right-sided chylous effusion, and damage above this level to an effusion on the left.

Elective exposure of the thoracic duct in its early course is most easily achieved by a right-sided approach when it may be found lying on the vertebral column between the aorta and the azygos vein. If a left-sided approach has to be used, the aorta must be mobilized to gain access to the duct, which may be reached either in front of or behind the aorta.

Any operation in or about the mediastinum carries with it the risk of damage to the main thoracic duct or a major tributary, but the duct is particularly vulnerable in the upper part of the chest in any procedure involving mobilization of the aortic arch, left subclavian artery, or oesophagus. Here the duct lies along the left border of the oesophagus, being crossed by the aortic arch, and comes to lie behind the beginning of the left subclavian artery close to the mediastinal pleura. It is important for the surgeon operating in this area to be aware of a structure that he seldom sees, and which usually only manifests its presence once it has been cut.

Phsyiology of the thoracic duct

The thoracic duct is a muscular endothelial-lined tube containing multiple valves. The forward, or upward flow of chyle within the duct is maintained chiefly by rhythmic contraction of the duct wall. Flow is also augmented by the inflow of chyle into the lacteal system (*vis a tergo*) which in turn is governed by the intake of food and liquid into the intestine, and by negative intrathoracic pressure on inspiration (*vis a fronte*).

Both the volume and the flow of chyle vary enormously with meals, and are particularly affected by the fat content of food, being increased when the fat content is high.

Volumes of up to 2500 ml of chyle have been collected from the cannulated human thoracic duct in a 24-hr period, and the flow rate has been shown to vary between 14 and 110 ml/hr. In the presence of a chylous fistula, aspiration of the chest may yield between 2 and 3 litres of chyle daily. Water taken by mouth can increase the flow of chyle by 20 per cent and an ordinary hospital meal can cause a three-fold increase in flow. Starvation reduces flow to the merest trickle of clear lymph.

The pressure within the thoracic duct at the height of maximum flow is between 10 and 28 cm of water.

The thoracic duct as a metabolic pathway

Thoracic duct lymph contains 0·4 to 6 g per cent of fat, and 60 – 70 per cent of ingested fat is conveyed to the bloodstream by way of the thoracic duct. This is made up of neutral fat, free fatty acids, phospholipids, sphingomyelin, and cholesterol esters. Neutral fat is found in the form of minute globules, or chylomicrons, 0·5 μm or less in diameter. The rate of passage of ingested fat from the intestine to the cervical end of the thoracic duct is between 1 and 2 hr, and if neutral fat in the form of radio-active labelled olive oil is given by mouth, peak radio-activity in the venous blood occurs within 6 hr in normal individuals.

It is likely that any protein which passes unchanged through the intestinal mucosa enters the lymphatics and not the blood capillaries, although the capacity to absorb quantities of unchanged protein of large molecular size (colostrum protein) disappears within the first few days of life. Thoracic duct lymph contains about 4 per cent of protein, consisting of albumin, globulin, fibrinogen and prothrombin, and with an albumin-globulin ratio of 3:1.

The thoracic duct and cellular elements of the blood

The lymphocyte count of human chyle varies between 400 and 6800/mm^3, and the duct is known to be an important pathway for the entry of lymphocytes into the circulation. Erythrocytes are also found in thoracic duct lymph, the count varying between 50 and 600/mm^3.

Physiological effects of thoracic duct fistula

First, such a fistula results in the loss of water and electrolytes, the electrolyte content of chyle being, for all practical purposes, that of the blood plasma; the volumes that are lost have already been mentioned.

The loss of fat and fat-soluble vitamins, which can be considerable, and results in a serious metabolic deficit, is better tolerated than the protein loss, which leads to a steadily falling plasma protein level, wasting, and famine oedema. Circulating lymphocytes are greatly reduced in number and antibodies are probably also lost. The total effect of a thoracic duct fistula is disastrous, and death is inevitable once supportive treatment fails, unless the fistula closes spontaneously or is surgically closed.

Physiological effects of thoracic duct ligation

It has been shown repeatedly, both experimentally and clinically, that ligation of the thoracic duct at any point in its course is surprisingly well-tolerated, and is not followed by the extravasation of chyle distal to the point of ligature. This is due to the richness of the lymphatic collateral circulation. The intraduct pressure can rise to surprising heights after ligation, pressures as high as 50 mmHg having been recorded after obstruction of the human thoracic duct: the pressure falls with the opening-up of collateral vessels.

Ligation of the thoracic duct is followed by no outward sign of nutritional disturbance, but the blood fat level falls within 3 hr of the duct being tied, normal levels being regained by the sixteenth day following ligation.

The lymphocyte count in the peripheral blood falls dramatically within a few hours of the thoracic duct being tied to a value 50 to 60 per cent of normal, becoming normal again within 7 – 11 days.

Surgical pathology of the thoracic duct and aetiology of chylothorax

Congenital

Single or multiple thoracic duct fistulae can be found soon after birth. In the absence of notable birth trauma, this occurrence may either be due to congenital weakness in the thoracic duct, which only becomes apparent once the infant is being fed, or may be due to failure of junction of the multiple segmental components of the embryonic duct, which is most likely to be the case when multiple fistulae are found at operation for chylothorax early in infancy.

Traumatic

Damage to the thoracic duct may follow closed chest injury, or may be the result of penetrating injury or operative procedures in its vicinity.

Non-penetrating injury. The commonest form of non-penetrating injury to the thoracic duct is that due to sudden hyperextension of the spine with rupture of the duct just above the diaphragm. Sudden stretching over the vertebral bodies may alone be enough to tear the duct, but some believe that duct fixation as the result of prior injury or disease is responsible for making it susceptible to such violence. The less the severity of the closed trauma, the more likely it is that some other factor is involved. Blast and crush injuries of the chest, vomiting, or a violent bout of coughing may be associated with tearing of the thoracic duct.

There are two remarkable facts about a chylous fistula following closed chest trauma which demand attention – one is that there is nearly always a latent interval, usually of from 2 to 10 days, but sometimes of weeks or months, between the time of injury and the onset of the chylous pleural effusion. The other feature is the reluctance of such fistulae to close spontaneously.

The latent interval is due to the fact that, following rupture of the duct, chyle accumulates in the posterior mediastinum – the so-called 'chyloma' – and finally ruptures the mediastinal pleura, usually on the right side at the base of the pulmonary ligament.

Thoracic duct fistulae do not obey the law that fistulae tend to close in the absence of distal obstruction. Spontaneous sealing of thoracic duct fistulae after closed chest injury may be expected in only 50 per cent of such cases, and death may be expected in the remaining 50 per cent unless the fistula is surgically closed.

Penetrating injury. Although gunshot and stab wounds of the thoracic duct have been described, they are apt to be overshadowed by damage to other structures of more immediate importance in the vicinity.

Chylothorax has been reported following almost every known thoracic operation. Here, two main sub-groups may be identified. First are those procedures in which the main thoracic duct is clearly at risk, including such procedures as resection of coarctation of the aorta, Blalock's procedure, and oesophagectomy. Secondly, and frequently baffling to the surgeon are those occasions when chylothorax complicates operations far removed from the main duct itself, including lung resection and operations on intrapericardial structures, including open-heart surgery: here it has been shown that the chylous leak may occur within the anterior mediastinum in relation to thymic tissue, when it is a mediastinal rather than a pleural complication. However, the author has seen one instance of a classical left-sided chylous effusion following an open-heart procedure in a child, and other examples have been reported in the literature. Other examples of postoperative chylous leaks occurring at sites remote from the main duct must follow injury to unrecognized thoracic duct tributaries capable of allowing chylous reflux.

Circulatory

Thrombosis of the great veins into which the thoracic duct drains has been held responsible for chylous effusions, and aneurysms of the thoracic aorta may erode the duct with subsequent fistula formation. Thrombosis of the great veins may be secondary to malignant involvement of the duct and vessel walls, and in this, as well as other malignant chylous leaks, the pericardial sac may be filled with chyle.

Inflammatory

As the thoracic duct carries lymph from the intestine and peritoneum, it is responsible for passing on micro-organisms absorbed from the gut and peritoneal cavity, and may itself become secondarily inflamed in the process. The duct wall can be directly involved by intrathoracic tuberculosis, and the lumen may become obstructed in filariasis: both can be associated with chylous fistulae.

Neoplastic

Benign intrinsic cysts and tumours. Degenerative thoracic duct cysts are nearly always found in the elderly, and are usually incidentally discovered at necropsy, degenerative changes in the duct wall having been likened to the changes seen in ageing peripheral veins. These cysts may be multiple. Benign lymphangiomata arising in the thoracic duct may also produce single or multiple cyst-like spaces filled with chyle, a more extensive variant being the mediastinal hygroma with multiple chyle-containing channels forming a tumour-like mass in the mediastinum. Such cysts are more likely to rupture into the pleura than the degenerative ones, and this is a rare cause of 'spontaneous' chylothorax. They are found as a rule in younger people.

The thoracic duct and malignant disease. Primary malignant tumours of the thoracic duct have not been described.

The thoracic duct may become secondarily involved by the lymphatic spread of primary abdominal and intrathoracic cancer, either by the invasion of the lumen by direct lymphatic permeation in continuity from the primary growth, or by direct invasion of the duct wall from without, or by way of small lymphatics found in the areolar tissue surrounding the duct. Once tumour enters the lumen, dissemination may occur by further permeation or by embolism, or both.

The frequency with which the thoracic duct is involved in malignant disease has been assessed at between 3·6 and 30 per cent.

The practical importance of malignant involvement of the thoracic duct in this context is that a proportion of those involved will eventually leak chyle, the mechanism of the leak being either the rupture of a distended tributary, or of erosion of the duct wall itself. The resulting chylous effusion may be unilateral or bilateral, and may be the presenting sign of an unsuspected underlying tumour (e.g. retroserous lymphosarcoma). Chylous ascites followed by chylothorax is a sinister progression, strongly suggesting a primary retroperitoneal tumour.

Primary malignant tumours of the pleura may be associated with chylous effusions arising from multiple fistulae, so that the lungs appear to weep chyle, and may be complicated by pneumothorax.

Spontaneous chylothorax

This is a misleading term, and has been loosely applied to chylothorax after childbirth, after closed chest injury, and to those cases secondary to malignant disease. There remain some examples for which no underlying cause can be found, but these are uncommon.

Complications of chylothorax

In addition to the nutritional changes already described that follow a thoracic duct fistula, and apart from complications related to the pathology of the underlying cause, there are few complications peculiar to chylothorax. Empyema is rare because chyle is bacteriostatic. In some, fibrinous deposition on the surface of the lung results in 'trapping' of the lung by a fibrinous rind, but this is an inconsistent happening. Spontaneous pneumothorax and chylothorax may occur together and chyle may be coughed up.

Diagnosis of chylothorax

This depends upon the recognition of chyle once it has been removed from the chest by aspiration or by drainage tubes. Initially it is commonly mistaken for pus. In traumatic chylothorax, the chyle is frequently blood-stained at first, and this may be misleading. The characteristics and composition of chyle are set out in Table 1. The simplest test to confirm the diagnosis is by adding ether to the aspirate in a test tube when the fat dissolves and the milky fluid clears. Clinically the history may be valuable, particularly in the case of chylothorax following closed chest injury when the latent interval and sudden onset of a shock-like state and breathlessness, with the appearance of a large effusion, are characteristic. Low-grade fever is very often found in all varieties of chylothorax.

Table 1

Composition	
Total protein	22·0 – 59·8 g/l
Albumin	12·0 – 41·6 g/l
Globulin	11·0 – 30·8 g/l
Fibrinogen	1·6 – 2·4 g/l
Total fat	4·0 – 60 g/l
Total cholesterol	1·7 – 5·6 mmol/l
Cholesterol esters	0·6 – 4.8 mmol/l
Sugar	2·6 – 11·0 mmol/l
Urea nitrogen	1·3 – 2·9 mmol/l
Non-protein nitrogen	1·0 – 2·4 mmol/l
Electrolytes	
Na	104 – 148 mmol/l
K	3·8 – 5·0 mmol/l
Cl	85 – 130 mmol/l
Ca	3·4 – 6·0 mmol/l
Inorganic phosphate	0·3 – 1·8 mmol/l
Lymphocytes	0·4 – 6·8 x 10^9/l
Erythrocytes	50 – 600 x 10^6/l

The diagnostic triad of a rapidly accumulating pleural effusion, low serum protein level, and a falling lymphocyte count may be of use.

If confirmation is needed that the fluid is chyle and not 'pseudochyle' the patient may be given fat to eat, stained with a lipophilic dye, e.g. Sudan III or Sudan IV, followed by further chest aspiration. Lymphangiography may be valuable, particularly when the chylothorax is 'spontaneous' and the underlying cause obscure.

THE MANAGEMENT OF CHYLOTHORAX

Although there is some evidence that traumatic lymph fistulae in general tend to close spontaneously, the fact remains that spontaneous closure of a thoracic duct fistula is unpredictable and, as already stated, those following closed chest injury may only be expected to resolve spontaneously in 50 per cent of cases. A single pleural aspiration may be followed by cure, but a crucial decision in the management of chylothorax is how long to carry on with the trial of conservative treatment before resorting to operative intervention.

No rigid plan can satisfy the demands of all circumstances in which chylothorax can occur, but there is a choice of three courses that can be followed which may be effective singly or in combination.

First, there is much to be said for the operative control of a chylous leak as soon as possible after establishing the diagnosis, if morbidity and mortality are to be kept to a minimum. Early operation is indicated if the chylothorax is loculated and contains fibrin clot, and in all instances where the lung is restricted and requires decortication. Early exploration is also indicated if there is uncertainty about the exact pathology of the underlying condition, when waiting might postpone appropriate treatment for a previously unsuspected underlying neoplasm.

Secondly, if a period of conservative treatment is decided upon, thoracic duct flow must be reduced to a minimum. The most efficient way of achieving this is to stop all feeding by mouth, maintaining the patient's nutrition intravenously and replacing observed chyle loss volume for volume with plasma. Alternatively, the patient may be given a strict fat-free diet, and be kept on a restricted oral fluid intake, with intravenous fluid supplement to achieve the daily fluid requirements. The method of chest drainage during this period should be by intercostal catheter, or by drainage tubes remaining after operation, together with gentle suction from the outset. This will ensure that the lung is given every chance to remain fully expanded all the time, instead of intermittently, as is the case with periodic aspiration.

A period of 7 days is suggested as the maximum time to follow this conservative plan, unless there is evidence that the volume of drainage is becoming progressively less. If during this 7-day period, the fistula appears to have closed spontaneously, oral feeding should be started before removing the chest tube, to confirm that closure is complete. During the conservative trial period, daily plasma protein and serum electrolyte estimations, white blood cell counts and chest radiographs should be made. If lymph continues to drain steadily, then thoracotomy should be undertaken without delay.

Thirdly, circumstances may strongly contra-indicate thoracotomy and demand prolonged conservative treatment. If this is so, for example, in a patient with vertebral or multiple injuries, or immobilized following anterior fusion of the thoracic spine, then the fat-free diet regime with continued chest drainage should be used from the outset, with daily assessment of the patient's nutritional state. Re-infusion of aspirated chyle has been achieved on a large scale, but is not recommended owing to the risk of anaphylactic shock.

Neonatal chylothorax and that occurring post-operatively in small babies presents a special problem. Conservative treatment for as long as 3 weeks has been recommended but the problem of maintaining a small infant with chylothorax in a satisfactory metabolic state must be very great. The good results of early surgical closure of the fistula may indicate, particularly in places where the most skilled supportive treatment is not available, that operative treatment carries the lesser risk.

In chylothorax complicating malignant disease, even when this is advanced, thoracic duct ligation may be the kindest and quickest way of ridding the patient of a most uncomfortable complication.

SURGICAL TECHNIQUE

In unilateral chylothorax, the chest should be opened on the side of the effusion. This applies particularly in postoperative cases when the aim should be to control the chylous fistula at the site of the duct damage, rather than to carry out a formal ligation of the duct lower in the chest. The many advantages of operating on the involved side outweigh the arguments in favour of routine right-sided approach, of which the sole merit is the ease of access to the main duct just above the diaphragm. When the effusion is bilateral, it is sensible to explore the right side first, with duct ligation, although it may prove necessary to explore the left side later.

The simplest way to find the thoracic duct fistula is to give the patient butter or cream by mouth 3 – 4 hr before operation. A lipophilic dye may be added to the fat if desired, or a 1 per cent aqueous solution of Evans Blue (0·7 – 0·8 mg/kg) may be injected into the leg once the chest is opened, but the whiteness of chyle is usually sufficiently striking without the addition of colour, and dyestuffs tend to cause extensive tissue staining if there is free escape of chyle.

As already stated, the main principle of operation for chylothorax is to find the site of the fistula and to close it. It is stating the obvious that the best time to achieve closure of a fistula is at the time it is created, if the duct is damaged during a mediastinal operation. If the duct is at risk, the surgeon should be aware of this possibility, and alert to the sudden presence of clear, slightly grey fluid in the operative field, this being the appearance of thoracic duct lymph in the fasting patient. This event should immediately stimulate a search for the thoracic duct, followed by its ligation with non-absorbable material.

When dealing with an established chylothorax, there are three techniques which can be used to control a chylous leak. These are direct control of the fistula, suture of the leaking mediastinal pleura and supradiaphragmatic ligation of the thoracic duct (*see* Surgical Anatomy of the Thoracic Duct, page 349).

As indicated, the best method is to find the actual point of leakage and to ligate the duct on either side of the breach. If this is not possible, particularly when the mediastinal tissues are extensively soaked in chyle, or when there are multiple leaks, it may be sufficient to suture the mediastinal pleura at the point or points where the chyle is leaking. Either of these methods may be combined with the third technique, that of ligation of the thoracic duct low in the chest, which alone has proved effective in many instances when no attempt has been made to gain direct control of the fistula. In cases of chylothorax complicating advanced malignant disease, there may be a place for iodized talc pleurodesis, particularly if the situation is one where chyle is weeping from all serous surfaces.

References

Blalock, A., Robinson, C. S., Cunningham, R. S. and Gray, M. E. (1937). *Archs Surg. (Chicago)* **34**, 1049

Garamella, J. J. (1958). *A.M.A. Archs Surg.* **76**, 46

Joyce, L. D. *et al.* (1976). *J. thorac. cardiovasc. Surg.* **71**, 476

Lampson, R. S. (1948). *J. thorac. Surg.* **17**, 778

Little, J. M., Harrison, C. and Blalock, A. (1942). *Surgery* **11**, 392

Meade, R. H. (1952). *A.M.A. Archs intern. Med.* **90**, 30

Watne, A. L., Hatiboglu, I. and Moore, G. E. (1960). *Surgery Gynec. Obstet.* **110**, 339

Yoffey, J. M. and Courtice, F. C. (1956). *Lymphatics, Lymph and Lymphoid Tissue*, 2nd edition. London: Arnold

Pectus Excavatum

Mark M. Ravitch, M.D.
Professor of Surgery, University of Pittsburgh and
Surgeon-in-Chief, Montefiore Hospital of Pittsburgh

PRE-OPERATIVE

Indications

Deep deformities of this kind are associated with an unattractive kyphotic posture and a protuberant abdomen. Almost all adolescents have some modest decrease in exercise tolerance and all of them have electrocardiographic evidence of cardiac displacement and rotation. Severe cardiorespiratory embarrassment does occur but is extremely rare. The deformity is usually noted in infancy and tends to be progressive. If the deformity is deep or is reliably known to be progressing, operation at any age is advised, even as young as 3 months. Infants tolerate the operation well and respond to precisely the same operative technique, although since the deformity is less marked a less extensive resection is required. We do not operate beyond adolescence except for extremely deep deformities which are either totally unacceptable socially or cause significant symptoms. A pleasant reward of the operative procedure is frequently an increase in vigour and appetite in a child previously not realized to have been deficient in these respects. The indications for the operation are then: (*1*) prophylactic against progression; (*2*) correction of the thoracic and postural deformity; (*3*) correction or prevention of physiological deficit; and (*4*) sociopsychological. Appropriately-directed physiological measurements in Sweden and in the United States have demonstrated very real physiological defects even in patients with deformities considered to be asymptomatic. This last is a valid indication for operation not to be dismissed.

Choice of technique

A good many operative techniques have been described. The one portrayed here has been in use with slight progressive modifications for 30 years with satisfactory immediate and long-term results. It seems to us the simplest effective operation. The 'limited' operation, merely dividing several of the lower cartilages, will not achieve satisfactory results. Preservation of the cartilages with multiple incisions in them is in fact a more difficult and bloodier operation. Failure to disengage the perichondrium and the intercostal bundles from the sternum seems to us to invite recurrence. External traction is unnecessary and may lead to infection. The autoplastic operation shown here is entirely satisfactory for the vast majority of patients. In adults, in rapidly growing six-foot teenagers with an extremely long gladiolus and in patients operated upon for recurrence, we may employ metallic fixation as indicated in *Illustration 8*.

Position of patient

In infants particularly it is useful to place a folded towel the length of the dorsal spine to elevate the chest somewhat.

THE OPERATION

1

The incision

The incision in males, and in all adults, is mid-line from well up on the sternum to well down on the epigastrium. The dotted line indicates the portion of the incision which is hidden from view in the projection shown. In girls we employ a transverse submammary incision arching upwards in the mid-line. This yields a superior cosmetic result but involves a dissection of the skin and subcutaneous fat separate from the dissection of the pectoral muscles, and there is, additionally, some risk to the vascular supply of the edge of the upper flap. Some loss of time and of blood is involved as well.

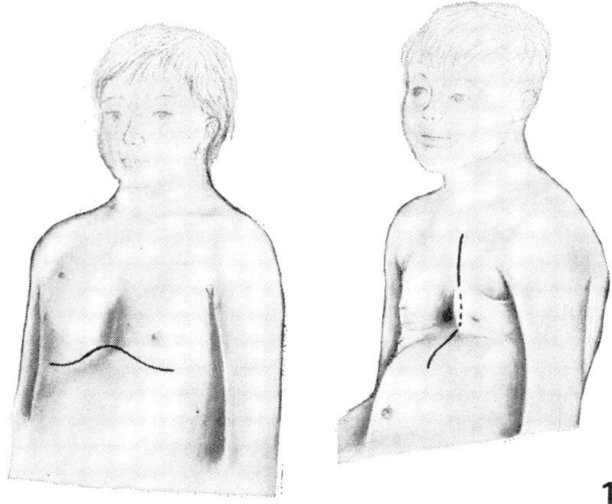

1

Exposure of costal cartilages

2

Vertical incision

Traction on the skin and subcutaneous fat is transmitted to the pectoralis major, the muscular slips of which are divided from the sternum and costal cartilages preferably with the electrocautery. If this is done carefully, and if the assistant is alert to see and clamp the perforating branches of the internal mammary before they have been divided, there will be no blood loss. The clamps may be left on the perforators until they have thrombosed, or electrocoagulation may be employed. Inferiorly the obliquity of the lower cartilages and the direction of the fibres of the rectus abdominis require one to slit the sheath of the muscle and to lay bare the cartilages by splitting the muscle fibres. All of the involved cartilages are exposed for the full extent of their deformity which, particularly in older children, may be beyond the costochondral junctions. Superiorly the lowest apparently normal costal cartilage is laid bare and the sternum in the interspace above this.

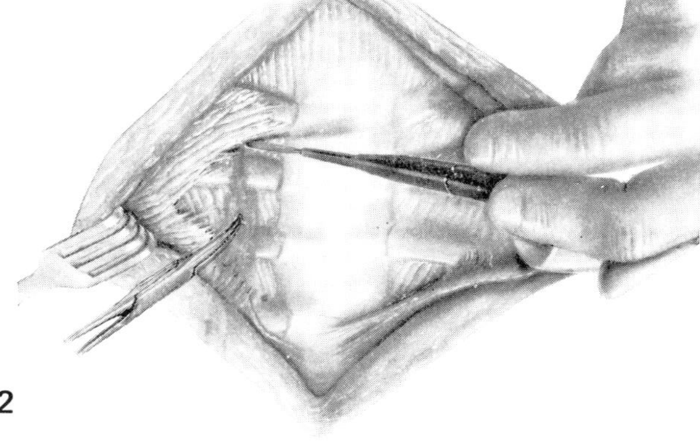

2

Transverse incision

Precisely the same technique is employed, after the skin flaps have been developed.

3

Resection of deformed cartilages

A longitudinal incision is made through the perichondrium with scalpel or the cautery knife. A transverse incision through the perichondrium at either end allows rectangular perichondrial flaps to be reflected. Curved clamps are applied to the upper edge of the incised perichondrium. If these clamps are correctly applied, scraping across the cartilage as they are closed, the stripping of the perichondrium will be well started by this manoeuvre alone. We usually strip the perichondrium of the upper flap before applying the clamps to the lower flap. A thin, blunt elevator of the kind (Freer) employed in submucous resections works well. The perichondrium is tougher than the cartilage and the elevator is best placed, to begin with, with the curve towards the perichondrium. The perichondrium is thinnest at the upper edge of the cartilage and it is not difficult to perforate it at this point in the dissection. The inset shows the cartilage lifted up until an opening can be dissected under it. A blunt elevator (for example, a Brophy right-angled palate elevator), will now strip the cartilage clean. The medial edge is usually divided from the sternum with a small Doyen elevator (not shown) although the scalpel is satisfactory.

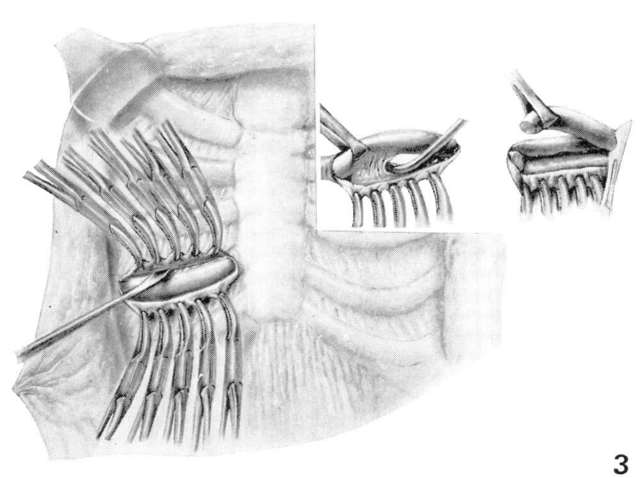

3

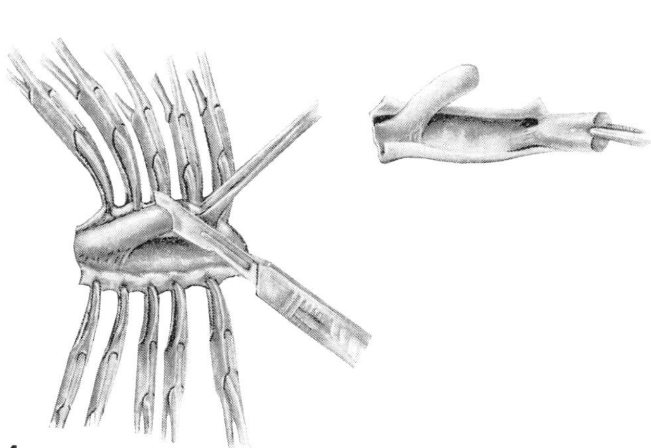

4

4

Alternative method

When the posterior perichondrium does not strip well, or in older children, or in adults in whom the ribs tend to take a triangular cross-section with an increased anteroposterior diameter so that stripping is difficult or impossible, stripping is frequently facilitated if the cartilage is grasped with a Kocher clamp, lifted up and cut through; the grasped portion of the cartilage pulling away from the perichondrium underneath. The two halves of the costal cartilage are then separately removed.

5

Division of xiphoid

All of the deformed costal cartilages have been removed subperichondrially for the full extent of the deformity. In this instance four cartilages have been removed. Often five are removed, infrequently six, and rarely three. The xiphoid is divided from the sternum with heavy scissors. There is usually a vigorous arterial spurter which must be seized on each side of the xiphoid.

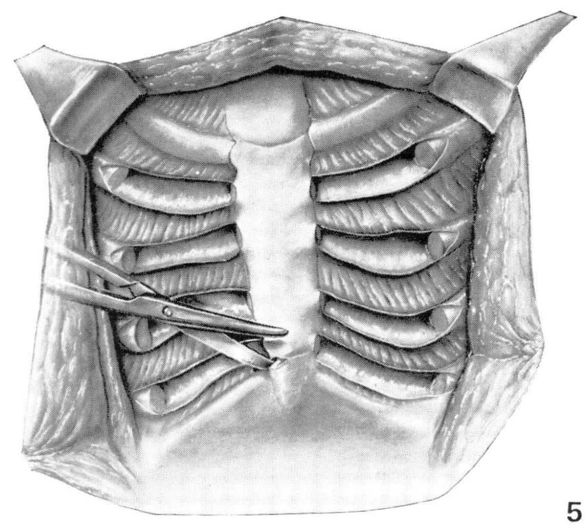

5

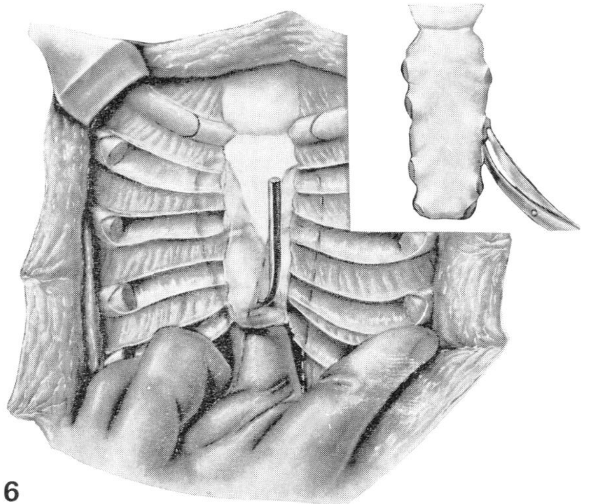

6

6

Freeing the sternum

The finger is inserted in the mediastinum and moved from side to side behind the sternum as indicated by the transparent rendering, displacing the pleural envelopes to either side. The intercostal bundles and perichondrium are now cut away from the sternum with heavy scissors. With care and good fortune the internal mammary vessels can be avoided, lying as they do lateral to the line of division of the intercostal bundles. The oblique incision, made from in front and medially to behind and laterally in the first normal cartilage encountered, is actually made after the intercostal bundles have been divided. It is not uncommon to injure an intercostal artery in this manoeuvre.

7

Sternal osteotomy and repair

A wire is passed around the sternum to serve as a guide for the osteotomy which is made by drawing the sharp corner of a slender osteotome across the sternum until the sternum fractures anteriorly, remaining supported at this point only by a greenstick fracture in the anterior table and by the posterior periosteum. It is important that the line of the osteotomy be exactly transverse. A small segment of bone is cut from one of the exposed rib ends. If the cartilage has been divided medial to the costochondral junction, the bony rib fragment is obtained through a separate incision in the costal periosteum. The rib fragment is placed as a chock block in the osteotomy, wedging it open, and is maintained there either by a mattress suture placed across the osteotomy, around the chip of bone, by a suture passing through the chip of bone and through the anterior periosteum and tied anteriorly, or more commonly by both. In small patients, the heavy silk sutures which we use can be passed through the bone with heavy cutting needles. In larger patients, we tend to employ a saddler's awl. If the bone block is not employed, as in infants, the mattress sutures through the bone must be so placed as to increase the angulation when they are tied. The medial ends of the divided cartilages just below the level of the sternal osteotomy now overlap the lateral ends and are maintained in this way with a single through-and-through silk suture on each side.

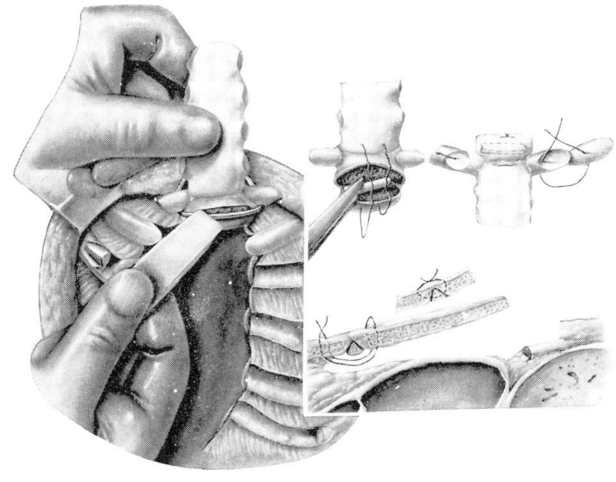

7

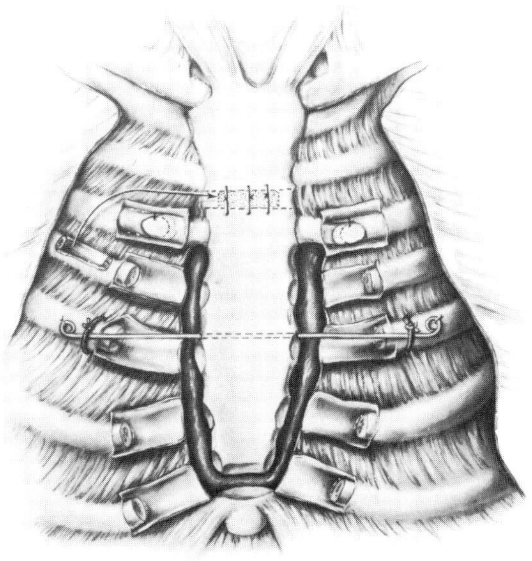

8

8

Wire internal fixation

In very tall adolescents whose long gladiolus would exert too much leverage on the osteotomy, in adults, in patients operated upon for recurrent deformity after a previous operation, and in patients with associated problems (as in one adult simultaneously operated upon for bullous emphysema, or a child with congenital absence of one lung), we often resort to internal fixation. The simplest technique in our hands involves the use of a heavy Kirschner wire placed through the sternum parallel to the chest wall. The ends are closed in a circle to eliminate the risk of perforation if the wire migrates and to facilitate the fixation of the wire to the rib on which it rests. The suture placed through the ring is substantially heavier than is shown. The sutures in the overlapping third cartilage ends are similarly usually of 0/0 silk. Occasionally, if the gladiolus is very long, it will seem appropriate to employ two wires. The pectoral muscles are pulled over the wires and sutured to each other and to the sternal mid-line. Ordinarily, the wire is left in place permanently. If it migrates enough to cause a subcutaneous bulge or discomfort, it may be removed any time after 6 months and this has occasionally been necessary.

9

Closure

The pectoral muscles are tacked back to each other and to the sternal mid-line with silk sutures, completely covering the sternum except for the distal portion of the gladiolus. The intercostal bundles are not tacked back to the sternum since this tends to pull on the sternum and to re-create the defect. Care is taken to place at least two layers of subcutaneous sutures to effect a good closure before the skin is closed either with subcuticular sutures or with skin sutures of nylon.

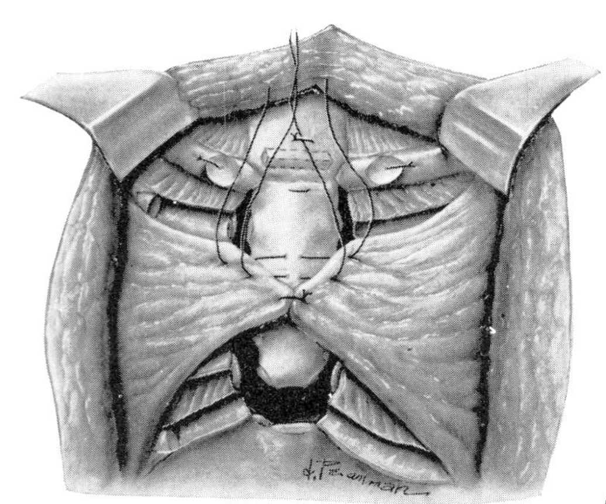

9

SPECIAL POSTOPERATIVE CARE AND COMPLICATIONS

A little more frequently than in former years, we employ a portable plastic suction drain (Hemovac) for the mediastinum or deliberately incise the right pleura to allow mediastinal blood to be absorbed from the pleural cavity. As frequently perhaps, we aspirate the mediastinum as necessary with syringe and needle. No protective dressing is required and there is no restriction on normal activities after 3 weeks, although older boys are asked to avoid contact sports for 3 months. It has become a rarity to transfuse a child at all, but most adults and large adolescents may require a unit or two of blood. Paradoxical motion of the sternum may be conspicuous for 4 or 5 days after operation, but need cause no concern, and interference with respiratory efficiency in the postoperative period has not been a problem. In 400 patients operated upon over the last 30 years, only two patients have received respiratory assistance, for the night after operation.

References

Bevegard, Sture (1962). 'Postural circulatory changes at rest and during exercise in patients with funnel chest, with special reference to factors affecting the stroke volume.' *Acta Med. Scand.* **171**, 695

Beiser, G. D., Epstein, S. E., Stampfer, M., Goldstein, R. E., Noland, S. P. and Levitsky, S. (1972). 'Impairment of cardiac function in patients with pectus excavatum, with improvement after operative correction.' *New Engl. J. Med.* **287**, 267

Ravitch, M. M. (1976). 'Disorders of the sternum and the thoracic wall.' In *Gibbon's Surgery of the Chest*, Third Edition, Edited by D. C. Sabiston and F. C. Spencer.' Philadelphia: W. B. Saunders

Ravitch, M. M. (1977). *Congenital Deformities of the Chest Wall and their Operative Correction*. Philadelphia: W. B. Saunders

[*The illustrations for this Chapter on Pectus Excavatum were drawn by Mr. I. Pearlman.*]

Pectus Carinatum

Mark M. Ravitch, M.D.
Professor of Surgery, University of Pittsburgh and
Surgeon-in-Chief, Montefiore Hospital of Pittsburgh

PRE-OPERATIVE

Indications

This is a deformity which tends to show many more variants than one sees in pectus excavatum. The name of the deformity would suggest that the sternum is principally at fault. However, it has been our observation that in most cases the deformity is actually one of the costal cartilages on either side of the sternum, the incurvation of which produces a deep gutter or runnel. At times the sternum may also be involved either (and most commonly) by a posterior angulation of the tip of the sternum which requires additional correction, or by an increased prominence of its upper portion. We have chosen in the first instance to correct the posterior angulation by an anterior cuneiform osteotomy, and in the second instance to saw away the anterior table of the sternum, removing the prominence and leaving only the posterior table of the sternum, since this prominence is usually associated with an anterior bowing of the sternum and a very great thickening of the anterior cortical lamella. There seems to be no justification for freeing up the sternum and dropping it back into the chest. The decision for operation is made on the basis of the severity of the deformity. In instances in which this deformity is combined with a sharp tilting of the sternum to one side or the other, necessitating a mobilization of the sternum as well, the operation has been done in stages so that the chondral beds can be tautly attached to a stable sternum. In several instances patients who had not previously admitted to limitation of exercise tolerance stated that after operation their exercise tolerance had been greatly increased, presumably because of the increased intrathoracic capacity and the better motion of the chest with respiration.

THE OPERATION

1

The incision

A long transverse incision is required with some upward bowing in the centre, partially for cosmetic reasons, partially to decrease the length of the mid-portion of the upper flap and partially to provide maximal exposure. The skin and fat are dissected superiorly, inferiorly and laterally to expose the deformed costal cartilages for the full extent of their deformity. This is highly variable.

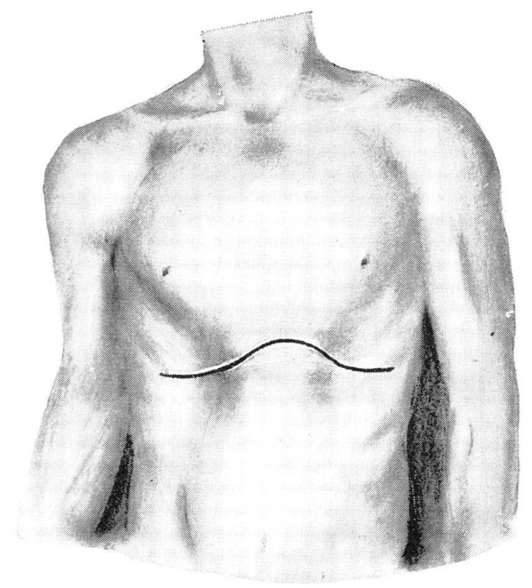

1

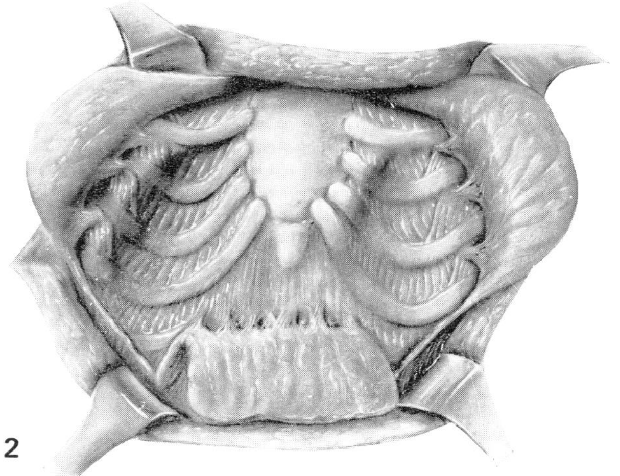

2

2

Reflection of muscles

The pectoral muscles are detached, as in the operation for pectus excavatum (*see* page 356), to expose the deformed cartilages completely. The recti are dissected free and reflected inferiorly. This yields a remarkable exposure of the deeper structures of the chest wall.

3

Smoothing off chondrosternal prominence

If, as illustrated, there is a prominent chondrosternal knob this may be shaved away. In two cases we have found the articulations within the cartilage indicated here. The cartilages are then restored subperichondrially for the full extent of their deformity, almost invariably into bony rib, just as in the operation for pectus excavatum.

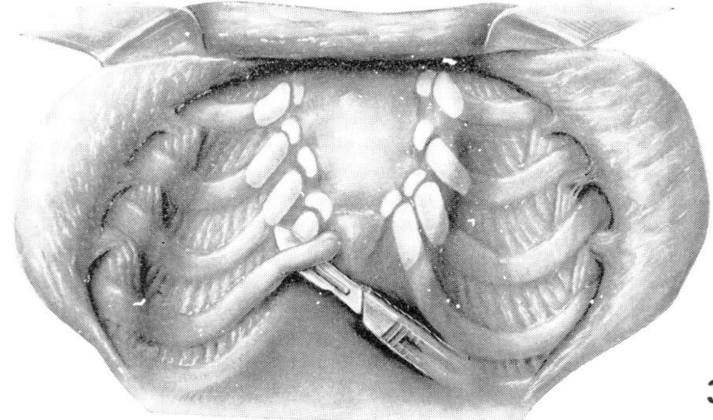

3

4

Reefing the perichondrium

The perichondrium is now redundant, since as soon as the cartilages have been removed the pleura and intercostal muscles move forward and the perichondrium which has dipped downward and posteriorly now can take a much more direct course from the lateral end of the cartilage to the sternal end. The perichondrium is reefed up in this way with interrupted silk sutures. At times, as in this instance, so small a segment of the superior-most rib resected has been removed as to permit re-approximation of the ends.

At times the distal end of the sternum will be found to be angulated sharply posteriorly and a transverse wedge osteotomy is then made in the anterior cortical lamella and this backward displacement of the tip and lower portion of the sternum corrected by mattress sutures closing the cuneiform osteotomy. This is not shown here.

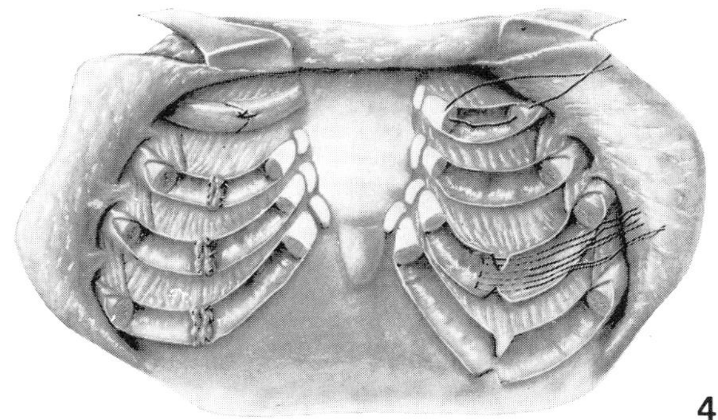

4

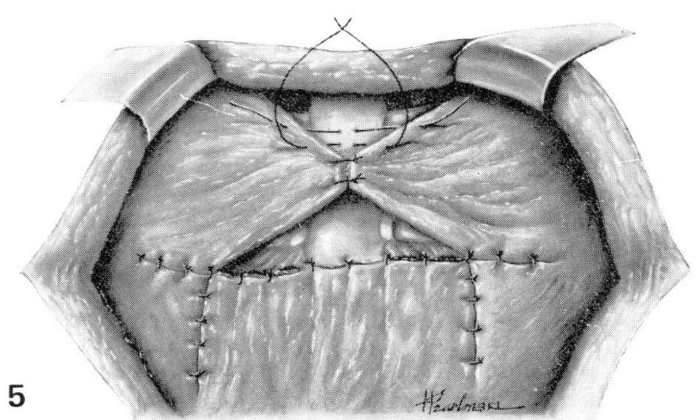

5

Re-attachment of muscles

The pectoral muscles are re-attached to the sternum and the pectoral muscles drawn together in the mid-line, to each other and to the sternum, and laterally re-attached to the recti. The usual shape of the rectus muscle when resutured is actually remarkably transverse at its upper end, as shown. No drains or tubes are necessary and fluid re-accumulation has not been a problem.

Reference

Ravitch, M. M. (1977). *Congenital Deformities of the Chest Wall and their Operative Correction*. Philadelphia: W. B. Saunders

[*The illustrations for this Chapter on Pectus Carinatum were drawn by Mr. I. Pearlman.*]

Tracheostomy

Mary P. Shepherd, M.S., F.R.C.S.
Consultant Thoracic Surgeon, Harefield Hospital, Middlesex

INTRODUCTION

Tracheostomy should always be carried out as a planned procedure under general anaesthesia in an operating theatre using aseptic technique with good lighting and assistance.

Provision of an airway in an emergency can be achieved by endotracheal intubation. In the very rare instance when this, or passage of a rigid bronchoscope, is not possible, immediate laryngotomy or tracheotomy may be required.

An airway provided by a plastic endotracheal tube may be safely maintained for several days. A blue line Portex or Jackson-Reece nasotracheal tube is useful in *infants*. In many cases tracheostomy will not be required. If, however, an artificial airway is needed for a longer period, tracheostomy is necessary.

The technique of fashioning a permanent tracheostomy will not be described here.

Indications

Where chest trauma has resulted in an unstable, paradoxically moving segment of chest wall and respiratory embarrassment is evident. There may or may not be underlying lung damage. Intermittent positive pressure respiration (IPPR), with frequent aspiration of secretions, may be required for several weeks.

Where pulmonary infection requires assisted ventilation and/or frequent aspiration of secretions.

Where, following lung resection, patients continue to be unable to clear retained secretions despite bronchoscopic aspiration.

When *infants* or *children* with severe congestive cardiac failure, or postoperative cardiac surgical patients require prolonged respiratory support.

Where separation of the pharynx and larynx is necessary, such as patients with Guillain-Barré syndrome, severe head injury or bulbar poliomyelitis.

Equipment

1&2

Tracheostomy tubes

Tubes, varying in shape, are available in graded lengths and diameters.

Silver tracheostomy sets include inner and outer silver tubes with obturator and special forceps for insertion.

Red rubber tubes can still be obtained. These are irritant to the trachea and are not recommended.

Plastic tracheostomy tubes are the type of choice.

Tracheostomy tubes, except the silver variety, are made with or without cuffs, and may possess one or two cuffs.

A selection of sterile, cuffed and uncuffed plastic tracheostomy tubes must be available.It is wise to use a cuffed tube for *adults* and uncuffed for *infants* and *children* in the first instance. The largest tube which will pass easily through the surgical stoma in the trachea should be the one chosen.

The appropriate sterile connections for maintenance of anaesthesia and oxygenation after insertion of the tracheostomy tube must be ready for use.

Diathermy should be available if possible, to ensure meticulous haemostasis throughout the procedure.

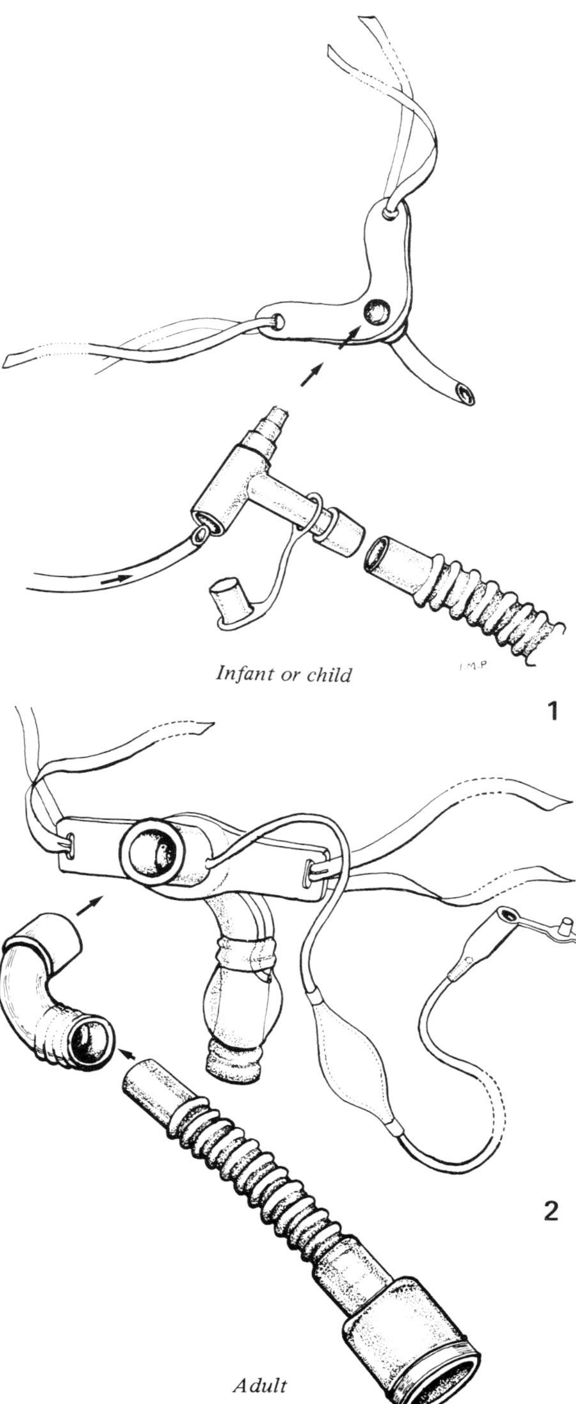

Infant or child

1

Adult

2

Anaesthesia and position of patient

After suitable premedication a general anaesthetic is given.

3

The intubated patient is placed supine on the operating table.

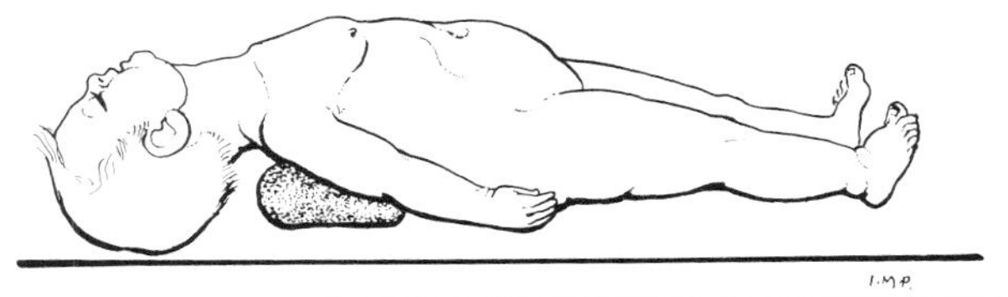

3

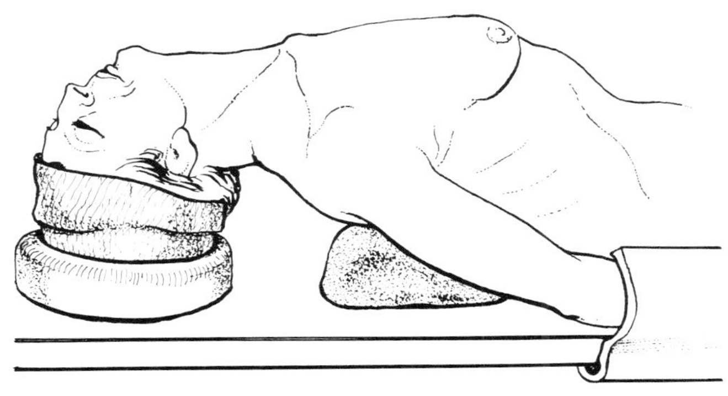

4

4

Full extension of the neck is facilitated by placing a sandbag under the shoulders. The head may be stabilized by a padded ring under the occiput.

THE OPERATION

The incision

5

A transverse, skin-crease incision is made half-way between the sternal notch and the cricoid cartilage. It is made 2 – 3 cm long in the *adult*, and 1·5 cm long in the *infant* or *child*.

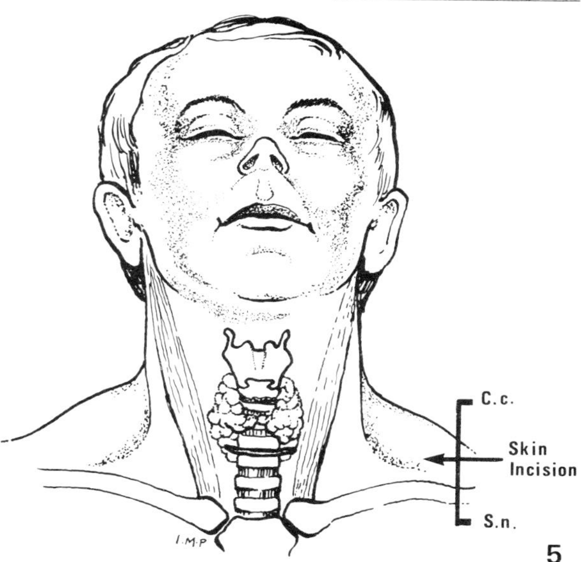

5

6a&b

The deep fascia and strap muscles are separated in the mid-line. The thyroid isthmus is identified and either retracted, or if necessary divided between ligatures or clamped and sutured. Exposure is facilitated by the use of a self-retaining retractor.

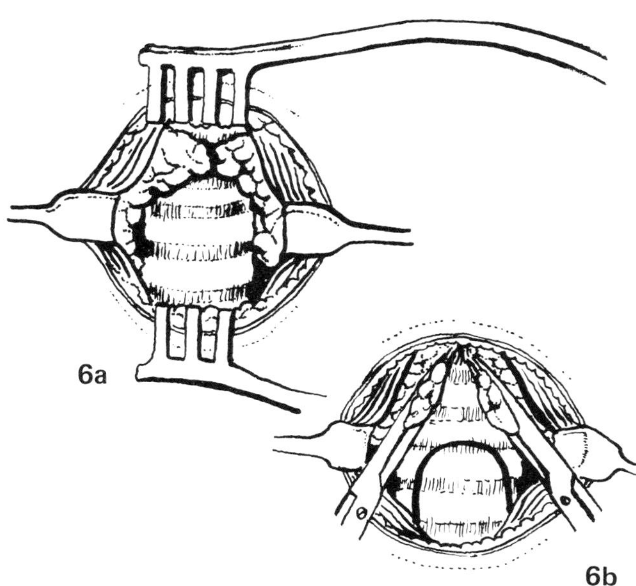

6a

6b

7a&b

In the adult

(*a*) A transverse stitch is inserted into the anterior wall of the trachea immediately above the second tracheal ring.

(*b*) The trachea is incised horizontally above the stitch, but below the first tracheal ring, dividing the central two-thirds of the trachea.

(*c*) Both ends of this incision are extended vertically downwards through the second and third tracheal rings. Great care must be taken not to puncture the cuff of the endotracheal tube.

(*d*) The free edge of the ∩ shaped flap (after Bjork) of the anterior wall of the trachea is sutured securely to the subcutaneous tissue at the centre of the lower skin edge. This facilitates insertion of the tube into the trachea and prevents faulty re-insertion.

(*e*) A plastic, cuffed tracheostomy tube of appropriate size is selected and the cuff tested.

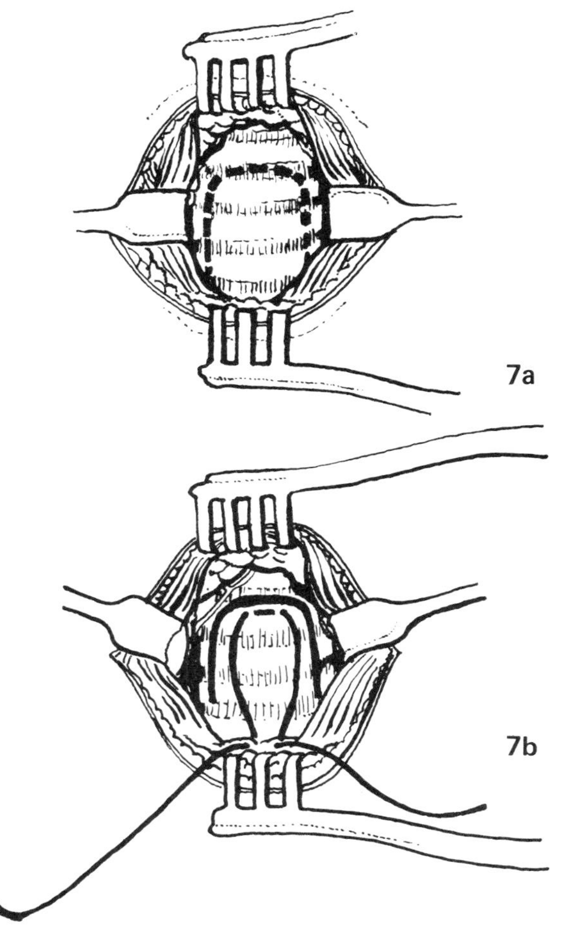

7a

7b

8&9

In the infant or child

(*a*) The trachea is stabilized with a skin hook.

(*b*) It is incised vertically, *exactly* in the mid-line, through the second, third and fourth tracheal rings. No cartilage is removed or displaced.

(*c*) The edges of the tracheal incision are held apart by McIndoe's forceps to allow insertion of the tube.

(*d*) An uncuffed plastic tube with a diameter of about 1·5 mm less than that of the trachea is selected.

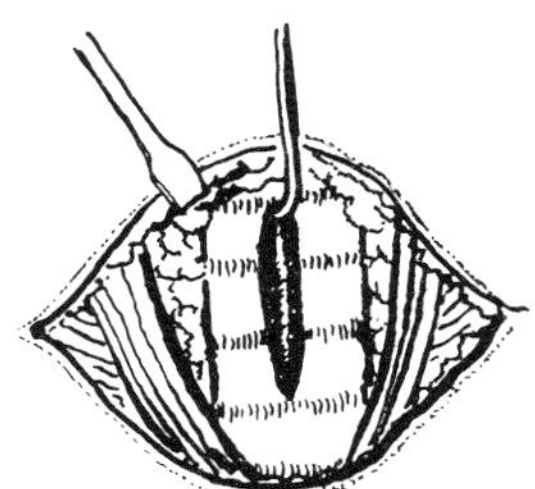

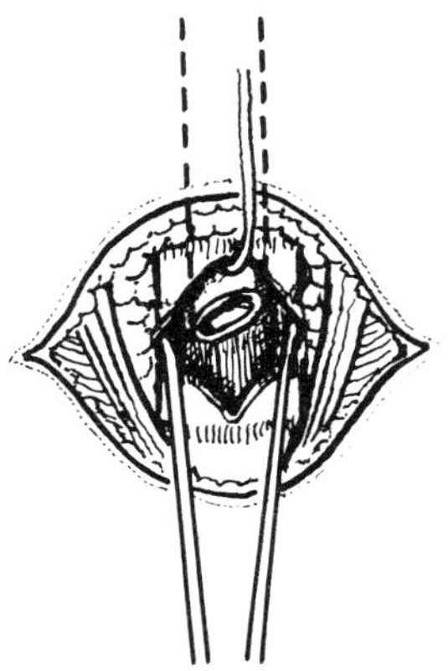

8

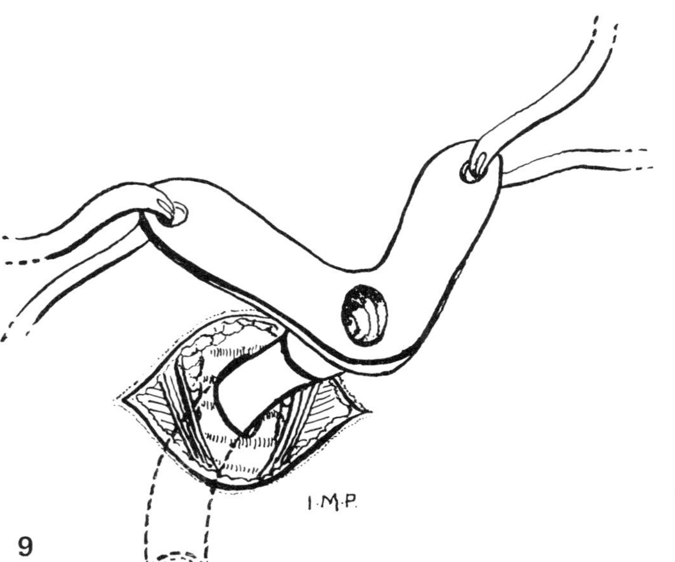

9

10&11

The anaesthetist slowly withdraws the endotracheal tube. When the tip reaches a point immediately above the tracheal stoma, the moistened tracheostomy tube is slipped into the trachea. In the *adult* the cuff is inflated so that the trachea is just occluded around the tube. In the *infant* or *child,* it may be necessary to change to a larger tracheostomy tube.

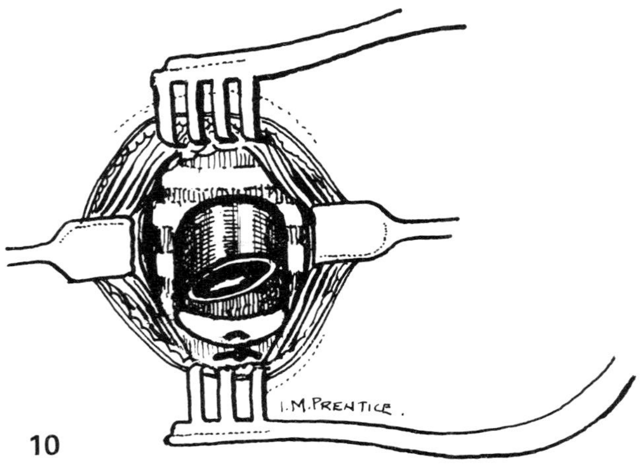

10

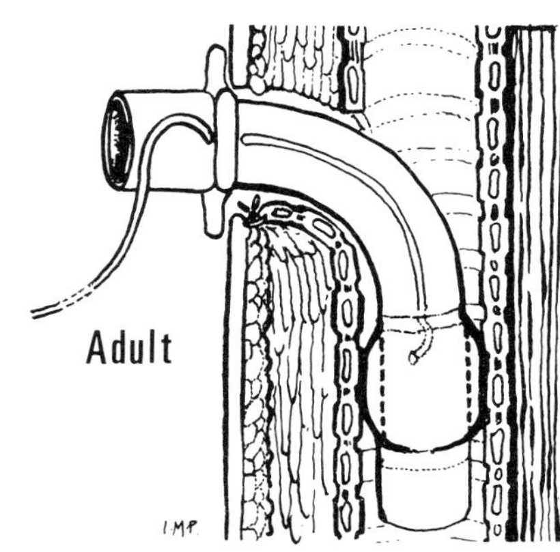

11

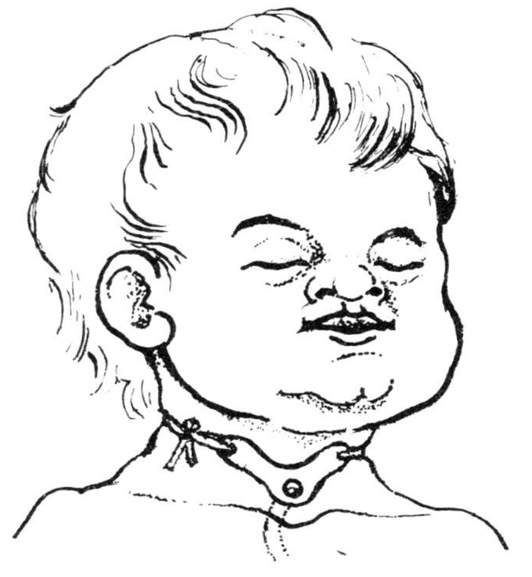

12

12 & 13

While the tracheostomy tube is held in place by an assistant: (*a*) the trachea is aspirated through the tube; (*b*) the sterile anaesthetic connections are attached to restore the ventilating system; (*c*) the sandbag is removed from behind the patient's shoulders; (*d*) skin sutures are inserted.

Frequently no skin sutures are necessary. If they are required, the skin edges should be only loosely approximated around the tracheostomy tube.

The tracheostomy tube is held securely in place by tying the tapes firmly behind the neck, using a knot and not a bow.

Inflation of both lungs must be ascertained. In the *infant* or *child* it is possible for the tracheostomy tube to enter the right main bronchus. The tube can be withdrawn slightly by elevating it from the skin surface with a plastic foam pad.

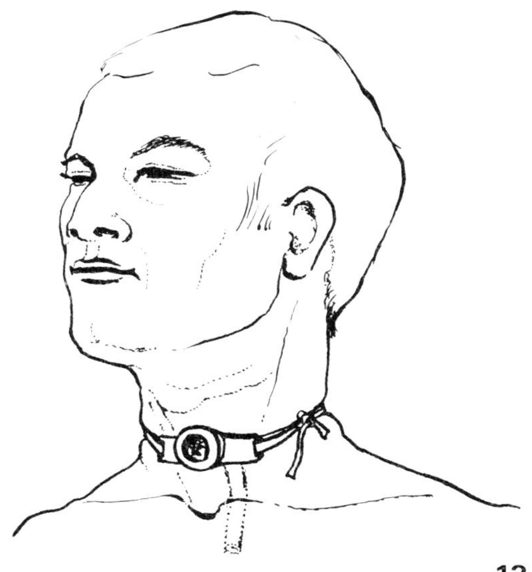

13

POSTOPERATIVE CARE

A patient with a tracheostomy should be nursed in an area allowing close observation. An *infant* or *child* must be attended by a special nurse at all times.

Scissors, to release the tracheostomy tube in an emergency, and a sterile replacement tube of the same size and shape must always be available at the bedside.

While a patient has a tracheostomy, frequent reassurance must be given that the loss of voice is temporary only. Pencil and paper should be provided.

The well-placed tracheostomy tube should be kept as still as possible to minimize the effects of movement and traction on the trachea. This applies particularly when IPPR is used.

Tracheal aspiration is carried out as often as necessary.

(*a*) A mask is worn and a sterile, soft catheter used for each aspiration.

(*b*) Using sterile disposable gloves, a catheter is inserted gently as far as it will readily go. This may be 12 – 18 cm. Following lung resection, however, the catheter should be introduced only to a point in the trachea just beyond the end of the tracheostomy tube, approximately 8 – 10 cm.

(*c*) Suction is applied only when the catheter is in position and being withdrawn. A Y connection is useful in this respect.

(*d*) The left main bronchus may be entered if the head is turned gently well to the right.

(*e*) The aspiration procedure should only take 10 – 15 sec, i.e. as long as a person can comfortably hold their breath.

Prophylactic antibiotics are not given. It is possible for sterile secretions to be kept so if the aseptic techniques of management are strictly adhered to. Tracheal aspirate is cultured regularly and the appropriate antibiotic given systemically and/or by direct instillation into the trachea if necessary.

Cuff management

(*a*) The cuff of a tracheostomy tube should only be inflated if IPPR is required or if there is a risk of aspiration of secretions or food.

(*b*) The volume of air used to inflate the cuff should be the *smallest* which occludes the trachea around the tube. A small air leak is often acceptable; over-inflation must be avoided.

(*c*) The practice of intermittent cuff deflation is hazardous as it can lead to over-inflation which in turn can cause pressure necrosis of the trachea, tube collapse or cuff prolapse.

Changing the tracheostomy tube

(*a*) It may not be necessary to change the tube for a week or more.

(*b*) Changing the tube is always preceded by pharyngeal aspiration and tracheal aspiration after deflation of the cuff.

(*c*) If difficulty is experienced in passing the suction catheter, or a rise in IPPR infation pressure is noted, the tube must be changed and checked immediately. These observations may mean a decrease in the lumen of the tube by crusting, kinking or cuff prolapse.

Extubation in the adult

(*a*) A cuffed tracheostomy tube is replaced with an uncuffed plastic tube of the same size.

(*b*) The practice of using a spiggot to obstruct the tracheostomy tube is not advocated although it allows the return of speech. Airway obstruction of a degree relative to the size of the tube *in situ* is produced.

(*c*) After 1 – 2 days the uncuffed tube is changed for one a size smaller.

(*d*) This is repeated until an uncuffed tube of about 1 cm in diameter is reached (size 33 Ch approximately).

(*e*) Finally this tube is removed and a firm, sterile dressing is applied to the stoma in the neck. Speech is restored. Should tracheal aspiration be required, this is readily carried out through the stoma, employing the same aseptic technique.

(*f*) The stoma will close spontaneously during the course of about a week. Formal closure, even after the Bjork flap type of tracheostomy is seldom required.

Extubation in the infant and child

(*a*) The tracheostomy tube is changed for one a size smaller.

(*b*) After 3 – 4 days the tube is again changed for one a size smaller. This is repeated until a tube size 3·5 mm approximately is reached.

(*c*) This tube is removed and a firm sterile dressing applied to the stoma in the neck.

(*d*) Immediately following extubation, bronchoscopy is advisable to confirm that the airway is clear.

COMPLICATIONS

14, 15 & 16

Infection of the tracheostomy and/or tracheo-bronchial tree.

Haemorrhage resulting from pressure effects or infection.

Pneumothorax.

Obstruction of the tracheostomy tube due to: (*a*) crusting with dried secretions; (*b*) collapse of the tracheostomy tube due to an over-inflated cuff; (*c*) herniation of an over-inflated cuff over the end of the tube (*see Illustration 14*); (*d*) detachment of the cuff from the tube (*see Illustration 15*); (*e*) displacement of the tube from the trachea into the tissues, also producing surgical emphysema (*see Illustration 16*).

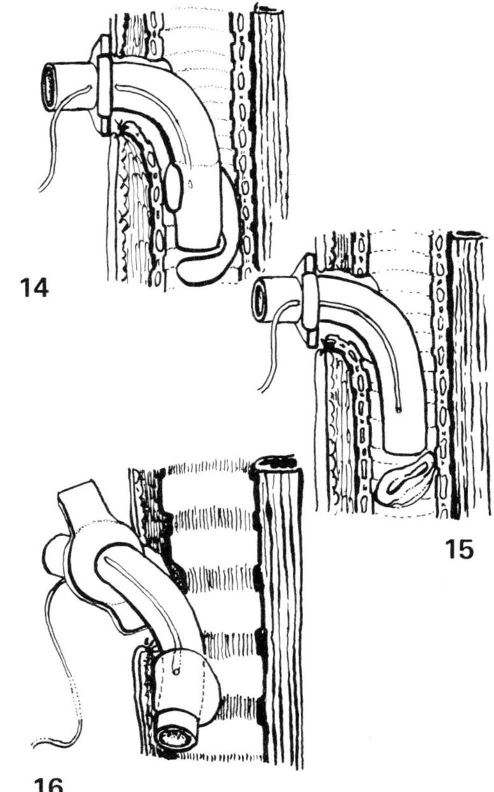

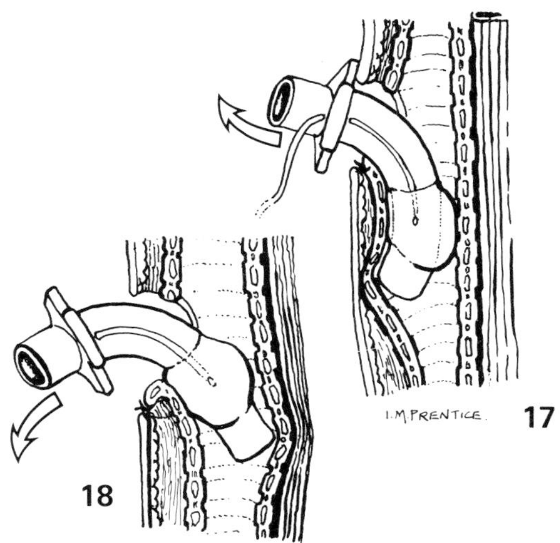

17 & 18

Trauma to the trachea due to: (*a*) inappropriate type of suction catheter; (*b*) inappropriate technique of tracheal suction; (*c*) over-inflation of the tracheostomy cuff; (*d*) inadequate fixation or inappropriate shape of the tracheostomy tube allowing: (*i*) pressure necrosis of tracheal cartilage around the stoma or in the region of the cuff; (*ii*) the tip of the tube to impinge on the anterior tracheal wall which can result in innominate artery erosion (*see Illustration 17*); (*iii*) the tip of the tube to impinge on the posterior tracheal wall which can result in tracheo-oesophageal fistula (*see Illustration 18*).

19 & 20

Tracheal stenosis

(*a*) Subglottic stenosis can occur, especially in infants or children, if the tracheostomy is too high.

(*b*) Stomal stenosis occurs, especially in infants or children, and is due to: (*i*) removal of tracheal cartilage; (*ii*) pressure necrosis and/or infection of tracheal cartilage; (*iii*) granulomatous polyps (*see Illustration 19*); (*iv*) forward angulation of the trachea (*see Illustration 20*).

(*c*) Infrastomal stenosis due to: (*i*) mucosal ulceration and/or infection at the level of the cuff on the tube; (*ii*) mucosal ulceration and/or infection at the level of the tip of the tube.

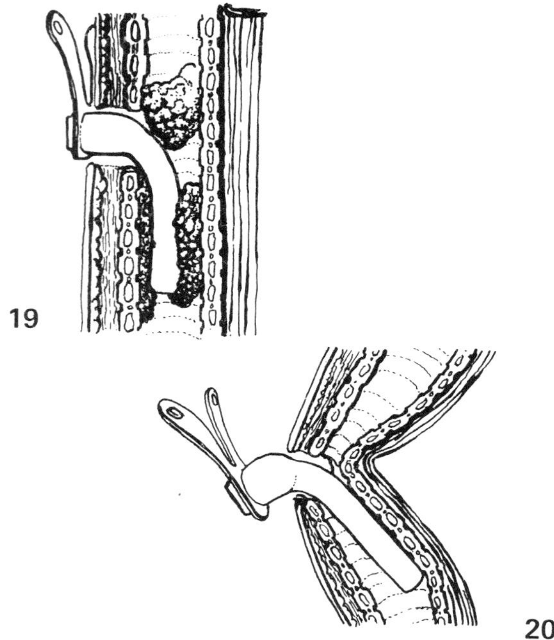
19

20

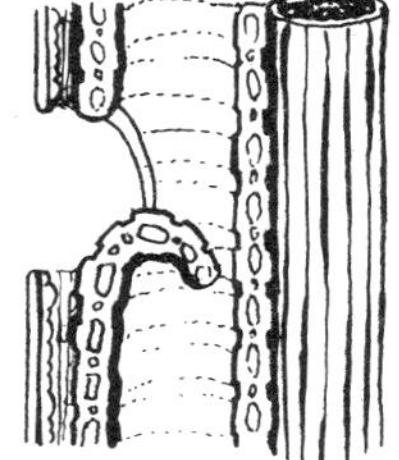
21

21

In adults the Bjork type flap of anterior tracheal wall may fall back into the tracheal lumen when the tube is changed or removed unless securely sutured to the subcutaneous tissue.

References

Collis, J. L., Clarke, D. B. and Abbey Smith, R. (1975). *d'Abreu's Practice of Cardiothoracic Surgery*, 4th Edition, pages 41 – 43

d'Abreu, A. L., Brian Taylor, A. and Clarke, D. B. (1968). *Intrathoracic Crises*. 1st Edition, pages 224 – 229. London: Butterworths

Feldman, S. A. and Crawley, B. E. (1971). *Tracheostomy and Artificial Ventilation*, 2nd Edition.

Harley, H. R. S. (1971). 'Laryngotracheal obstruction complicating tracheostomy or endotracheal intubation with assisted respiration: A critical review.' *Thorax* **26**, 493

[*The illustrations for this Chapter on Tracheostomy were drawn by Mrs. I. M. Prentice.*]

Resection of the Trachea for Stricture

F. G. Pearson, M.D., F.R.C.S.(C.), F.A.C.S.
Professor of Surgery, University of Toronto and
Head, Division of Thoracic Surgery, Toronto General Hospital

Indications

Diseases of the trachea requiring segmental resection and reconstruction by primary anastomosis are relatively uncommon. The lesions most frequently encountered are postintubation strictures, primary tumours of the trachea and the sequelae of blunt or penetrating trauma.

POSTINTUBATION STRICTURES

The commonest indication for tracheal resection today is stricture due to injury from a cuffed tracheostomy tube or endotracheal tube. Strictures may develop at the level of the tracheostomy stoma in the cervical trachea, or at the level of the inflatable cuff in the mediastinum (Pearson, Goldberg and DaSilva, 1968; Grillo, 1970). The pathogenesis of these lesions is well summarized in a monograph by Grillo (1970).

Postintubation strictures are usually short–no more than 2–4 cm in length, and extensive mobilization techniques to achieve a tension-free primary anastomosis are infrequently required.

Certain features of the pre-operative assessment are critical to obtaining optimal results. The precise length and level of the stricture should be determined by rigid bronchoscopy, and tomography or contrast tracheograms. Such definition will avoid resection of unnecessary segments of healthy, adjacent trachea. Whenever possible, the tracheal mucosa should be free of inflammation and ulceration at the levels of transection and subsequent anastomosis. During the early acute stages in the evolution of postintubation strictures, inflammatory changes may extend for some distance on either side of the actual site of ulceration and wall destruction. In this situation, it is desirable if possible, to delay resection and reconstruction until the adjacent inflammatory changes have resolved. On occasion, this may be achieved by extubating the patient and allowing the tracheostomy stoma to close, and maintaining the airway by intermittent endoscopic dilatation.

THE OPERATION

1

The airway between the hyoid bone superiorly and the junction between middle and lower thirds of the mediastinal trachea below, is easily accessible through a generous collar incision in most patients. Resection of strictures at these levels (unshaded area) rarely requires a median sternotomy, except in patients with a very short neck, or in older patients with a dorsal kyphus and a rigid inelastic trachea. With the neck extended, a bolster between the shoulders, and a traction suture placed in the anterior tracheal wall below the stricture, it is almost always possible to elevate a long segment of mediastinal trachea into the operative field afforded by a collar incision.

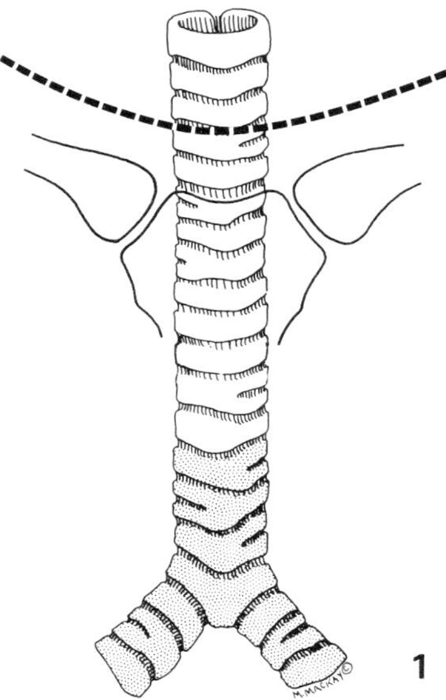

1

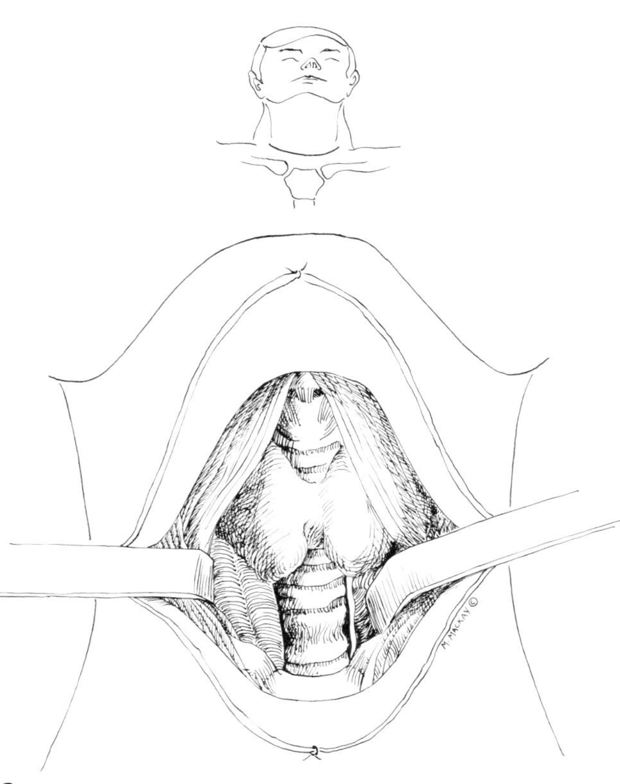

2

2

Skin flaps are elevated in the plane deep to the platysma, and retracted to expose the airway from the level of thyroid cartilage to the suprasternal notch. The strap muscles have been separated in the mid-line and retracted to expose the anterior tracheal wall. With the neck in full extension, the upper mediastinal trachea is elevated into the operative field and the stricture is identified at the level of the seventh tracheal cartilage. At the level of the stricture, the tracheal wall if often deformed, and enveloped by fibrous tissue which may be densely adherent to adjacent structures. The strictured segment is mobilized circumferentially by sharp dissection which is maintained as close to the tracheal wall as possible, particularly at the tracheo-oesophageal angles in which the recurrent laryngeal nerves run. No effort is made to identify the recurrent nerves in most cases.

3

The stenotic segment is freed circumferentially, but circumferential mobilization should not extend for more than 1 cm above and below the segment to be resected (*see* dotted lines) in order to preserve maximum blood supply. The anterior and lateral walls of the trachea may be freed from the cricoid cartilage above to the bifurcation below without jeopardizing the circulation.

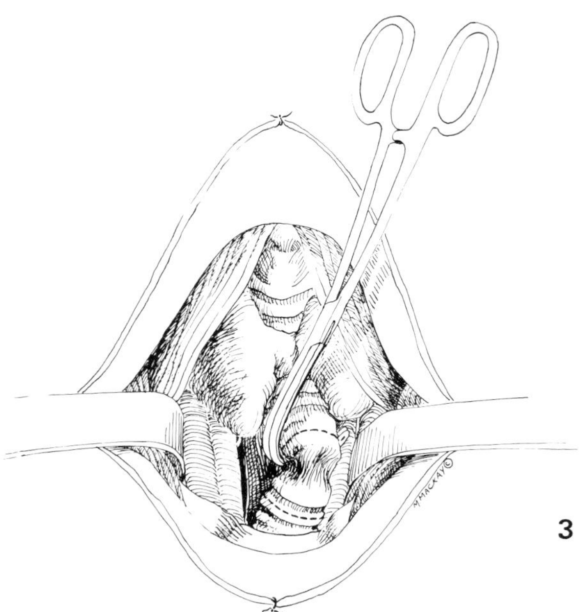

3

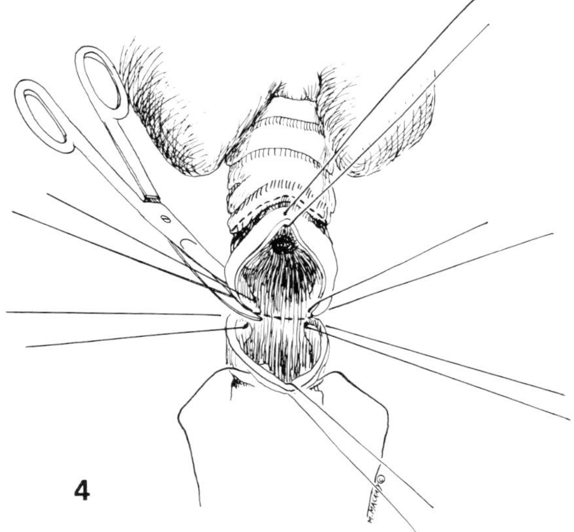

4

4

The airway is divided transversely through healthy trachea immediately below the damaged segment. Following incision of the cartilaginous wall anteriorly and laterally, stay sutures are placed in the mid-line anteriorly, and on each side at the junction between cartilaginous and membranous trachea. Traction on these sutures will accurately display the tracheal lumen and membranous tracheal wall, which may otherwise be deformed and contracted. These stay sutures also prevent retraction of the distal tracheal stump into the mediastinum once the membranous trachea is divided.

5a,b&c

Following division of the airway distal to the stricture, anaesthesia is maintained with sterile connections carried across the operative field. The distal stump is intubated with a cuffed, armoured endotracheal tube.

The anastomosis is begun by placing a row of interrupted sutures in the posterior membranous trachea. These sutures are spaced at 2–3 mm intervals, taking a generous bite of trachea on each side of the anastomosis, and the entire posterior row is placed before any suture is tied. In this case, the membranous trachea was sutured with fine gauge (No. 35) stainless steel wire suture with the knots on the inside. This technique permits precise approximation of the posterior tracheal wall under direct vision. Using appropriate traction on the stay sutures, all tension is removed from the tracheal ends while the posterior sutures are being tied.

The anastomosis is completed using similarly spaced, interrupted sutures of 2/0 or 3/0 chromic catgut in the anterolateral cartilaginous wall. Once the sutures in the membranous trachea have been tied, anaesthesia may be maintained by advancing the original orotracheal tube across the anastomosis from above. Tension on the completed anastomosis should be minimal, and approximation should be easily maintained by relatively fine suture material. Unfortunately, there is not yet a practical method to quantitate tension at the anastomosis, and this evaluation must be learned through experience.

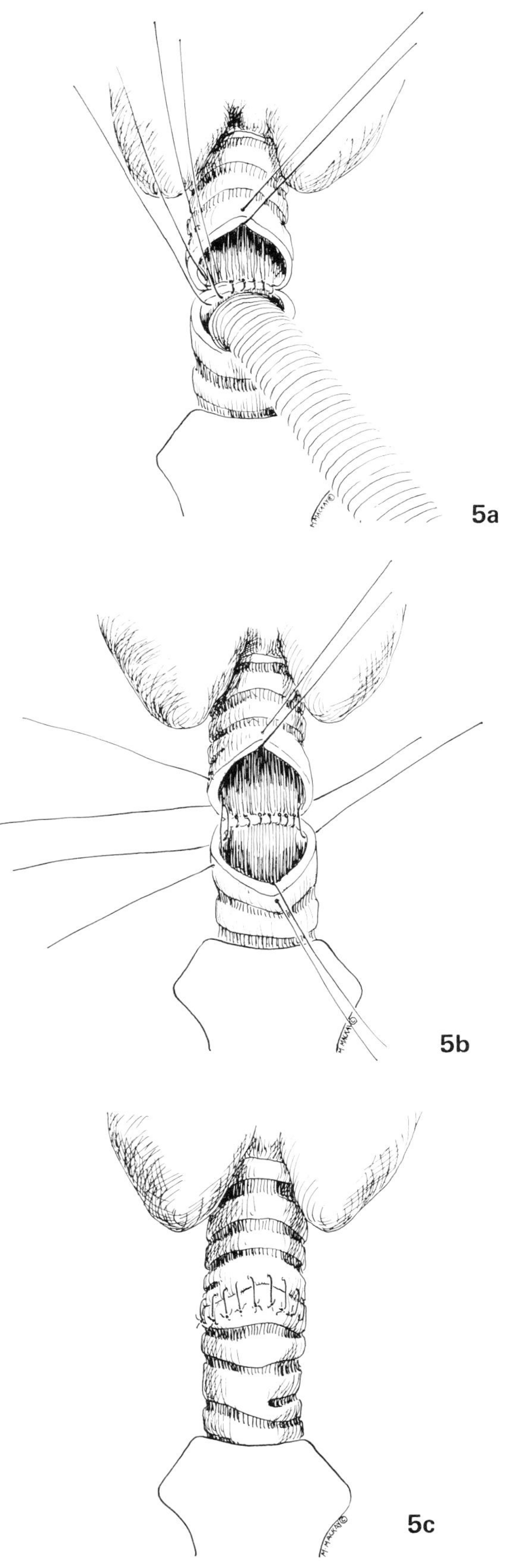

5a

5b

5c

6

The wound is closed and the operative area drained with a closed system. Cervical flexion undoubtedly reduces tension at the anastomosis, and is maintained for 7–10 days after operation. Neck flexion can be very effectively maintained with a stout silk suture tethering the skin of the chin to the skin of the chest. This apparently barbaric technique is remarkably well tolerated by the patient and is completely dependable in maintaining flexion at all times.

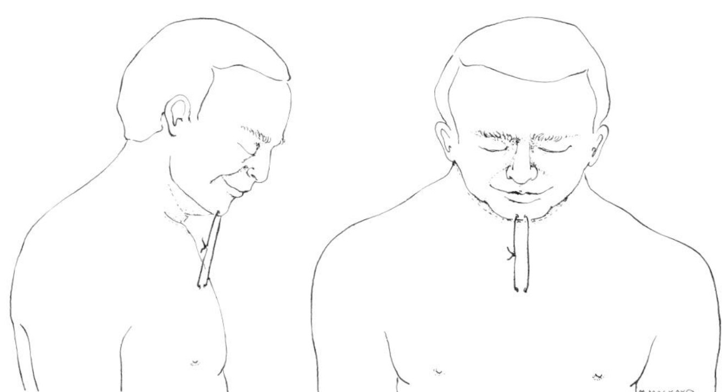

6

RESECTION OF TRACHEA FOR TUMOUR

Most primary tumours of the trachea are malignant. Squamous cell carcinoma and adenoid cystic carcinoma are the cell types most frequently encountered (Grillo, 1970; Houston *et al.*, 1969). In most instances squamous cell carcinoma of the trachea is inoperable at the time of presentation due to invasion of local structures and mediastinal lymph node metastases. Adenoid cystic carcinoma of the trachea infrequently invades vital structures adjacent to the airway, mediastinal lymph node metastases are less common than with squamous cell carcinoma, and this tumour is more often amenable to resection and reconstruction (Pearson *et al.*, 1974).

Tracheal tumours are rarely recognized before the patient develops significant symptoms of upper airway obstruction. At this stage most such tumours have grown to a dimension which requires resection of extensive segments of trachea, and mobilization procedures are almost always required to reduce tension on the subsequent anastomosis. In most individuals it is possible to resect up to 3 cm of trachea and obtain a primary anastomosis with minimal tension without the addition of special mobilization techniques. The laryngeal release operation described by Dedo and Fishman (1969) permits resection of an additional 2–3 cm of trachea by dropping the larynx and reducing tension at the anastomosis. Mobilization of the right pulmonary hilum permits resection of a further 2 cm. With the addition of these techniques it is therefore possible to resect circumferential segments up to 7 cm in length and approximate the divided tracheal ends without undue tension or critical interruption of the tracheal blood supply.

THE OPERATION

Primary adenoid cystic carcinoma of the lower cervical and upper mediastinal trachea

7

Exposure is obtained through a collar incision with the addition of median sternotomy. The strap muscles are separated and retracted exposing the trachea from the level of the thyroid cartilage to the aortic arch. The innominate artery is retracted inferolaterally. The gross boundaries of the tumour on the external aspect of the trachea are defined above and below. The dotted lines represent the initial levels for the proposed segmental resection, and lie about 1 cm beyond the gross limits of the tumour. Since adenoid cystic carcinoma may extend well beyond the visible and palpable limits of the tumour, the resection lines must be assessed by frozen section.

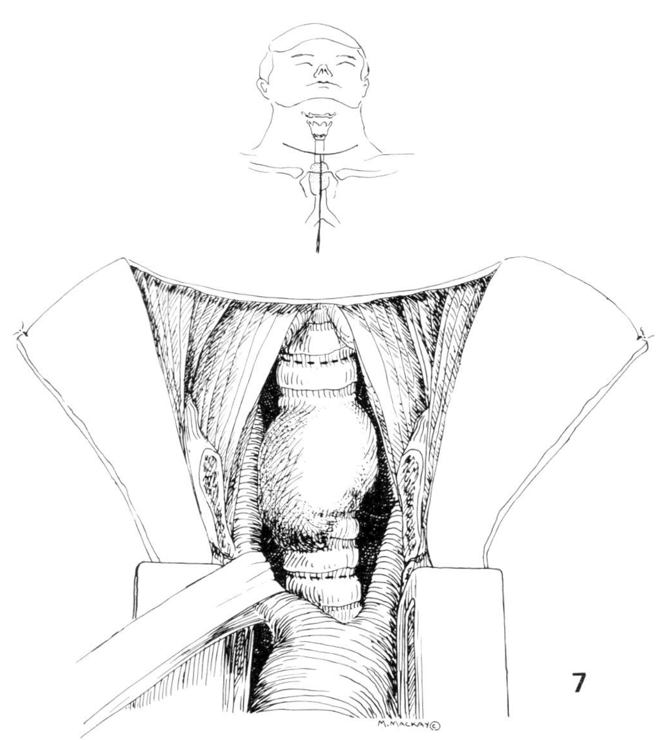

7

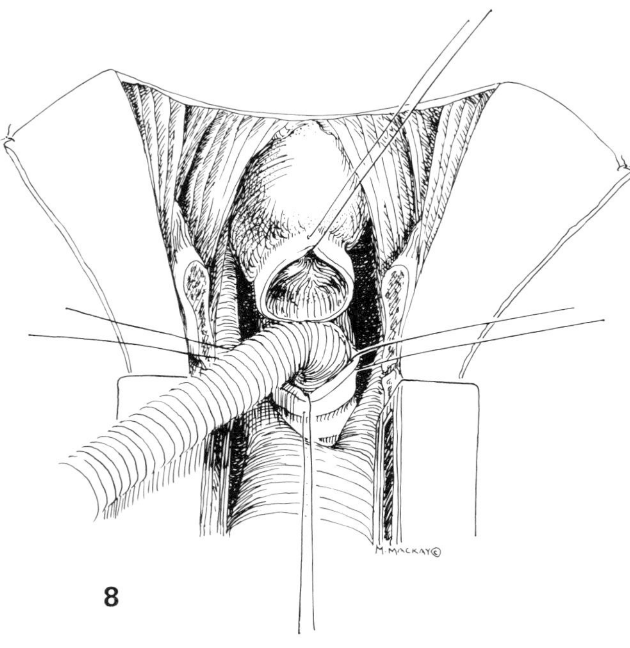

8

8

The mediastinal trachea is divided transversely on the distal side of the tumour, three stay sutures are placed in the distal stump to provide control of the lumen and prevent retraction inferiorly. The distal stump is intubated with a sterile armoured orotracheal tube for maintenance of ventilation and anaesthesia.

9

The trachea has been divided proximally above the tumour, completing segmental resection of a 7 cm length of trachea. This represents approximately half of the length of the average adult trachea. If either resection line is found to be involved by tumour on frozen section assessment, then an additional segment of trachea is resected whenever possible.

At this stage in the procedure the bolster is removed from between the shoulders and the neck flexed in order to shorten the trachea and reduce tension. If after applying appropriate traction on the stay sutures which have been placed in the upper and lower tracheal stumps, it is evident that the ends cannot be approximated without excessive tension, additional mobilization of the trachea is required.

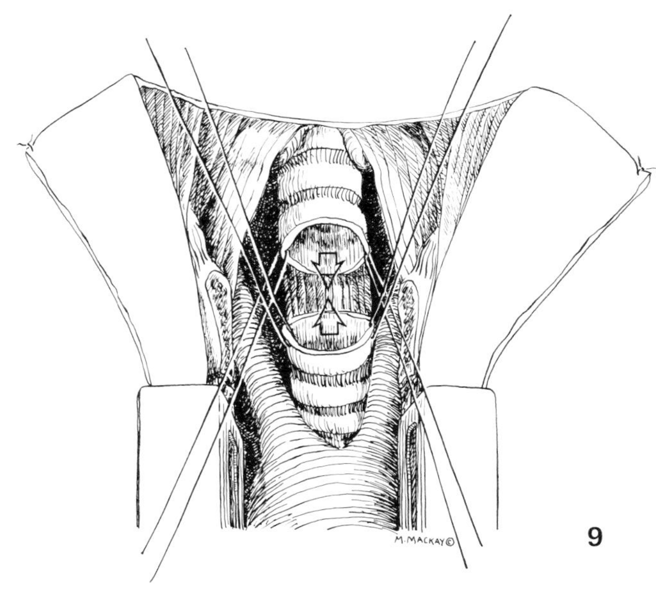

9

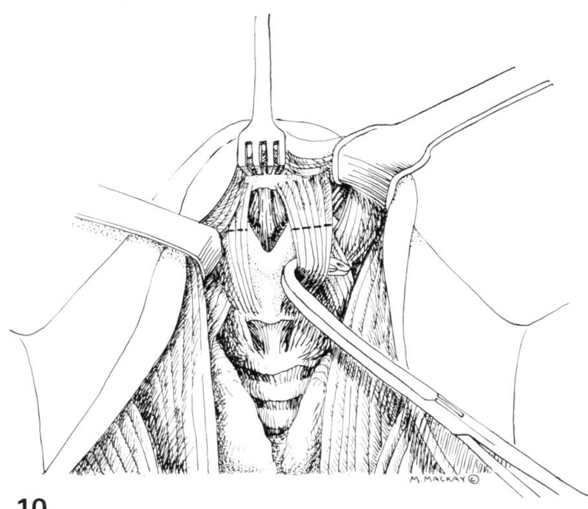

10

10

The upper cervical skin flap has been elevated to the level of the hyoid bone above. In the illustration, the sternohyoid muscles have been retracted laterally exposing the underlying soft tissues behind the hyoid and thyroid cartilages. The thyrohyoid muscles on each side are freed and divided transversely (*see* dotted lines).

11a&b

Following division of the thyrohyoid muscles, the thyrohyoid membrane and central thyrohyoid ligament are exposed. The membrane and ligament are divided anteriorly and laterally between the superior cornua of the thyroid cartilage. The tips of the superior cornua are amputated, taking care to avoid injury to the superior laryngeal nerves and their accompanying vessels which are usually readily identified on each side.

After division of the thyrohyoid membrane and ligament, the submucosa of the anterior pharyngeal wall is exposed. It is easily recognized from the rich submucosal plexus of vessels which it possesses. It is now possible to 'drop' the larynx for at least 2–3 cm inferior to its original position. It is then possible to anastomose the divided tracheal ends without excessive tension. The anastomosis is done in the same fashion illustrated for the benign tracheal stricture.

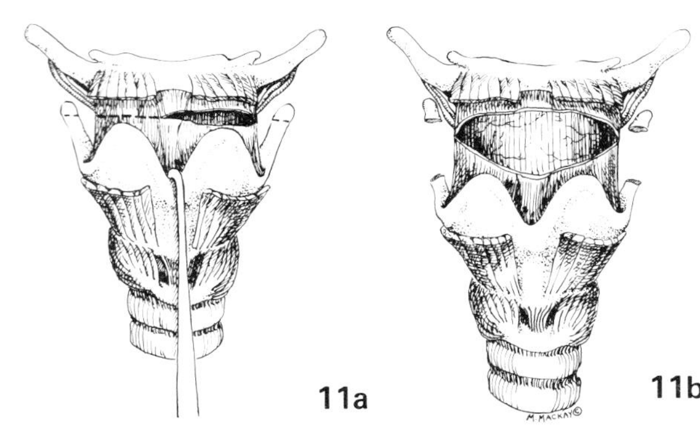

11a 11b

Recent experience (Grillo; Payne) suggests that the *suprahyoid* laryngeal release originally described by Montgomery (1973) results in a laryngeal 'drop' of similar magnitude, and avoids the common complication of transient difficulty in swallowing which is associated with the thyrohyoid release described here.

The wound is closed leaving a large bore catheter in the anterior mediastinum behind the sternotomy for closed drainage. A stout suture between the skin of the chin and the anterior chest wall is used to maintain neck flexion for 7–10 days after operation.

If the upper resection line lies at or above the level of the inferior border of the cricoid cartilage, there is a significant hazard from laryngeal or subglottic obstruction due to haematoma or oedema. In such cases, a small bore tracheostomy tube may be inserted distal to the anastomosis to ensure a safe airway during the early postoperative period. In most cases, however, a tracheostomy is neither necessary nor advisable.

References

Dedo, H. H. and Fishman, N. H. (1969). 'Laryngeal release and sleeve resection for tracheal stenosis.' *Ann. Otol. Rhinol. Laryngol.* **78**, 285

Grillo, H. C. (1970). 'Surgery of the trachea.' *Curr. Probl. Surg.*, July

Grillo, H. D., Personal communication

Houston, H. E., Payne, W. S., Harrison, E. G., Jr. and Olsen, A. M. (1969). 'Primary cancers of the trachea.' *Archs Surg.* **99**, 132

Montgomery, W. W. (1973). *Surgery of the Upper Respiratory System*, Vol. II. Lea and Febiger

Payne, W. S., Personal communication

Pearson, F. G., Thompson, D. W., Weissberg, D., Simpson, W. J. K. and Kergin, F. G. (1974). 'Adenoid cystic carcinoma of the trachea.' *Ann. thorac. Surg.* **18**, 16

Pearson, F. G., Goldberg, M. and DaSilva, A. J. (1968). 'A prospective study of tracheal injury complicating tracheostomy with a cuffed tube.' *Ann. Otol.* **77**, 867

[*The illustrations for this Chapter on Resection of the Trachea for Stricture were drawn by Miss M. Mackay.*]

Thymectomy

M. F. Sturridge, M.S., F.R.C.S.
Consultant Thoracic Surgeon, The Middlesex Hospital, London;
Consultant Surgeon, London Chest Hospital;
Honorary Consultant Thoracic Surgeon, The National Hospital for Nervous Diseases, London

Thymectomy is indicated in the treatment of myasthenia gravis and in the majority of these cases the gland is macroscopically normal. Tumours of the thymus present early and are relatively small if they are associated with myasthenia whereas they otherwise present late with pain in the chest and signs of mediastinal compression when they are large. The first section of this chapter will deal with thymectomy in relation to myasthenia gravis and the second with the treatment of thymic tumours without myasthenia.

MYASTHENIA GRAVIS

This disease which affects both sexes and all age groups is generally most severe and dangerous in young women aged 15–35 years and it is this group that responds best to thymectomy. A short history and generalized manifestations of the disease are good prognostic signs but the operation should be considered in all but the mildest cases and certainly in patients with important bulbar myasthenia affecting swallowing and respiration.

The differential diagnosis of myasthenia can be difficult and is usually made by a neurologist. It is confirmed by intravenous injection of edrophonium 4 mg which produces short-lived relief of symptoms and signs. Muscle antibodies are usually absent when the thymus is not enlarged and are commonly present if there is a thymic tumour. All patients should have chest radiography performed with postero-anterior and lateral views and lateral tomography of the anterior mediastinum. If a mass is visible on these films a tumour can be expected.

Pre-operative preparation

The aims of this preparation are to present the patient for the operative procedure in an optimal state for a smooth uncomplicated recovery. Attention is particularly directed to diaphragmatic breathing exercises to increase ventilation without inducing pain postoperatively and to careful regulation of anticholinesterase agents to avoid overdosage. Most patients are less active in hospital and are still less active after operation so that the dosage of drugs can be substantially reduced to a level that leaves them mildly myasthenic through most of the day. If the myasthenic symptoms are severe and affect breathing, the dosage may need to be maintained but consideration may be given to pre-operative steroid therapy with the expectation that this can be discontinued after full surgical recovery. Repeated assessment of vital capacity can greatly assist pre-operative management. Oral medication should continue up to the time of operation.

THE OPERATION

1

The patient is placed horizontally in the supine position and the skin is prepared and towels placed as for cardiac surgery. A mid-line incision is made from the sternal notch to the lowermost point of the xiphisternum and is carried down to the periosteum of the sternum. The mid-line of the sternum is noted by palpation of the lateral margins between the costal cartilages and the sternum is divided longitudinally along all its length. Periosteal bleeding is controlled by diathermy and bleeding from the bone by plugging with bone wax.

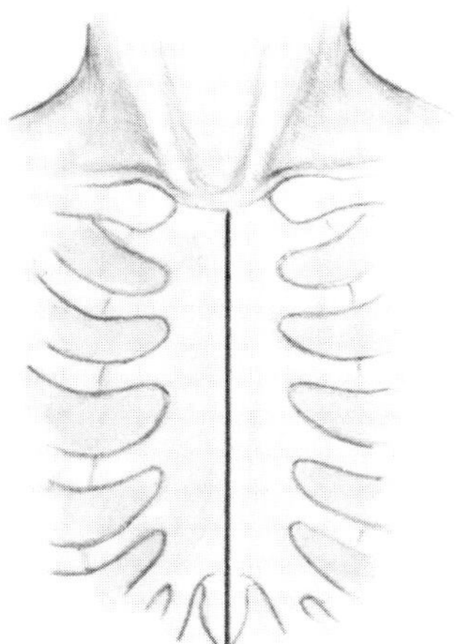

1

2

A sternal retractor is inserted and is opened gradually to avoid fracture of the upper ribs which would cause postoperative pain below the clavicles. Fatty tissue behind the sternum is cleared laterally with a swab and the pretracheal fascia, extending down from the neck, deep to the sternothyroid muscles is exposed. Inferiorly it is attached in an inverted horseshoe line to the anterior pericardium and laterally it blends with the extrapleural fascia. It forms the anterior capsule of the gland and is the key to the operation.

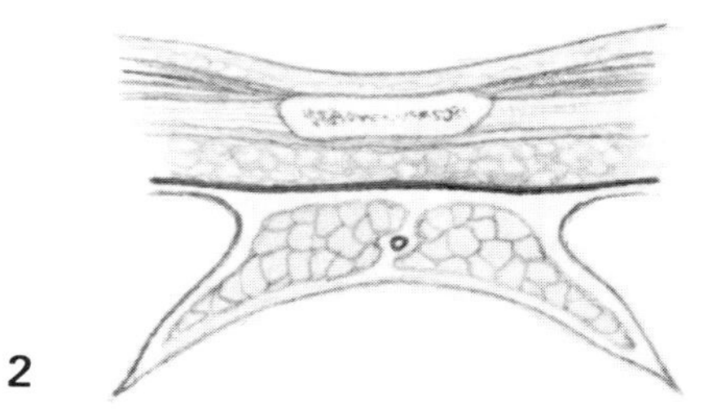

2

3

The thin fascia is incised in the mid-line and held either side in a clamp for identification. By blunt dissection, the thymus is separated from its posterior surface and the fascia divided from its pericardial attachment to expose the lower poles of the gland on each side. The thymus differs from extrapleural fat in its texture, which is larger and smoother in its lobulation, and in its colour, which is pinker. The lower pole can usually be easily mobilized and is held in a small tissue forceps. The gland can then be separated from the pericardium by blunt dissection and laterally from the pleura. Mobilization is continued upwards until the small arterial branch from the internal mammary artery is identified and divided between ligatures and the process is repeated on the contralateral side.

By retraction of the upper end of the wound the two upper poles of the gland are identified lying anterior to the left innominate vein and passing upwards into the neck. Blunt dissection and gentle traction will deliver these into the wound but a small arterial branch usually enters the uppermost end of these and this can be caught in a clamp and ligated before the upper poles are finally freed.

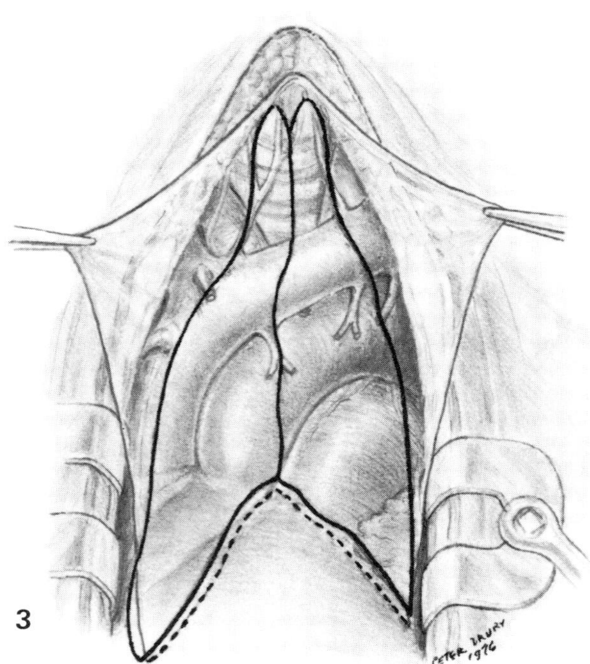

3

The gland is then separated from the innominate vein and its own venous drainage identified and ligated as it enters the inferior surface of that vein.

Haemostasis is not usually difficult. Special attention should be given to avoid undue clearance of extrapleural fat in the upper mediastinum as this may lead to damage to the phrenic nerves which enter the chest much more anteriorly than they are usually seen during thoracic surgery. Small accidental perforations of the thin parietal pleura do not require separate drainage since this thin pleura is relatively avascular and air can be expelled anteriorly before the chest is closed. Wider transgression of the pleura particularly through fatty tissues requires pleural drainage.

The sternum is approximated securely with wire sutures and the wound is closed in layers leaving a suction drain (Redivac) in the anterior mediastinum.

POSTOPERATIVE CARE AND COMPLICATIONS

The postoperative management of patients after thymectomy for myasthenia is best arranged in an intensive care area with full anaesthetic staffing since serious complications are most commonly associated with the patient's ability to breathe.

Ideally on leaving theatre a pernasal endotracheal tube should be present and artificial ventilation is continued probably for the first 24 hr. A nasogastric tube should also be present to enable the crushed anticholinesterase drugs to be given by the most effective route in a small quantity of water.

Anticholinesterases should not be restarted postoperatively until the patient's condition requires it. This can be assessed from time to time by intravenous injections of edrophonium 4 mg and observing whether this does or does not help the patient. Vital capacity is measured at intervals during the day using a Wright's respirometer or similar apparatus attached to the end of the endotracheal tube and artificial ventilation can usually be discontinued if the patient's airway remains uninfected and the vital capacity is greater than 1·5–2 litres. The endotracheal tube should be left *in situ* as long as there is doubt about the patient's safety without it—commonly for 3–4 days—and it is usually well tolerated. Intragastric feeds via the nasal tube can be started when bowel sounds return.

Complications

Haemothorax and pneumothorax are rare complications of thymectomy. A chest radiograph should be taken immediately after the patient's return from the operating theatre to demonstrate the presence of air or blood in the pleura. Small collections require no treatment but larger collections may require aspiration or water seal drainage of the affected pleura. Most complications are associated with the patient's myasthenia and include respiratory infection and weakness of the muscles of respiration and coughing. It seems best always to overcome these by respiratory assistance and tracheal aspiration rather than recourse to additional medical therapy in the first instance. Difficulty in swallowing may prevent administration of drugs and require replacement of the nasogastric tube.

THYMIC TUMOURS AND CYSTS

Benign tumours and cysts of the thymus may be discovered during routine chest radiology or when they give rise to pulmonary symptoms. Malignant tumours are usually 'silent' until they are large and then cause pain and symptoms and signs of mediastinal compression.

4

Small tumours with a well demarcated edge that present to one side of the mediastinum may be excised through a lateral thoracotomy incision so long as it is not intended to excise the entire thymus. Cysts, intrathoracic dermoids and the benign lympho-epithelioma are suitable for this approach which is dealt with in this section.

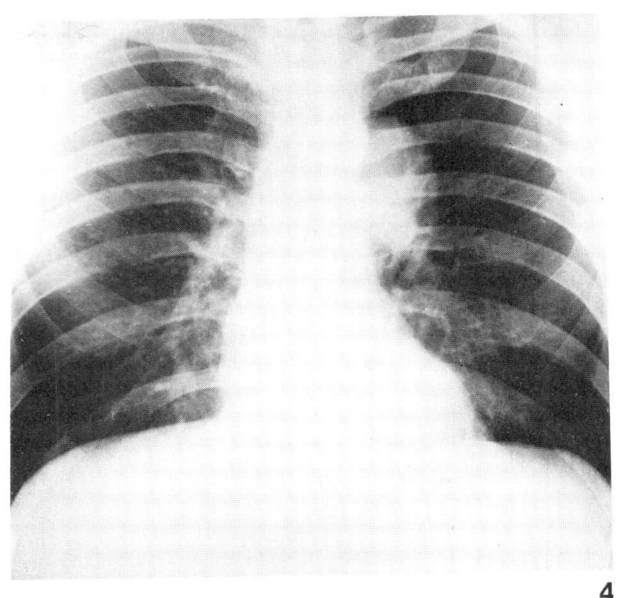

4

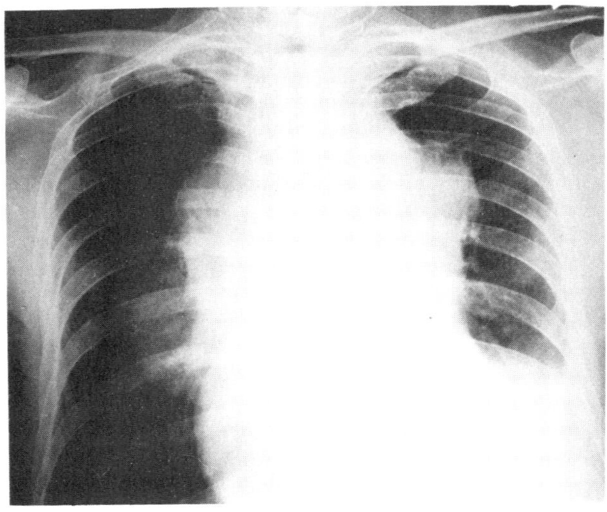

5

5

Large tumours with a diffuse outline presenting to both sides of the mediastinum should be suspected of malignancy. Histological evidence of their nature is sought by needle biopsy under radiographic screening control. Radiotherapy is usually the treatment of choice for these tumours.

Transpleural approach

With the patient supported in the right lateral position, the left chest is opened by an incision through the periosteum of the upper border of the fifth rib and the left lung is retracted posteriorly.

6-9

The tumour presents either anterior or medial to the phrenic nerve which may be stretched over it and then requires careful dissection to avoid damage to its fibres or its blood supply which runs with it. The overlying mediastinal pleura is incised and the tumour is mobilized from its bed noting any signs of invasion of the surrounding tissues which would indicate a more radical form of excision. The tumour is mobilized with the lower pole of the thymus until normal thymic tissue is encountered above it and is then excised. Bleeding is controlled by diathermy and the mediastinal pleura is not repaired.

The lung is re-expanded by the anaesthetist and a basal drainage tube inserted before closing the chest in layers in the routine manner.

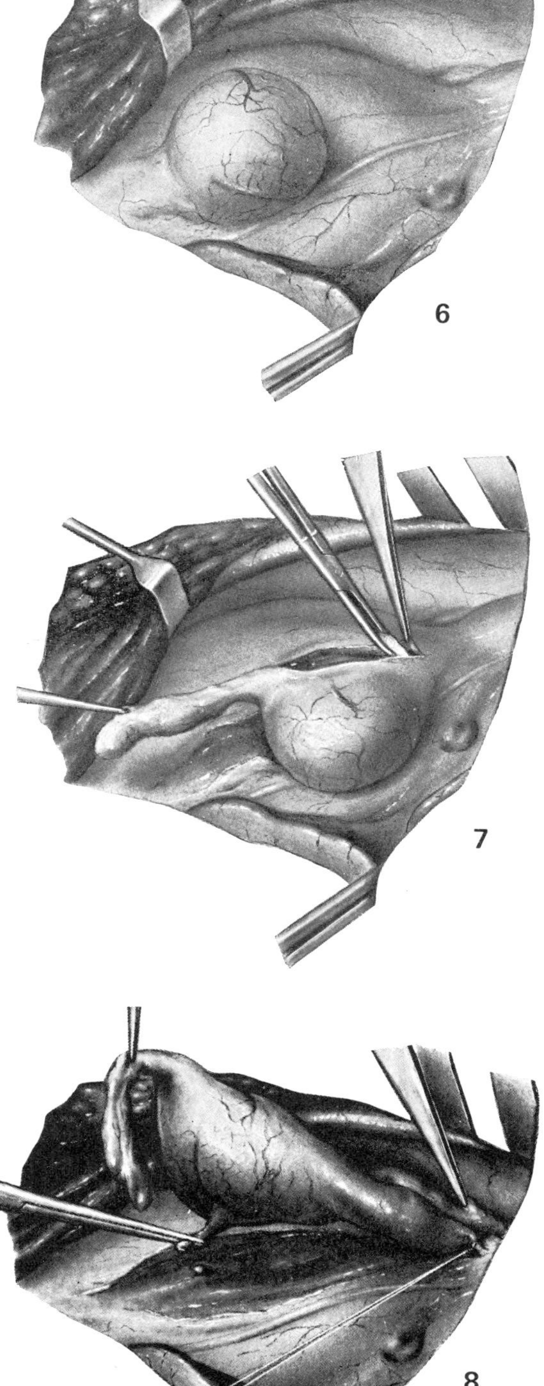

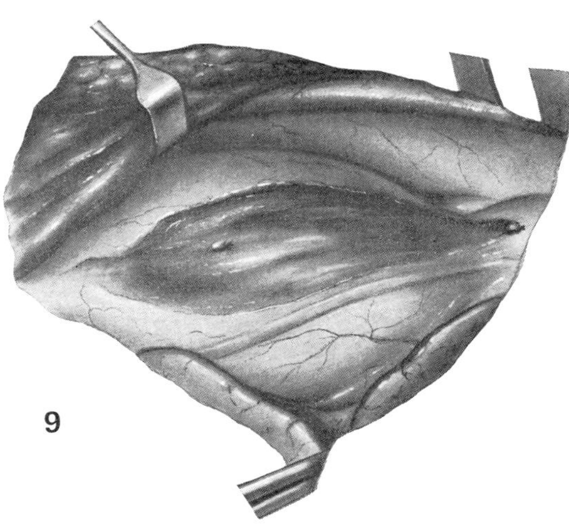

Special complications

Lung tissue that has been affected by the presence of the tumour, particularly after removal of an infected dermoid may take a long time to return to a normal radiographic appearance but this need not delay the patient's convalescence if all other features of recovery are satisfactory.

Damage to the phrenic nerve may be temporary if the nerve was involved in the tumour or permanent if the nerve has to be excised with a malignant tumour. This may seriously interfere with the patient's ability to keep his chest clear of secretions after operation but should ultimately produce little disturbance to normal respiration.

[*The illustrations for this Chapter on Thymectomy were drawn by Mr. P. Drury and Mr. D. P. Hammersley.*]

Oesophagoscopy

M. Meredith Brown, F.R.C.S.
Thoracic Surgeon, Milford Chest Hospital, Godalming, Surrey

PRE-OPERATIVE

Indications

Diagnostic

To complement or replace radioscopy with an opaque medium. To observe and record intrinsic and extrinsic lesions and take biopsies.

Therapeutic

Especially for Removal of foreign bodies
Dilatation of strictures.
Palliative intubation of carcinoma.

Contra-indications

Very few.

A small hazard of perforation is always present, particularly if dilatation is performed.

The rigid instrument cannot be introduced if the jaw is fixed or the cervical spine ankylosed. The lower oesophagus cannot be visualized if there is a marked thoracic kyphosis.

1

Hazards of osteophytes

Cervical osteophytes may risk damage by compression of the posterior oesophageal wall.

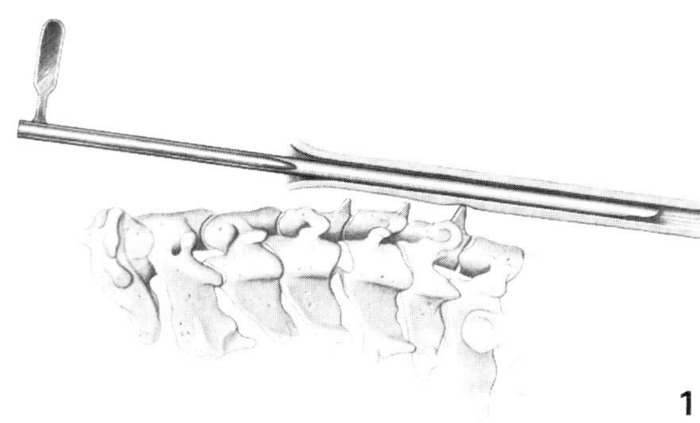

1

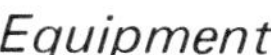

Preparation for oesophagoscopy

(*1*) Adequate clinical examination. Note (*a*) state of lungs, (*b*) cardiovascular system, (*c*) glands in neck and, (*d*) spinal column.

(*2*) Recent chest x-ray essential–may be needed for comparison.

(*3*) Estimate haemoglobin.

(*4*) Attend to dental hygiene. Extract loose teeth.

(*5*) Oesophageal washouts if oesophagus dilated with food residues. A clean empty oesophagus carries no danger of overflow into the bronchial tree, and allows the surgeon a good view.

Equipment

The rigid oesophagoscope allows good suction, removal of foreign bodies, dilatation and adequate biopsy.

The flexible oesophagoscope can be passed even when the spine is rigid, general anaesthesia is not essential, the view is better and the stomach can be examined.

Ideally both instruments should be available.

2

Rigid oesophagoscope

Negus pattern recommended.

Fibre light desirable, but low voltage acceptable.

For adult, must be at least 40 cm long to reach the cardia. Diameter should not exceed 20 mm—smaller adequate for routine use. Thirty centimetre instrument convenient for upper oesophagus.

Scaled down instrument for children. (Bronchoscope a possible substitute.)

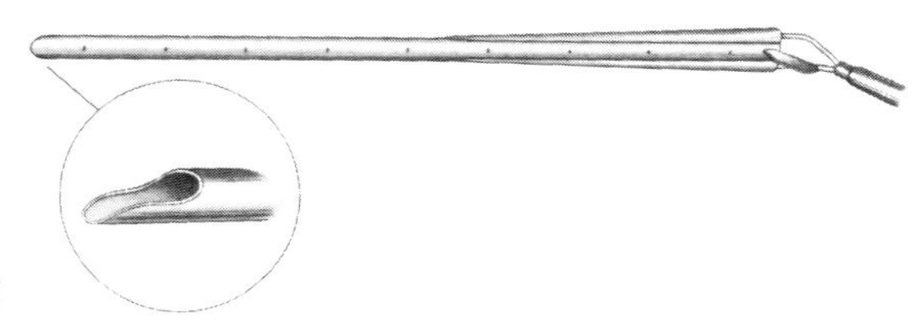

2

Suction

Adequate power essential.
Spare source desirable.

3

Aspirating tubes are best longer than an oesophagoscope, with a side hole to avoid obstruction by mucosa.

A secretion collector gives specimens for bacteriology, biochemistry or cytology.

Litmus paper offers simple confirmation of gastric reflux.

A tube and funnel facilitates a washout if preparation inadequate.

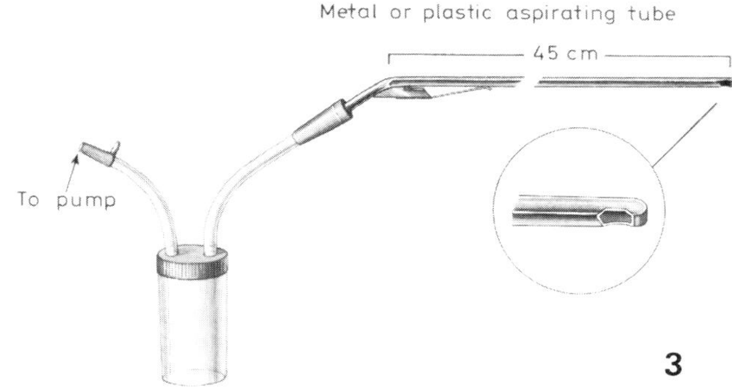

3

4a

Bougies

A set of graduated Chevalier-Jackson gum-elastic bougies, mounted on rigid wire stems, for assessment of an obstruction and dilatation under vision.

A set of Hurst mercury loaded bougies, originally designed for self-passage in the treatment of achalasia, can also be used as dilators, perhaps with a smaller hazard of perforation.

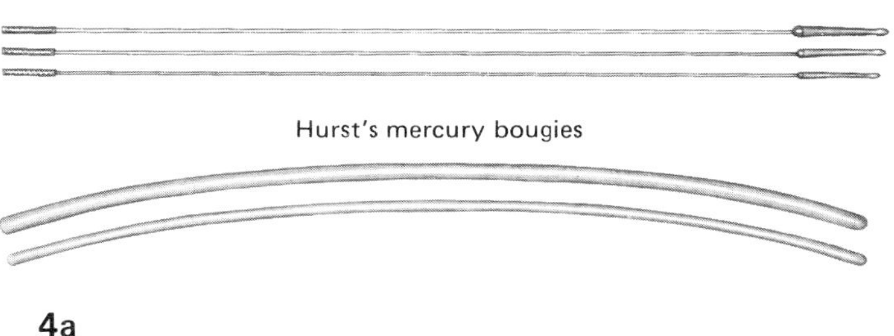

4a

4b

Biopsy and grasping forceps

Brock's angled bronchus biopsy forceps.
Souttar's cup forceps.

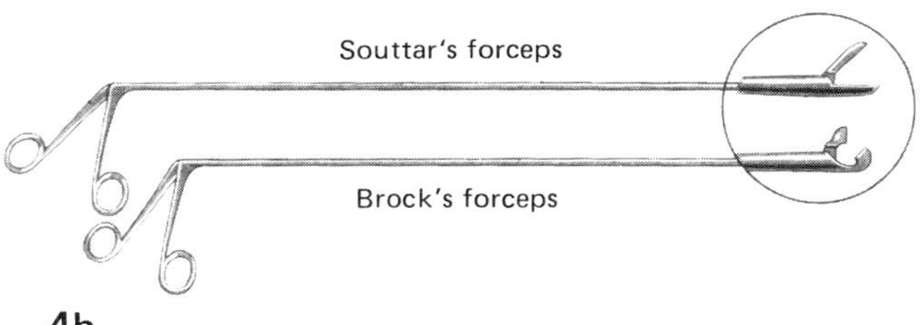

4b

5

Flexible oesophagoscope

With fibre view as well as fibre light. Must look forward, directly or obliquely. (A side-viewing lens, useful in the stomach, will be obscured by the mucosa.)

Single-plane angulation of the distal end, combined with rotation of the whole instrument, allows inspection of all fields.

Although the stomach cannot be fully examined, useful information can often be gained.

A suction channel allows aspiration of mucus and the passage of a fine biopsy forceps.

A water jet cleans the lens.

A camera can make a permanent record.

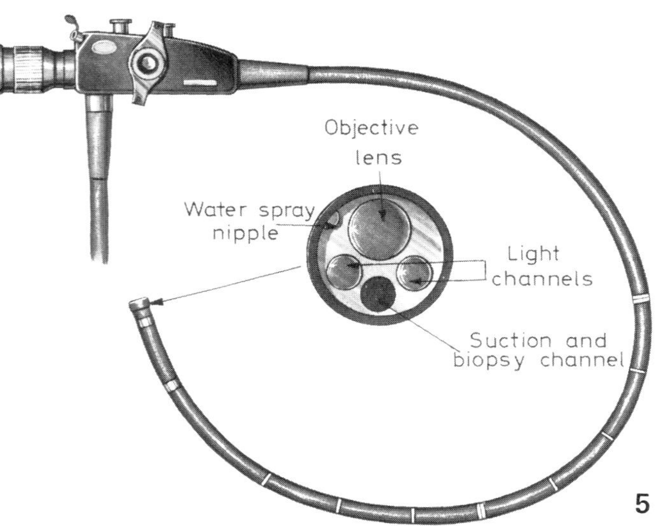

5

Laryngoscopy and bronchoscopy equipment

Concomitant examination of the air passages may be indicated, particularly in carcinoma of the upper oesophagus.

Equipment for intubation

Instruments for cervical gland biopsy

Anaesthesia

Local anaesthesia may be sufficient, but the discomfort associated, especially with the rigid instrument, makes general anaesthesia desirable.

Many patients are old and frail.

Local anaesthesia

Preliminary sedation may be supplemented by intravenous Diazepam.

A pastille to suck is followed by surface application of 2 per cent lignocaine to lips, oropharynx and cricopharyngeal inlet.

General anaesthesia

The anaesthetist must be alert to the danger of overflow of oesophageal contents into the tracheobronchial tree.

He will insert an endotracheal tube, without which the oesophagoscope may compress the trachea. The Oxford type is convenient.

He must provide complete relaxation of the cricopharyngeal sphincter, to reduce the hazard of perforation at the moment of introduction. Subsequently the patient may resume gentle respiration.

Position of patient

Rigid instrument

Supine, on an operating table with a flap allowing extension of the neck. The head supported on a grommet ring or rest.

A feet down tilt reduces gastric reflux and maintains the field of view at a comfortable eye level.

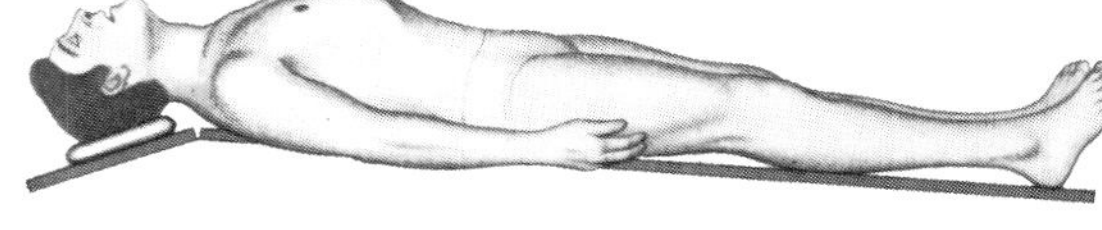

6

Flexible instrument

Supine or lateral, on any firm surface.

THE OPERATION

Introduction of the rigid oesophagoscope

The well lubricated distal end of the instrument lifts the tongue forward, avoiding damage to lips or teeth, or the use of the upper jaw as a fulcrum. Under direct vision, the cricopharyngeal inlet is found behind the larynx as the neck is flexed: the tip of the oesophagoscope slides in without force, almost by its own weight. As the instrument advances the neck is extended to maintain alignment.

If there is any difficulty, a Jackson bougie should be dropped through the cricopharyngeus as a guide, to be followed by the oesophagoscope, always keeping the wire stem in the centre of the field of view.

If there is a pharyngeal pouch, the instrument may enter the pouch rather than the oesophagus. It must then be withdrawn before it causes damage.

7a-d

The examination

Take advantage of anaesthetic relaxation to palpate the abdomen carefully.

Observe (*a*) the contents (*b*) the calibre of the lumen (*c*) rigidity or displacement of the wall (*d*) abnormalities of the mucosa.

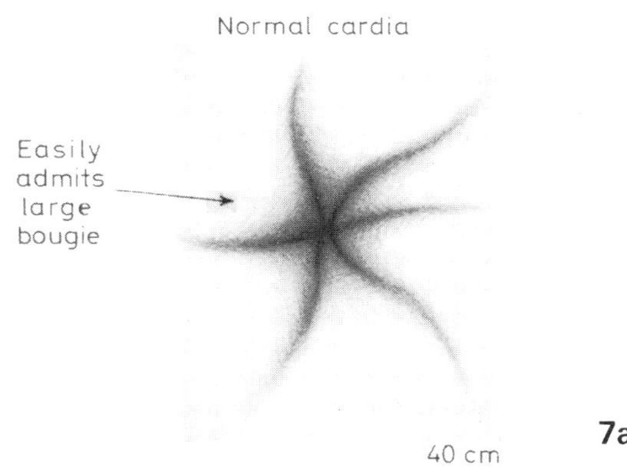

7a

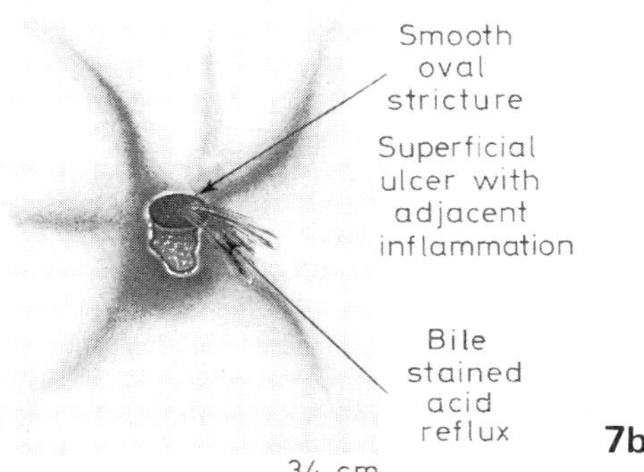

7b

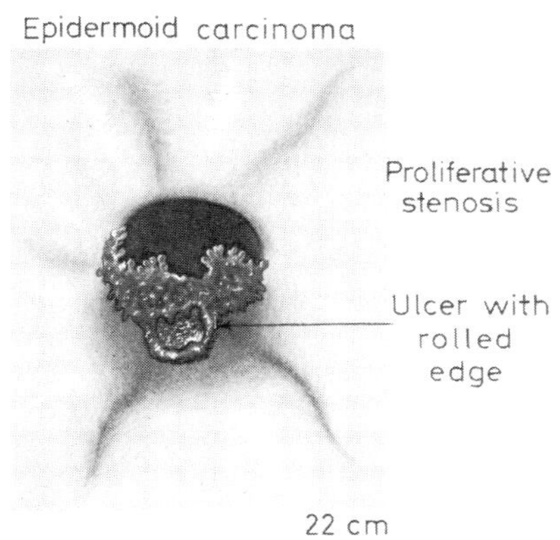

7d

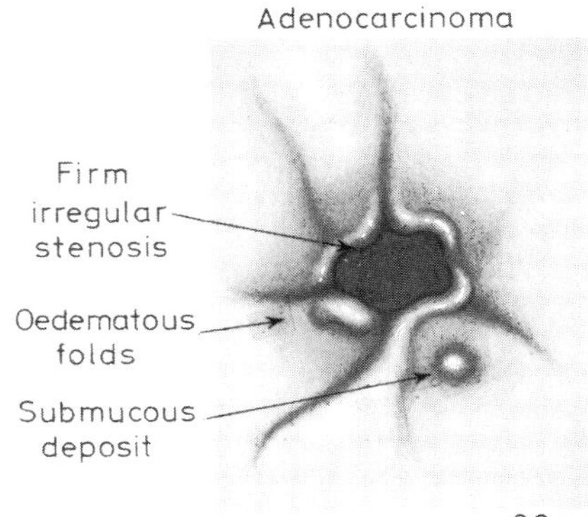

7c

8

Normal oesophageal levels

The position of lesions should be recorded in centimetres from the upper jaw, as indicated on the instrument.

Inspection should be repeated as the instrument is withdrawn.

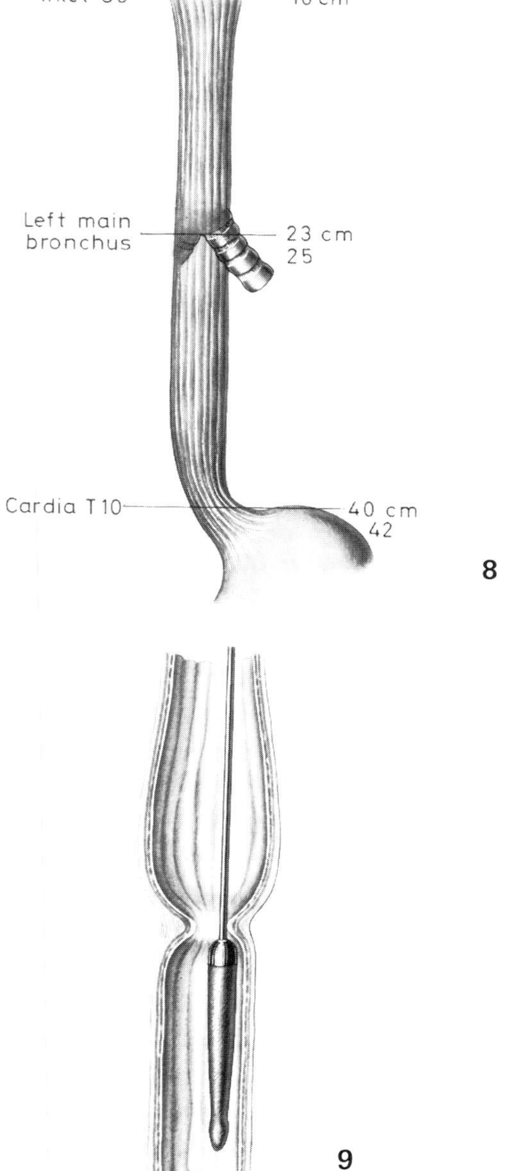

Assessment of obstruction

The diameter of an obstruction can be assessed by passing a Jackson bougie, and its length by withdrawal until the shoulder impinges.

Biopsy

Obtain an adequate specimen by accurate placement of the forceps.

Avoid large bites from normal mucosa, which may cause perforation.

Introduction of the flexible oesophagoscope

Check the controls, lubricate the tip, and leave the distal end in the free position. Pass through a plastic ring between the teeth, if any. Preliminary passage of a mercury bougie opens the cricopharyngeus and confirms that there is no upper obstruction. The instrument follows gently, guided by a finger or depressor blade lifting the tongue. The conscious patient should be asked to swallow.

Once entered, the oesophageal contents may be aspirated and air introduced to cause sufficient distension for a good view. These procedures are repeated as the instrument advances into the stomach, and on withdrawal.

THERAPEUTIC PROCEDURES

The rigid instrument is usually required.

Removal of foreign bodies

Seldom immediately urgent, but do not delay if spikey. Sometimes it is wise to prepare for external oesophagotomy (usually by thoracotomy).

If radio-opaque, repeat x-ray on way to theatre.

Grasp with suitable forceps—biopsy forceps often adequate. Dislodge by firm gentle traction. If large, withdraw oesophagoscope while maintaining grasp of the object at its tip.

Injection of varices

Submucosal injection of a sclerosant through a special long needle may be of temporary value in the treatment of varices associated with portal hypertension.

Cauterization

Persistent oesophageal fistulae may be cauterized with 20 per cent sodium hydroxide applied on a pledget. Any excess must be neutralized with 30 per cent acetic acid.

10

Dilatation of strictures

Dilatation is achieved by the sequential passage of graduated bougies, each of diameter only slightly greater than the preceding. Each should be well lubricated, and introduced without force.

There is an inevitable hazard of perforation, by rupture or false passage: especially through necrotic carcinoma.

Hydrostatic dilatation

Achalasia is usually treated by Heller's cardiomyotomy, but if this is contra-indicated forcible dilatation of the cardia by oesophagoscopy may be performed. This is achieved by introducing a hydrostatic dilator, placing the centre of the bag at the level of the cardia, and distending the bag with saline.

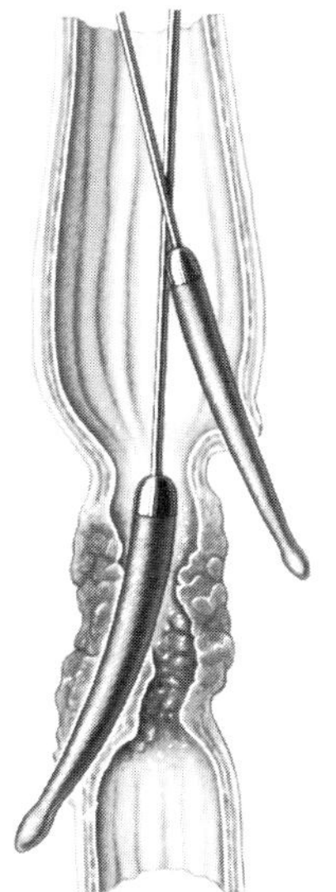

10

11

Palliative intubation of inoperable carcinoma

Intubation is preferred to gastrostomy: it allows natural swallowing to continue, and avoids overflow of saliva. It is most effective in the mid-oesophagus, but can be used at the cardia; a tube too high impinging on the inlet, cannot be tolerated. The patient and his attendants must be instructed always to take a liquid or semisolid diet that will easily pass through the inert segment. Inadvertant food impaction can sometimes be relieved by drinking soda water or hydrogen peroxide.

A Symond gum-elastic or Souttar spiral wire tube can be inserted through an oesophagoscope after dilatation. The tube can be mounted on a Jackson bougie, and held in place with a biopsy forceps as the bougie is withdrawn. Special instruments are available for Souttar's tubes.

To insert the larger—and more effective—tubes, such as Mousseau–Barbin, Celestin or Gourevitch, an additional short upper laparotomy is made. This allows a limited exploration, and a gastrotomy through which the tube is drawn into position.

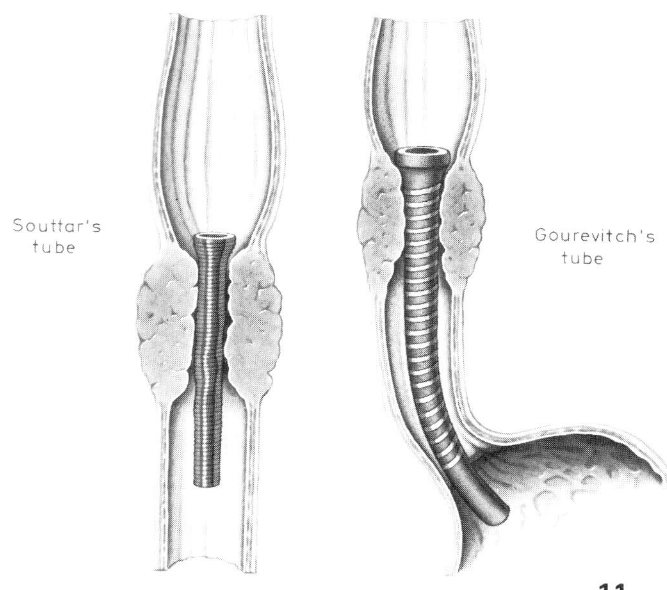

11

COMPLICATIONS

Haemorrhage

Small bleeds cease spontaneously, or may be controlled by application of adrenaline 1:1000. Diathermy, with an insulated rod, must be used with caution for fear of perforation. Pressure, applied by a Sengstaken tube, may succeed. Transfusion may be necessary.

There should be no hesitation in performing an emergency operation, particularly if the responsible lesion is one properly treated surgically, such as a neoplasm.

Bronchial aspiration

Overflow into the air passages should be treated by prompt bronchial toilet with suction and perhaps bronchoscopy. Atelectasis and bronchopneumonia may follow, demanding physiotherapy and antibiotics.

Oesophageal perforation

If recognized early, again an emergency major operation may be indicated, combining repair with treatment of any underlying obstructive lesion (*see* Chapter on 'Management of Distension Ruptures and Instrumental Perforations of the Oesophagus', pages 395–403).

POSTOPERATIVE CARE

Careful observation desirable for at least several hours.

Some surgeons withold all oral intake, and take a routine x-ray. Neither precaution is essential, provided nurses are alert to report unexpected pain—rather than soreness—or subcutaneous emphysema.

Allow only clear fluids by mouth until a doctor has seen the patient.

[*The illustrations for this Chapter on Oesophagoscopy were drawn by Mr. M. J. Courtney.*]

Management of Distension Ruptures and Instrumental Perforations of the Oesophagus

H. R. S. Harley, M.S., F.R.C.S.
Consultant Surgeon, University Hospital of Wales
and Llandough Hospital

Terminology

Rupture and perforation of the oesophagus are not synonymous. Rupture is a bursting injury; perforation is caused by foreign bodies, instruments, ulcerative processes or penetrating injuries.

Aetiological classification

Distension rupture or 'burst' oesophagus

(*1*) Muscular violence, such as unco-ordinated vomiting, defaecation or weight lifting, the first of which accounts for 85 per cent of cases.

(*2*) Exposure of mouth or nose to compressed gases.

(*3*) Compression injuries of the abdomen or lower chest.

(*4*) Hydrostatic bag dilatations for achalasia.

Perforation

(*1*) Ingested foreign bodies.

(*2*) Instrumentation, such as endoscopy, bougienage, intubation of malignant strictures, or removal of foreign bodies.

(*3*) Acute penetrating ulcers.

(*4*) Para-oesophageal operations, especially vagotomy, right pneumonectomy and repair of hiatus hernia.

(*5*) Penetrating wounds.

Sites and nature of ruptures and perforations

About 90 per cent of distension ruptures other than those caused by distension bags, affect the lower end of the thoracic oesophagus, usually at its left posterior aspect. A few occur in the mid-thoracic oesophagus, nearly always on the right side and a very few affect the abdominal or cervical oesophagus. The tears are characteristically single, longitudinal and cleanly cut, but are occasionally bilateral or transverse.

Hydrostatic dilators rupture the cardia into either the chest or abdomen. Ingested foreign bodies usually perforate the region of the cricopharyngeal sphincter, less often the thoracic oesophagus near the aortic arch or above a stricture. Oesophagoscopes usually perforate the region of the cricopharyngeal sphincter posteriorly, often to the left of the mid-line if the endoscopist is right-handed. Bougies usually perforate just above a stricture, more rarely below it, while intubation usually causes perforation at or just above a new growth. Para-oesophageal operations result in perforation, often delayed for days, weeks, months or even years, at the site of operation.

Pathology

Ruptures and perforations may be:

(*1*) Mucosal (*a*) local; (*b*) dissecting.

(*2*) Whole thickness (*a*) mediastinal; (*b*) pleural; (*c*) peritoneal; (*d*) pericardial.

Mucosal injuries caused by foreign bodies usually form localized intramural pockets, while those caused by distension or instrumentation are more liable to dissect the oesophageal wall in the submucous layer, this being increased by bleeding and swallowed material. Either variety may subsequently become full thickness. Full thickness rupture or perforation of the thoracic oesophagus may enter primarily the mediastinum or one or both pleural cavities, or rarely the lesser sac of the peritoneum, or the pericardium if it is adherent to the oesophagus.

Endoscopes usually perforate the posterior cervical oesophageal wall and the buccopharyngeal membrane into the retro-oesophageal space, particularly in kyphotic and elderly subjects. This extends from the base of the skull to the tracheal bifurcation. Sagittal septa cross this space and prevent the spread of infection laterally in the neck, but not downwards into the mediastinum. Rarely a perforation more anteriorly enters the prevertebral space from which infection may spread either laterally into the neck or downwards into the mediastinum.

Extra-oesophageal factors which predispose to distension rupture

Co-ordinated vomiting probably never bursts a normal oesophagus. However, a full stomach and inco-ordinated vomiting are common associates. These two in combination lead to sudden powerful ejection of gastric contents into an oesophagus, the upper end of which is closed by an unrelaxed cricopharyngeal sphincter, resulting in a high intraluminal pressure. This may follow the copious intake of food and alcohol.

Neurological disease, especially affecting the hypothalamus or its pathways, predisposes to distension rupture by causing oesophagomalacia, due to vasospastic ischaemia and by causing inco-ordinated vomiting.

Diagnosis of distension rupture

Pain is usually of sudden onset and may be felt in the epigastrium, behind the sternum, in the back, in the lower chest or in the shoulder. It persists and worsens, despite narcotics and may be accompanied by a feeling of impending death or of something bursting or tearing in the lower part of the chest. If initiated by vomiting or retching these often cease with the onset of pain. Shock, sweating, cyanosis, thirst and rapid grunting respirations are common features and the patient tends to be restless and to sit up and lean forwards, clasping the lower part of his chest with his arms. Upper abdominal rigidity is the rule, often with tenderness and diminished peristalsis. Haematemesis is uncommon and scanty when it does occur. Surgical emphysema occurs in about 50–65 per cent of cases, developing early when rupture is intramediastinal, later when it is intrapleural. Signs of hydrothorax or hydropneumothorax may develop on one or both sides, but are often not obvious until a late stage. Mediastinal emphysema may give rise to Hamman's sign (systolic mediastinal crunching sound), a nasal or high-pitched voice, cardiac or tracheal displacement, distal heart sounds and loss of retrosternal dullness. As time passes, chest symptoms tend to overshadow abdominal ones.

Diagnosis of cervical perforation after instrumentation

Pain on swallowing after endoscopy is of little diagnostic value. Suspicious features are dysphagia, pain in the neck aggravated by flexion, sometimes also felt in the retrosternal or scapular regions, and tenderness, especially along the anterior border of the sternomastoid muscle, or in the supraclavicular fossa. Later, subcutaneous emphysema appears in the neck. Pain persists from the time of endoscopy. Tenderness, fever and leucocytosis may develop within 6 hr and cervical or mediastinal infection occur if treatment is delayed.

Diagnosis of intrathoracic and intra-abdominal instrumental perforations

The endoscopist is often unaware that he has damaged the oesophagus. The symptoms and signs resemble those of distension rupture but are less fulminating because gastric contents under high pressure are not expelled through the rent. The most constant clue is again the acute onset of severe pain which persists for more than an hour after endoscopy and is aggravated by swallowing. It may be felt in any of the sites mentioned for distension rupture and followed by any of the features of that condition. Pain, pyrexia and crepitus form a diagnostic triad, but crepitus occurs in only 50 per cent of cases.

DIAGNOSTIC PROCEDURES

Radiological examination

In cervical perforations postero-anterior films and penetrating lateral films, with the neck in hyper-extension, will show gas bubbles behind the oesophagus before crepitation can be felt.

For intrathoracic leaks anteroposterior radiographs should be taken of the abdomen, chest and neck and lateral ones also of the latter two sites. Mediastinal air is best shown by over-exposed films. Air is rarely seen under the diaphragm in distension ruptures. Features include mediastinal emphysema, widening or displacement, hydrothorax, hydropneumothorax or occasionally pneumothorax on one or both sides, an air bubble or liquid level behind the heart and surgical emphysema in the neck. Mediastinal emphysema due to perforation of a gastric or duodenal ulcer, will be accompanied by air below the diaphragm.

Contrast swallow

Whatever the level of the oesophageal leak a contrast swallow is mandatory, Dionosol being the best contrast medium.

The contrast swallow will usually diagnose both the presence and site of an intrathoracic leak, but may place a distension rupture too low if the contrast leaks only through the lower end of a long rent. When the contrast swallow is negative, it should be repeated in 1 hr if the diagnosis is still in doubt.

Oesophagoscopy

For suspected intrathoracic distension ruptures oesophagoscopy is essential whether the contrast swallow is negative or positive, in order to determine accurately the site and length of the rupture and to exclude the presence of a second tear.

TREATMENT

Treatment depends upon the site and nature of the injury, the time since it occurred and the presence or absence of other disease of the oesophagus, especially if obstructive.

Treatment of instrumental perforations of cervical oesophagus

These perforations are rarely associated with concomitant disease of the cervical oesophagus, though there may be a lesion, obstructive or otherwise, lower down. A non-obstructive lesion, or an obstructive one which has been successfully dilated, will not influence the immediate treatment.

About 75 per cent of cases respond to non-operative management, but the safest method of treatment is immediate cervical mediastinal drainage by an incision along the anterior border of the sternomastoid, combined with wide-spectrum antibiotic therapy in conventional doses, intravenous feeding, nasogastric suction and expectoration of saliva. Any foreign body present must be removed, but there is no need to suture the oesophageal rent unless it is large. Fistulae heal rapidly unless there is distal obstruction. Concomitant obstruction must be relieved at the time or later. If perforation has occurred through a pharyngeal pouch, the rent should be sutured and diverticulopexy performed or the pouch excised.

If diagnosis is uncertain, expectant treatment with close observation is permissible. Should a cervical abscess or mediastinitis develop, drainage must be instituted without delay. It remains difficult to act promptly, yet never to act unnecessarily.

Postoperative care

Feeding intravenously or by nasogastric tube is continued until the fistulous track is sealed off or contrast radiography shows that the oesophageal tear is closed, the first study being performed after about 5 days. Provided there is no distal obstruction, the fistula will close even if the drains are removed.

Treatment of full thickness distension ruptures of thoracic oesophagus

Pre-operative care

Rapid and profound deterioration of the general condition occurs. Immediate supportive measures must be followed by thoracotomy as soon as possible. The aphorism 'the patient is too ill not to operate' is apt.

Fluids and electrolytes are administered intravenously, blood loss is replaced as necessary, massive doses of broad-spectrum antibiotics are given intravenously and nasogastric suction is instituted. Profound shock demands intravenous steroid therapy. Methyl prednisolone sodium succinate, 5 mg/kg is administered forthwith and continued in the same dosage every 12 hr for 36 hr after surgery. If a large hydropneumothorax or hydrothorax is embarrassing respiration, intercostal drainage should be instituted before thoracotomy.

OPERATION FOR SUTURE-CLOSURE OF DISTENSION RUPTURES OF THORACIC OESOPHAGUS WITHOUT ASSOCIATED OESOPHAGEAL LESIONS

Anaesthesia

The patient is anaesthetized with the aid of a double-lumen endotracheal tube, so that the lung on the side of operation can be kept deflated when the chest is open.

THE OPERATION

1

Oesophagoscopy is performed and the patient is then placed in lateral decubitus with the operation side uppermost and the arm held forwards and supported on a rest at right angles to the trunk. The position of the inferior angle of the scapula is illustrated.

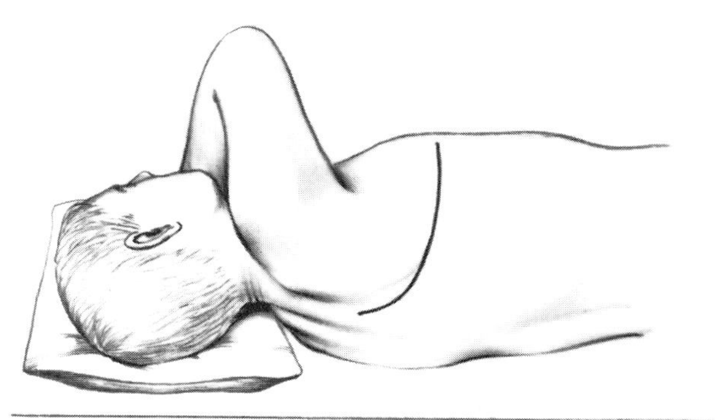

1

The pleura is opened by dividing the sixth or seventh rib bed while the anaesthetist is asked to deflate the lung. A clear pleural effusion suggests an intact mediastinum, while a sour one indicates that it has been ruptured or perforated.

2

The mediastinum over the oesophagus is exposed by lifting the lung forwards. If the mediastinal pleura is intact, the mediastinum will be distended with blood, gastric contents, saliva and air. It will be the site of acute necrotizing and gangrenous mediastinitis and may look dark purple. A clear pleural effusion of exudative type may be present on one or both sides. If the rupture is intrapleural there will be a hydro-pneumothorax, the liquid being acid, brownish and sour smelling and often containing partially digested food, but the mediastinitis tends to be less severe.

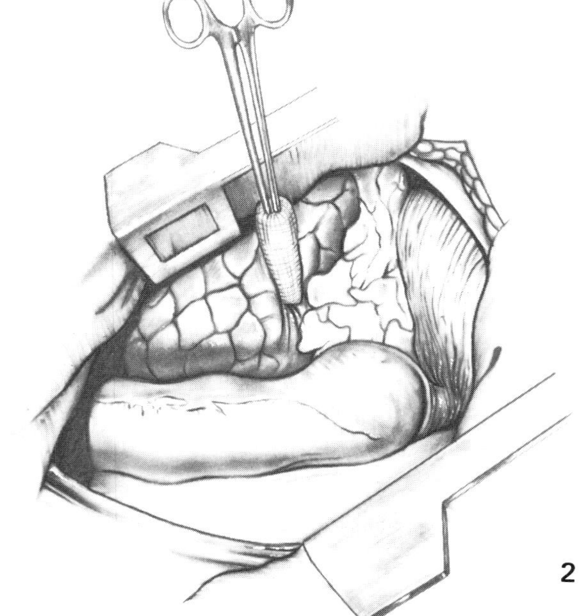

2

3

The oesophagus is exposed and the tear examined. The rents may be long and the mucosal tear may be longer than the muscular one. Elongation of the muscle tear is required if there is doubt about this. A careful search is made for associated oesophageal disease. If present, especially if obstructive, treatment and prognosis may be influenced. Fortunately, 80 per cent of distension ruptures affect a normal oesophagus. The decision must be made whether or not to suture the rent. The success rate of suture declines with time, but no arbitrary time limit can be set and surgical judgement is required. If the oesophageal wall appears to be healthy, particularly during the first 24 hr, the rent is closed with two layers of interrupted non-absorbable sutures and is re-inforced by suturing adjacent lung to it, or by wrapping it with a pedicled graft of pericardium. Complete debridement of the mediastinum and pleural cavity is essential. If the tissues look oedematous, necrotic or digested, primary suture is omitted in favour of one of the other procedures described later.

4

The chest is closed with drainage by two or three tubes. One is inserted into the apex of the pleural cavity and one to the base. If the latter is not near the oesophageal rent, a third tube is placed close to it but should not touch it. The three tubes are attached to water seal bottles. The skin is closed with interrupted sutures. If the oesophageal tissues are doubtfully viable, double gastrostomy may be advisable.

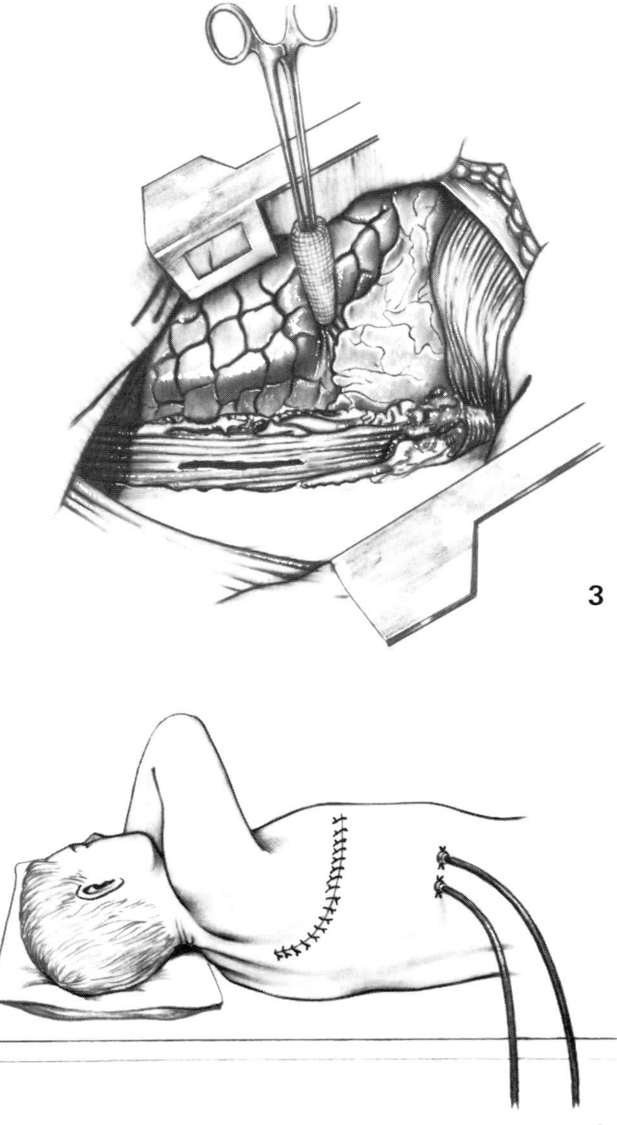

3

4

Postoperative care

The water seal bottles are connected to suction, which is maintained continuously until the tubes are withdrawn. An x-ray film of the chest is taken at once to exclude a pneumothorax or hydropneumothorax on either the operated or the opposite side. If found, it must be corrected by adjustment of the intercostal tubes or the insertion of another tube. Intravenous steroid therapy, if used, is maintained for 36 hr after operation. Massive intravenous antibiotic therapy continues for at least 48 hr. Thereafter, if progress is satisfactory, dosage is reduced and the intravenous route abandoned. Suction drainage is maintained until the tubes have been quiescent and the lung fully expanded for 48 hr. A tube near the oesophageal rent may be left in longer. Intravenous alimentation should be maintained for a week or until serial Dionosil studies, the first after about 5 days, show the oesophageal leak to be sealed. Drained fistulous tracks seal off quite rapidly from the surrounding tissues and then drinking of bland liquids is safe.

ALTERNATIVES TO PRIMARY SUTURE CLOSURE

In cases unsuitable for primary suture-closure the alternatives are to close the rent by other methods, to leave it open and rely on mediastinal and pleural debridement with pleural suction drainage, or to exclude the thoracic oesophagus.

5

Closure of rupture by Thal fundal patch graft

Late cases can sometimes be closed successfully by this technique, provided the rupture is at the lower end of the oesophagus and in its left or anterior wall (Thal, 1968, 1970). The phreno-oesophageal ligament is divided in its anterior two-thirds, the peritoneal cavity entered, the diaphragm divided laterally from the hiatus for about 5 cm and the fundus of the stomach brought up well above the defect. The margins of the defect are sutured to the fundus of the stomach with interrupted or running lock sutures of 2/0 chromic catgut, to form a roof over which the squamous epithelium of the oesophagus can spread. A valve is then made by enfolding two-thirds of the circumference of the oesophagus with gastric fundus so that the previous line of sutures is completely covered and at least 5 cm of the length of the oesophagus is enfolded by a series of interrupted 4/0 Tevdek or silk sutures which do not enter the lumen of the stomach. A resident large oesophageal tube prevents inadvertent narrowing of the oesophagus as this is done. The valve may be left in the chest or in the abdomen. It prevents subsequent gastro-oesophageal reflux.

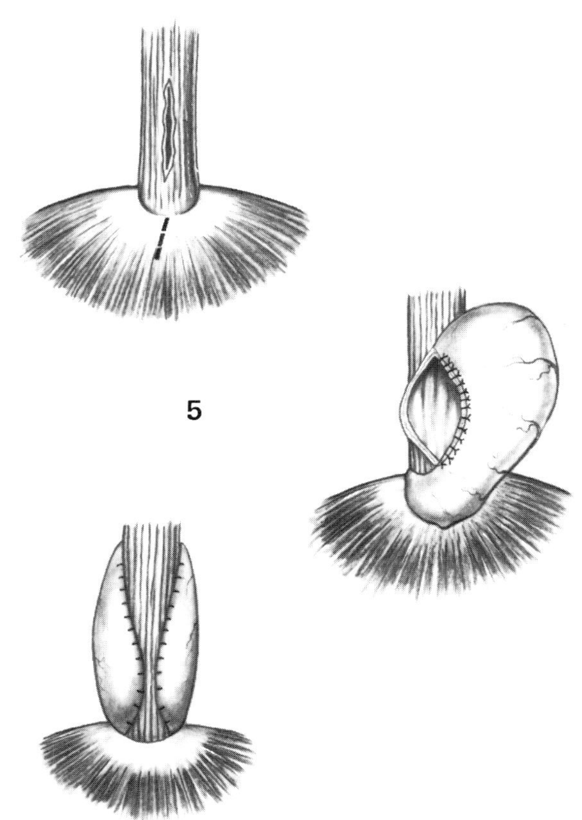

Debridement of pleura and mediastinum and pleural drainage

The technique is as described for suture-closure except that the rent is left unsutured. This method is accompanied by a high mortality (30–50 per cent) and morbidity and by prolonged convalescence. Double gastrostomy at the time of thoracotomy or later may improve results. One gastrostomy tube is passed through the pylorus into the jejunum for feeding, while a second is passed up towards the fundus and attached to suction. This keeps the stomach empty and prevents reflux of gastric juice.

6

Oesophageal exclusion with subsequent resection and reconstruction (Johnson et al., 1956; Johnson and Schwegman, 1967)

This operation can be used as an alternative to drainage for very late cases unsuitable for any type of closure of the rupture, whether the lower or the middle third of the oesophagus is affected. A two-stage procedure is preferable to the three-stage one originally described. An end-cervical oesophagostomy with closure of the distal end is constructed through an incision along the anterior border of the right sternomastoid muscle, the abdominal oesophagus is divided through an upper mid-line abdominal incision, both its ends being closed and a feeding gastrostomy is made. At stage two the excluded oesophagus is excised and replaced with left colon through a left thoraco-abdominal incision by the technique of Belsey (1965). The colon is anastomosed to the oesophagus in the right side of the neck.

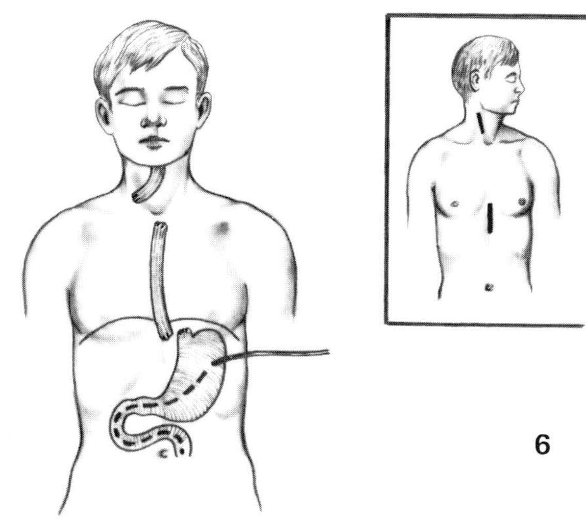

6

TREATMENT OF FULL THICKNESS INSTRUMENTAL PERFORATION OF THE THORACIC OR ABDOMINAL OESOPHAGUS

Most instrumental perforations of the thoracic or abdominal oesophagus occur at or immediately above an obstructive lesion. For the very few without such a lesion, treatment is as for distension ruptures. The presence of unrelieved obstruction makes suture of the perforation futile.

Four groups will be discussed: (*1*) operable carcinoma; (*2*) inoperable carcinoma; (*3*) a benign stricture; (*4*) achalasia of the cardia.

Operable carcinoma

One-stage oesophagectomy and oesophagogastrostomy

This is the treatment of choice when the patient is fit enough. It is best done within 8 hr of perforation, but can be successful later, even in the presence of established mediastinitis if the anastomosis is made high in the chest or in the neck where the oesophagus and its surrounding tissues are healthy.

Oesophageal exclusion

For late cases or when the general condition is poor, oesophageal exclusion is performed followed by subsequent excision and reconstruction of the excluded oesophagus, as previously described (*see Illustration 6*).

Inoperable carcinoma

The only procedure likely to be of benefit is the insertion of a Celestin or other suitable tube.

Benign stricture

Several possibilities are available:

Primary suture closure of the perforation

This can only be done in the unlikely event that the stricture was adequately dilated at the time of oesophagoscopy.

Closure of the perforation and correction of the stricture by the Thal fundal patch procedure

This operation can succeed for a perforation suitably sited at or just above a short stricture near the lower end of the thoracic, or in the abdominal oesophagus. The technique is as described previously (*see Illustration 5*), except that the rent is enlarged downwards through the stricture before the repair.

7

If necessary and if the health of the tissue allows, the strictured area may be widened by transverse approximation on the aspect opposite to the tear. Intraperitoneal perforation can be treated through an upper abdominal incision. Truncal vagotomy allows 8–10 cm of oesophagus to be delivered into the abdomen, but requires pylorotomy, with the risk of its complications.

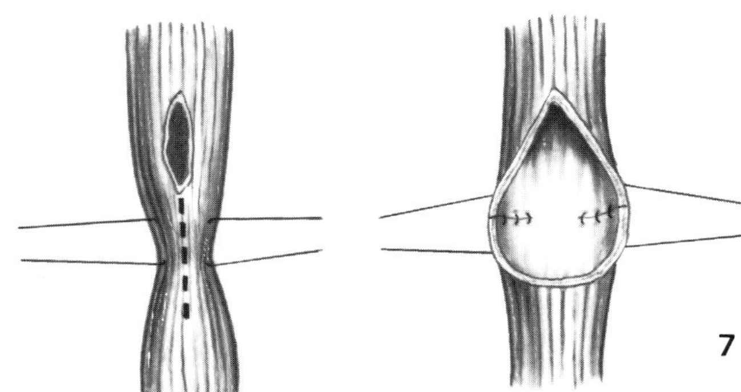

7

Resection of the perforation and stricture

If the general condition is suitable, the injured and strictured portions of the oesophagus are excised and replaced with an interposed segment of left colon or jejunum. Kerr's two-stage operation is quicker (Kerr, 1968). Through a left thoracotomy incision, the perforated and strictured part of the oesophagus is excised and the proximal end anastomosed to the gastric fundus. Elective reconstruction with left colon or jejunum is performed later to avoid gastric reflux.

Oesophageal exclusion

For late cases or when the general condition is bad, this operation is performed as previously described (*see Illustration 6*).

Cases with achalasia of the cardia

An immediate left thoracotomy is performed through the sixth or seventh intercostal space, the rent is closed by two-layered suture and a Heller's myotomy is performed. The prognosis is good.

COMPLICATIONS AFTER INTRATHORACIC RUPTURE OR PERFORATION

These are most frequent after distension rupture because of digestion of the oesophageal and pleural tissues by gastric juice.

Fulminating anaerobic or gram negative infection is liable to occur, especially after burst oesophagus and may overwhelm the patient. This is prevented and treated by massive intravenous antibiotic therapy as detailed under pre-operative management.

Breakdown of the oesophageal suture line after primary suture-closure is common and probably occurs in at least half the cases of distension rupture. The later the closure the more likely is breakdown to occur. The consequence is an oesophagopleural or oesophagopleurocutaneous fistula. Early breakdown leads to increased discharge through the intercostal drains, later breakdown to air and a liquid level in the pleural cavity and fever. These fistulae often heal spontaneously, provided they are well drained, the lung is kept expanded, there is no distal obstruction and nutrition can be maintained. The patient is treated with antibiotics and intercostal pleural suction drainage, while nutrition is maintained by intravenous feeding, or later, by nasogastric tube or double gastrostomy if necessary. If the fistula does not close reasonably soon the opening in the oesophagus is sutured in two layers, an inner of interrupted chromic catgut and an outer of interrupted Tevdek sutures and is re-inforced by suturing lung over it. Any thickened visceral or parietal pleura is removed and efficient intercostal suction drainage established.

Any of the complications of thoracotomy or of the special operations discussed, may occur and should be treated appropriately.

References

Belsey, R. H. R. (1965). 'Reconstruction of the oesophagus with the left colon.' *J. thorac. cardiovasc. Surg.* **49**, 33

Johnson, J. *et al.* (1956). 'Oesophageal exclusion for persistent fistula following spontaneous rupture of the oesophagus.' *J. thorac. cardiovasc. Surg.* **32**, 827

Johnson, J. and Schwegman, C. W. (1967). 'Iatrogenic and spontaneous perforation of the oesophagus.' *Am. J. Gastroent.* **47**, 365

Kerr, W. F. (1968). 'Emergency oesophagectomy.' *Thorax* **23**, 204

Thal, A. P. (1968). 'A unified approach to surgical problems of the oesophagogastric junction.' *Ann. Surg.* **168**, 542

Thal, A. P. (1970). Discussion of Abbott, O.A. *et al.* (1970)

[The illustrations for this Chapter on Management of Distension Ruptures and Instrumental Perforations of the Oesophagus were drawn by Mr. G. Lyth.]

Congenital Oesophageal Atresia and Tracheo-oesophageal Fistula

Keith D. Roberts, Ch.M., F.R.C.S.
Consultant Paediatric Cardiothoracic Surgeon, The Children's Hospital, Birmingham;
Senior Clinical Lecturer in Surgery, University of Birmingham

Gross (1953) grouped congenital oesophageal obstructions and fistulous communications with the respiratory tract into six types (*see* Table 1).

Table 1
Clinical Features in the Various Types of Oesophageal Abnormality

Clinical feature	*Group A*	*Group B*	*Group C*	*Group D*	*Group E*	*Group F*
Excess oral mucus	Always	Perhaps	Always	Perhaps	No	Perhaps
Cough and cyanosis with feeds	Always	Always	Always	Always	Perhaps	Perhaps
'Wet' bronchial tree	Usually	May be severe	Usually	May be severe	Perhaps	Perhaps
Abdominal distension	Never	Never	Frequent	Frequent	Frequent	No

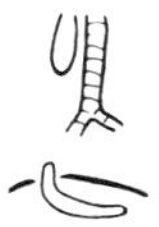

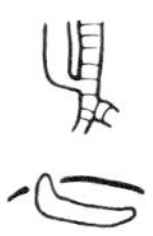

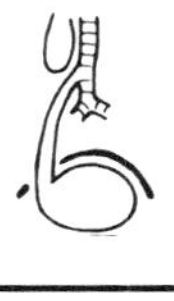

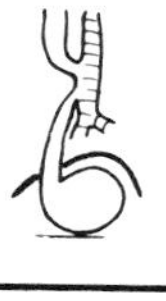

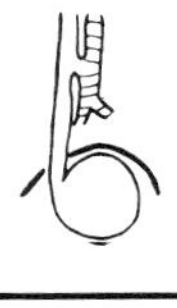

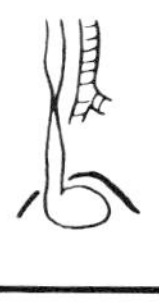

Group A. Oesophageal atresia without tracheo-oesophageal fistula, the upper oesophagus ending blindly, and the lower oesophagus beginning blindly with a considerable gap between the two segments.
Group B. Oesophageal atresia with a fistula between the upper pouch and the trachea, but the lower oesophagus not in communication with the respiratory tract.
Group C. Oesophageal atresia, the upper pouch being blind and the lower oesophageal segment communicating with the trachea. This is the common variety and constitutes about 90 per cent of all cases. Variation occurs between those with the two portions of the oesophagus overlapping with some degree of muscular continuity, to those with a considerable gap between the segments, the upper oesophagus lying in the neck and the tracheo-oesophageal fistula being connected to the trachea in the region of the right bronchus.
Group D. Oesophageal atresia with both segments communicating with the trachea by separate fistulae.
Group E. A tracheo-oesophageal fistula but without atresia (so called 'H-fistula').
Group F. Congenital stenosis of the oesophagus.

The clinical features of congenital oesophageal atresia are primarily those of complete obstruction, namely the inability of the infant to swallow his saliva so that a characteristic fine frothy mucus is continually produced in his mouth, while there may be episodes of choking and cyanosis particularly if the diagnosis has not been suspected and a feed is given with 'spill-over' into the larynx. It cannot be too strongly emphasized that the diagnosis should always be suspected and made *before* any feed is given. In oesophageal atresia an important clue is the presence of maternal hydramnios in the antenatal history, this being present in well over 50 per cent of the cases. In Group C and D cases contamination of the lungs is possible not only from inhalation of infected saliva but also from regurgitation of gastric juice through the distal fistula into the bronchial tree. 'Paradoxical haematemesis' may occur (Lecutier, 1955), and the pharyngeal contents may be bile stained owing to regurgitation of alimentary contents into the trachea and so into the mouth. Respiratory obstruction with stridor may be due to a fold of mucous membrane in the trachea at the site of the fistula (Franklin and Graham, 1953). Occasionally air may be forced into the stomach in large volumes when the infant cries so that the abdomen is distended and tympanitic, with embarrassment of diaphragmatic movement and pulmonary ventilation. Other congenital defects (high intestinal atresia, imperforate anus, renal abnormalities and congenital cardiac defects) may be present, comprising 20 per cent in one series (Roberts, 1958), although not necessarily life-threatening.

Group E cases form a special group in that the symptoms of coughing and choking with feeds, and abdominal distension, may not be very marked in the first few days after birth, so that only episodes of recurrent pneumonitis may lead to the suspicion of a tracheo-oesophageal communication.

PRE-OPERATIVE CARE

Diagnosis

Congenital obstruction of the oesophagus is demonstrated by passage of a 10 Ch plastic radio-opaque catheter (such as the Argyle* feeding tube) through the mouth and into the oesophagus. In atresia it will usually be held up 10 cm from the alveolus, and a radiograph will demonstrate the level of obstruction, together with the presence of gas in the stomach and intestines showing that a distal tracheo-oesophageal fistula is present. In duodenal atresia gas will not, of course, pass beyond the point of duodenal obstruction, and this is an important diagnosis to make since this condition may readily be treated at the same time as the oesophageal one. There is no virtue and severe disadvantage in introducing radio-opaque material such as iodized oil into the blind pouch, even if done under direct screening observation, because of the risk of 'spill-over'. Oesophagoscopy (which does not require an anaesthetic in the neonate) will confirm the diagnosis and may reveal the presence of a Group B or Group D upper fistula. A Group E abnormality ('H-fistula') can be difficult to demonstrate by oesophagoscopy and/or bronchoscopy, but may be facilitated by positive pressure ventilation by the anaesthetist, when gas bubbles can be seen to enter the oesophagus. The most useful diagnostic aid is the use of cine-radiography and the introduction of an aqueous opaque contrast medium with the child prone. This has the advantage that other conditions, such as pharyngeal or oesophageal inco-ordination which may mimic tracheo-oesophageal fistula, can be excluded.

Preparation

Although urgent operation is required this need not, and in many cases should not, be *immediate.* Time should be allowed for the infant's temperature, often low on admission, to be restored to normal. The infant should be nursed in a humidified oxygen-enriched atmosphere in an incubator with a 10° head down tilt, and his position changed from side to side every 30 min. The pharynx must be aspirated repeatedly (or continuously via a Replogle* tube (1963) attached to low suction). Antibiotic therapy is commenced and vitamin K_1 is given by intramuscular injection in view of the normal fall in prothrombin level during the first few days of life. In the case of an H-fistula a nasogastric tube may be required to decompress a distended stomach, but only rarely in other groups is a preliminary gastrostomy required for this purpose.

*Sherwood Medical Industries, Inc., St. Louis, Missouri, U.S.A.

Choice of operation

In Group C and D whenever possible oesophageal continuity should be restored by primary oesophageal anastomosis. If the gap between the oesophageal segments is too great for an immediate anastomosis then either the tracheo-oesophageal fistula is closed and a gastrostomy performed, so that growth of the upper pouch will permit a delayed anastomosis as described by Howard and Myers (1965); or the fistula is closed, a cervical oesophagostomy is done together with a gastrostomy, reconstruction of the oesophagus using colon (Waterston, 1967) being delayed until the infant has grown to about 6 kg weight.

In Group A and B the multiple stage plan of cervical oesophagostomy, gastrostomy and an oesophageal replacement procedure is usually employed.

Group E patients require separation of the oesophagus and trachea at the site of the fistula with repair of both structures, and (in all but the highest communications which are explored through a cervical incision) this is done through a thoracotomy.

Anaesthesia

No premedication is required. An intravenous infusion of dextrose/saline is given via a percutaneous cannulation and a paediatric microset. The infant is kept on a heat-controlled water mattress and a thermistor probe is inserted into the rectum and one applied to the skin of the abdomen. ECG electrodes are applied to the limbs. Endotracheal intubation is carried out without anaesthesia; the tube is aspirated and then connected to a nitrous oxide/oxygen gas mixture with added halothane if necessary. Where there is a fistula between the distal oesophagus and trachea the infant is allowed to breathe spontaneously to avoid the distension of the stomach resulting from positive pressure ventilation, until the intercostal space is about to be entered when an intravenous relaxant is given and intermittent positive pressure ventilation commenced. It is important that the surgeon then controls the distal oesophagus *as soon as possible* to avoid anaesthetic gases passing down it into the stomach.

PRIMARY OESOPHAGEAL ANASTOMOSIS

1

The incision

The infant is positioned on his left side with a rolled towel or sorbo-rubber pad under the thorax towards the axilla. The skin incision is almost transverse in line with the ribs (not truly periscapular) and is positioned just below the inferior angle of the scapula extending from the lateral border of the trapezius to the nipple line. Apart from the skin itself all cutting is with surgical diathermy so that blood loss is minimal. The periosteum on the upper border of the fifth rib is incised and at this point the anaesthetist gives the intravenous relaxant. The periosteum and intercostal muscles are stripped from the rib and the thorax is entered through the fourth intercostal space. The transpleural approach is preferred as it gives more rapid control of the fistula and renders the anaesthetist's task much easier.

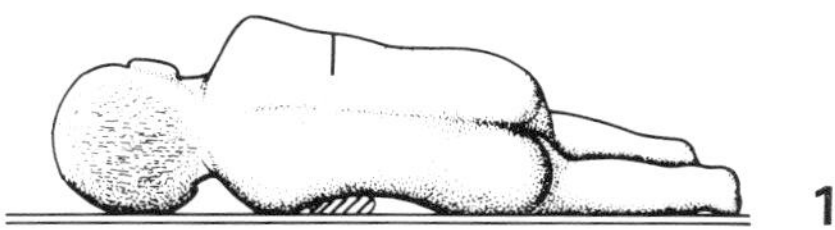

1

2

Control of the fistula

The lung is retracted exposing the mediastinal pleura, which is opened below the vena azygos arch to display the distal oesophagus which distends with gas as the anaesthetist inflates the lungs. A tape is passed around the oesophagus (taking care not to injure the vagi) and gentle traction on this prevents further gas leak into the stomach.

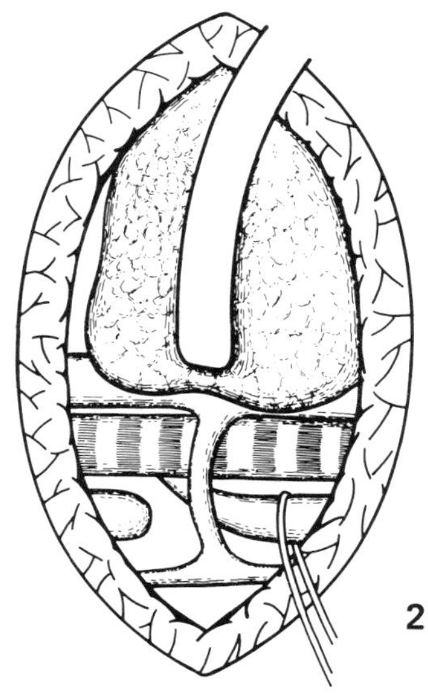

2

3

Closure of the fistula

The incision in the mediastinal pleura is carried upwards to the apex of the thorax, the azygos arch being divided between ligatures. The distal oesophagus is carefully dissected with scissors to the point where it enters the membranous portion of the trachea as the tracheo-oesophageal fistula, which is then divided parallel to and close to the trachea. The lower oesophagus is allowed to lie free in the wound, while the tracheal end of the fistula is closed with interrupted 6/0 sutures on atraumatic needles (synthetic material is preferred to silk which can provoke excessive fibrous reaction).

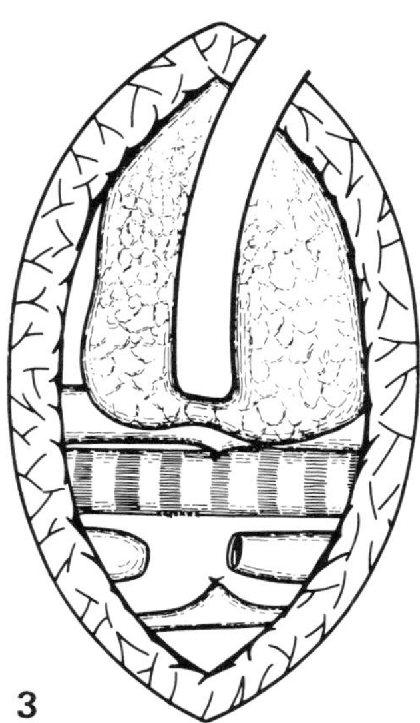

3

4

Mobilization of the blind upper segment

This, unless very high, can usually be seen as a pale pink-white bulge at the apex of the pleura lying behind the trachea. If difficulty in recognition is encountered the anaesthetist can pass a plastic catheter through the mouth into the pouch. Two 6/0 stay sutures are inserted into the lower border of the pouch, and by traction on these and careful dissection the pouch is freed. Much caution is required in separating the upper segment from the membranous portion of the trachea, and care must be exercised not to injure this. With full mobilization the pouch can be drawn down into the thoracic cavity to a variable extent.

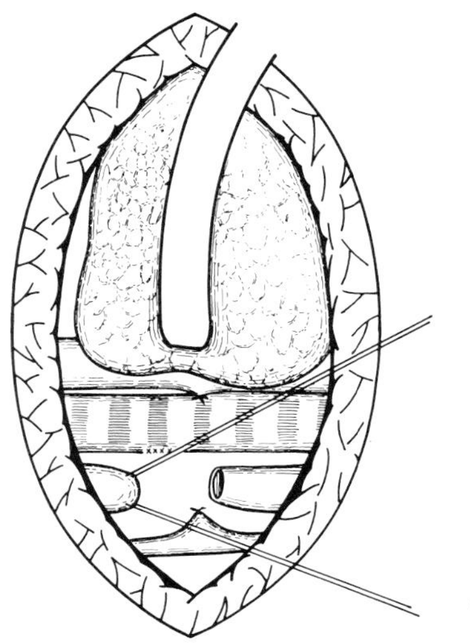

4

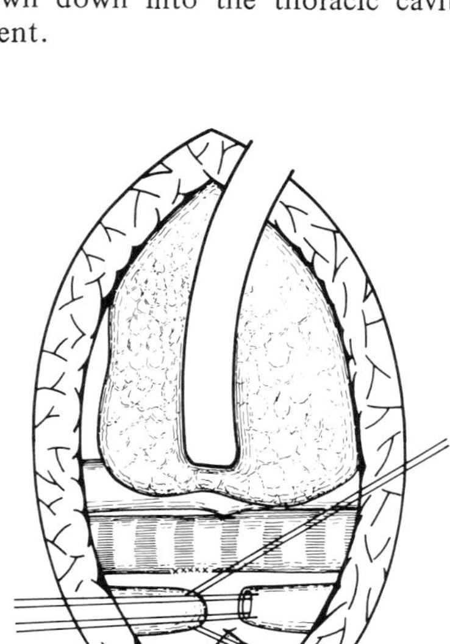

5

5

Mobilization of the lower segment

This is freed from its mediastinal bed, if necessary as far as the oesophageal hiatus, segmental oesophageal arteries being coagulated and divided, until by *gentle* traction on two 6/0 stay sutures the upper and lower segments can be approximated without undue tension. The muscular coat of the lower segment is thin, and its blood supply is easily imperilled by rough handling which must be avoided.

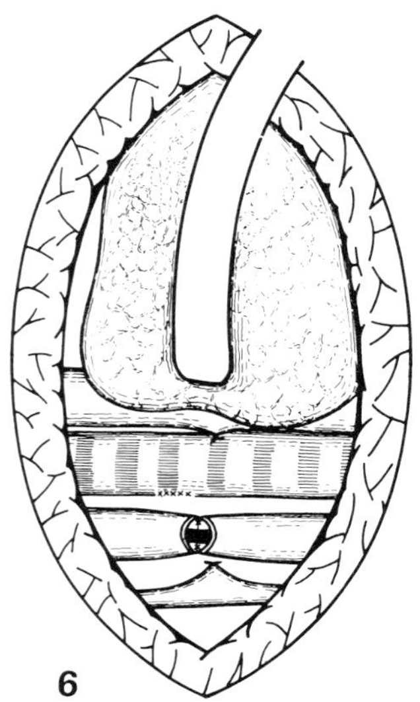

6

6

Beginning the anastomosis

The blind upper segment is opened at its apex, a relatively *small* opening being made in view of the disparity in size between the large upper and smaller distal segments. The muscle coat of the upper pouch is thick, in contradistinction to that of the distal segment. A posterior layer of interrupted 6/0 atraumatic synthetic fibre sutures is introduced and tied, care being taken to pick up the muscle coat and mucosa of each segment. The anaesthetist now passes an 8 Ch Argyle feeding tube through the nose into the upper oesophagus, and it is guided into the distal oesophagus and so on into the stomach; the tube is left open to allow gas to escape from the stomach. The nasogastric tube is fixed firmly to the face with adhesive tape.

7

Completion of the anastomosis

An anterior row of interrupted 6/0 sutures is inserted and tied over the indwelling nasogastric tube; the mediastinal pleura is then sutured over the repaired oesophagus and trachea with fine interrupted sutures.

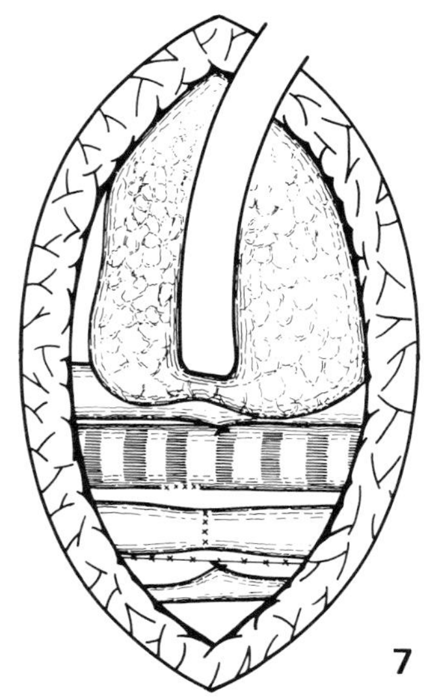
7

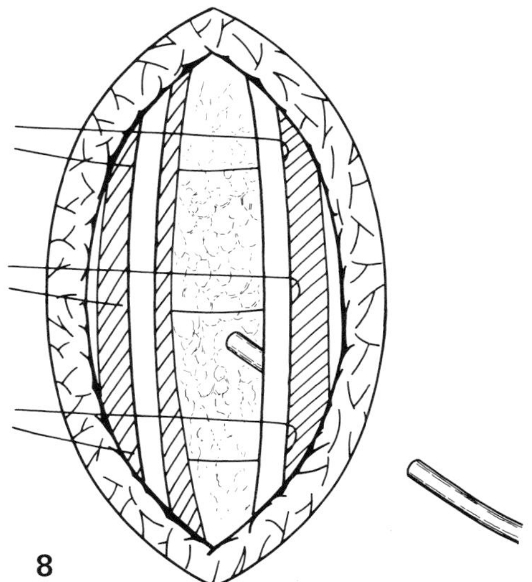
8

8

Closure of the chest

An intercostal drainage tube attached to an underwater seal and gentle suction is introduced and the lung re-expanded fully. Three non-absorbable pericostal sutures are inserted and tied. The muscle layers and fat are closed with continuous Dexon* sutures and the skin by a continuous Dexon subcuticular stitch.

*Davis and Geck, Cyanamid of Great Britain, Gosport, Hampshire.

DELAYED OESOPHAGEAL ANASTOMOSIS

This procedure, first described by Howard and Myers (1965), may be used in Group C patients in whom immediate anastomosis is not possible because the gap between the segments is too great. The fistula is disconnected as described previously and the upper pouch mobilized, but if the two segments cannot be approximated the distal oesophageal segment is closed with interrupted sutures and then anchored as high as possible to the prevertebral fascia. It is useful to mark this site by a metal haemostatic clip as suggested by Hamilton (1966).

A gastrostomy is done for feeding purposes and the upper blind oesophagus is kept empty by continuous gentle suction on a Replogle catheter. Elongation of the upper segment may be facilitated by introducing a mercury-filled bougie twice daily, and most growth is to be expected in the first 2–3 weeks, with progressively smaller increments of lengthening up to 6–8 weeks. Reduction of the gap can be judged radiologically by measuring the distance between the end of the bougie and the metal clip. After suitable lengthening has been achieved, the chest is re-opened and the anastomosis carried out as described previously.

Although of most use in Group C patients, success from the above technique has also been reported in Group A cases (Hayes, Woolley and Snyder, 1966) although these are usually considered more suitable for a colon interposition.

TRACHEO-OESOPHAGEAL FISTULA (GROUP E)

Very high communications are better closed through a cervical incision, but the lower ones (including instances of recurrence of tracheo-oesophageal fistula following repair of Group C patients) are dealt with at thoracotomy.

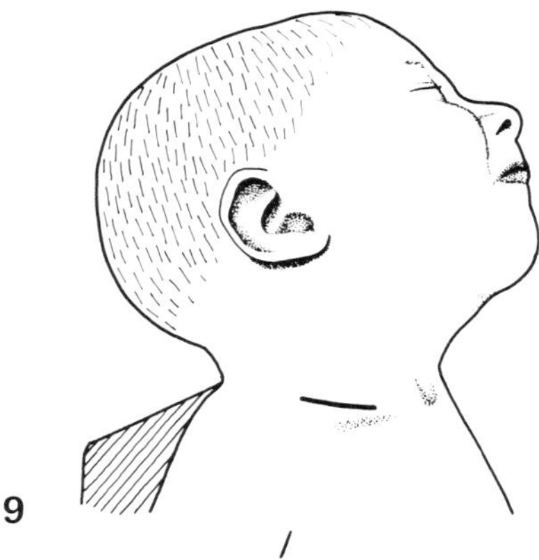

9

The cervical operation

9

Position of patient

The infant is placed on his back with his head to the left and a folded towel under the right shoulder. The right side is operated on to avoid risk to the thoracic duct, and an incision is made 1 cm above the clavicle parallel to its medial half.

10

Identification of the fistula

The sternal head of the sternomastoid is divided, the carotid sheath is identified and the plane behind the sheath is opened up. Dissection is carried out posterior and parallel to the trachea, and care is taken to identify and preserve the right recurrent laryngeal nerve. The oesophagus is identified from its muscle fibres, and a tape is passed around it below the fistula.

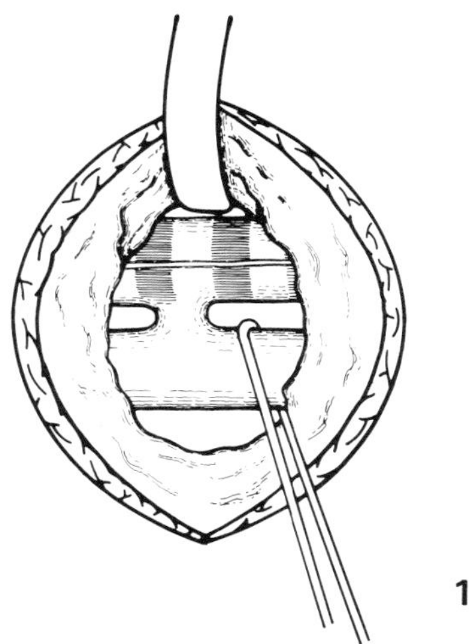

10

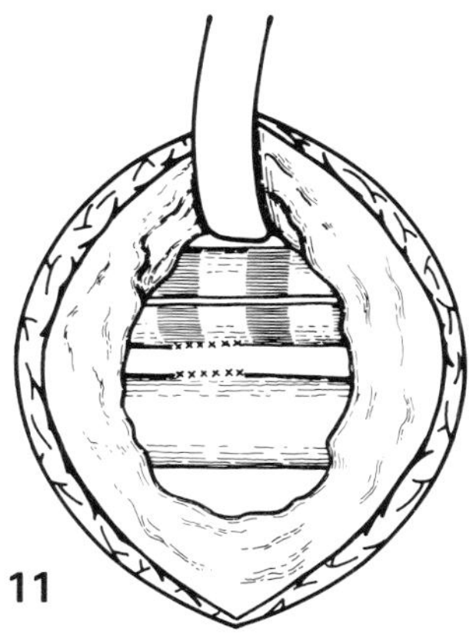

11

11

Division and closure of the fistula

Traction on the tape allows the fistula to be dissected. The upper and lower limits are defined and the fistula is then divided with a knife. The tracheal end is closed first with interrupted 6/0 synthetic atraumatic sutures, and then the oesophageal wound is similarly repaired taking care to pick up mucosa as well as muscle. An 8 Ch Argyle nasogastric tube is introduced for feeding purposes for the first 2–3 days, and a Redivac* drain is inserted through a small stab incision. The sternomastoid is repaired with interrupted Dexon sutures, and the wound is then closed in layers with continuous Dexon, a subcuticular suture being used to approximate the skin.

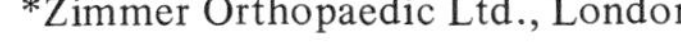

*Zimmer Orthopaedic Ltd., London

The thoracic operation

The initial stages of this are the same as for primary oesophageal anastomosis for oesophageal atresia.

12

Identification of the fistula

After opening the chest the oesophagus is taped below the fistula, as in the primary oesophageal atresia repair operation in order to control leak of anaesthetic gases into the stomach. The azygos vein is doubly ligated and divided, and the upper part of the oesophagus is also encircled by a tape.

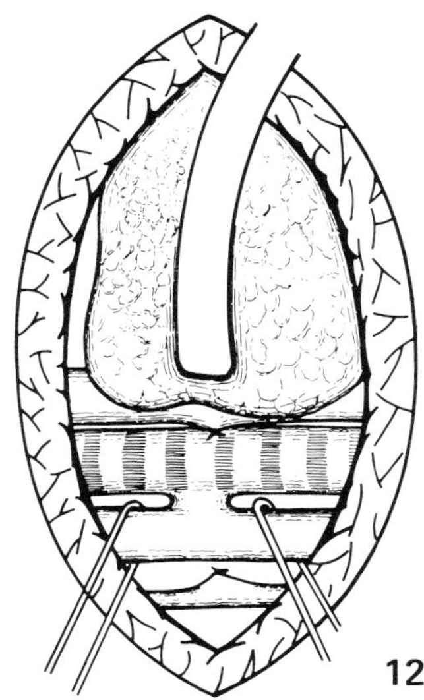

12

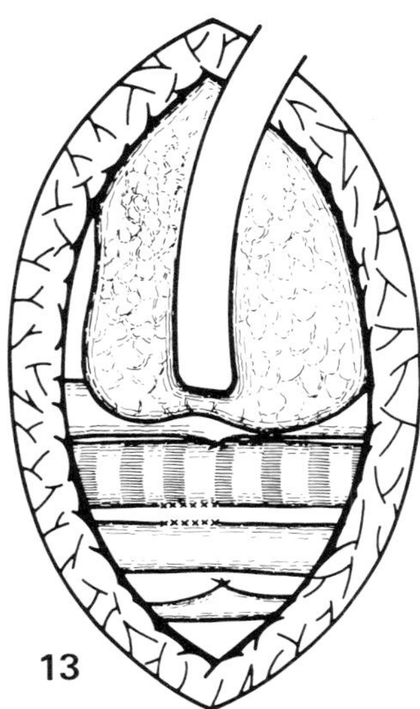

13

13

Closure of the fistula

By traction on the tapes and cautious dissection with scissors the oesophagus above and below the fistula is freed from the trachea to the upper and lower margins of the fistula. This is then incised with a knife parallel to the trachea and the tracheal end closed with interrupted 6/0 atraumatic synthetic sutures. The oesophagus is closed similarly, taking care to include both mucosa and muscular coats. An 8 Ch Argyle nasogastric tube is introduced and left *in situ* for 2–3 days.

The repair is covered with mediastinal pleura and the chest closure is as detailed in primary anastomosis.

OESOPHAGEAL REPLACEMENT WITH COLON

In Group A patients, and those Group C cases in whom it is decided not to proceed to primary or delayed oesophageal anastomosis, it is necessary to ensure that the baby will not die of inhalation pneumonia, and that he can be fed pending his reconstruction. Drainage of the blind upper oesophagus is achieved by cervical oesophagostomy, the pouch being exteriorized and opened just to the left of the mid-line above the suprasternal notch. The exposure for this is similar to that described in the cervical operation for Group E tracheo-oesophageal fistula, except that the operation is done on the left side of the neck. A Stamm gastrostomy is done through a small left transverse upper abdominal incision, the gastrostomy tube being brought through a separate stab incision in the abdominal wall above the laparotomy wound.

In Group A patients it is not necessary to open the chest, but this will have already been done in Group C patients in whom, in any case, it is necessary to disconnect the tracheo-oesophageal fistula and close both the tracheal and oesophageal ends.

It is important in such patients to preserve the mechanism of feeding and swallowing in response to hunger, so that food should be given by mouth at the same time as gastrostomy feeds, being allowed to discharge through the cervical oesophagostomy into a dressing.

Transverse colon is preferred in the intrapleural (left mediastinal) position, rather than in the retrosternal site. Retrosternal colon has to be anastomosed to the stomach and it is impossible to control reflux, so that a 'reflux' colitis can occur, with the possibility of peptic ulceration. In the intrapleural operation the cardio-oesophageal sphincter mechanism is preserved.

Prior to operation low-residue gastrostomy feeds are given, such as Vivonex*. The bowel is prepared with a pre-operative course of succinylsulphathiazole and neomycin, but enemata are unnecessary.

*Eaton Laboratories, London

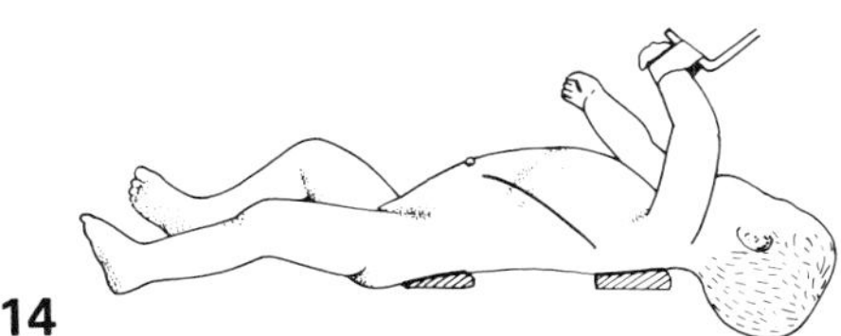

14

14

The incision

The baby is positioned on his right side with a slight backward inclination and a pad is placed under the right loin. The left arm is placed so that, with a pad under the shoulder and the head turned to the right, the left cervical oesophagostomy is accessible. Drapes are applied to leave an area exposed for an abdomino-thoracic incision, and also the suprasternal and left cervical region. The abdomen and chest are opened through an abdominothoracic incision passing below the gastrostomy stoma (the tube having been removed prior to operation), across the costal margin and into the eighth intercostal space. The diaphragm is incised radially in the line of the incision, but not across the lateral pillar of the right crus. A transverse incision is made in the neck below the oesophageal stoma and the sternal head of the sternomastoid is divided.

15

Mobilization of the colon

The lienorenal ligament is divided so that the spleen, tail of the pancreas and stomach can be retracted medially, exposing the kidney and suprarenal gland. The transverse colon is seen at the lower limit of the wound and the gastrocolic omentum is divided. The mediastinal pleura over the lower oesophagus is divided; the oesophagus is freed from its bed taking care to avoid injury to the vagi. It is convenient to pass a tape (not shown) around the oesophagus so that it can be drawn towards the surgeon when the anastomosis is being performed.

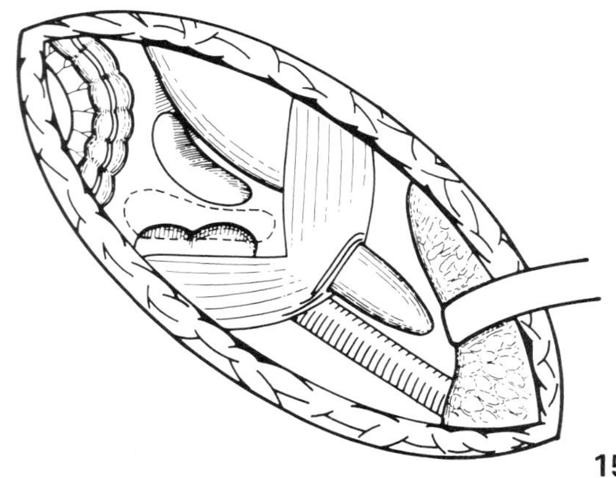

15

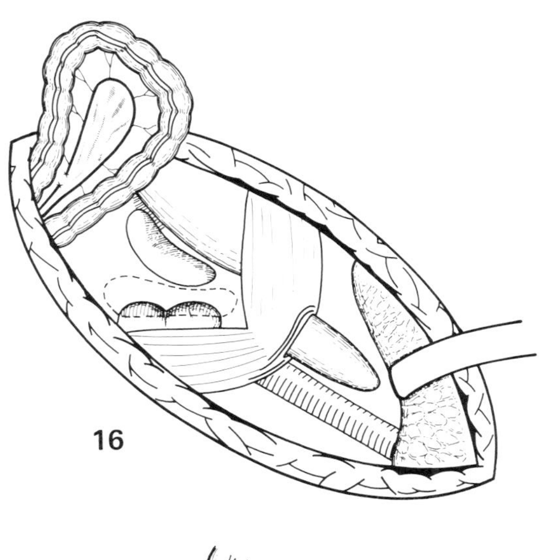

16

16

Preparation of the pedicled colon segment

The middle colic artery is ligated close to its origin and divided, taking care not to imperil the lumen at the bifurcation. Before dividing the colon a careful estimate is made of the length required to bridge the gap between the lower oesophagus and the neck. If necessary the right colic artery must be divided. The transverse colon is now supplied by the ascending branch of the left colic artery. The colon is divided in the region of the flexures. A tunnel is made from the apex of the pleura to the cervical incision, lying medial and anterior to the subclavian artery, care being taken to avoid injury to the subclavian vein and obstruction of the airway. It is convenient to pass a nylon tape through the tunnel in order to facilitate positioning of the colon.

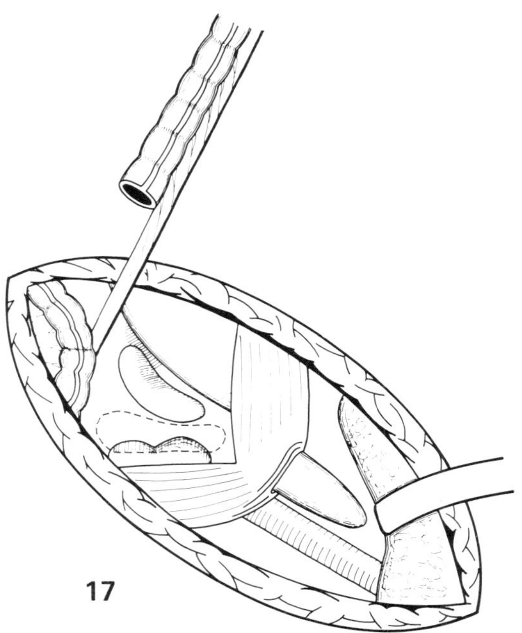

17

17

Positioning of the colon

Continuity of the colon is restored by end-to-end anastomosis in two layers using interrupted 6/0 synthetic atraumatic sutures. The proximal end of the pedicled colon is ligated and attached to the nylon tape. It is then carefully drawn behind the hilum of the lung until it appears in the neck. The pedicle *must* lie without tension in the space behind the displaced spleen and anterior to the kidney. The colon segment will be found to be too long distally, and redundant colon is carefully excised, preserving the left colic artery, so that an anastomosis without tension can be made to the distal oesophagus.

18

Distal oesophagocolic anastomosis

After trimming back the redundant colon an oblique incision is made in the distal oesophageal segment, which can conveniently be drawn towards the operator by an encircling tape (not shown). A one-layer anastomosis of interrupted 6/0 synthetic atraumatic sutures is made between the end of the colon and the oesophagus, care again being taken not to imperil the blood flow in the pedicle.

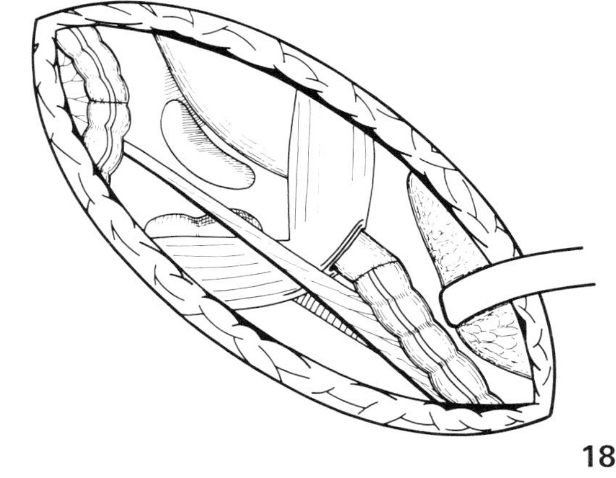
18

19

Closure of the wound

The diaphragm is carefully sutured with interrupted sutures in front of the pedicle so as not to compromise its blood flow; the closure is carried forwards to the costal margin and so on to the transversus abdominis/internal oblique/peritoneum layer. Two strong through-and-through sutures are passed through the divided costal margin and repaired diaphragm to be tied when the thoracic part of the incision is closed; this step is important in order to ensure that the diaphragm is securely attached at this point. Pericostal sutures are used to approximate the ribs and the wound is closed in layers, leaving an intercostal pleural drain inserted via a stab incision and attached to underwater sealed drainage with gentle suction. The gastrostomy tube is then re-inserted.

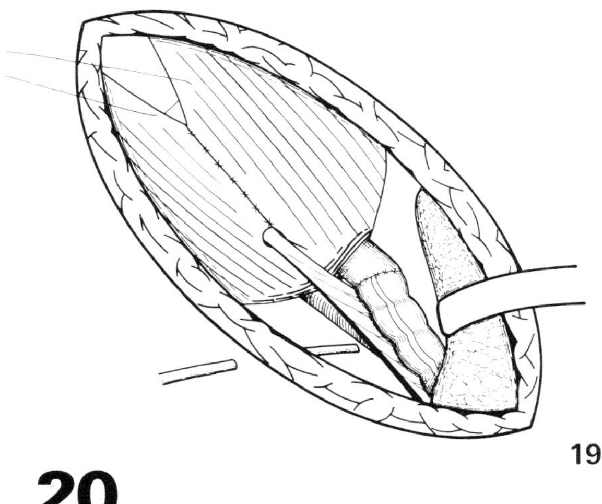
19

20

The cervical anastomosis

This may be done immediately or may be deferred for 1–2 weeks, which has the advantages that the viability of the colon is established without doubt, and peristaltic activity will have returned to it. If the delayed anastomosis is decided upon, the ligature attaching the colonic segment to the nylon tape is removed and the colon is anchored to the skin by interrupted sutures. When the anastomosis is done the oesophagus and colon are dissected free of any scar tissue so that after trimming back they lie together without tension. A posterior layer of interrupted 6/0 synthetic atraumatic sutures is inserted and tied and a 10 Ch Replogle tube is passed through the nose into the oesophagus and across the anastomosis into the colon. The anterior layer is completed and the wound is closed leaving a small corrugated or Redivac drain down to the anastomosis.

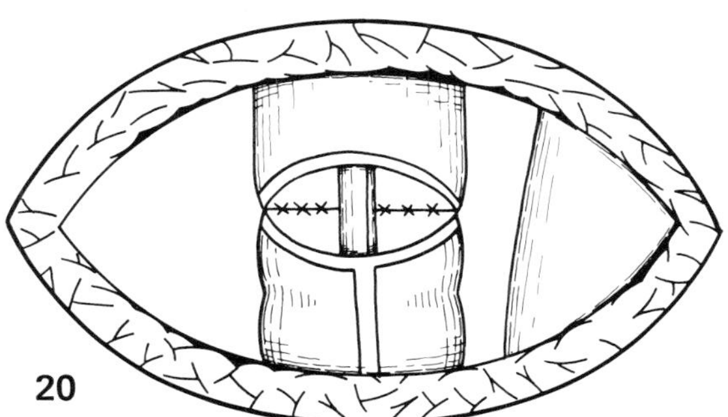
20

POSTOPERATIVE CARE

Infants who have had oesophageal anastomotic operations or repair of tracheo-oesophageal fistula are nursed in an incubator in a moist atmosphere which is oxygen-enriched if necessary. Antibiotic therapy will be needed for the first few days particularly if aspiration pneumonitis has been present pre-operatively. Lobar or lung collapse will require endotracheal intubation with suction and possibly bronchial lavage. Intercostal drainage is removed when chest radiographs show full lung expansion with no pleural fluid or air—usually in 24–48 hours. Nasogastric tube feeds are allowed after 48 hours, prior to which intravenous fluid is given, and, in the case of an oesophageal anastomosis radiological examination using a swallow of aqueous contrast medium is carried out on the seventh day in order to see if oral feeds may be commenced, supplemented at first by tube feeds.

Following oesophageal anastomosis with excessive tension the two most probable complications are leakage and stricture formation. An oesophago-pleural leak is initially managed by intercostal drainage, with nasogastric or gastrostomy feeding, and, if not excessive and the lung is kept expanded, will usually heal. A life-threatening huge leak will require a salvage procedure of ligation of the distal oesophagus, exteriorization of the proximal oesophagus on the neck, and a feeding gastrostomy; continuity is restored later by a colon interposition.

Stricture formation almost always responds to intermittent dilatation, but in the early stages difficulties with oral feeding may necessitate a gastrostomy.

In the case of staged colon replacement it is important to maintain the swallowing reflex by giving food by mouth while the infant is awaiting reconstruction. The infant does not require hospitalization during the waiting time as his mother can be taught to give his gastrostomy feeds. Stenosis of the oesophageal stoma in the neck may need periodic dilatation.

After the positioning of the colonic segment in colon reconstruction the gastrostomy tube should be drained, and intravenous fluids given until post-operative ileus has recovered and stools are being passed, when gastrostomy feeds can be resumed. The intercostal tube can usually be removed after 48 hr.

When the cervical anastomosis has been completed, the Replogle tube is kept on gentle suction to prevent distension of the colonic segment due to air swallowing. The neck drain is removed after 3 days, and, provided there is no anastomotic leak in the neck, the Replogle tube can be removed on the fourth day and oral feeds commenced in small amounts, supplemented by gastrostomy feeds. The gastrostomy tube is retained until oral feeding is well established, when it is removed and the sinus allowed to close.

References

Franklin, R. H. and Graham, A. J. P. (1953). 'Atresia of the oesophagus with an abnormal tracheal fold.' *Thorax* **8**, 102

Gross, R. E. (1953). *The Surgery of Infancy and Childhood*. Philadelphia and London: Saunders

Hamilton, J. P. (1966). 'Esophageal atresia: technical points in the staged procedure leading to esophageal anastomosis.' *J. pediat. Surg.* **1**, 253

Hayes, D. M., Woolley, M. M. and Snyder, W. H. (1966). 'Esophageal atresia and tracheo-esophageal fistula: management of the uncommon types.' *J. pediat. Surg.* **1**, 240

Howard, R. and Myers, N. A. (1965). 'Esophageal atresia: A technique for elongating the upper pouch.' *Surgery* **58**, 725

Lecutier, E. R. (1955). 'Paradoxical haematemesis in oesophageal atresia.' *Br. med. J.* **1**, 647

Replogle, R. L. (1963). 'Esophageal atresia: plastic sump catheter for drainage of the proximal pouch.' *Surgery* **54**, 296

Roberts, K. D. (1958). 'Congenital oesophageal atresia and tracheo-oesophageal fistula.' *Thorax* **13**, 116

Waterston, D. J. (1967). 'Colonic replacement of oesophagus (intrathoracic).' *Surg. Clins N. Am.* **44**, 6

[*The illustrations for this Chapter on Congenital Oesophageal Atresia and Tracheo-oesophageal Fistula were drawn by the Author.*]

Transabdominal Repair of Hiatus Hernia

J. W. P. Gummer, M.S., F.R.C.S.
Consultant Surgeon, Central Middlesex Hospital, London

PRE-OPERATIVE

Pre-operative considerations

The most important pre-operative consideration is the establishment of the diagnosis and the exclusion of other conditions as the cause of the symptoms. A careful history is essential and the diagnosis is mainly established by barium swallow and meal examination augmented, if thought necessary, by oesophageal pressure studies and oesophagoscopy. The possibility of associated conditions such as hyperacidity, duodenal ulcer and gall-stones should be remembered.

Indication for surgery

The usual reason for advising surgery for the treatment of a hiatus hernia is the failure of medical management to relieve the symptoms. Such measures as weight loss, regular meals, antacids and the avoidance of stooping are the usual ones adopted. Early evidence of stricture formation in the lower oesophagus is a definite indication for surgical repair and dilatation may have to be carried out at the same time.

Thoracic or abdominal approach?

The choice of approach is very largely influenced by the personal preference and training of the surgeon concerned. In the majority of cases it is the author's experience that it is easier to obtain a sound repair from below rather than from above. The abdominal approach also allows a full laparotomy to be performed and for associated intra-abdominal lesions to be dealt with. There are some cases where the transthoracic approach has advantages and a surgeon dealing with hiatus hernias should have a working knowledge of both approaches. It is sometimes difficult to obtain a good access to the hiatus via the abdominal approach in an extremely obese patient and the thoracic approach may have an advantage. The large fixed hiatus hernia should also be approached transthoracically and the assessment of these cases requires oesophagoscopy.

Object of operation

The object of the operation is the prevention of acid and peptic reflux from the stomach into the oesophagus. In the author's opinion this can best be achieved by obtaining a long length of intra-abdominal oesophagus and not just restoring the normal anatomy. The operative technique to be described is aimed at obtaining this objective.

Pre-operative preparation

The patient should be prepared in the usual way for a major upper abdominal operation. Opinions differ as to whether or not a nasogastric tube should be passed. A nasogastric tube may be necessary to empty the stomach of fluid and gas during the operation, but if it is left in for any time after the operation it may predispose to reflux and oesophageal damage. On the whole a nasogastric tube is not recommended.

Position of patient

The patient should be lying on the operating table in the ordinary supine position. The table should be tilted to raise the head and to lower the legs. This will improve access to the oesophagogastric region and drop the intestine and omentum, which is frequently large and fatty, away.

THE OPERATION

The incision

A long left upper paramedian incision gives a good approach to the hiatal region and should be made with the surgeon standing to the patient's right side. A full laparotomy should then be performed both to confirm the diagnosis and to exclude any other significant lesion.

1

Liver mobilization

Before it is possible to get a good view of the hiatal region it is necessary to mobilize and retract the left lobe of the liver. This is done by dividing the left triangular ligament in exactly the same way as for truncal vagotomy. Care should be taken to avoid damaging some large veins close to the diaphragm.

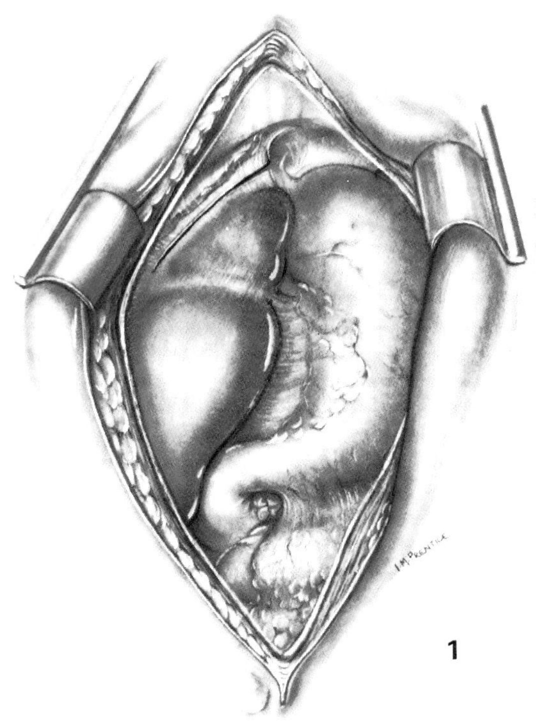

1

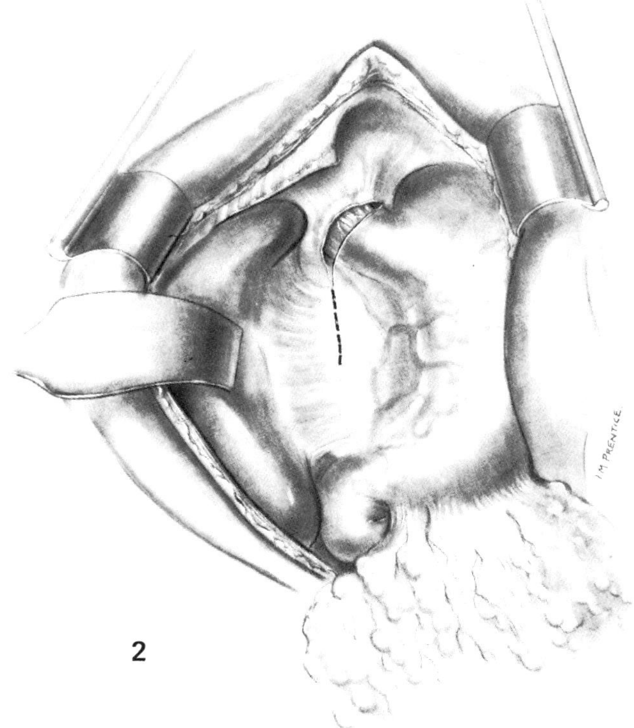

2

2

Peritoneal division

The stomach should now be drawn down as much as possible and this may be effective in reducing the hernia. The peritoneum at the hiatus should then be divided and again this is similar to the technique used in truncal vagotomy. There is, however, a slight difference because there may be two quite separate layers of peritoneum both of which have to be divided before it is possible to pass a finger up through the hiatus and mobilize the lower oesophagus. Care should be taken at this stage to avoid any damage to the vagi.

3

Oesophageal mobilization

Mobilization of the lower oesophagus is performed digitally through the hiatus and should be continued for at least half the length of the oesophagus. Unless this is done thoroughly it will not be possible to obtain a good length of intra-abdominal oesophagus. A rubber sling is passed round the lower oesophagus and this is helpful in both drawing down the oesophagus and in holding it to one side whilst performing the repair.

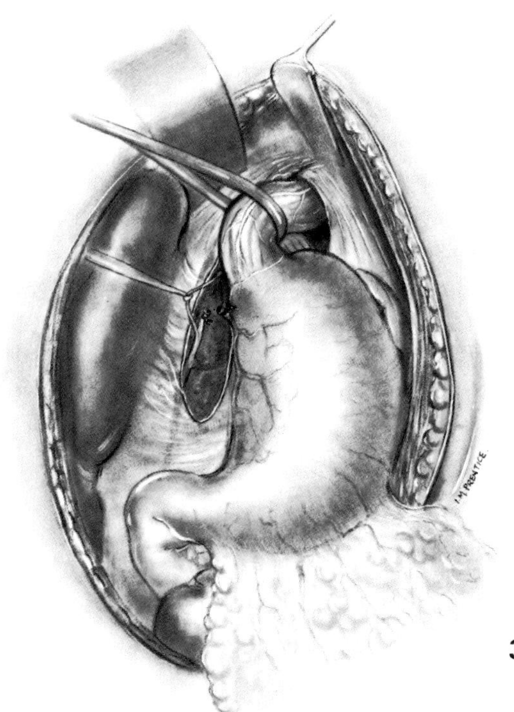

3

Identification of crura

There is usually no difficulty in exposing the left crus. The lower oesophagus and upper stomach are drawn across to the right. Some posterior parietal peritoneum may have to be dissected away and care is necessary to avoid any damage to the spleen.

The right crus may be more difficult to identify and a good view of it will only be obtained if the upper part of the lesser omentum is divided. The upper margin of this structure is defined by the oesophageal mobilization and it is a simple matter to push a finger through the omentum. The division should be performed between ligatures which are passed on an aneurysm needle as the omentum may contain quite a large branch from the left gastric artery. Once the omentum is divided the right crus becomes apparent and the deficiency through which the hernia has developed can be seen.

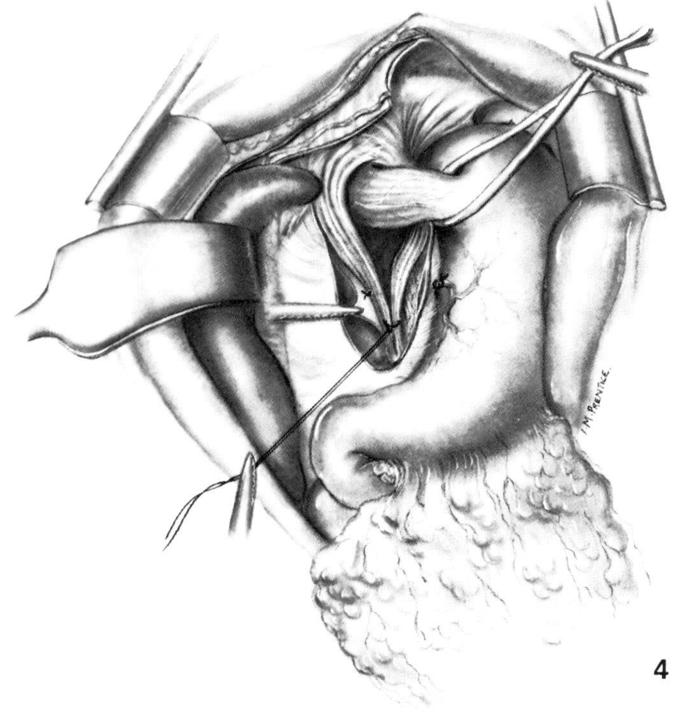

4

4,5&6

Repair

The repair is carried out by suturing the crura together behind the oesophagus until the opening just accomodates the oesophagus. If too many stitches are inserted and the repair made too tight dysphagia will result. The author uses interrupted braided nylon sutures for the repair and large bites should be taken but the stitches should not be tied too tightly.

There is often some difficulty in inserting the first stitch. The oesophagus should be drawn across to the left and a small needle in a long needle-holder is necessary. This stitch is inserted at the bottom of the V made by the two crura and after it has been tied it should be held in an artery forceps.

Traction on this stitch will facilitate the insertion of the remaining stitches.

After each stitch has been inserted the size of the hiatal opening should be checked.

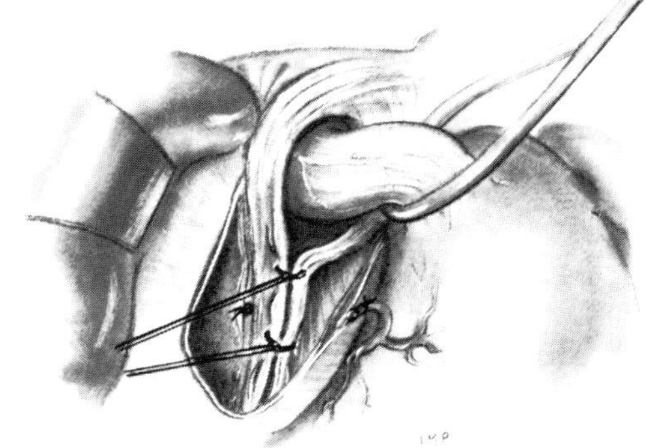

5

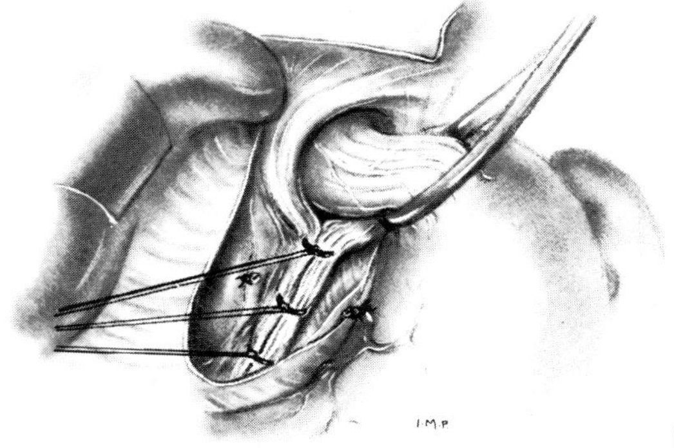

6

7

Oesophagogastric fixation

The final step in the operation is to attach the newly-formed intra-abdominal oesophagus to the fundus of the stomach. This serves to maintain the length of intra-abdominal oesophagus and also narrows the angle of oesophageal entry into the stomach which may be of importance in preventing reflux. To do this the oesophagus is drawn down firmly by the rubber sling. It is then a simple matter to insert three or four interrupted silk sutures between the left side of the oesophagus and the fundus of the stomach.

The rubber sling is now removed and the usual check of swabs, packs and instruments is made before closing the wound in layers. Drainage is not usually necessary.

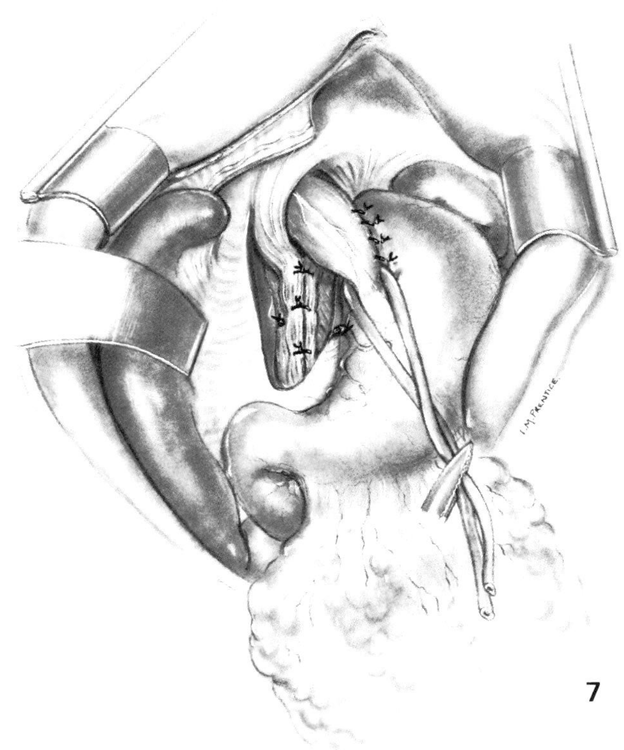

7

POSTOPERATIVE CARE

Unless gastric distension or postoperative ileus develop, nasogastric intubation and suction should be avoided. Only minimal quantities of fluids are allowed orally until normal peristaltic activity has returned after which the diet may be increased rapidly. Post-operative breathing exercises and encouragement to cough are both important as many of these patients are obese and it may be wise to give antibiotics postoperatively as a prophylactic against pulmonary infection.

MANAGEMENT OF ASSOCIATED OESOPHAGEAL STRICTURE

Many of the patients who require surgery for the treatment of their hiatus hernia have an associated stricture at the lower end of the oesophagus. In the early stages most of these strictures will settle provided the reflux is prevented by repairing the hernia. These strictures should be dilated at the time the repair is performed.

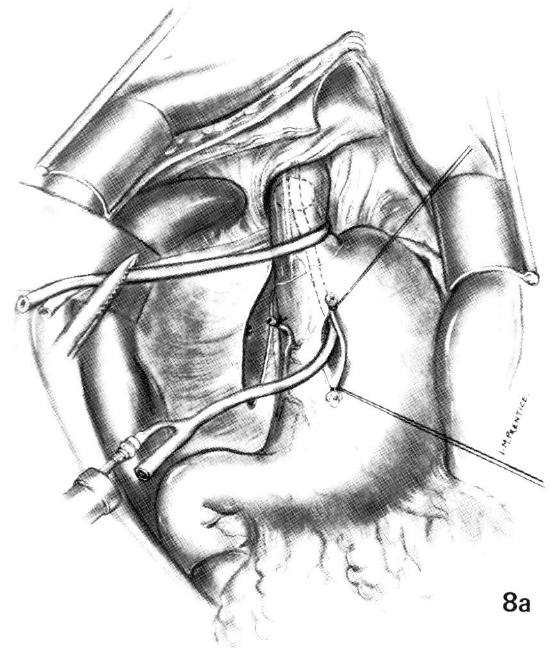

8a

8a&b

A simple and effective way of doing this is as follows. After the lower oesophagus has been fully mobilized a small opening is made in the upper stomach. The stricture can then be explored and stretched digitally after which a Foley catheter is passed up through the stricture. The bag of the catheter is distended with saline and the catheter is then withdrawn back through the stricture. The procedure is repeated two or three times with increasing volumes in the bag of the catheter. The catheter is removed and the opening in the stomach closed in two layers before going on with the repair of the hernia in the usual way.

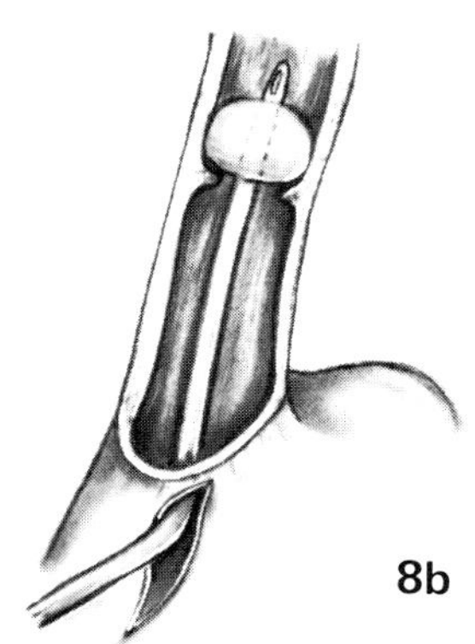

8b

[*The illustrations for this Chapter on Transabdominal Repair of Hiatus Hernia were drawn by Mrs. I. M. Prentice.*]

Thoracic Repair of Hiatus Hernia

G. Keen, M.S., F.R.C.S.
Thoracic and Cardiac Surgeon, United Bristol Hospitals and Frenchay Hospital, Bristol

INTRODUCTION

There are two distinct varieties of hiatus hernia, each with characteristic anatomical features and pathological consequences. By far the commoner (Type I), the so-called sliding hiatus hernia, is associated with failure of the barriers to gastro-oesophageal reflux and may be complicated by oesophagitis and stricture formation. A variant of this group is the syndrome of patulous cardia, in which a hernia is absent but the florid picture of gastro-oesophageal reflux and its consequences may be seen.

The second distinct group (Type II), that of para-oesophageal hiatus hernia (sometimes called rolling hiatus hernia) is not usually associated with gastro-oesophageal reflux. The intrathoracic portion of the stomach is prone to congestion and chronic bleeding, and patients with this condition frequently present with severe anaemia. Such a hernia is liable to incarceration, volvulus and acute dilatation within the chest. The last complication may follow a trivial injury or illness and has caused fatal respiratory embarassment in one elderly patient with a fractured fibula.

Rarely, the two distinct types of hernia may co-exist (mixed Type I and Type II). It is with the surgical treatment of the Type I hernia that this chapter is concerned.

PRE - OPERATIVE

Aims of surgery

(*1*) The correction of gastro-oesophageal reflux. (*2*) Preservation of the ability to belch or vomit when necessary. (*3*) Maintenance of normal swallowing mechanisms.

Anatomical and physiological barriers to gastro-oesophageal reflux

(*1*) The pinchcock effect of contraction of the crura of the diaphragm is undoubtedly contributory although this is an over-simplification of what is a complex mechanism.

(*2*) A lower oesophageal sphincter can be demonstrated manometrically and the point of transition between the negative intra-oesophageal pressure above and the positive pressure below is described as the pressure inversion point. This sphincter is a complicated and dynamic structure which responds to physical and humoral (gastrin) stimuli and provides part of the barrier to the reflux of gastric contents.

(*3*) The antireflux effect of the oblique entry of the oesophagus into the stomach has probably been overemphasized. Certainly, many patients with severe reflux have a normal angle of entry of the oesophagus and in others with an apparently wide angle no reflux can be demonstrated.

(*4*) An adequate length of intra-abdominal oesophagus is considered to play a major part in the prevention of gastro-oesophageal reflux. The positive intra-abdominal pressure flattens this segment against the supporting crura which prevents suction of gastric contents into the chest during inspiration or during changes in posture.

An adequate surgical operation seeks to correct or modify these mechanisms although it is unlikely that any surgical procedure can influence the function of the physiological lower oesophageal sphincter.

Pre-operative assessment

The repair of radiological hiatus hernia in the absence of specific symptoms related to this condition is not advised. Postoperative persistence of symptoms related to undiagnosed and untreated disease elsewhere serves only to discredit the surgical treatment of hiatus hernia.

In addition to eliciting the specific symptoms of gastro-oesophageal reflux, which are aggravated by postural changes and sometimes complicated by dysphagia, oesophagoscopy is required in all patients. This should be conducted using the conventional oesophagoscope or the fibre-optic instrument under local or general anaesthesia. Should general anaesthesia be used, it is important to maintain normal respiration in the patient to ensure that the negative pressure phase of respiration is maintained during which gastro-oesophageal reflux may be observed and the cardia examined under relatively normal conditions. Oesophagoscopy will furthermore ensure the accurate assessment of oesophagitis and biopsy may be undertaken. Barium studies should be carefully scrutinized, for in addition to the condition under discussion careful assessment of the stomach and duodenum is necessary. Evidence of hold-up at the pylorus, whether by spasm, ulcer or fibrosis, will indicate the need for pyloroplasty in addition to hiatal hernia repair. Manometric studies, although elegant, are not readily available in most centres.

Indications for transthoracic repair

The controversy concerning the choice of transthoracic or abdominal repair of hiatus hernia will subside as the specific indications for each become clear. As it becomes more universally recognized that gastro-oesophageal reflux can be controlled by specific local procedures, the wide variety of transabdominal manoeuvres and quaint gastric operations for the management of gastro-oesophageal reflux will be restricted to few situations. Although simple hiatus hernia is often repaired from below, either as a definitive procedure, or more frequently as an additional procedure during the course of another abdominal operation, care should be taken to avoid an inadequate repair offered as an after-thought with poorly-defined indications. There is no doubt that in patients with oesophagitis, oedema and fibrosis, the consequent shortening of the lower oesophagus will prevent adequate mobilization from below and such an operation is unlikely to produce an effective reduction and repair without tension. Furthermore, mediastinal adhesions frequently require accurate sharp dissection under direct vision which is unobtainable via the abdominal route. Inadequate reduction or reduction under tension is inevitably followed by recurrence of symptoms. It is claimed that the transabdominal approach is justified during other operations such as cholecystectomy or pyloroplasty but it is under these conditions that repair of the difficult hiatus hernia will fail. On the other hand, pyloroplasty is readily undertaken during transthoracic hiatus hernial repair when the operative exposure is extended into the left upper quadrant of the abdomen.

THE OPERATION

1

Position of patient

The patient is placed in the right lateral position with 45° backward rotation. This enables the thoracic incision to be extended, should this prove necessary, across the costal margin and into the upper abdomen.

The incision

The left chest is opened through the bed of the left sixth rib. Rib resection or rib division is usually unnecessary. The exposure enables adequate mobilization of the oesophagus to be undertaken and gives an excellent view of the cardia and subdiaphragmatic structures. Furthermore, this incision is readily extended across the costal margin to enter the upper abdomen, such extension being required when pyloroplasty is undertaken, or should reduction of the hernia prove impossible and resection be necessary.

The left lung is retracted upwards and forwards by an assistant and the diaphragm is retracted downwards. The oesophagus, cardia and diaphragm are thus exposed.

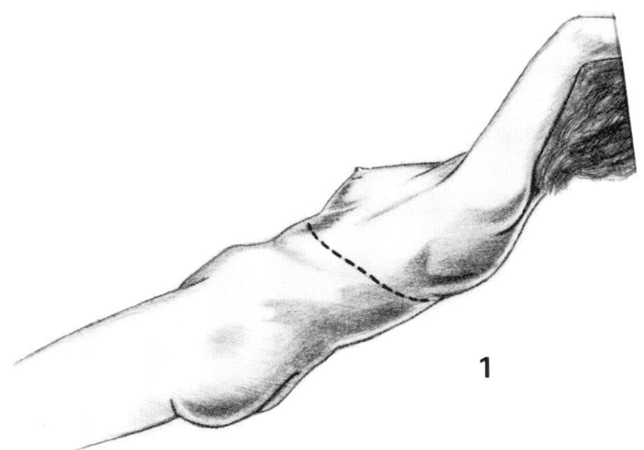

1

2

The lateral pulmonary ligament is divided and the oesophagus is dissected from its bed, ligating and dividing the aortic branches to the oesophagus as high as the aortic arch. The oesophagus is dissected with the left vagus nerve, which is readily palpated posteriorly and the oesophagus is encircled by a rubber sling.

The pleura at the junction between the oesophagus and cardia is incised circumferentially and by gentle traction on the rubber sling the hernia is drawn into the chest. Incision of the phreno-oesophageal ligament, the extraperitoneal fat and the lesser sac of the peritoneum anteriorly, enables the cardia to be freed in its entirety apart from musculovascular connections posteriorly. These latter contain arterial branches to the lower oesophagus from the inferior phrenic and left gastric arteries which must be carefully divided and tied.

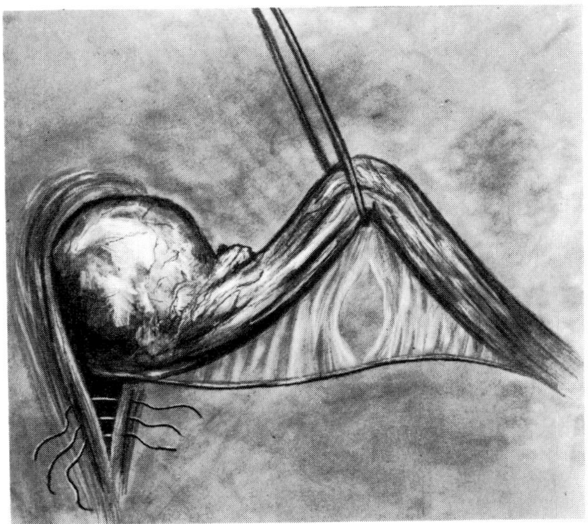

2

Following complete mobilization of the lower oesophagus and cardia, a trial of reduction is then undertaken by reducing the cardia into the abdomen as far as possible. In the majority of instances, this is readily accomplished but in patients with chronic and severe oesophagitis, or oesophageal fibrosis, shortening of the oesophagus may be so marked that reduction is impossible despite adequate mobilization. This situation must be recognized, for attempting hernial repair in these circumstances will result in the persistence of symptoms and may proceed to stricture formation. In these patients, resection of the lower oesophagus with short segment colon interposition should be undertaken. Oesophago-gastrectomy is employed as a last resort in those patients in whom colonic interposition is not possible for anatomical reasons and in the elderly, for the exchange of a natural hiatus hernia for a man-made hiatus hernia is followed in many cases by stricture formation some years postoperatively. Oesophago-gastrectomy is an operation best reserved as a palliative procedure in carcinoma and is to be avoided in patients with benign conditions.

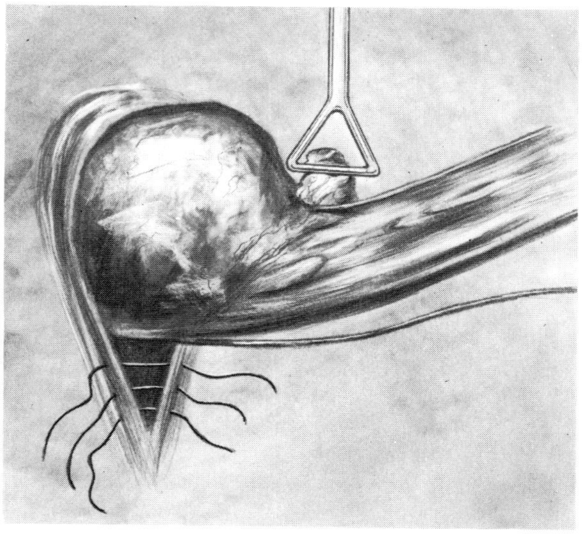

3

3

When it is clear that satisfactory reduction is possible, the operation is continued. The pad of fat which occupies the angle between the oesophagus and gastric fundus must be carefully removed, preserving the right vagus nerve which runs close to the stomach and oesophagus in this situation.

The gastro-oesophageal hiatus usually requires narrowing and the sutures for this procedure are placed at this stage of the operation but are not tied. Traction on the oesophageal sling holds the stomach and lower oesophagus forwards, and exposes the crura. Three or four linen sutures are placed and held by artery forceps, and these are to be tied later (*see Illustrations 2* and *3*).

Sutures are now placed at the cardia. The aim of these is twofold: (*a*) to restore the acute angle of entry of the oesophagus into the stomach (*see* cut away in *Illustration 5*); (*b*) to ensure the reduction into the abdomen of an adequate length (5 cm) of intra-abdominal oesophagus.

4

4,5&6

First layer

Mattress sutures are taken from the stomach to the oesophagus. These linen thread sutures pick up and secure the stomach wall 2 cm below the cardia and the oesophagus at the cardia. Although the bites should not be too superficial, care must be taken to avoid penetrating the full thickness of the oesophagus. Usually three or four such sutures are required and when these are tied the stomach embraces the lower oesophagus. Encircling the oesophagus with the stomach should be resisted for this has been shown to interfere with the mechanism of belching and may cause dysphagia. The ideal result is achieved by wrapping the oesophagus with the stomach over three quarters of a circle (270°).

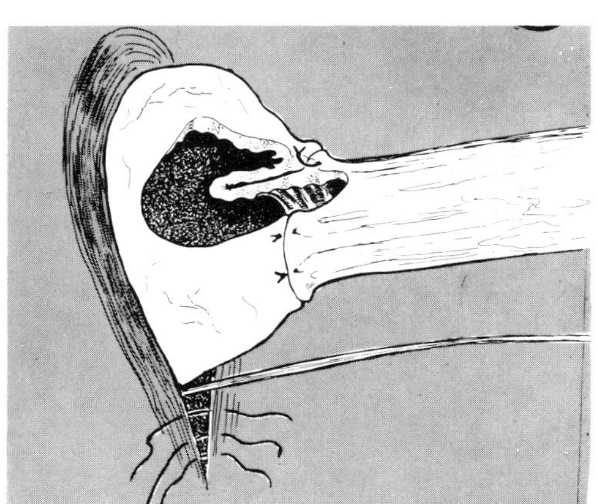

5

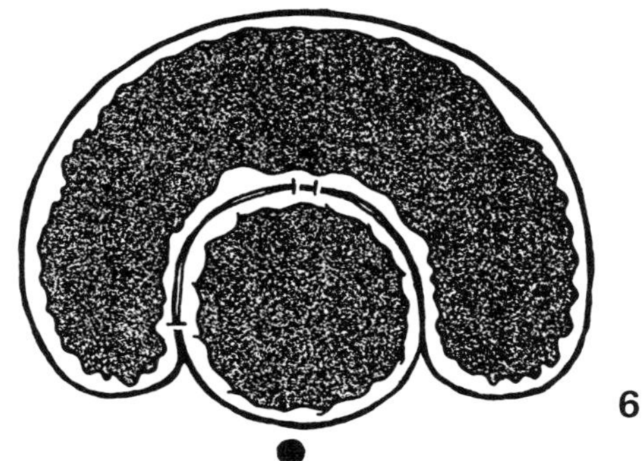

6

Second layer

7

The second layer of sutures enters the lower oesophagus and stomach and attaches this to the underside of the diaphragm 4 cm away from the hiatus which ensures reduction and fixation of the hernia. The diaphragmatic sutures are inserted with the aid of a spoon introduced through the hiatus from above (Belsey). This spoon ensures the safe passage of the sutures through the diaphragm whilst subdiaphragmatic structures are safely displaced. Again, three or four sutures are placed entering the diaphragm from above, the stomach 3 cm below the first row, and then the oesophagus, returning to the stomach and emerging again through the diaphragm.

Gentle traction on this row of sutures reduces the hernia and when these sutures are tied, fixation is complete. Adequate mobilization of the oesophagus and preparation of the cardia will result in a tension-free reduction and under these circumstances the oesophagus will be lax and freely movable. Should the oesophagus be as tight as a bow string the scene is set for postoperative recurrence and further mobilization of the oesophagus is necessary.

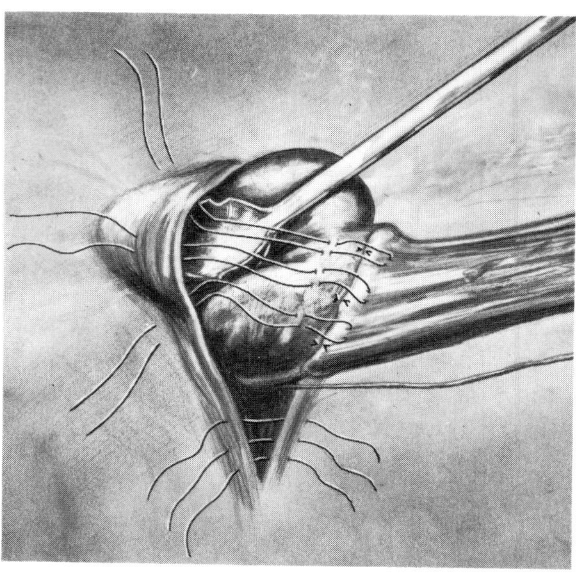

7

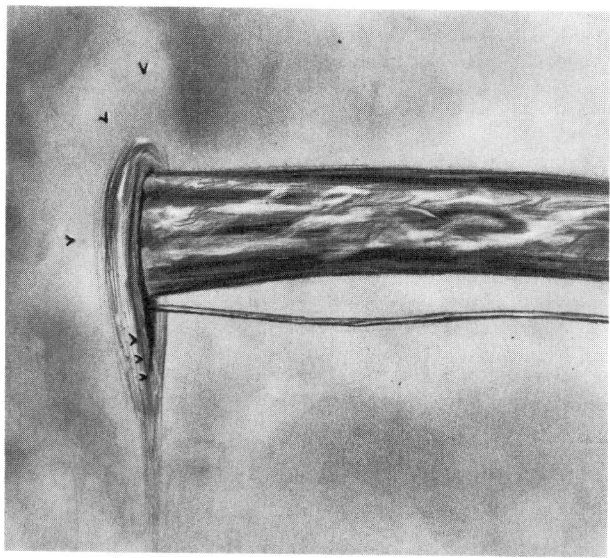

8

8

The previously-placed crural stitches are now tied, commencing with the most posterior. Tight closure of the hiatus should be avoided, as food needs to pass through the oesophagus. The sutures should be tied seriatim until the hiatus posterior to the oesophagus will take the first digit of the surgeon's forefinger and will have the feel of an anal sphincter.

The chest is closed with drainage. The passage of a nasogastric tube is unnecessary. Indeed, the presence of such a tube in the presence of oesophagitis may predispose to ulceration and stricture formation.

It is usually possible to remove the intercostal drainage tube on the first postoperative day, following which the patient is mobilized. Fluids by mouth are allowed after 24 hr if bowel sounds are present, gradually progressing to free fluids and a light diet over the subsequent 2 days.

Acknowledgement

The opinions and operation described here are based on the philosophy and teaching of R. H. Belsey at Frenchay Hospital, to whom the author is indebted.

[*The illustrations for this Chapter on Thoracic Repair of Hiatus Hernia were drawn by Mr. C. Tyrrell.*]

Nissen's Fundoplication

H. C. Nohl-Oser, D. M., F.R.C.S.
Consultant Thoracic Surgeon, Harefield, Hillingdon
and West Middlesex Hospitals

PRE - OPERATIVE

General considerations

Recent research into the sphincteric action at the cardio-oesophageal junction has stressed the importance of the physiological rather than the anatomical factors which control the competence of the valvular mechanism at the cardia. On the basis of these new concepts the emphasis has shifted away from the actual repair of the hiatus to other more effective methods which will abolish gastro-oesophageal reflux. Various types of fundoplication have, therefore, gained wider acceptance. In the past, stress has always been laid on the fact that an intra-abdominal segment of oesophagus was essential to achieve control of gastro-oesophageal regurgitation. In practice this may, of course, not be possible in the presence of a shortened oesophagus. It was, therefore, a real advance when it became apparent that a fundoplication in the chest can prevent reflux equally effectively. The potentialities of fundoplication became, therefore, more far reaching. Firstly it is well known that with effective control of reflux, many strictures, which occur especially in the elderly, will resolve without resection and oesophageal replacement. Secondly, severe strictures, which are unlikely to disappear on simple fundoplication, can be dealt with by an oesophagoplasty and a fundoplication covering the reconstituted area. This will not only prevent further reflux, but will also secure the operation site against possible leakage. Finally, gastro-oesophageal reflux and its sequelae are less likely to follow a Heller's myotomy or a local resection of the oesophagus with a gastro-oesophageal anastomosis, if they are combined with a fundoplication.

Pre-operative assessment of hiatus hernia and reflux

A very careful pre-operative assessment is necessary, especially as the symptoms are very similar to other frequently associated lesions, including peptic ulcers, cholelithiasis and coronary insufficiency. Barium studies of the oesophagus, stomach and duodenum are essential. The barium swallow and meal will give information as to normal or abnormal motility of the oesophagus and also whether there is shortening of the oesophagus. Radiological studies will further detect the presence and type of strictures, show the type of hiatus hernia present and demonstrate whether there is gross gastro-oesophageal reflux and whether there are associated lesions present in the stomach or duodenum. A pre-operative oesophagoscopy is essential as it will reveal the degree of oesophagitis and allow biopsies to be taken in the presence of strictures or any other abnormalities.

Indications

With this information available, the chief indications for surgery are: Severe symptoms, which fail to respond to medical treatment, the presence of definite oesophagitis and/or its sequelae, i.e. stricture formation, haematemesis, melaena and anaemia. Every para-oesophageal hiatal hernia should also be treated surgically, as they have a tendency to obstruct.

THE OPERATION

The operative approach can either be by an abdominal or a thoracic incision, provided that good access to the lower 5–8 cm of the oesophagus is obtained. In view of the fact that in many cases peri-oesophagitis can be gross and the oesophagus is often shortened, the thoraco-abdominal approach, to be described, is advised. This allows good access to both the chest and the upper abdomen, making it even possible to deal with lesions in the stomach, duodenum and gall-bladder.

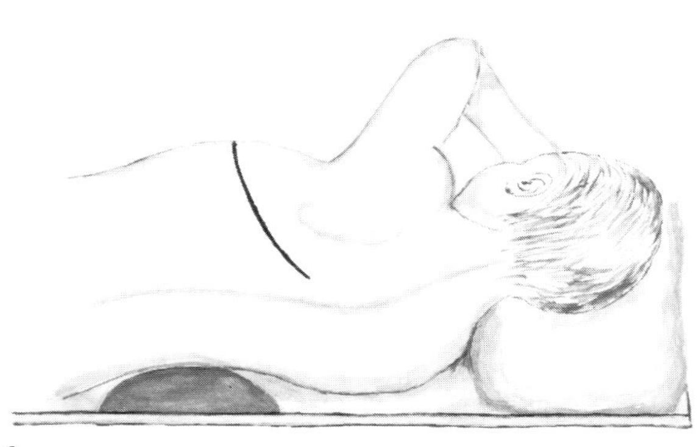

1

1

The incision

A posterolateral thoracotomy incision is made along the line of the eighth rib. The periosteum over the eighth rib is incised with the diathermy needle from the lateral edge of the sacrospinalis muscle at the back to the costal cartilage in front. The upper border of the rib is laid bare by raising the periosteum with a curved raspatory. The back end of the rib is divided by removing a small segment of the rib with the costotome. The pleural cavity is entered by incising through the rib bed. The incision is widely opened with a rib spreader.

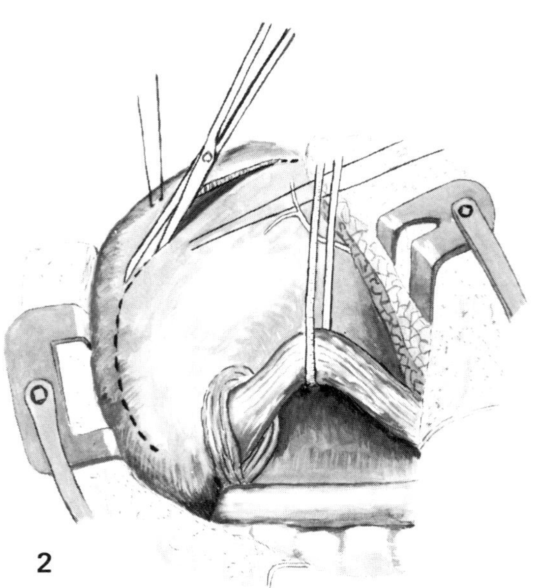

2

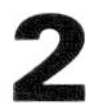

Exposure of the oesophagus and incision of the diaphragm

The pulmonary ligament is divided until the inferior pulmonary vein comes into view. The lung is retracted upwards and forwards. The mediastinal pleura is incised over the oesophagus. The oesophagus is mobilized and a nylon tape is passed around it, allowing the oesophagus to be elevated from its bed by gentle traction. The oesophageal arterial branches are divided between ligatures and the oesophagus is mobilized, if necessary, up to the arch of the aorta. The vagal nerves are preserved. At diaphragmatic level, the crural fibres of the hiatal margin are displayed. The diaphragm is now incised circumferentially, parallel with the eighth rib, approximately 5 cm from its attachment to the chest wall. This incision lies anteriorly in front of the phrenic nerve as it enters the diaphragm and extends backwards to well beyond the lateral extent of the spleen. This type of incision preserves the nerve supply of the diaphragm and gives excellent access to the upper abdomen without incising the abdominal wall. The incision can, however, be continued across the costal margin, should it be necessary, for instance, to deal with biliary disease.

3

Exposure of hiatal region and oesophagus from the abdomen

The left triangular ligament is divided, care being taken to avoid damage to the inferior phrenic vein. The stomach is pulled downwards by the assistant and the peritoneum incised transversely in front of the oesophagus. The anterior vagus nerve must not be damaged. The peritoneal incision is continued medially and downwards, opening the lesser sac. This will bring into view the caudate lobe of the liver and to the left, lying alongside it, will be found the right limb of the right crus of the diaphragm. Continuing the peritoneal incision in front of the oesophagus to the left, the left limb of the crus will be exposed. By passing a finger to the right of the oesophagus into the lesser sac and lifting the oesophagus forwards, the remaining peritoneum can then be incised from the left, thus entering the lesser sac from the left of the oesophagus. A nylon tape is now passed around the oesophagus and by traction, 5 cm of the oesophagus is drawn into the abdomen. At this stage a large Hurst's mercury bougie (size 45–48Ch, if possible) is passed into the stomach. Both limbs of the crus are now well defined and the enlarged hiatus can be narrowed. The right limb of the crus has a tendency to be a flimsy structure in the elderly and obese patient. The approximation of the two limbs behind the oesophagus can, therefore, be strengthened by a strip of Teflon felt (author's modification), as indicated in the diagram. One or two mattress sutures of linen thread will suffice, leaving enough room to accommodate the bougie and the tip of the small finger.

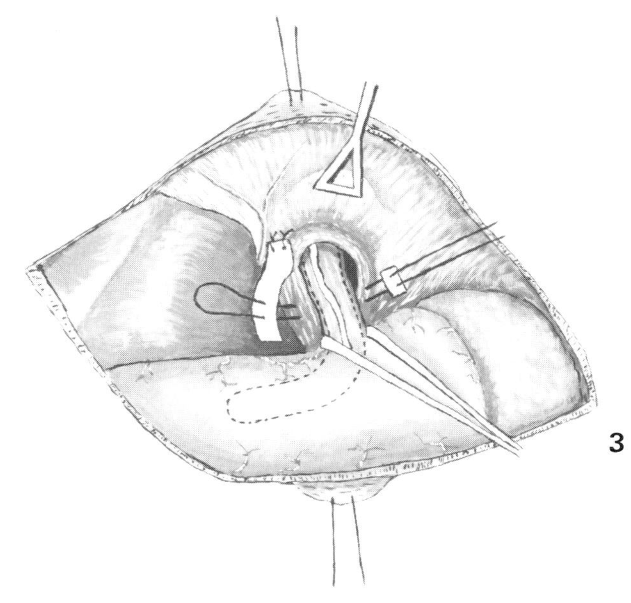

3

Fundoplication

4

The left gastro-epiploic and the short gastric vessels are divided, thereby mobilizing the upper third of the greater curvature and fundus of the stomach. Great care is taken not to injure the spleen. With the bougie still in the stomach, the right hand pushes the fundus of the stomach behind the oesophagus, so that a good part of it lies to the right of the oesophagus.

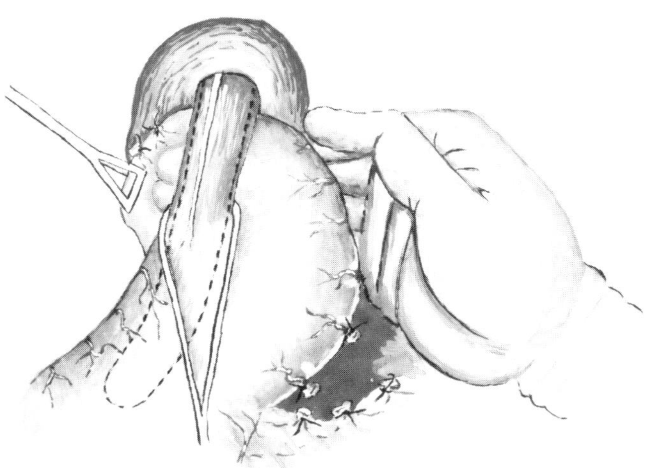

4

5

The two pouches of stomach now lying on either side of the oesophagus are brought together in front of it by linen thread sutures which pick up the oesophagus as well, thus preventing it from slipping out of the cuff that is created. The first and uppermost suture (*see* illustration) is a mattress suture, which passes first through the hiatal margin, then through one side of the stomach, then the oesophagus, then the other side of the fundus and then back through the hiatus. Similar hiatal sutures are passed on either side. The vertical row of seromuscular sutures in front of the oesophagus is buried by a second serosal suture.

At the completion of the fundoplication the mercury bougie is removed and a nasogastric tube passed into the stomach.

5

6

Closure of diaphragm

Meticulous closure of the diaphragm is essential to prevent herniation in the future. The first row of sutures consists of interrupted linen thread, placed as 'X' sutures as shown in the diagram. Every stitch must pick up the peritoneum and the diaphragmatic pleura. The second row is a continuous inverting suture of atraumatic catgut, burying the knots of the first row.

The chest is closed leaving a basal drainage tube, connected to an under-water seal.

6

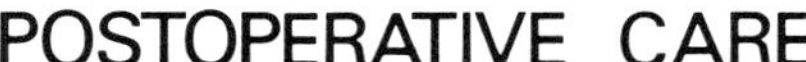

POSTOPERATIVE CARE

Physiotherapy, which was started before the operation, is continued to prevent pulmonary atelectasis due to sputum retention. The nasogastric tube is allowed to siphon into a bag for at least 48 hr, as gastric distension can occur. Intravenous fluids are given to supply the necessary fluid and electrolyte requirements. After this, oral feeding is steadily built up from fluids to semisolids to solid diet. There may be temporary dysphagia due to oedema at the cardia, especially with fish, chicken and fresh bread which are best avoided. There is evidence to suggest that the incidence of deep vein thrombosis and pulmonary embolism is greater in patients undergoing surgical treatment of hiatus hernia: postoperative anticoagulants and early ambulation are therefore advised.

References

Franklin, R. H., Iweze, F. I. and Owen-Smith, M. S. (1973). 'Fundoplication for hiatus hernia.' *Br. J. Surg.* **60,** 65

Kent Harrison, G. and Gompels, B. M. (1971). 'Treatment of reflux strictures of the oesophagus by the Nissen–Rossetti operation.' *Thorax* **26,** 77

Nissen, R. and Rossetti, M. (1963). 'Surgery of the cardia ventriculi.' *Ciba Symposium* **11,** 195

[*The illustrations for this Chapter on Nissen's Fundoplication were drawn by the Author.*]

Reflux Oesophagitis Treated by Gastroplasty

J. Leigh Collis, M.D., F.R.C.S.
Professor of Thoracic Surgery and Consultant Surgeon
to Queen Elizabeth Hospital, Birmingham;
Thoracic Surgeon to the West Midland Health Authority

PRE - OPERATIVE

Indications

This is a treatment for reflux oesophagitis where a simple plastic repair of the oesophageal hiatus is impracticable because of the shortness of the oesophagus. In this circumstance a considerable bulk of stomach and attached tissue will occupy the hiatus. In about three-quarters of these cases a stricture is present. This is due to a combination of spasm, oedema and fibrosis, and at least the first two will be eradicated if reflux of gastric acid is removed. Control of gastric reflux obtained by the operation of gastroplasty is therefore a treatment for stricture of the oesophagus. It is emphasized that no peptic stricture of the oesophagus is too fibrotic to be treated in this way, although some pre-operative and postoperative dilatation will be necessary. Using this method the stricture is not excised and no bowel resection is necessary. It therefore avoids the use of colon or jejunum for bridging the gap after resection of the stricture. It is a relatively simple operation and has a low mortality—this is important as many of the patients are elderly; the other group of patients are children and adolescents. For these it is undesirable to give them such an abnormal anatomy for the rest of their lives as a colon interposition. Gastroplasty leaves the organs in the right sequence and in any case gives excellent results in the young age group. Gastroplasty is only used when simple methods such as postural restriction and dilatation have failed.

Pre-operative preparation

Dysphagia may be severe. In these cases the stricture must be dilated and dietetic deficiency corrected. A milk drip into the oesophagus may help if oesophagitis is very acute. This may be given throughout every night for a week. The patient will be treated sitting up.

THE OPERATION

The patient is anaesthetized and placed on his back on the operating table. The left side of the patient is raised about 2 inches (5 cm) with sand-bags and a No. 10 English gauge catheter is passed via the mouth into the stomach.

1

The incision

An abdominothoracic incision is made in the seventh intercostal space and the diaphragm is separated from the costal margin before bringing the division centrally so as to avoid damage to the branches of the phrenic nerve (P).

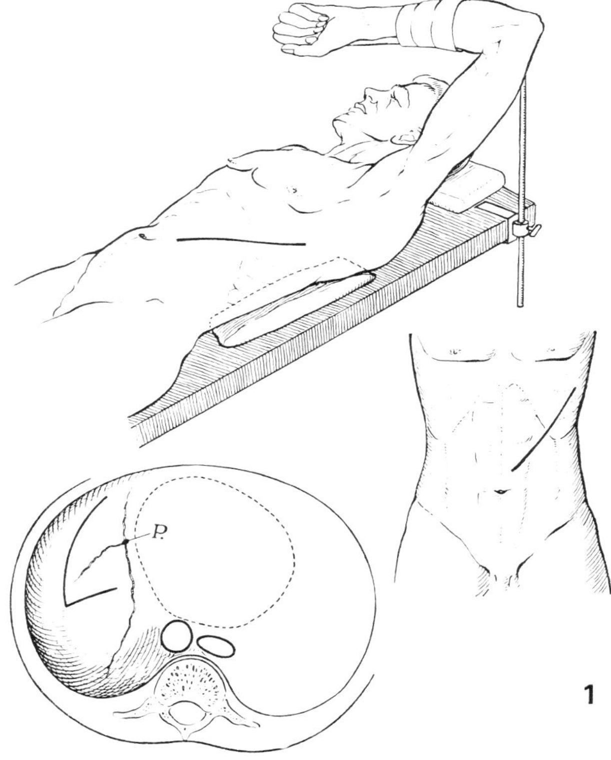

1

2

Dissection of the two halves of right crus

The area of the right crus (A) is now dissected so as to identify both halves of that muscle. Care must be taken to preserve the peritoneal covering on the right half of the right crus. If this simple precaution is not taken the muscle fibres separate and tear very easily in the later suturing. The herniated portion of the stomach is reduced as far as possible, but the actual stricture area (B) and the oesophagus above it is not mobilized.

The fatty and omental tissue lying on the stomach in the area of the right crus is cleared away so as to leave a smooth stomach wall in this area. This is important because if it is not done the subsequent invagination of the cut stomach will be bulky in this area and will interfere with the suturing of the two halves of the right crus.

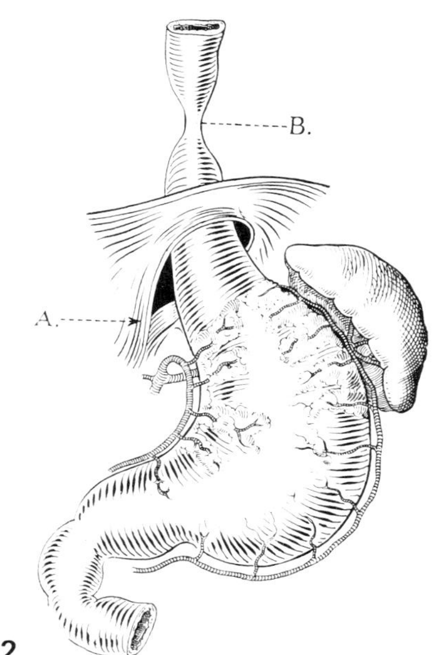

2

3 & 4

Placing of clamps

A finger is placed (B) under the left gastric vessels and up behind the stomach to the top of the lesser sac (A). The peritoneum is incised here and the finger passed through. The three upper gastrosplenic vessels are divided between haemostats. The stomach is thus mobilized and the front and back of it is now clear for positioning of the clamps.

One of the smaller pair of clamps is now applied to the stomach parallel to the lesser curve. The small rubber gastric tube is passed down into the stomach and its presence helps with the adjustment of the clamp. This clamp is put on from below the hiatus but at the same time drawing the stomach down from the chest as far as possible. With this clamp lightly applied it is easier to position one of the pair with longer blades. This is put down parallel to the lesser curve so that a tube (A) is left rather smaller than the normal oesophagus. The other large clamp (C) is then placed towards the fundus and parallel with the first clamp (B). The stomach is incised between these clamps (D).

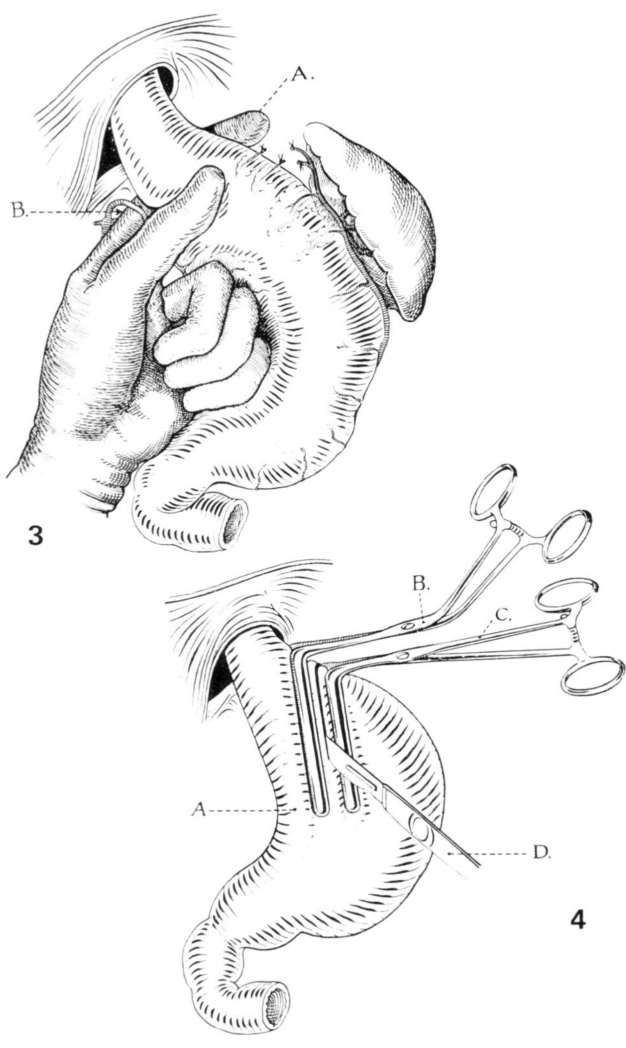

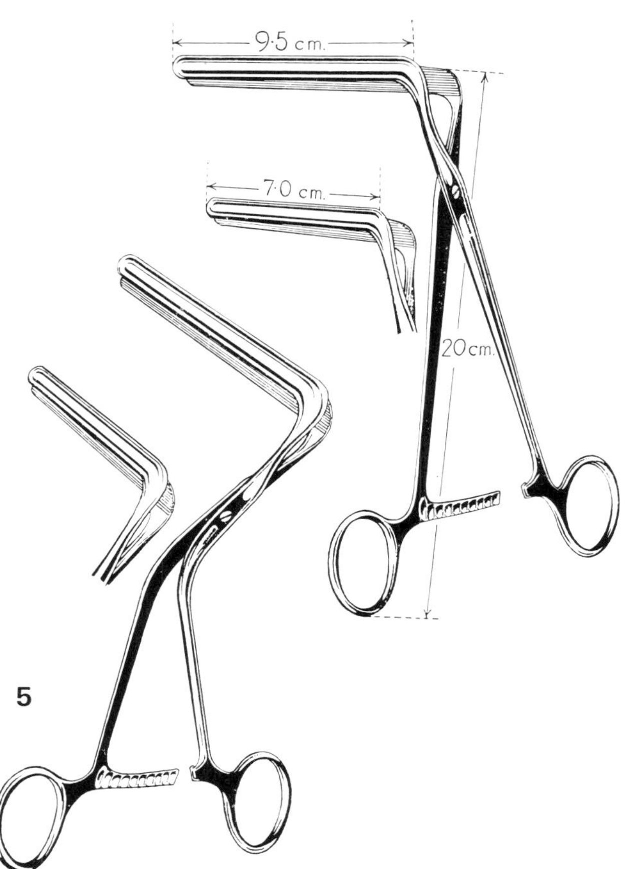

5

Gastroplasty clamps

These clamps were designed for the operation on the basis of the Aldridge clamps.

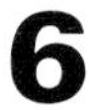

6

Forming the connecting link

The incised edges of the stomach are now sutured with continuous catgut and invaginated. This must be done as neatly as possible so as to avoid a bulky suture line. The connecting link has now been formed which extends from the stricture in the chest through the opening of the hiatus (A) and well down into the abdomen to enter the rest of the stomach (C) at an acute angle of implantation. The rest of the stomach (D) has been separated from this connecting link to make an enlarged fundus. The rubber gastric tube is now removed in preparation for the repair of the hiatus.

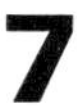

7

Repair of hiatus

The two halves of the right crus have already been dissected to their origin from the tendon of the right crus. The right half overlaps the left half at the bottom in the same manner as the two halves of a double-breasted waistcoat. The V between these two halves is opened up and the connecting tube attached with one stitch to the bottom of this.

The two halves of the right crus are now sutured together above and in front of the connecting link (H). The connecting link is now gripped firmly by this suturing and the acute angle of implantation (C) is also supported, making the general shape of the connecting link and the rest of the stomach similar to an inverted retort. This is the same general shape as the normal oesophagogastric junction.

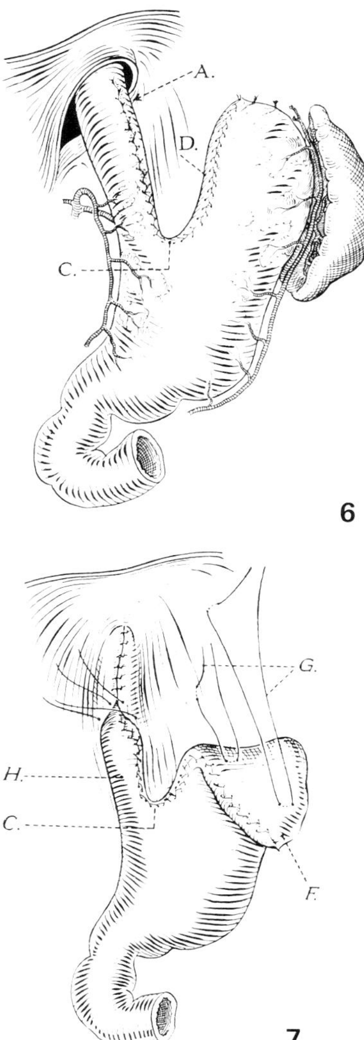

6

7

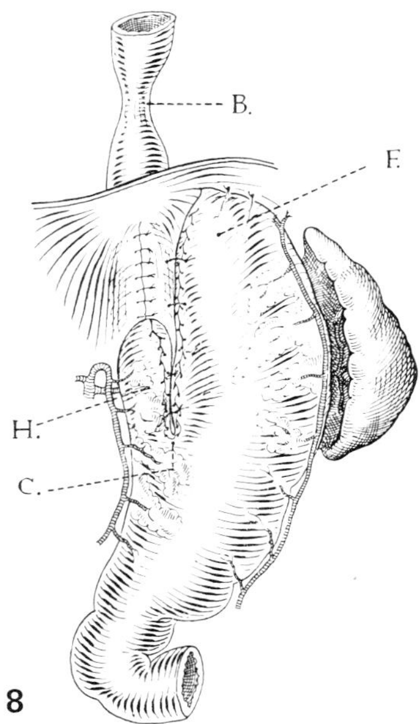

8

Fixing of fundus

The newly enlarged fundus is excessively mobile (F in *Illustration* 7). It must be attached to the undersurface of the diaphragm by suturing it to the area of the left crus by three thread stitches (G in *Illustration* 7). The highest stitch attaches it to the cut edge of the left triangular ligament.

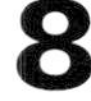

8

Stomach-to-stomach fixation

The connecting link (H) is now sutured with thread in three places to the adjacent part of the new enlarged fundus (F). The position is now complete with part of the connecting link in the chest, part gripped by the repair of the hiatus and part within the abdomen and entering the stomach at a very acute angle (C). The incision in the diaphragm is now sutured and the chest and abdomen closed with intercostal drainage.

POSTOPERATIVE CARE

The patient is given only ice to suck for 48 hr. After this oral feeding is steadily built up to full fluid requirement by mouth after 4 days. Intravenous fluids are given to maintain the necessary fluid and electrolyte balance. Ampicillin and streptomycin are given for 5 days. Semisolids are started on the sixth day and then the diet is rapidly built up. The intercostal tube is removed after 24 hr. A barium swallow x-ray examination is done to check the position on the ninth postoperative day and the patient goes home on the fourteenth day. In about a quarter of those cases who have dysphagia before operation some further oesophagoscopic dilatation will be necessary. It is rare for it to be required after a year. It may be many months before the full benefit is obtained and it is necessary to guard against disappointment by warning the patient about the likely position in the first few postoperative months.

[*The illustrations for this Chapter on Reflux Oesophagitis Treated by Gastroplasty were drawn by the late Mr. W. J. Pardoe.*]

Reflux Oesophagitis with Stricture: Alternative Methods of Management

W. Spencer Payne, M.D.
Head of Section of Surgery, Mayo Clinic and Mayo Foundation;
Professor of Surgery, Mayo Medical School, Rochester, Minnesota

INTRODUCTION

The exquisite sensitivity of oesophageal mucosa to the corrosive effects of certain digestive secretions has been implicated in the genesis of almost all the complications of gastro-oesophageal reflux. Gastro-oesophageal incompetence permits the free reflux of acid-peptic secretions and also corrosive biliary and pancreatic secretions from the stomach to the oesophagus. The oesophageal consequences of this reflux are directly related to the noxious effects of these secretions on the oesophagus and to the tissue response to chemical injury. Desquamation, erosion, ulceration, inflammation, pain, bleeding, motility disturbances, oesophageal shortening, and stricture formation, as well as columnar epithelial lining of the lower oesophagus (Barrett), are the recognized consequences of such injury. Such complications occur in varying intensity from patient to patient, and the pathological processes are often reversible once physical contact between corrosive secretions and oesophagus is eliminated.

Two surgical techniques currently provide the chief means of control of the complications of gastro-oesophageal reflux: (*1*) surgical restoration of gastro-oesophageal competence, and (*2*) surgical alteration of the quality of secretions present in the stomach so that they are no longer corrosive to the oesophagus when they reflux. In the management of benign strictures of the oesophagus due to gastro-oesophageal reflux, rehabilitation of oesophageal function additionally entails restoration of oesophageal lumen size or patency. The majority of such benign strictures readily respond to simple dilatation by the passage of sounds or bougies of appropriately graduated sizes. Subsequent stabilization of luminal diameter can usually be achieved if continued oesophageal contact with corrosive secretions can be eliminated by one of the two surgical means to be described.

When oesophageal stricturing has progressed to an irreversible stage as the consequence of the deposition of dense hypertrophic collagen scar, stricture resection with restoration of oesophagogastric continuity provides long-term rehabilitation of function, provided that recurrent reflux oesophagitis is prevented by one of the two aforementioned surgical techniques.

The two operative techniques to be described demonstrate alternative methods employed by the author, under a variety of circumstances, in treating benign strictures of the oesophagus due to gastro-oesophageal reflux: (*1*) when the stricture can be dilated adequately and an antireflux procedure can be accomplished, (*2*) when the stricture is intractable to mechanical dilatation, and (*3*) when the stricture can be dilated but previous surgery precludes the performance of an antireflux procedure.

OESOPHAGEAL DILATATION AND RESTORATION OF COMPETENCE BY COLLIS-BELSEY PROCEDURE (PEARSON)

1

Pre-operative assessment

All adult patients who are candidates for surgical treatment should undergo roentgenographic examination and preliminary oesophageal dilatation to 50 Ch. The passage of graduated Plummer bougies through the strictured oesophagus over a previously swallowed thread as a guide provides valuable information about the reversibility of the stricture, and it usually restores oesophageal function temporarily. Oesophagoscopy should be performed to define the type and severity of associated complications and to obtain cytological and biopsy material to rule out malignancy. Manometric studies of oesophageal motility provide diagnosis of unsuspected motility disturbance. The liberal use of oral antacids and the slanted head-up oesophageal bed minimize reflux during the evaluative period.

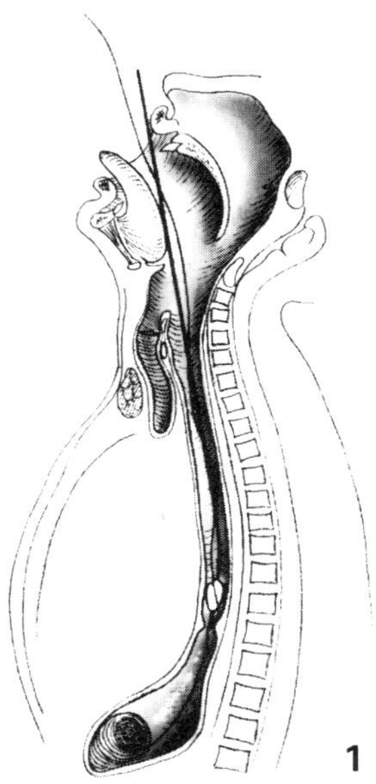
1

THE OPERATION

Prevention of respiratory aspiration during anaesthetic induction is achieved by orotracheal intubation under topical anaesthesia with the patient awake. General anaesthesia is immediately induced after the anaesthetic tube is in place and the airway is sealed with an inflated cuff. The patient is then placed in the right lateral decubitus position (*see Illustration 2*) and stabilized in position with appropriate bolsters.

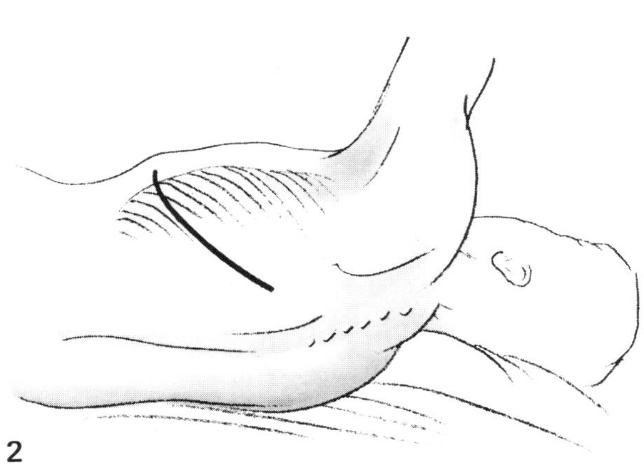
2

2

The incision

A left thoracotomy is performed, and the pleural space is entered through the periosteal bed of the non-resected left eighth rib.

3

Exposure

Appropriate spreading of the intercostal incision provides easy access to the pleural cavity. After division of the inferior pulmonary ligament, the lung is retracted cephalad and the pleural leaves of the inferior pulmonary ligament are dissected anteriorly and posteriorly to expose the distal oesophagus. A Penrose drain is passed around the oesophagus and vagi to elevate the oesophagus from its mediastinal bed. The intrathoracic protrusion of proximal stomach and oesophagogastric junction is usually apparent.

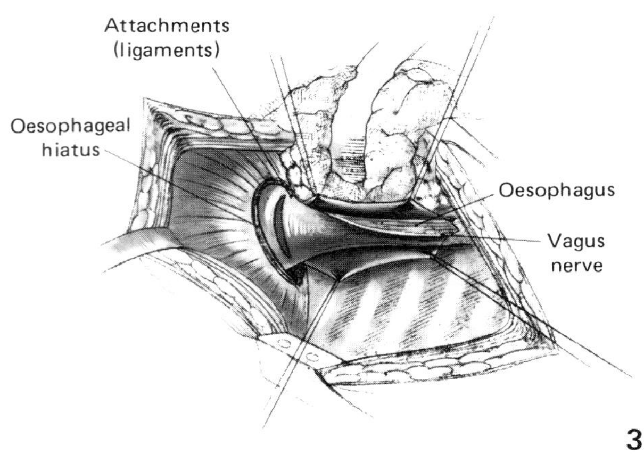

3

Dissection of oesophageal hiatus

4

A transverse incision is made in the phreno-oesophageal ligament and contiguous layers of pleura and peritoneum, creating a tunnel between chest and abdomen through the oesophageal hiatus. A small Richardson retractor is passed through this defect and the oesophageal hiatus is retracted laterally.

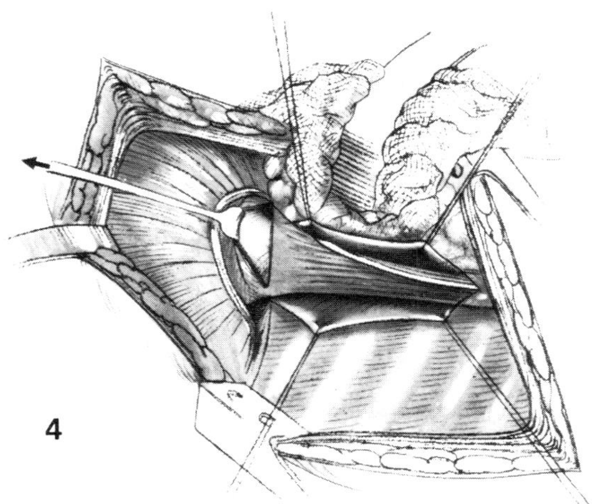

4

5

By placement of the fingers of the left hand astride the attachments between the oesophagogastric junction and the crura of the diaphragm, these attachments can be safely divided; this completely frees the cardia circumferentially from all hiatal attachments.

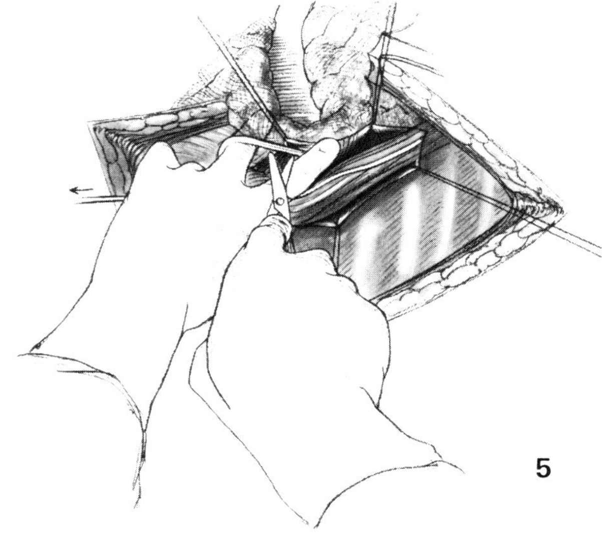

5

6&7

Dissection of oesophagogastric fat pad

Vagal trunks are identified and preserved. The highly vascular fatty connective tissues at the oesophagogastric junction is carefully dissected from lateral medialward. The anterior vagal trunk is preserved by sweeping it medially with the fat pad. Meticulous ligation of multiple gastric nutrient vessels is required not only to reflect this fat pad but also to clear the gastric serosa for subsequent steps of the operation.

Prolapse of stomach into chest

It is now possible to allow the proximal stomach to prolapse into the thorax through the oesophageal hiatus. It is usually unnecessary to divide short gastric vessels to gain access to the lesser peritoneal sac behind the stomach.

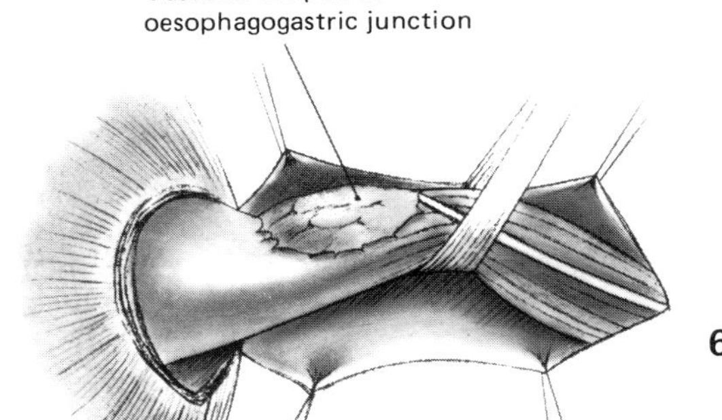

6

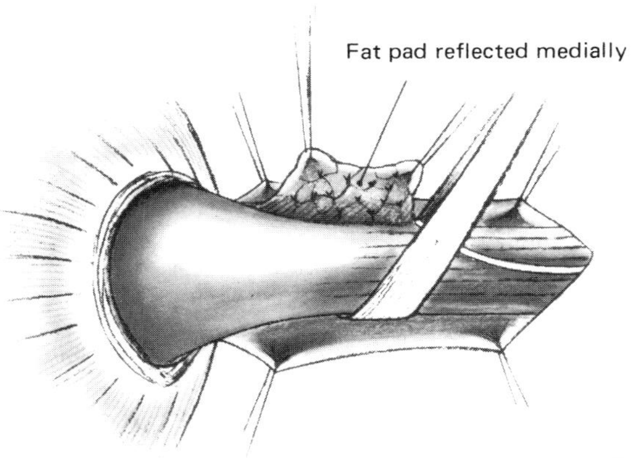

7

8, 9 & 10

Collis' gastroplasty

A 50 Ch mercury-weighted rubber dilator (Maloney) is advanced through the mouth down the oesophagus and into the stomach, dilating the oesophageal stricture and providing a mandrel about which a tubular extension of the oesophagus will be fashioned from the lesser curvature of the stomach. This is accurately and simply achieved by applying a GIA stapling device (U.S. Instrument Co.) parallel to and snugly against the indwelling mandrel. Activation of the cutting blade of this device not only incises the portion of stomach between the jaws of the clamp but also lays down parallel double rows of metallic staples, effectively closing each side of the 5 cm long incision. The rows of staples on the neo-oesophagus and fundus are then buried beneath a single row of interrupted silk sutures.

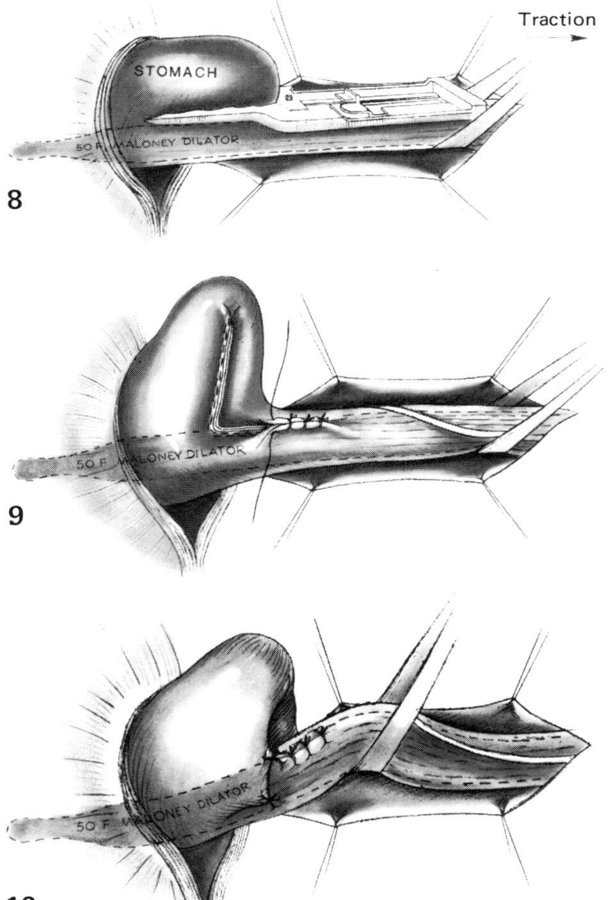

8

9

10

11–13

*Belsey-type repair**

The neofundus is now imbricated onto the neo-oesophagus with two rows of seromuscular mattress sutures. The imbrication encompasses 180° of the circumference of the neo-oesophagus on its antero-lateral aspect. The second row incorporates a rim of perihiatal diaphragm. Approximating crural sutures are placed posterior to the oesophagus if the hiatus is found to be too patulous. A snug but not tight hiatus is sought. When the repair is completed, the mandrel is removed and a nasogastric tube is passed for overnight suction-drainage. The tape is removed from around the oesophagus, the mediastinal pleura is re-approximated, and the lung is re-expanded. The chest is closed in layers with a single catheter brought from the pleural space to the outside for postoperative suction-drainage. The end result is a valve-competent Belsey-type repair without tension and with a long intra-abdominal segment of oesophagus held in place with sutures between stomach and stomach rather than stomach and oesophagus.

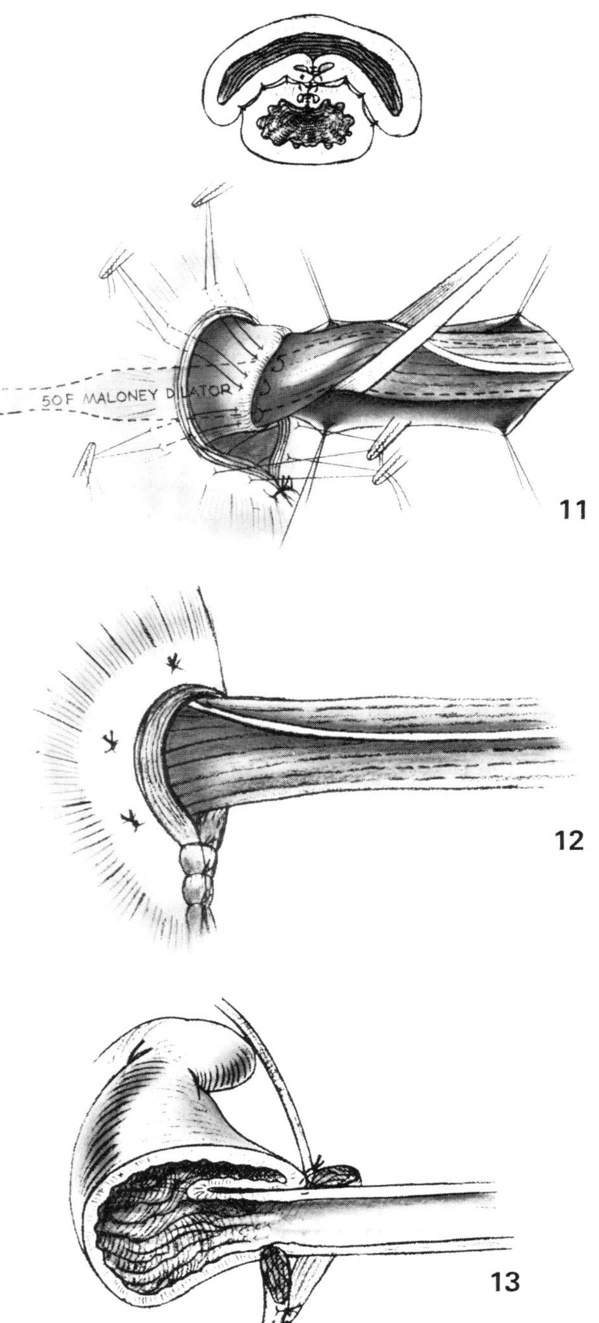

POSTOPERATIVE CARE

Chest tube and nasogastric tube are removed the morning after surgery and the patient is ambulated. Oral feedings are progressed rapidly over the ensuing 48–72 hr from liquid to a general diet as tolerated.

**Addendum.* Alternatively a Nissen fundoplication may be used.

THE UNDILATABLE STRICTURE: MANAGEMENT BY RESECTION AND ROUX-EN-Y GASTRIC DRAINAGE PROCEDURE (LARGE)

On rare occasions, benign oesophageal strictures do not yield to mechanical dilatation, and it becomes necessary to resect the strictured portion of oesophagus to restore function. Such resection removes not only the oesophageal obstruction but also the intrinsic oesophageal sphincter. Reconstruction by oesophago-gastrostomy results in permanent incompetence of the cardia with considerable risk of recurrent oesophagitis and stricture. To obviate this complication, a variety of procedures have been suggested. One, which the author has employed with success, alters the quality of secretions present in the stomach so that they are not corrosive to the oesophagus when they reflux. Essentially, gastric achlorhydria is effected by vagotomy and antrectomy, and alkaline biliary and pancreatic reflux is prevented by means of a long-limb Roux-en-Y gastric drainage procedure.

On occasion, the effects of previous surgical procedures about the oesophageal hiatus and stomach preclude surgical restoration of gastro-oesophageal competence by standard means. Under such circumstances, if the associated oesophageal stricture proves amenable to dilatation, permanent control of oesophagitis and stricture can be obtained by similarly rendering the stomach achlorhydric and preventing biliary reflux by Roux-en-Y gastric drainage.

In either of the aforementioned circumstances, gastro-oesophageal incompetence is permanent, and bland reflux occurs without oesophageal irritation or reaction. Nonetheless, it should be apparent that special postoperative postural precautions may be required for those patients who experience nocturnal respiratory aspiration.

Pre-operative care

Resection of a benign oesophageal stricture due to reflux oesophagitis should not be undertaken until a diligent pre-operative attempt at dilatation over a previously swallowed thread has been repeatedly attempted without success.

Complete vagotomy is an essential feature of the long-limb Roux-en-Y gastric drainage procedure. Gastrojejunal stomal ulceration occurs frequently when gastric vagotomy is incomplete. If stricture resection is not contemplated and previous vagotomy is to be depended on, a Hollander test is helpful to surgical planning.

In patients who are malnourished, it is usually desirable to start parenteral hyperalimentation via a subclavian vein on the day before surgery and to continue such postoperative nutrition until an adequate oral diet can be taken. Such hyperalimentation minimizes negative nitrogen balance and enhances anastomotic healing in depleted patients.

THE OPERATION

14

Anaesthesia, positioning, and surgical exposure of distal oesophagus are accomplished as previously described. Access to the proximal part of the stomach and the oesophageal stricture for resection and anastomosis is gained through a radial diaphragmatic incision that passes through the oesophageal hiatus.

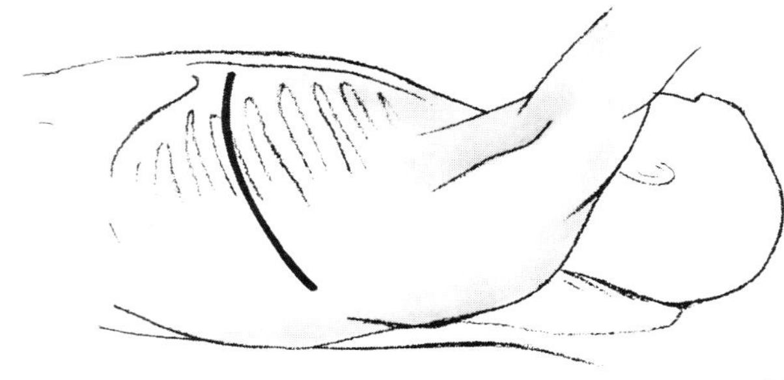

14

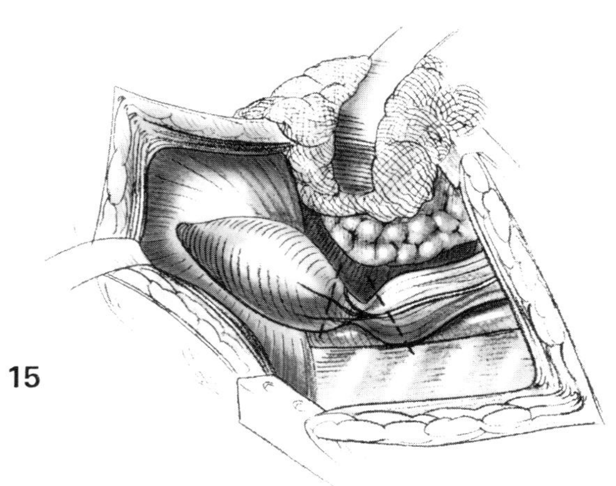

15

15

Resection of oesophageal stricture

Proximal transection of the oesophagus is carried out at a site well above the diseased tissue. Distally, minimal resection of the proximal portion of the stomach is effected with preservation of left gastric vessels. The stomach at the site of oesophageal resection is closed. Vagal trunks are resected along with the stricture.

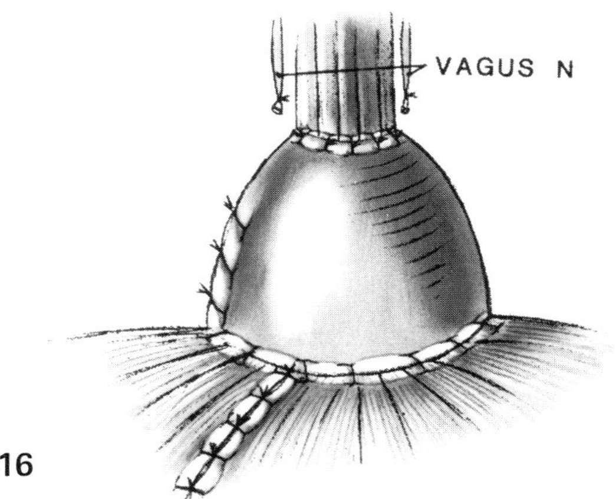

16

16

Oesophagogastrostomy

End-to-side oesophagogastrostomy is performed between the cut end of the oesophagus and the gastric fundus, which is brought into the chest. It is desirable to complete the anastomosis with a 50 Ch catheter in place. Depending on gastric mobility, several short gastric vessels may need to be divided to avoid anastomotic tension. Occasionally it is possible to invaginate the oesophageal anastomosis into the stomach to obtain some element of competence. The diaphragmatic incision is closed around the stomach, creating a snug hiatus to which the stomach is anchored with sutures. The lung is re-expanded and the chest is closed and drained as previously indicated.

Transabdominal procedure

17

The patient is turned and placed supine on the operating table, and the abdomen is explored through an upper mid-line incision.

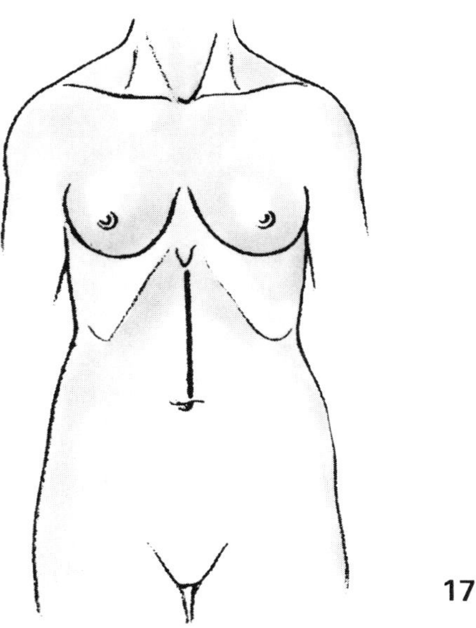

17

18

If it has not previously been done, a standard hemigastrectomy or antrectomy is performed, with preservation of the left gastric, left gastro-epiploic, and short gastric vessels. The duodenal stump is closed.

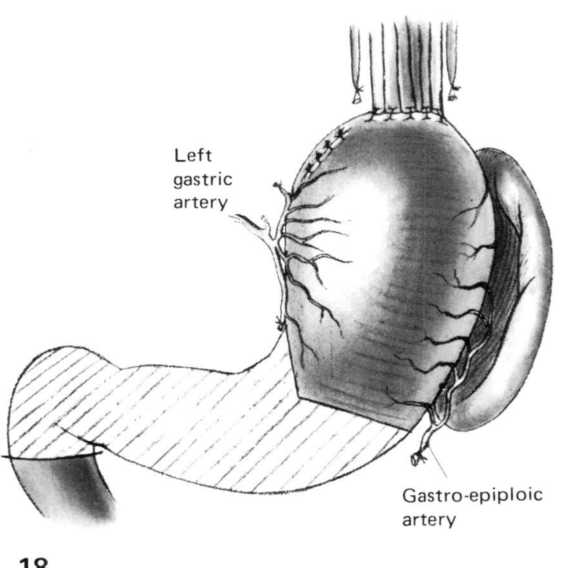

18

19

Long-limb Roux-en-Y gastric drainage

A long-limb Roux-en-Y is developed by dividing the jejunum at a point 9 inches (23 cm) distal to the ligament of Treitz.

The distal end of the transected jejunum is anastomosed end to end to the resected end of the stomach as a postcolic isoperistaltic gastric drainage.

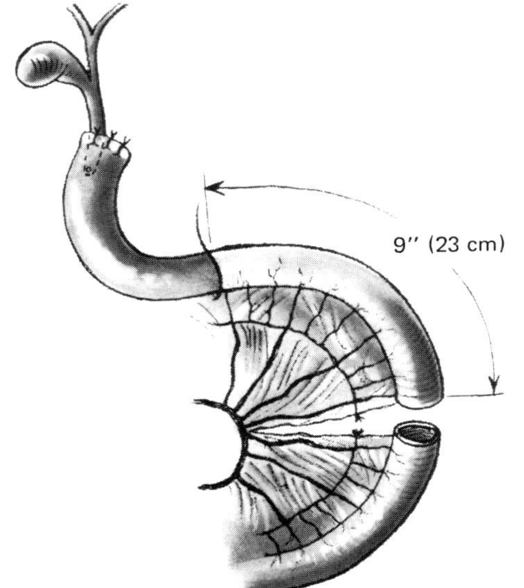

19

20

The Roux-en-Y anastomosis is completed by joining the proximal end of the transected jejunum end to side to the distal segment 18 inches (45 cm) below the gastrojejunostomy. This proximal jejunal segment is approximately half the length of the long-limb gastric drainage segment and passes behind and to the left of the latter to prevent distortion of the radian of small bowel mesentery. The 18 inch (45 cm) long limb of the Roux-en-Y provides an effective peristaltic barrier against reflux of bile and pancreatic secretions into the stomach and oesophagus. Intersecting mesenteries are closed to prevent internal herniation.

The abdomen is closed in layers in the usual fashion, two soft-rubber Penrose drains being brought from the duodenal stump to the outside through a right upper quadrant anterior abdominal wall stab wound. A nasogastric tube is passed and threaded into the upper reaches of the long-limb Roux-en-Y for postoperative suction-drainage.

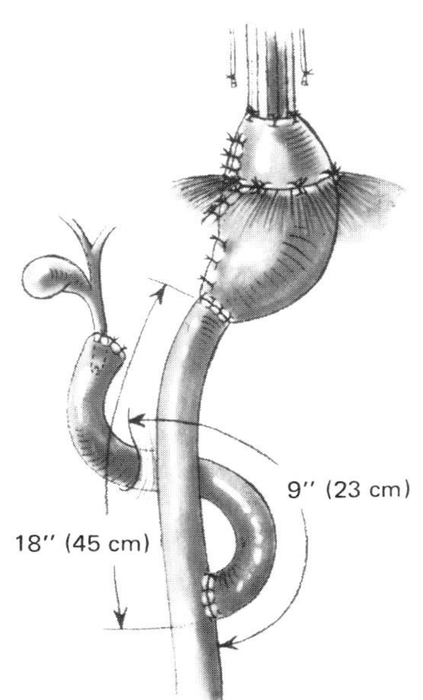

20

POSTOPERATIVE CARE

Patients are kept in a slanted, head-up oesophageal bed initially. Patients are ambulated the day after operation. Nasogastric suction is usually continued until bowel function returns on the fourth or fifth day. The chest tube is removed the day after operation.

Oral feeding is not resumed until a fluoroscopic examination of the oesophagus is obtained, using Gastrografin, to demonstrate patency without leakage at the oesophageal anastomosis. If leakage is apparent, the patient is not allowed oral intake; parenteral hyperalimentation is continued for 2 weeks, at which time the radiographic examination is repeated before oral feeding is begun.

Oral diet, when resumed, is rapidly advanced to solids over 4 to 5 days. Abdominal drains are removed by the eighth day, and patients are usually dismissed from the hospital 10–14 days after operation. Use of the oesophageal slant bed is continued only if nocturnal reflux with respiratory aspiration is experienced.

Surgical Treatment of Achalasia of the Cardia

Diffuse Oesophageal Spasm—'Corkscrew Oesophagus' and Periphrenic Diverticulum

A. W. Jowett, F.R.C.S.
Consultant Thoracic Surgeon, The Royal Hospital, Wolverhampton

ACHALASIA OF THE CARDIA

PRE-OPERATIVE

Diagnosis

Clinical suspicion is confirmed by barium swallow examination. In mild cases manometric tests may be helpful.

Oesophagoscopy should be carried out to exclude an unsuspected carcinoma either in the oesophagus or involving the cardia. Anaesthetic induction should be in a semisitting position to reduce over-spill risks before the cuff of the endotracheal tube can be inflated. In all but the mildest cases, the dilated oesophagus contains a large volume of secretions and decomposing food and there is frequently some oesophagitis. The cardia is usually further from the incisor teeth than normal for the patient's size. However, if long enough, the oesophagoscope can usually be passed into the stomach without encountering much resistance especially if a bougie is used to indicate the forward direction to be followed.

Indications

Surgery is indicated in all cases except when the general condition and especially the respiratory function cannot be adequately improved. In these, daily self-bougienage using a Hurst mercury bougie may be considered. Endoscopic procedures aimed at rupturing the circular muscle at the cardia, using instruments such as Plummer's hydrostatic bag or a Henning dilator cannot be recommended.

Heller's myotomy is the treatment for all uncomplicated cases but must always be accompanied by a definitive hiatus hernia repair to prevent the risk of subsequent complications from gastro-oesophageal reflux. In cases with gross mega-oesophagus or where a previous Heller's operation has failed, partial or total excision of the thoracic oesophagus should be considered. Direct anastomosis between the dilated oesophagus and the fundus of the stomach must never be contemplated as this can result in severe reflux.

HELLER'S MYOTOMY *(and repair of hiatus hernia)*

The operation consists of complete division of the circular muscle at the oesophagogastric junction.

The length of this division must always be adequate. Below, it should extend for a short distance onto the stomach and above, it should be continued until no more hypertrophied circular muscle is encountered. In cases which show little muscle hypertrophy, the division should extend for at least 5 cm up the oesophagus. A thoracic, thoraco-abdominal or entirely abdominal approach can be used. The operator may select the approach normally preferred for repair of the hiatus, which must always be performed as a formal procedure after the myotomy. However, a thoracic approach allows better exposure than does laparotomy, especially when the myotomy requires to be carried further up the oesophagus.

Pre-operative preparation

Even in cases with little oesophageal dilatation, careful clinical and radiological assessment should be made to exclude 'spill-over pneumonitis'. When the oesophagus is large and oesophagoscopy reveals much debris, this should be cleared completely, washing out if necessary. Following this, the patient should be allowed a fluid diet only and must not be permitted to lie flat. Physiotherapy and appropriate antibiotic treatment may be required for some days before the pneumonitis is adequately controlled.

THE OPERATION

Care should again be exercised during anaesthetic induction. Oesophagoscopy is performed to thoroughly clean the oesophagus. For the thoracic approach, the patient is placed in the true lateral position with a sandbag under the lower ribs in preparation for a left thoracotomy.

Exposure of the lower end of the oesophagus

The thorax has been opened by stripping the periosteum from the upper border of the left seventh rib. The pleura over the lower oesophagus is incised vertically and carefully dissected to form flaps for subsequent reconstitution.

Dissecting with care to avoid the adjacent right pleura, the oesophagus is lifted out of its bed and a tape passed around it. Further dissection around the hiatal margin allows the cardia and some stomach to be pulled up into view. Any fat in this area is carefully removed and the vessels just below the cardia identified.

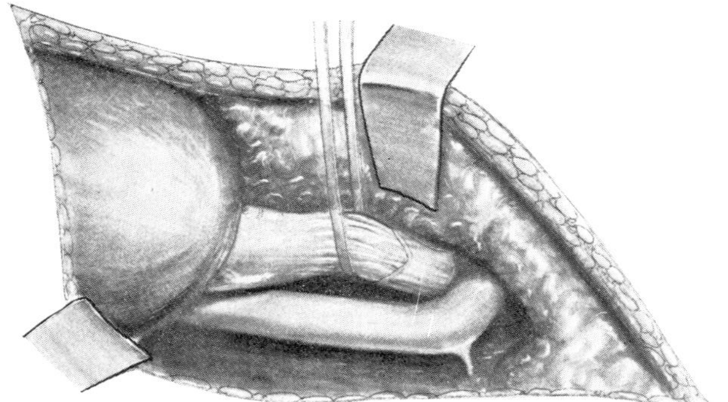

1

2

Division of the muscle at the oesophagogastric junction

The incision along the line of the oesophagus should be started some distance above the oesophagogastric junction. It is deepened until the mucosa is exposed. The submucosal venous plexus is a guide to this plane, but diathermy of these vessels risks mucosal damage. Once identified, this plane is followed downwards across the junction onto the stomach. At the oesophagogastric junction, the risk of opening the mucosa is greatest. Vessels on the stomach may require to be ligated and divided. The incision is then extended upwards on the oesophagus until the circular muscle no longer appears hypertrophied. The use of scissors rather than a knife decreases the risk of mucosal damage. It is unwise to have an oesophageal tube *in situ* during the myotomy as this also may increase the risk of mucosal damage. However, a tube gently introduced at this stage will demonstrate even the finest fibres of any residual circular muscle requiring division. Accidental perforation of the mucosa is immediately obvious and should be carefully repaired using fine interrupted sutures, and the postoperative regime will require modification.

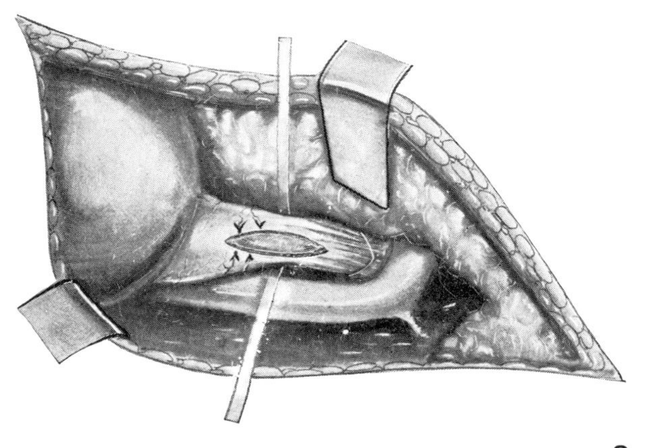

2

HIATUS HERNIA REPAIR

Methods of repair are described elsewhere (*see* pages 417–432) but whatever technique is used, including those where a thoraco-abdominal or laparotomy approach has been employed, a formal and complete repair of the hiatus will guard against reflux complications and does not appear to impede oesophageal emptying. Placing the cardia well below the hiatus also helps to correct the often sigmoid deformity of the oesophagus and will further assist function.

Postoperative care

Prevention of chest complications

Because of chronic lung damage from over-spill, special care needs to be taken.

Resumption of feeding

Oral fluids can normally be started on the day following operation. However, if the mucosa has been damaged and repaired, antibiotics should be given and oral intake delayed until mucosal integrity has been checked by Gastrografin swallow on the fifth to seventh day.

DIFFUSE OESOPHAGEAL SPASM ('CORKSCREW OESOPHAGUS')

Diagnosis

Barium swallow examination reveals the condition and usually demonstrates the presence of a hiatus hernia with gastro-oesophageal reflux. Manometric studies are also helpful.

Surgical treatment

This should be considered when the symptoms are very severe and do not respond to a strict medical hiatus hernia regime. Some cases benefit from repair of the hiatus hernia. In a few cases, an extended Heller's myotomy is indicated. The technique is similar to that described for the standard myotomy except that the muscle division is extended upwards on the oesophagus as far as the level of the aortic arch. Again, care should be taken to perform an efficient repair of the hiatus.

PERIPHRENIC DIVERTICULUM

Should the symtoms from a periphrenic diverticulum indicate the need for surgical intervention, simple excision of the diverticulum alone is liable to be followed by breakdown of the suture line. A Heller's myotomy at the cardia should also be carried out to prevent this complication.

[*The illustrations for this Chapter on Operations for Achalasia of the Cardia were drawn by Mr. G. Lyth.*]

Colon Replacement of the Oesophagus

R. H. F. Brain, F.R.C.S.
Consultant Thoracic Surgeon, Guy's Hospital, London

GENERAL

Skin tubes, the stomach, the jejunum, the ileocaecal region and the colon have all been successfully used to replace the oesophagus. Plastic tubes have been tried without success.

The advantages of using the colon are:

(*1*) Excepting the very rare instances of a grossly abnormal blood supply it can be used to bridge any sized gap between the pharynx and the duodenum.

(*2*) It has a better and more easily mobilized blood supply than the jejunum so that the risk of avascular necrosis is very much less.

(*3*) Its calibre and natural tone seem ideally suited to oesophageal replacement within the chest and, at the same time, it occupies minimal volume (*cf.* the stomach, which may be grossly space-occupying. This is important in the elderly and in those with limited respiratory reserve).

(*4*) Like the jejunum the colon is free of the effects of gastro-intestinal reflux on itself and prevents any such reflux from causing oesophagitis above the anastomosis. This is important because invariably the cardia and sometimes the pylorus have to be removed.

(*5*) Its use permits the stomach to be retained within the abdomen to function normally as a food reservoir, co-ordinating with the remainder of the alimentary tract, and thus ensuring that postoperational nutritional disturbances are absent.

Disadvantages:

(*1*) The rate of transmission of food through a colon transplant is slower than with the jejunum so that sometimes meals have to be taken at a slower than normal rate.

(*2*) The absence of a cardiac sphincter permits reflux from below with the rare late risk of gastric ulceration on the distal side of the cologastric anastomosis with secondary stricture formation.

(*3*) It is a longer and more complicated operation than stomach replacement.

Indications for use

(*a*) *Gastro-oesophagopharyngeal*—malignancy.

(*b*) *Simple peptic strictures* from reflux oesophagitis.

(*c*) *Caustic strictures.*

(*d*) *Simple tumours* where extensive or multiple, e.g. leiomyomata, where simpler measures are inapplicable.

(*e*) *Atresia of the oesophagus* where a primary anastomosis is impossible or impracticable.

(*f*) *Achalasia*—on rare occasions when cardiomyotomy either fails or is complicated by malignancy.

(*g*) *Bleeding varices*—portal hypertension, when 'shunting' fails or when stricture formation follows disconnection operations (e.g. Tanner's).

(*h*) *Ruptured oesophagus*—where conservative repair fails or is impossible.

GENERAL PRINCIPLES OF THE OPERATION

The site or level and extent of the pathology determines both the level of the anastomosis required and the incision or incisions necessary for adequate access. The oesophagus is subdivided into three important levels. (All distances measured from the incisor teeth.)

Low. From 30–40 cm, or even lower when varying amounts of stomach have to be removed at the same time.

Middle. From 20–30 cm levels.

High. From cricopharyngeus downwards to the 20 cm level.

Oesophagoscopy is essential for accurate siting and diagnosis of the pathology. Multiple biopsies, preferably using an open Negus type of oesophagoscope, are recommended.

Routing of the colon

For the 'low' and 'middle' replacements the colon is taken via the normal hiatus and the posterior mediastinum. In 'high' replacements the anterior mediastinal, or preferably the presternal subcutaneous route is favoured; this is taken just to the left of the midline, avoiding a right thoracotomy incision.

The use of the presternal route involves the formation of a hernia in the upper end of the abdominal wall incision sufficient to allow the easy passage of the colon without constricting its pedicled blood supply.

In children, Waterston prefers to make a deliberate incision in the dome of the left diaphragm. The colon is then brought up through this to the neck, passing via the left pleural space behind the lung hilum, and through its apex, anterior and medial to the left subclavian artery.

Anastomoses

Two-layer techniques are used for all anastomoses, an outer interrupted seromuscular and an inner watertight continuous which passes through all layers. The importance of a complete absence of tension cannot be over-emphasized; the organs must not only lie naturally in apposition before suturing, but must be sufficiently lax afterwards to allow free rotation of the gut, so that the outer interrupted suture layer can be inserted after the inner continuous one.

Anastomoses are end to end for oesophagus and colon, and end to side when the stomach is used. The latter anastomosis should be sited well down on the body of the stomach near the greater curvature on either its anterior or posterior walls. Continuity of the colon is restored by an end-to-end anastomosis.

Mediastinal dissection

The amount required depends upon the pathology. Carcinoma requires a complete clearance from the pericardium in front, from the aorta and the vertebral column behind, and from both pleurae laterally. *Gland* clearance should include groups around the coeliac axis, the oesophagus itself and the lung hilum: the *thoracic duct* is always at risk and is preferably deliberately divided, resected and ligated.

Simple strictures require minimal disturbance of the mediastinum.

The vagal nerves below their recurrent branches can be ignored and resected below the lung hila. In high oesophageal resections branches to the lung hila should be preserved as far as possible.

Pyloroplasties

Experience has shown that obstruction does not follow vagotomy in cases where the duodenum is healthy and unscarred; an intact sphincter is important in controlling the reflux of bile and pancreatic juices which can damage the oesophagus.

Gastrostomies

For feeding purposes, these are not advised since they function poorly, often with regurgitation upwards through the oesophagus or the transplant. However, a gastrostomy used for the introduction of a nasogastric type tube which is then threaded down through the duodenum into the jejunum will provide an excellent feeding stoma.

Mobilization of colon and preservation of its blood supply

1a,b&c

Even as shown in text books in common use, the anatomy of the blood supply to the colon is not constant. The operator must concentrate on the preservation of adequate inosculations between the primary arcades.

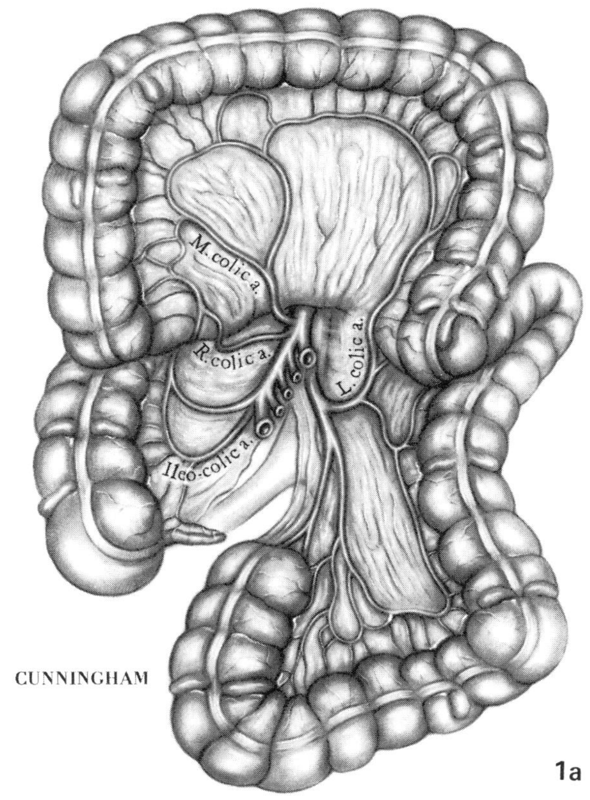

1a

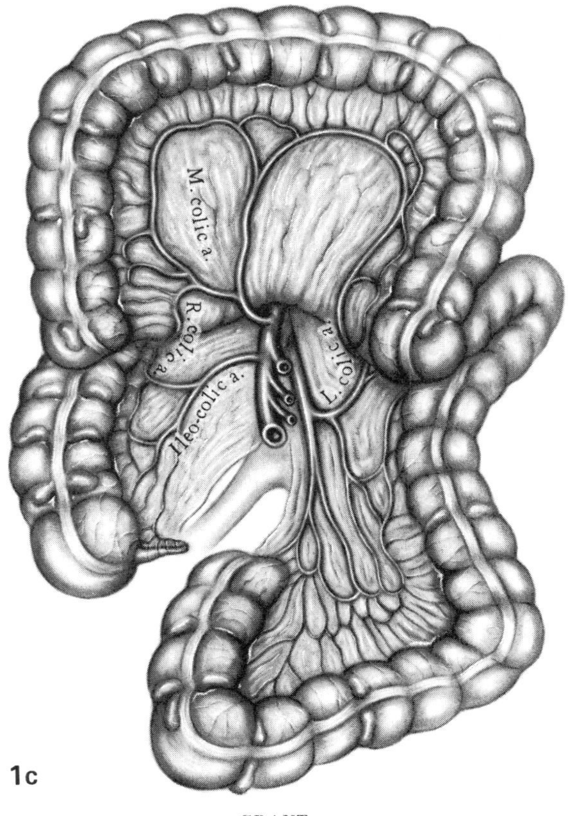

1c

GRANT

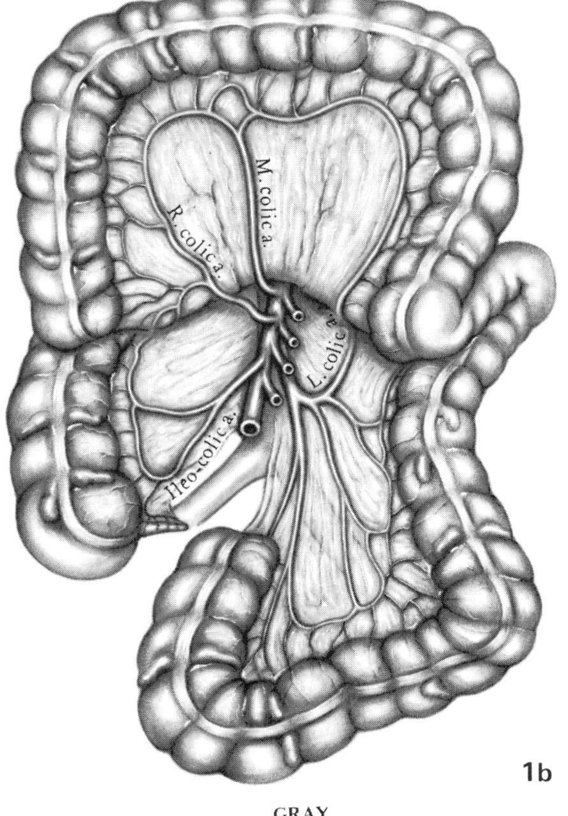

1b

GRAY

2

Depending upon the length of the colon required and the individual anatomical arrangement of the vessels, one, two or even three main vessels may have to be divided providing varying lengths of colon. Anastomotic sites at either A, B, C, D or even E may be chosen. On very rare occasions 'critical areas' with an inadequate para bowel circulation are found limiting the length available so that the proposed operation may be impossible. The importance of retaining adequate venous drainage, in particular that of the inferior mesenteric drainage into the splenic vein, is emphasized.

The colon is mobilized by the dissection of either or both of the paracolic peritoneal 'gutters' and excision of as much of the great omentum as is necessary with separation of the mesocolon from the lesser sac. Transillumination is a very useful technique when selecting vessels for division. Mobilization early in the operation, before excision of the oesophagus, is recommended so that imperfections in the blood supply will become obvious before the colon is used.

All clamps are avoided for bowel division where suture will be required later. Soiling is kept to a manageable minimum by the combination of an adequate pre-operative preparation of the bowel, ligature of the oesophagus immediately above the obstruction preventing reflux, and suction through an indwelling tube in the oesophagus above. The tape serves later as a landmark in malignant patients when the oesophagus has to be divided at least 4 cm above the tumour.

Transnasal intubation

Towards the end of the colo-oesophageal anastomosis and at whichever level this has been made, a firm but pliable tube is introduced through the nose, across the transplant, as far as the distal organ, usually the stomach, for the following reasons.

(*a*) It will act as a 'splint' to the transplant, maintaining its rectitude during the first few days.

(*b*) It will facilitate the regular, intermittent removal of *air* by suction and will thus prevent both dilatation of the colon transplant at a time when its tonus is minimal, and any general distension of the abdomen. The latter may cause both ileus and embarrassment of diaphragmatic ventilation. *Fluid* is aspirated until it becomes normal intestinal juice, after which it can be returned following the removal of air. The type and amount of fluid is carefully noted—the continuation of foul or old blood-stained aspirate after 48 hr may be the earliest sign of bowel necrosis. Such a calamity can thus be diagnosed early, and appropriate measures taken before the patient becomes moribund.

The usual time for removal of the tube is at the end of the third day.

Pre-operative preparation of the patient

Care at this time, particularly in the elderly and in the debilitated, will improve results.

(*a*) *A general health assessment* includes baseline measurements of the patient's biochemical, respiratory and cardiovascular systems, including E.C.G. and a straight chest film.

(*b*) *The details of the nutrition of the patient* will depend upon the pathology, the degree of obstruction present and its duration. Fluid, calorie and protein deficiencies may need pre-operative correction, if necessary by the intravenous route. Occult vitamin C and B deficiencies are common and must be supplemented.

(*c*) *Colon preparation*—an empty, almost sterile colon in good tone is needed and can be achieved by:

(*1*) A non-residue diet.

(*2*) A 5-day preparation with twice daily veripaque enemata (Oxyphenisatin 50 mg).

(*3*) A 5-day course (15 g/day) of an insoluble sulpha drug given by mouth, if necessary in the form of an emulsion.

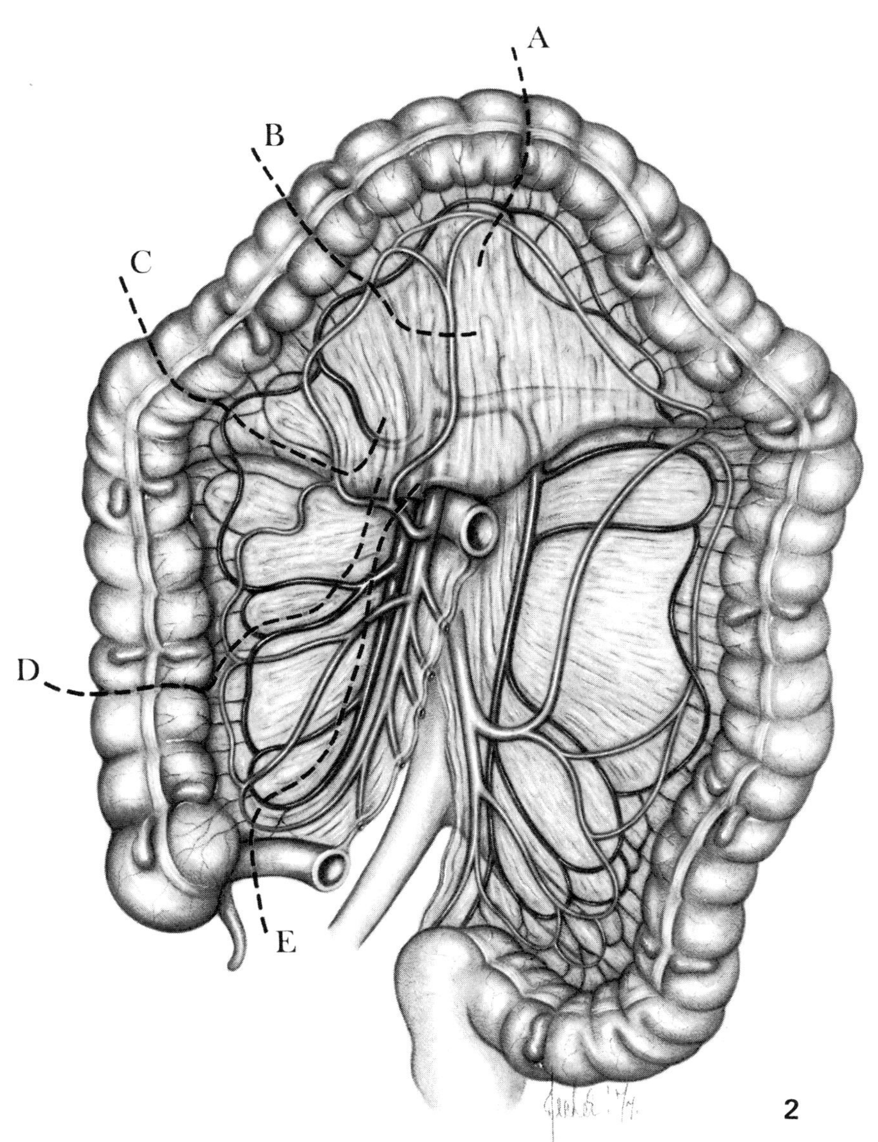

2

THE OPERATIONS

LOW STRICTURES (up to 30 cm)

3

The incision

This is through the left lower chest, eighth rib bed, with the patient in the full left lateral thoracotomy position. Rarely, it may have to be prolonged across the costal margin.

4

Exposure

Abdomen, through a circumferential incision in the diaphragm 1 cm from its costal attachment.

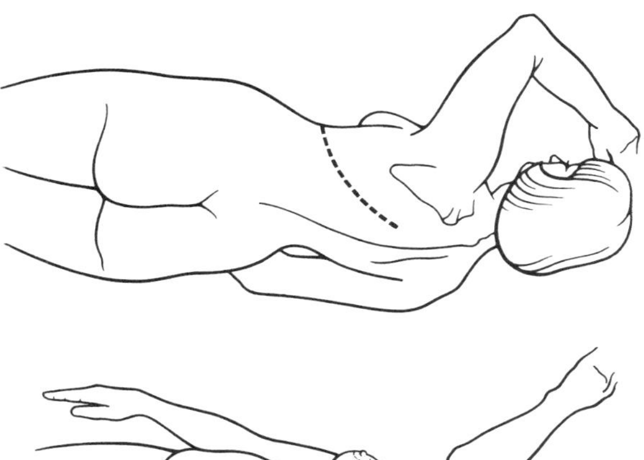

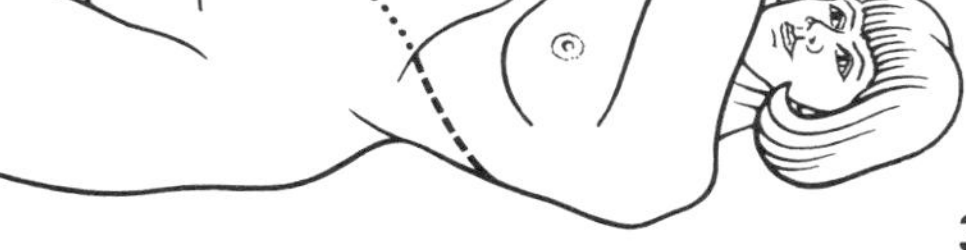

3

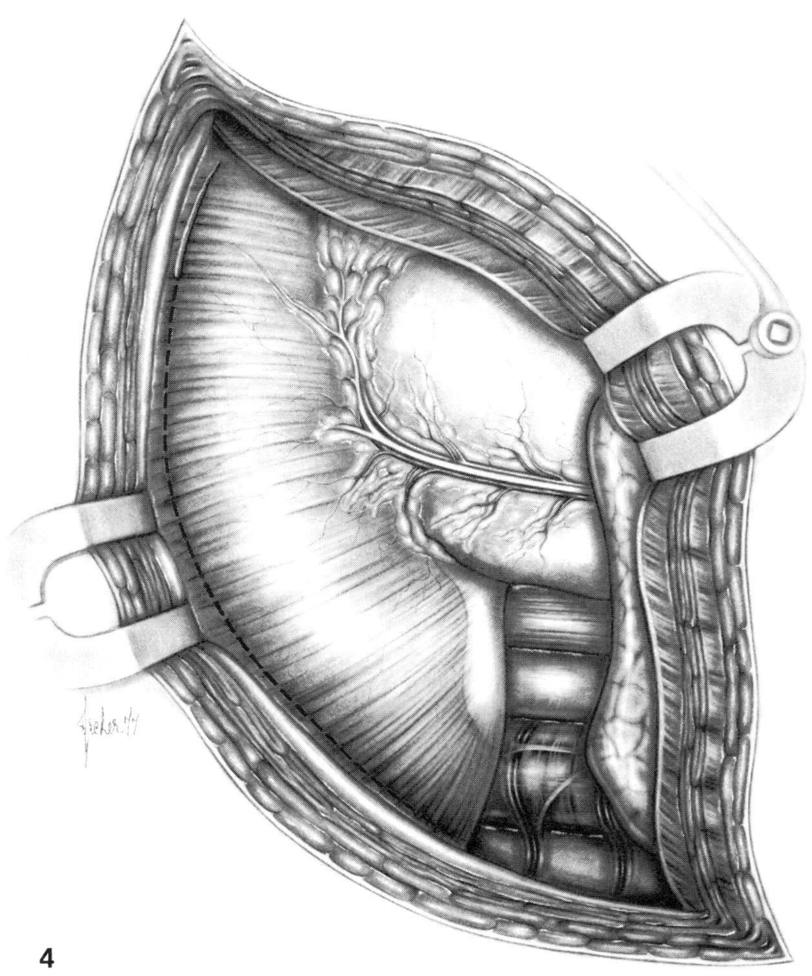

4

5

Providing there are no adhesions from previous operations or disease the left half of the colon can be pulled up into the chest quite easily. The great omentum has been detached.

Details of operation

(*1*) Complete division of the left coronary ligament with the left lobe of the liver folded back to the right aids access to the cardia, right crus and coeliac axis.

(*2*) Splenectomy is carried out routinely for easy access and for routing the transplant posteriorly through the lesser sac anterior to the pancreas.

(*3*) Colon mobilized (as in *Illustration 1*) and divided at levels A or B and hinged on the left colic artery (*see Illustration 2*).

(*4*) Anastomoses–above and later below the colon, well down on the posterior surface of the body of the stomach near the great curve (*see* page 452).

(*5*) In order to prevent herniation alongside the transplant, immediately prior to closure of the abdomen the fundus of the stomach is sutured to the remnant of the left coronary ligament on the undersurface of the diaphragm.

(*6*) Intubation (*see* page 454).

(*7*) Drainage–left pleural space.

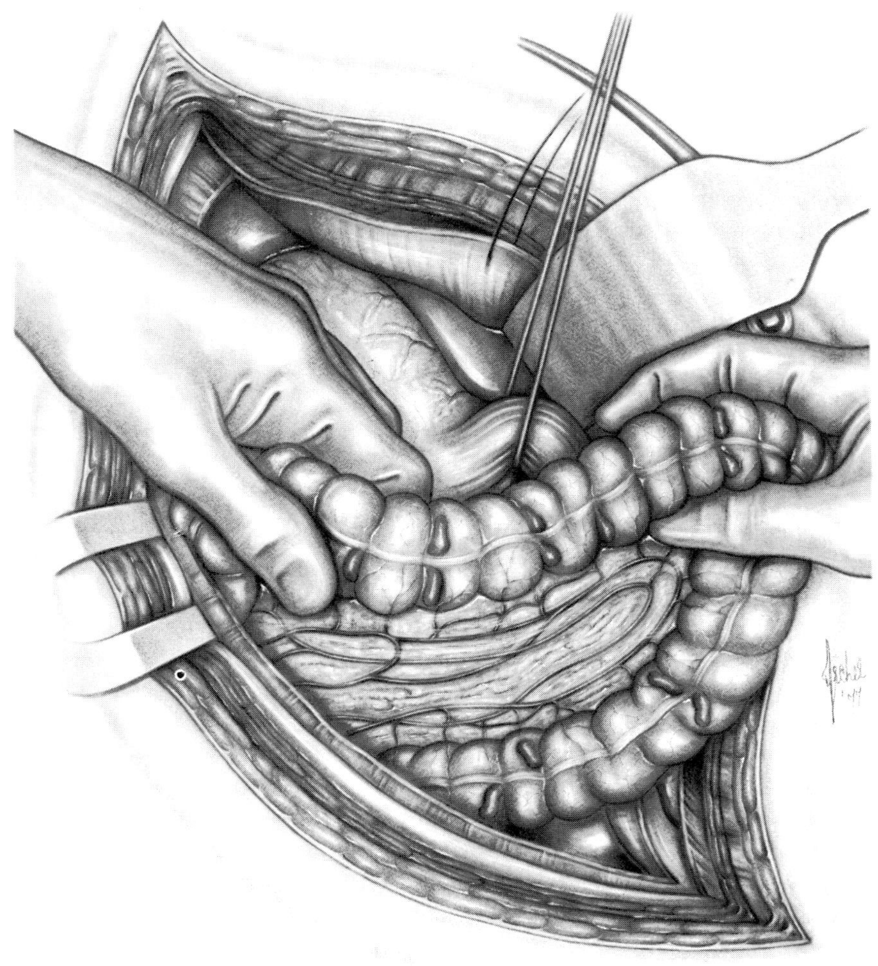

5

6
THE COMPLETED OPERATION

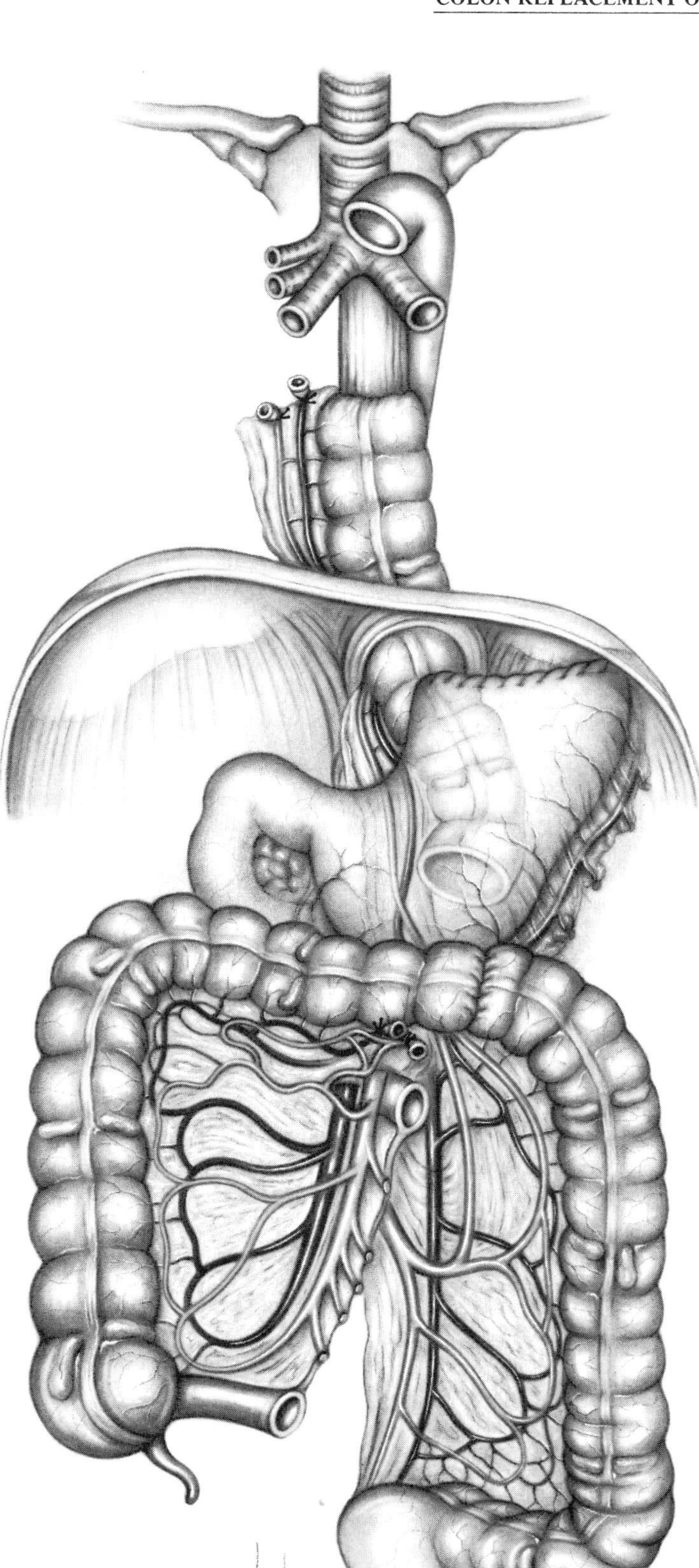

6

MIDDLE STRICTURES (20–30 cm)

7

These require excision and replacement through the right chest because of limited access due to the presence of the aortic arch on the left side. Separate abdominal and chest incisions, which preserve an intact costal margin, are preferred to a combined abdominothoracic one (through either of the fifth, sixth or seventh rib beds). The latter extends from the transverse processes behind to the costosternal junction in front. The use of a laterally rotating table facilitates a rapid transfer from one incision to the other.

8

Important details of operation

(*1*) The abdomen is explored first. Complete division of the left coronary ligament and retraction of the left lobe of the liver to the right aids access both to the cardia and the left gastric pedicle.

(*2*) The colon is mobilized for division later at points C or D (*see* page 454).

(*3*) The oesophagus is detached below, and the cardia closed.

(*4*) The abdominal wound is left open.

(*5*) The chest is explored, and the oesophagus mobilized and excised.

(*6*) The colon is pulled up from below, through the hiatus.

(*7*) The anastomosis above the diaphragm is usually made first, followed by the lower one into the anterior wall of the stomach (*see* page 452).

(*8*) Intubation of the transplant (*see* page 454).

(*9*) Right pleural drainage.

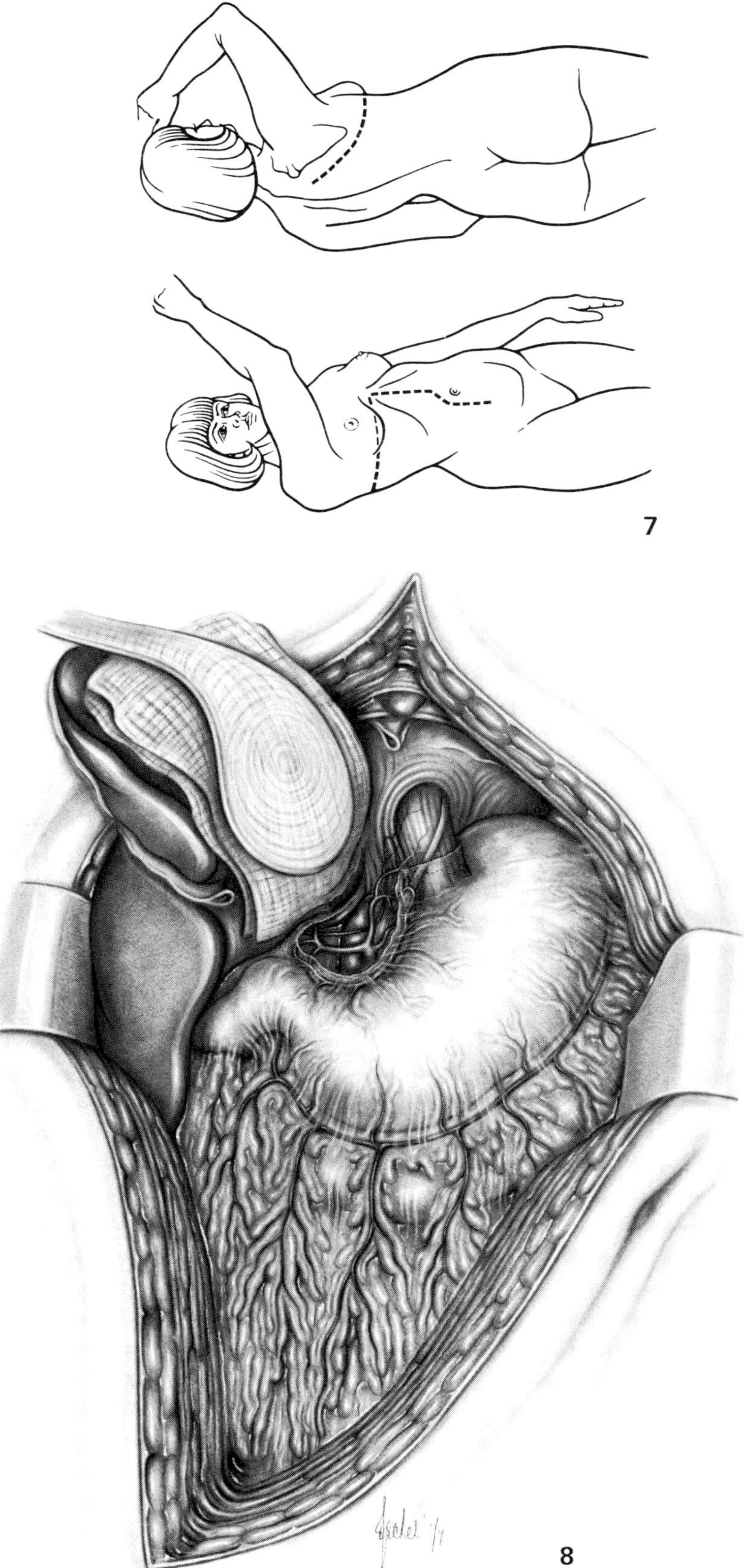

7

8

9

THE COMPLETED OPERATION

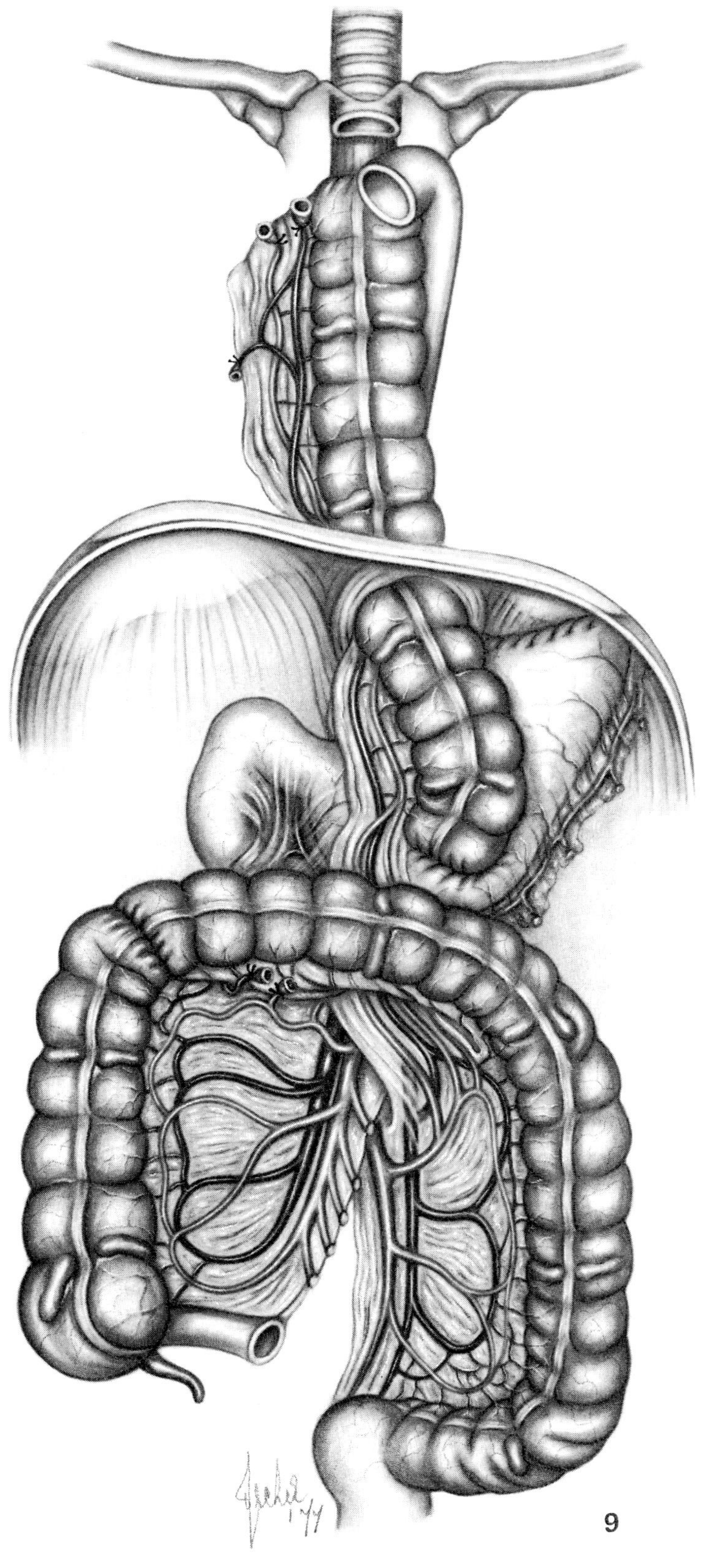

9

HIGH STRICTURES (down to 20 cm level)

Those within the thorax have to be managed on their individual merits including their pathology; but it is not usually possible to make a satisfactory anastomosis within the chest. Nevertheless the right thorax may have to be opened for an adequate mobilization and an excision which includes the lymph drainage.

10a&b

The incisions

Cervical, abdominal and possibly a right thoracotomy may be required. Alternative incisions in the neck are required depending upon the need for an accompanying laryngectomy.

Important details of operations

Depending upon the pathology and the site of the obstruction the abdomen or right chest is explored first. With lesions of the cervical oesophagus or pharynx, the right chest may or may not have to be explored depending on whether or not a sufficient clearance of the cancer can be made from above (3–4 cm).

(*1*) Right lateral thoracotomy–lateral position (fifth or sixth rib bed).

(*2*) Abdominal and cervical incisions– supine position.

(*3*) The oesophagus is divided in patients with intrathoracic lesions either at the thoracic inlet or closely below it, leaving a 'stump' to be brought out later through the cervical incision.

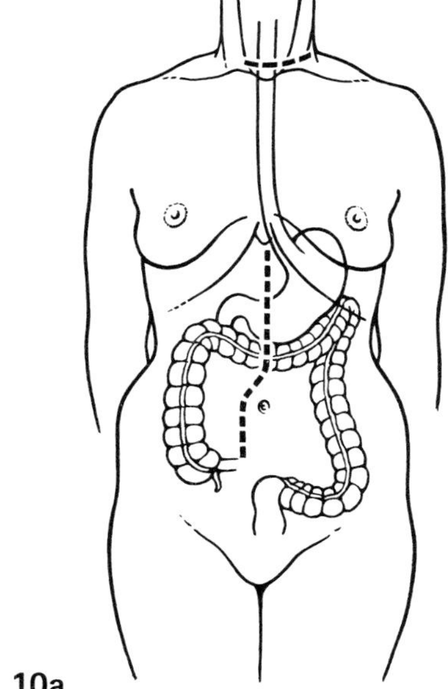

10a

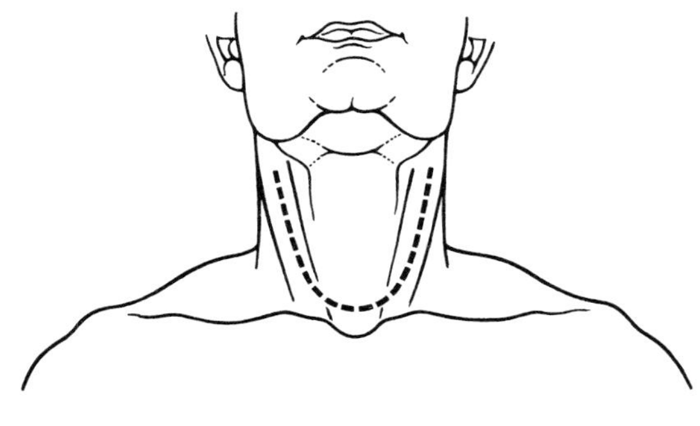

10b

11, 12 & 13

(*4*) The colon is mobilized in accordance with general principles (*see* page 454) at either site D or E and brought upwards through the abdominal incision and a presternal skin tunnel either as far as the oesophageal stump in the neck or to the pharynx (following laryngectomy).

(*5*) Intubation (*see* page 454).

(*6*) Drainage. This is from the right thorax, if opened, otherwise from the neck. If the chest is opened, the neck can be closed, as it will drain through the mediastinum into the pleura.

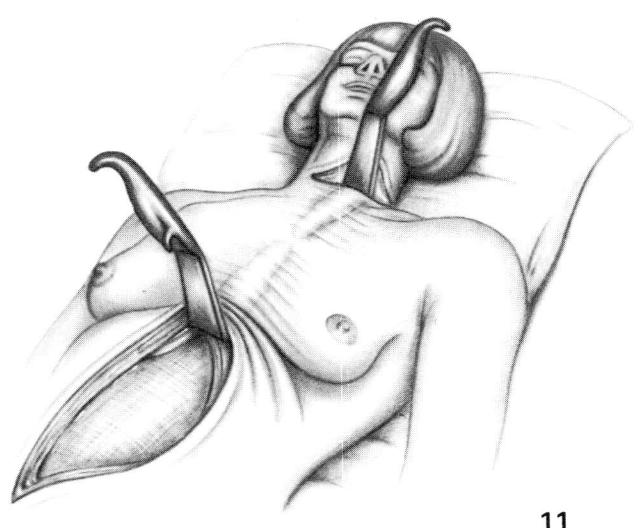

11

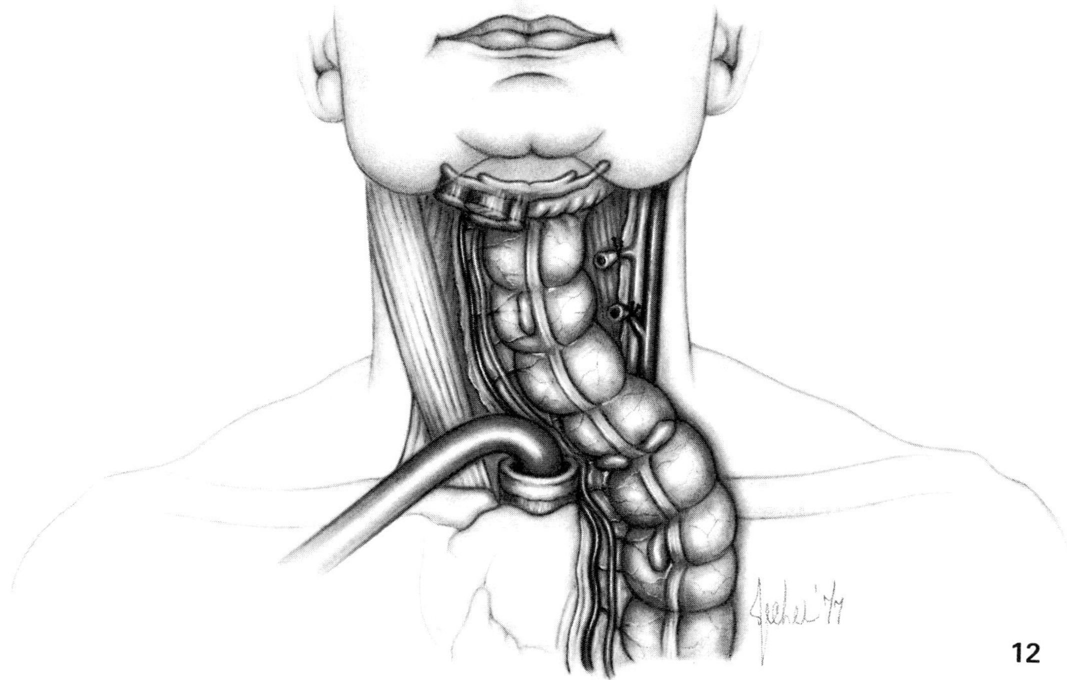

12

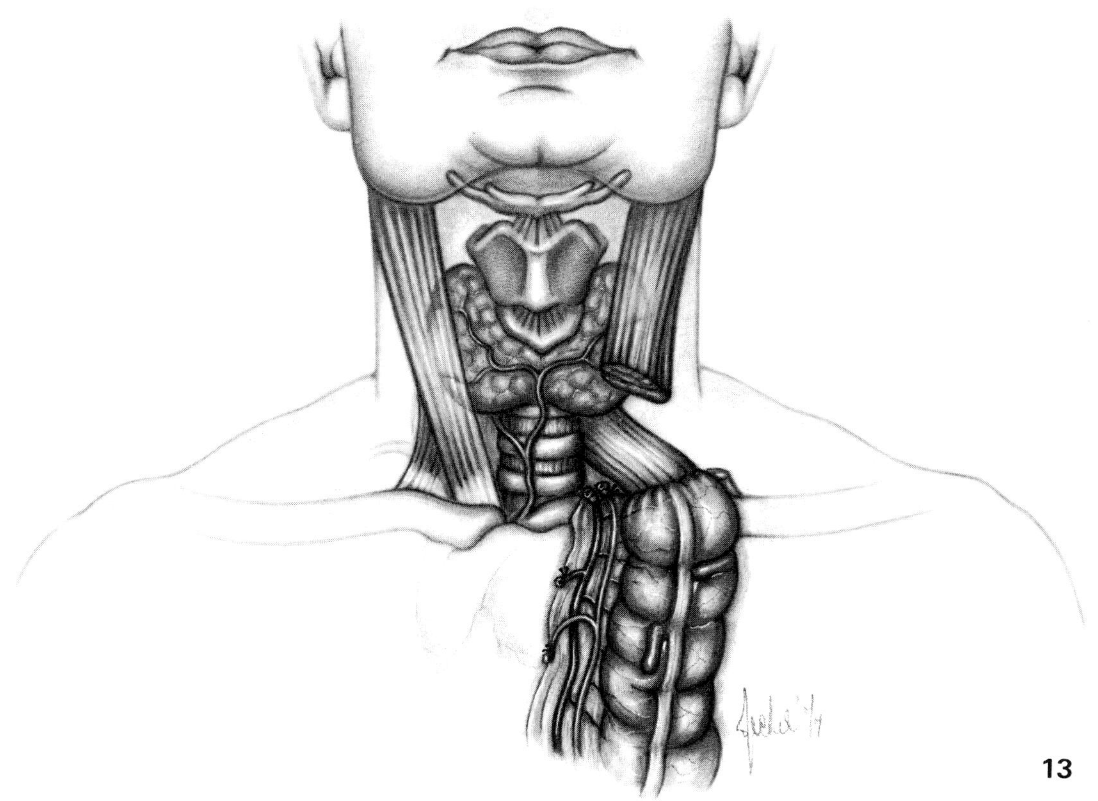

13

14a,b&c

THE COMPLETED OPERATION

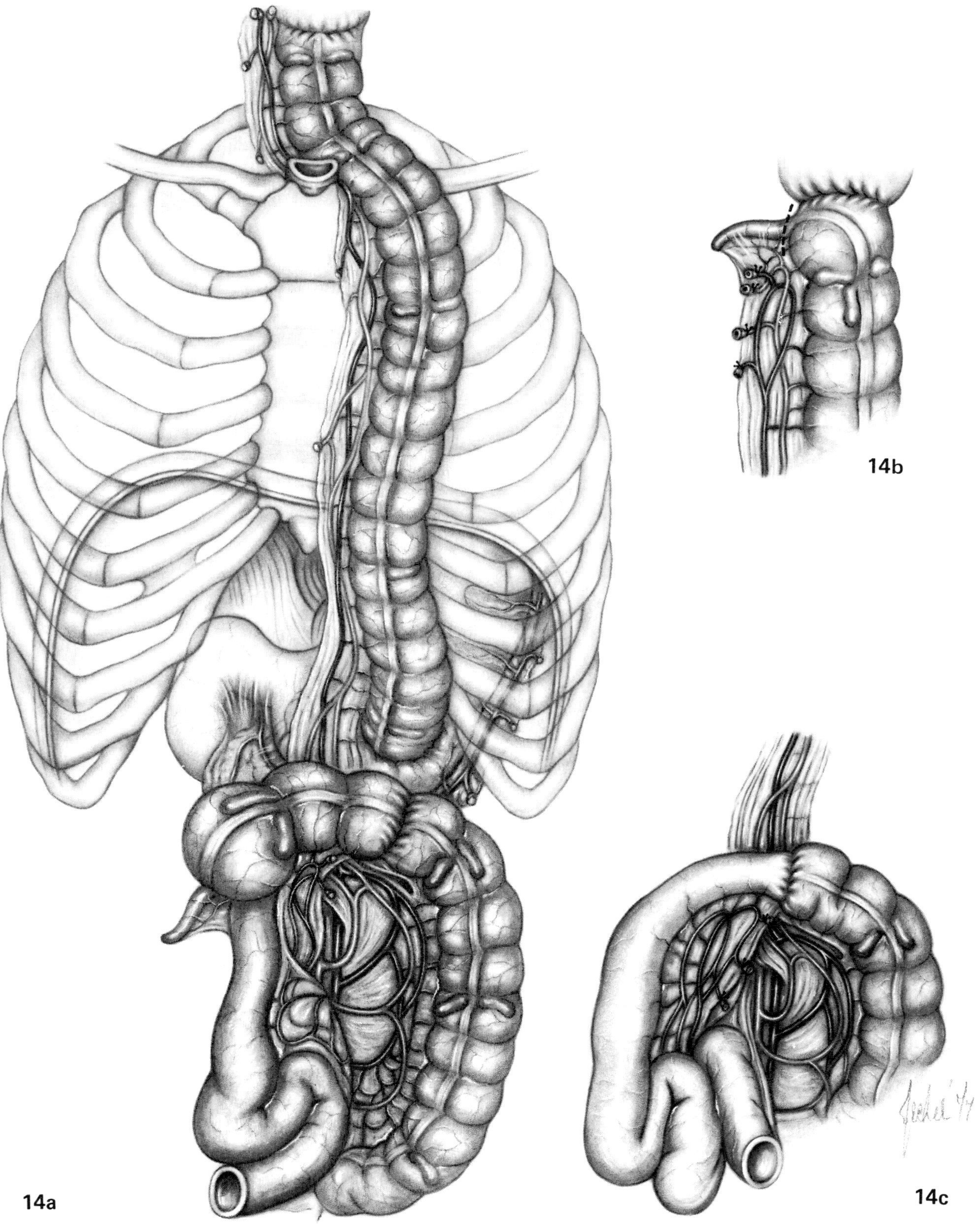
14a
14b
14c

POSTOPERATIVE CARE

This consists of:

(*1*) Intravenous alimentation over the first 10 days, during which time nothing will be taken by mouth.

(*2*) Bladder catheterization with a check on the hourly output of urine and its osmolarity.

(*3*) Regular checking of the usual parameters of fluid/electrolyte balance, including the blood urea and the measurement of the central venous pressure.

(*4*) Hourly aspiration of the nasogastric tube—with measurement of fluid and air aspirates, together with details of the type of fluid found. When clean, this is returned (*see* page 454).

(*5*) Chest supervision with physiotherapy and daily x-rays.

(*6*) A routine Gastrografin swallow on the tenth day checks the patency of the new oesophagus and its anastomoses.

If all is well, oral fluids, up to 4 ml hourly, can now be taken and the intravenous drip removed. The swallowing of normal food is re-instituted by the fourteenth postoperative day.

COMPLICATIONS

Early

These are surprisingly few, once a satisfactory technique has been established by the surgeon and his staff. Nevertheless, important likely causes of trouble are:

(*1*) *The problems of ventilation/oxygenation* common in minor forms may assume major proportions leading to a rapid death, particularly in the elderly, the grossly overweight and those who already have poor respiratory reserve. Sputum retention causing varying degrees of ventilatory obstruction, with or without collapse of lung tissue, is the main cause of respiratory failure at this time. Additional aggravating factors are pain, recurrent laryngeal nerve palsies and possible denervation of the bronchial tree after extensive high mediastinal dissections. If sputum retention occurs, early bronchoscopic aspiration of the bronchial tree is recommended, with tracheostomy and mechanical ventilation in extreme cases.

(*2*) *Poor vascularity* leading to minor necrosis of the colon is rare, but may occur particularly at the proximal anastomoses of the higher transplants. Massive necroses can be diagnosed early (*see* page 454) with early intervention and a more likely recovery. Minor leakages with fistula formation in the neck may follow but simple drainage usually resolves the problem. Delayed oral feeding may be necessary with continuance of the intravenous route; longer periods may require the use of jejunal feeding through a gastrostomy and intubation via the pylorus well down into the small intestine (*see* page 452).

Late

These are rare but the following have been seen in a very small percentage of patients.

(*1*) Fibrous stricture at the cologastric junction.

(*2*) Gastric ulceration just proximal to the cologastric anastomosis near the lesser curve. For this reason anastomosis well down on the greater curvature is advised.

(*3*) Redundancy of the colon above the diaphragm leading to stasis and slower transmission rates. At operation the need for an adequate opening for the colon through the diaphragmatic hiatus is emphasized, particularly in patients who have had previous operations for hiatal herniae where the hiatus has been sutured.

[*The illustrations for this Chapter on Colon Replacement of the Oesophagus were drawn by Miss P. Archer.*]

Operations for Carcinoma of the Thoracic Oesophagus and Cardia

John W. Jackson, M.Ch., F.R.C.S.
Consultant Thoracic Surgeon, Harefield Hospital, Middlesex

Age alone is not a bar to surgery for these lesions, the majority of patients are in the seventh decade and a number are over 80 years of age.

Increasing dysphagia at first to solids and then subsequently to soft foods and finally fluids leads to weight loss inanition and dehydration.

The tumour is locally invasive and may have extended beyond the normal confines of the oesophagus and stomach to become adherent to adjacent structures in the chest and abdomen, sometimes causing early peritoneal metastases. Spread by the lymphatics in the mediastinum to the neck and abdomen is often slow and spread by the bloodstream to the liver and elsewhere unpredictable. Neither local invasion nor limited lymphatic spread are contra-indications to surgical excision but peritoneal and hepatic metastases suggest that a palliative procedure would be more appropriate.

The prime aim of operation should be to restore swallowing and to remove the ulcerating fungating growth that lies in direct communication with the mouth. If at the same time a satisfactory cancer excision is obtained it should be regarded as a bonus. The mortality of 10 per cent is surgically acceptable and the extension of life by 1 or 2 years a real benefit to an elderly person. Operation has to be a once only procedure, there is seldom time for staged operations at this age. If dysphagia is complete operation should be carried out as soon as anaemia, dehydration and electrolyte imbalance have been corrected.

A careful clinical examination is essential to exclude other contra-indications to radical surgery, e.g. metastases to the neck glands, liver and peritoneum. A rectal examination is carried out to exclude pelvic metastases and assess the prostate. Severe constipation often made worse by recent barium studies may need attention so as to avoid faecal impaction after operation.

Investigations

Diagnosis is established by barium swallow, if possible the distal oesophagus, stomach and cardia should be outlined in the examination. A chest x-ray is necessary to exclude carcinoma of the bronchus as the next common cause of dysphagia and to detect any pneumonic change due to spill from the oesophagus.

Oesophagoscopy is essential to determine the level and extent of the lesion and to obtain material for histology. The examination should be followed by bronchoscopy in every case to exclude direct or indirect involvement of the carina or a main bronchus.

With intravenous alimentation there is now no need for a feeding gastrostomy or jejunostomy.

The oesophagus may be replaced by stomach, colon or small intestine. If the growth is confined to the oesophagus the author uses stomach and if the cardia and lower oesophagus are involved jejunum is preferred. The use of colon is described in the Chapter on 'Colon Replacement of the Oesophagus', pages 451–472.

Pre-operative treatment

It may be possible to improve the patient's swallowing temporarily by removing impacted food or fungating tumour at the time of oesophagoscopy. Usually dehydration and electrolyte imbalance need to be corrected by intravenous therapy. Anaemia should be corrected by blood transfusion.

Simple dental treatment should be carried out during this period–scaling and the removal of loose teeth which might be dislodged at operation. Oral candidiasis is common and antifungal agents may be required.

Chest infection, often associated with oesophageal spill-over, may call for a period of treatment with physiotherapy and antibiotics.

Generally these patients do not benefit by having their operations deferred.

THE OPERATION

OESOPHAGECTOMY WITH GASTRIC REPLACEMENT (IVOR LEWIS)

Anaesthesia

The patient is anaesthetized and a double-lumen tube inserted so that the right lung can be excluded from the circuit for part of the operation.

An intravenous drip, using a central venous line, is set up and a urinary catheter passed so as to monitor urinary output.

Stage I. Abdominal

1

With the patient supine laparotomy is made using a transverse incision mid-way between the xiphoid process and umbilicus dividing the rectus muscles. This affords good access to the pylorus and to the spleen and cardia. The abdomen is explored to exclude metastases or other pathology. If growth is palpable at the cardia a left-sided approach (*see* page 479) may be preferred and the incision can be extended into the chest along the eighth rib.

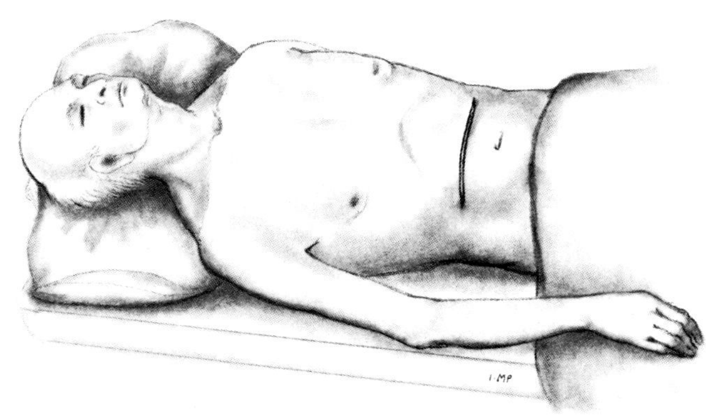

1

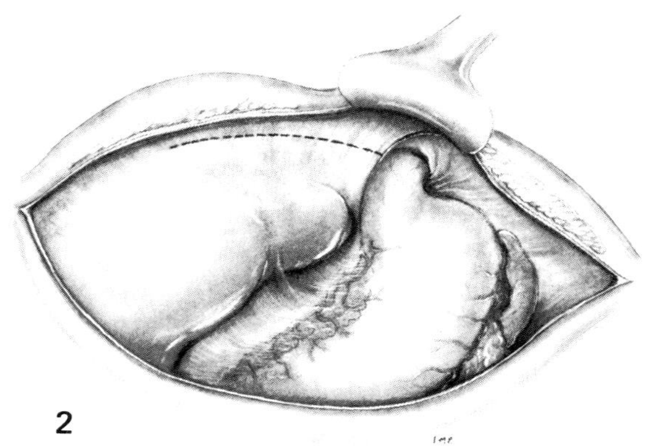

2

2

The left triangular ligament is divided at an early stage and the left lobe of the liver retracted so as to expose the oesophageal hiatus.

3

The stomach, omentum and transverse colon are delivered into the wound, an opening is made in the gastrocolic omentum on the greater curve so as to gain access to the lesser sac. The gastrocolic omentum is divided or separated from the colon preserving the right gastro-epiploic arch. The short gastric and left gastro-epiploic vessels are divided. If the spleen is in the way or bleeds it should be removed. The gastrohepatic omentum is divided. It frequently carries a sizeable hepatic branch from the left gastric artery. This may be divided provided there is an adequate main hepatic artery. The right gastric vessels are preserved and the left gastric pedicle is cleared and the artery and vein tied separately close to the coeliac axis. Any enlarged glands are removed and sent for histological examination. The hiatus is defined by sharp dissection but need not be enlarged. The oesophagus is freed from the mediastinum by blunt dissection using swabs and a finger. The lower end of the tumour may be palpable. Pyloroplasty is usually carried out. The peritoneum lateral to the duodenum may be divided to improve mobilization. When haemostasis is satisfactory the abdomen is closed.

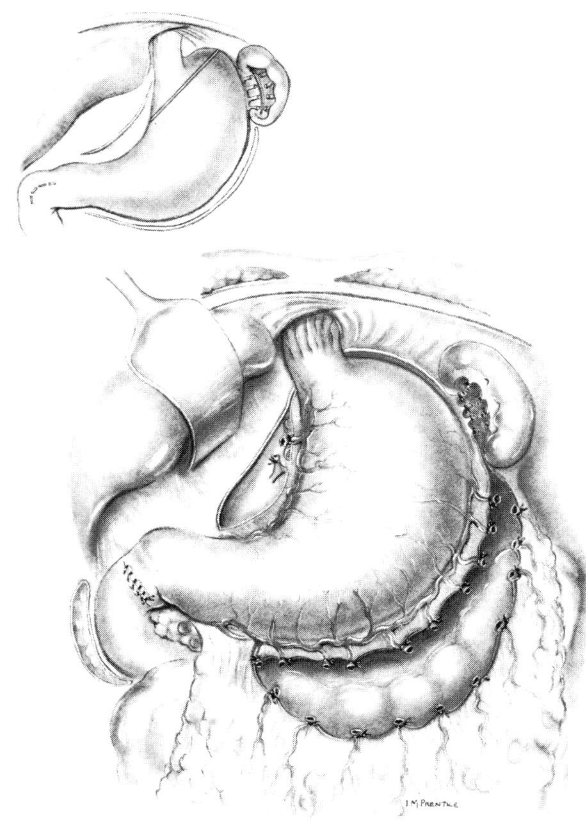

3

Stage II. Thoracic

Anaesthesia

A double-lumen tube with exclusion of the right lung for part of this stage is a distinct advantage.

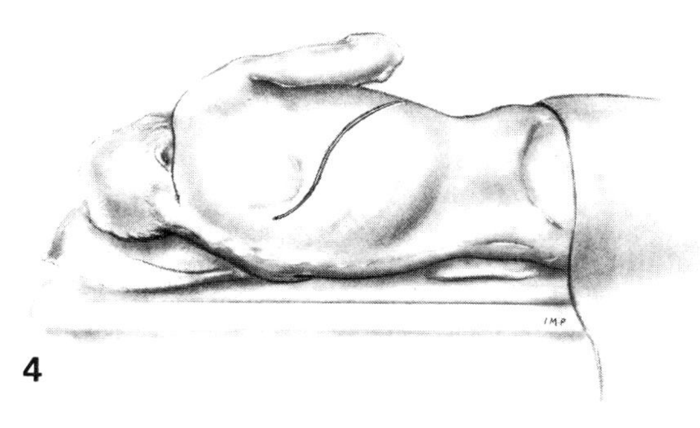

4

4

Position of patient

The patient is turned on to the left side and secured to the table. (The face down position is preferred by some surgeons.) A right thoracotomy is carried out along the upper border of the sixth rib.

5

The lung is freed to the hilum, retracted anteriorly, and allowed to collapse. The lesion in the oesophagus is inspected and palpated. The azygos vein is ligated and divided and the mediastinal pleura opened along the length of the oesophagus. Tapes are passed round the oesophagus above and below the tumour. By sharp dissection the pericardium, lower trachea and both main bronchi are separated from the oesophagus taking the subcarinal and mediastinal lymph nodes with the oesophagus. A plane is then opened between the oesophagus and the spine and aorta. The tumour may be densely adherent to any one of these structures, as if by direct extension, it must be separated by a process of sharp dissection, stealth and persuasion. Clean and intact mobilization is not always possible. One or two sizeable vessels from the aorta may need to be ligated or secured with a suture.

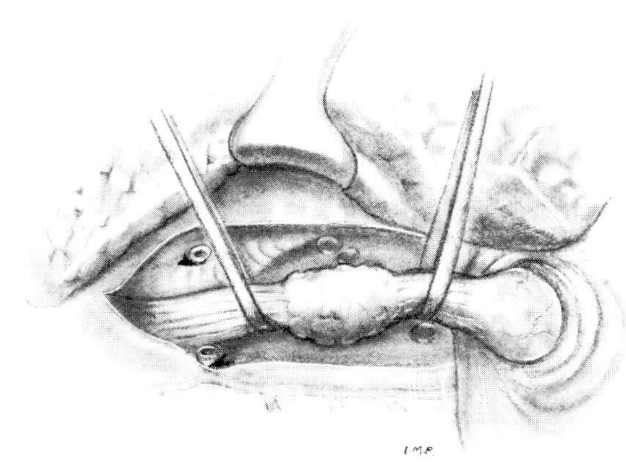

5

6

As soon as the oesophagus and its tumour are free the stomach is delivered into the chest, its initial presentation is noted so as to avoid subsequent rotation—the greater curve should be along the mediastinum. The pylorus may present through the hiatus. The oesophagus is mobilized to the base of the neck.

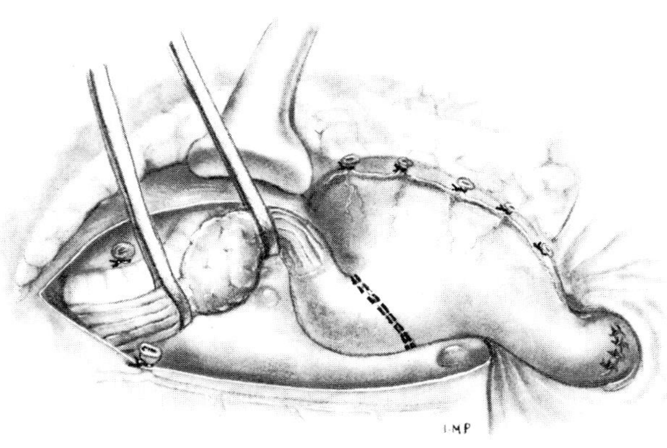

6

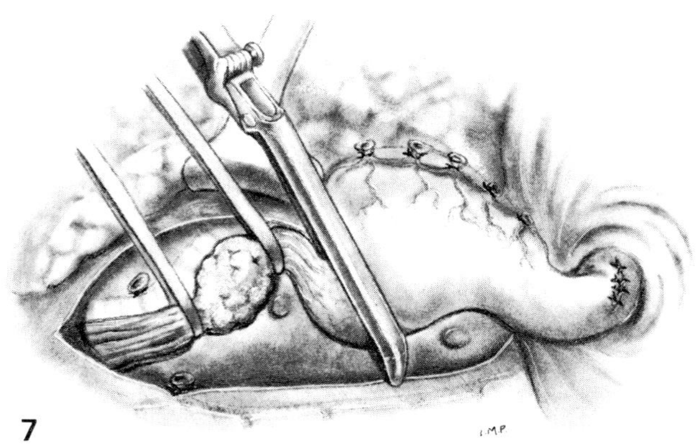

7

7

A Petz clamp is applied obliquely across the cardia and the stomach divided with diathermy between the rows of staples. The stomach edge is oversewn with catgut (2/0 chromic) and inverted with a row of interrupted Lembert sutures (3/0 linen).

8

The stomach is laid in the oesophageal bed and should reach the root of the neck—indeed if the oesophageal tumour is high anastomosis can be effected in the neck by a separate incision after the chest is closed.

A site is chosen near the fundus of the stomach for anastomosis with the oesophagus. It should be away from the suture line closing the cardia so as to avoid leaving an ischaemic bridge of tissue.

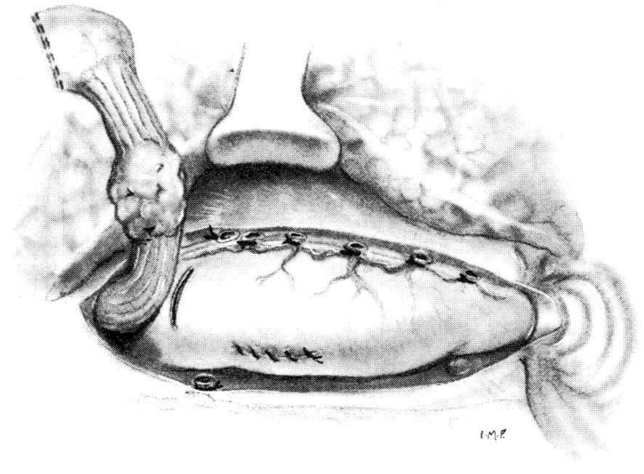

8

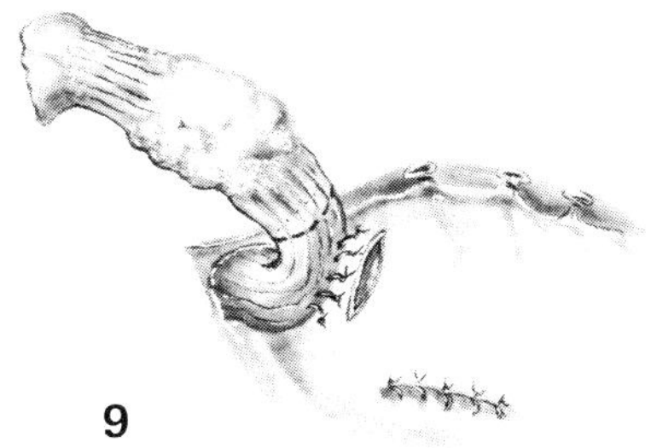

9

9

The oesophagus is attached to the stomach by a series of interrupted seromuscular type stitches (3/0 linen).

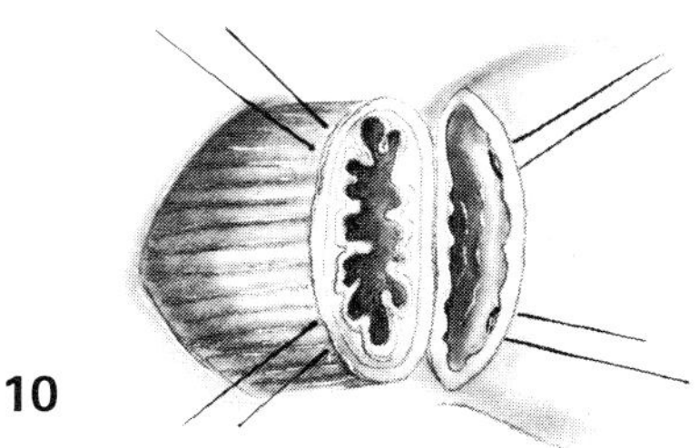

10

10

An opening is made in the stomach and two through-and-through marker sutures placed on the free edge to hold the stoma open. The oesophagus is divided level with the stoma. A clamp may be applied to the distal oesophagus only. Two matching marker sutures are applied to hold the mucosa on the free edge of the divided oesophagus.

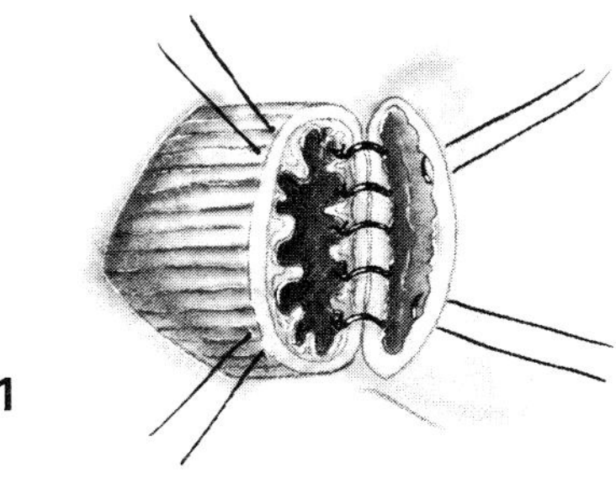

11

11

A row of interrupted, all-layers sutures is applied between the stomach and oesophagus posteriorly.

12

A nasogastric tube with a radio-opaque marker line is passed by the anaesthetist to the stomach and its tip located near the hiatus. The angles and front row of the anastomosis are completed using a series of interrupted Connell all-layers sutures which invaginate the mucosa. Each stitch starts and finishes on the outside of the stomach or oesophagus with loops on the mucosa of each. When tied the knots of this row are outside the lumen of the anastomosis.

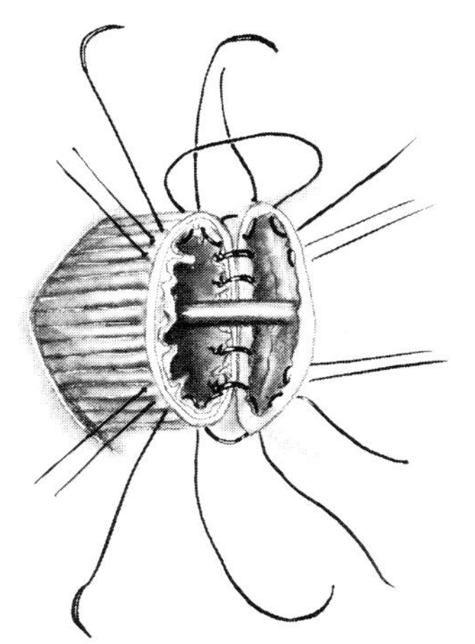

12

13 & 14

A row of seromuscular-type sutures between the stomach and the oesophagus draws a cuff of stomach up over the previous layer and hides it from sight.

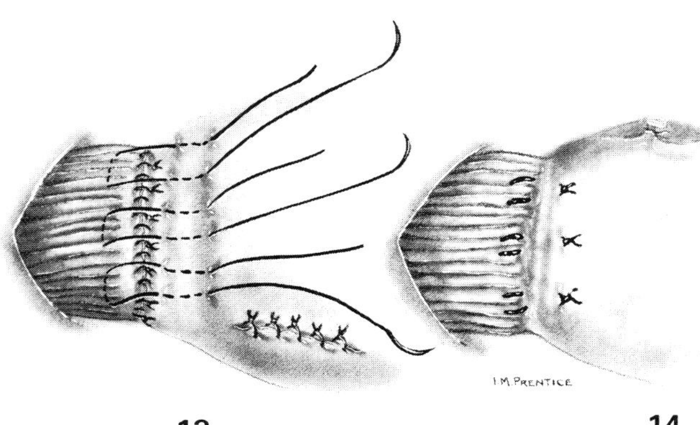

13 14

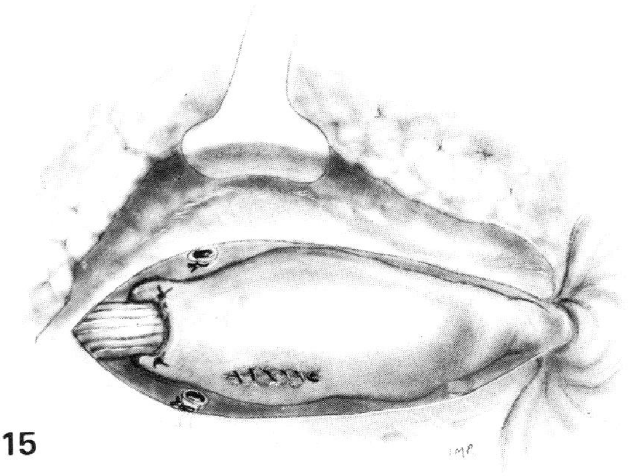

15

15

There should be no tension and any surplus of stomach may be returned to the abdomen. The anastomosis and the tube of stomach take their place in the mediastinum in the bed of the excised oesophagus.

The pleura is loosely closed over the anastomosis and the stomach confined to the mediastinum by a cradle of (2/0) catgut stitches placed loosely as interrupted loops or continuous zig-zag between the divided edges of the mediastinal pleura.

The lung is re-inflated and the chest closed with a basal drain (36 Ch). A separate mediastinal drain (32 Ch) is rarely indicated.

OESOPHAGOGASTRECTOMY WITH JEJUNAL REPLACEMENT, ROUX-EN-Y

The aim of this operation is to remove the entire stomach and as much as possible of the oesophagus above the tumour (10–12 cm) along with the spleen and omentum, the left gastric glands and part of the body and tail of the pancreas if it is involved.

Anaesthesia

The patient is anaesthetized and a double-lumen tube inserted so that the left lung can be excluded from the circuit for part of the operation.

An intravenous drip, using a central venous line, is set up and a urinary catheter passed so as to monitor urinary output.

The abdomen is opened first between the mid-line and the costal margin dividing the left rectus muscle. The extent and operability of the lesion are assessed. Free fluid, peritoneal seedlings and liver and pelvic metastases suggest that a palliative procedure may be preferable. Fixation near the hiatus or involvement of coeliac axis glands are unfavourable signs but need not constitute a bar to resection and a trial mobilization may be deemed worthwhile, bearing in mind Grey Turner's dictum: 'No tumour shall be deemed inoperable until it has been proved to be so at operation'.

Having decided to proceed, the skin incision is continued over the chest dividing the latissimus dorsi and serratus muscles as far as the trapezius. The periosteum on the entire length of the upper border of the seventh or eighth rib is stripped and the pleura opened and a chest spreader inserted. A block of costal margin (2–3 cm) is excised and the musculophrenic vessels secured.

16

Position of patient

The patient is secured on the operating table in a semilateral position with the pelvis at 45° and the chest nearly vertical.

The full incision extends from the mid-line anteriorly between the xiphoid and the umbilicus obliquely across the costal margin and along the seventh or eighth ribs, to the interval between the rip of the scapula and the spine.

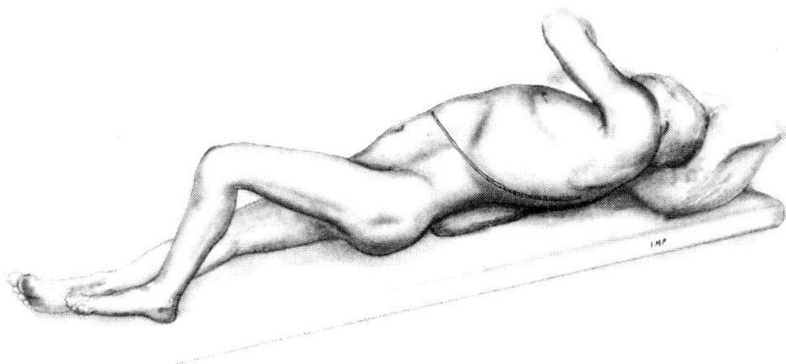

16

17

The diaphragm is divided circumferentially leaving a short cuff attached to the ribs. The anaesthetist allows the left lung to become deflated and retracted. The pulmonary ligament is divided and the mediastinal pleura opened and the oesophagus mobilized in the mediastinum as far as the aortic arch.

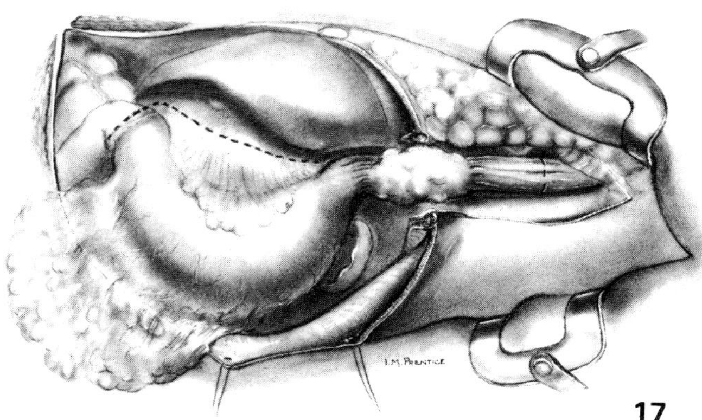

17

18

The lienorenal ligament is divided and the perinephric space entered so as to approach the splenic vessels from behind. The splenic artery and veins are dissected out, tied and divided. The stomach and omentum are separated from the colon as far as the pylorus, sometimes this is a completely avascular plane. Lesser sac adhesions are divided and mobilization completed to the hiatus taking the spleen with the stomach. Sometimes the oesophagus may be mobilized without dividing the crus at the hiatus. If the tumour is adherent at the hiatus the diaphragm should be divided to this point and the lesion mobilized by including part of the muscle of the crus. The left gastric vessels are cleared between the coeliac axis and the lesser curve of stomach and divided. The gastrohepatic omentum is divided.

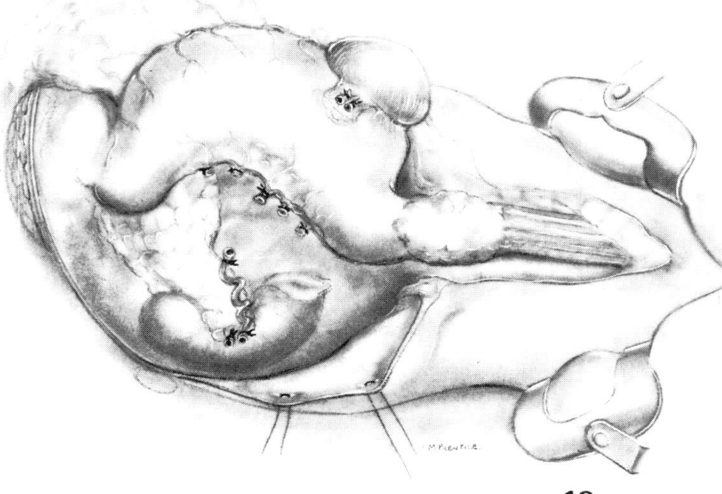

18

If tumour is adherent to the tail of the pancreas this should be mobilized with the splenic vessels and divided close to the superior mesenteric vein. The splenic and left gastric arteries are then ligated flush with the coeliac axis.

Before dividing the right gastric and gastro-epiploic vessels and closing the duodenum it is wise to leave the stomach and prepare the jejunum for the Roux-en-Y reconstruction. Occasionally a suitable length of jejunum cannot be obtained and a decision will then have to be made as to whether to use a segment of colon interposed between the oesophagus and the duodenum or fashion a tube from the greater curve of stomach.

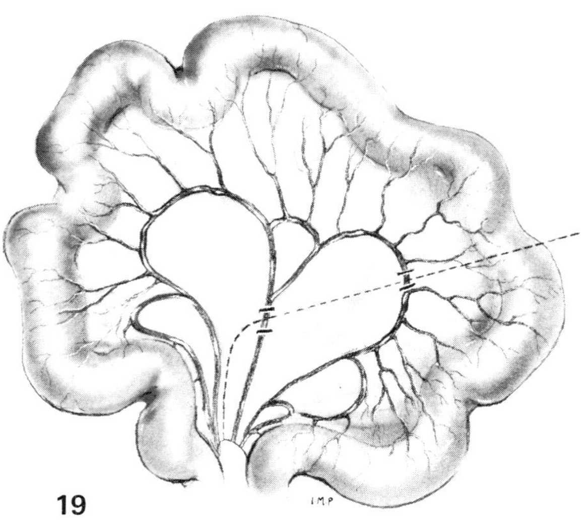

19

The jejunal segment

19

The jejunum below the duodenal flexure is inspected and a portion selected where the mesentery is beginning to lengthen and the vascular pattern becomes more easily discernible. The vessels in the mesentery may be more readily identified by turning off the room and overhead lights and transilluminating it like a leaf with a beam from a horizontal spot lamp. From the proposed point of division the arteries and veins are tied and divided individually so as to preserve the vascular arcades to a length of distal jejunum, the pulsations close to the bowel are observed as each major vessel is clamped. With patience and by making radial slits on either side of the mesentery a loop of 25–30 cm is made available. The bowel is then divided between non-crushing clamps and the ends covered and returned to the abdomen while the oesophagogastric excision is completed.

20

The right gastric and gastro-epiploic vessels are now secured and the duodenum divided and closed beyond the pylorus.

The entire stomach with spleen and if necessary tail of pancreas are now freed with the tumour and lower oesophagus. The oesophagus is mobilized in the mediastinum to above the level of the inferior pulmonary vein and sometimes to the aortic arch. The distal jejunum is drawn up posteriorly through the mesocolon and hiatus to lie in the oesophageal bed.

End-to-end anastomosis is effected between the oesophagus and jejunum below the aortic arch by the method described for oesophagogastric anastomosis (*see Illustrations 9–14*).

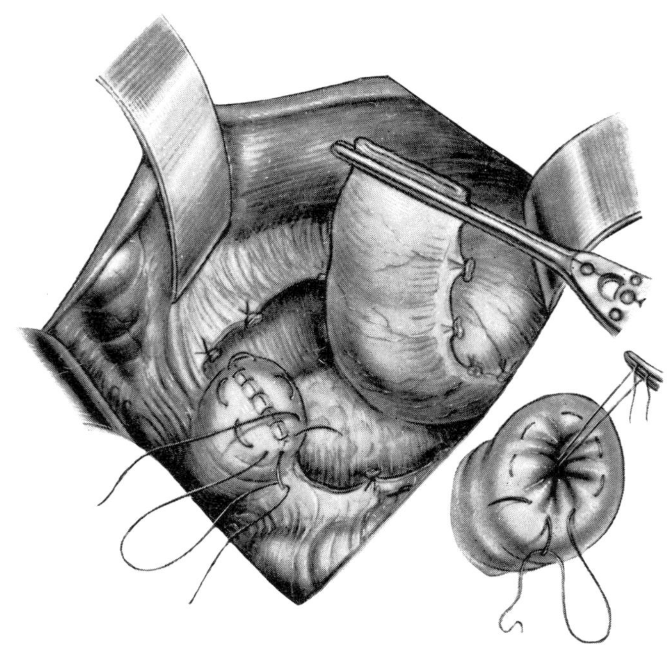

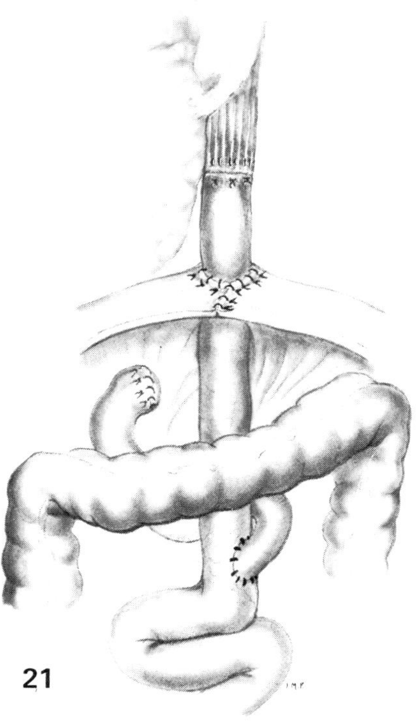

21

21

It may be necessary to shorten the jejunal loop or do an end-to-side anastomosis if extra length is required. The tip of the nasogastric tube is located below the opening in the mesocolon at the site of the end-to-side jejunojejunal anastomosis that completes the Roux-en-Y. The mediastinal pleura is repaired over the jejunum and the anastomosis, and the whole buried in the mediastinum. The oesophageal hiatus and the opening in the mesocolon are closed around the jejunal segment and the free edges of the mesentery are attached to peritoneum so as to prevent internal herniation.

The diaphragm and costal margin are repaired with non-absorbable sutures. The chest is drained and the abdomen and chest wall closed.

POSTOPERATIVE CARE AND COMPLICATIONS

Blood transfusion is continued to match the estimated blood loss. During the operation the patient may loose imperceptably a considerable volume of fluid from the exposed viscera in the chest and abdomen and this must be replaced intravenously. Central venous pressure should be recorded and maintained at +4 cm of water. Haemoconcentration must be avoided. A steady flow of urine is a satisfactory index of adequate fluid replacement.

Antibiotics are administered as indicated.

The nasogastric tube is allowed to siphon into a bag and may be aspirated occasionally. As soon as bowel sounds return oral feeding–sips of water, tea or ice cream are allowed and progressively increased. Warm and cold feeds each stimulate peristalsis.

The chest drain is removed as soon as drainage is minimal and the x-ray satisfactory and often before commencing feeding. It is not left longer just in case of a leak at the anastomosis.

Leaks from the anastomosis become less common with experience. They should be suspected when there is undue pain or fever or if a pleural effusion develops and they must be confirmed immediately by Gastrografin swallow as immediate resuture is the only hope of salvation. Some surgeons insist on a satisfactory Gastrografin swallow before commencing oral feeding.

Barium studies are necessary if dysphagia develops postoperatively: sometimes the anastomosis will need dilatation and this may have to be repeated but usually an adequate diet maintains a satisfactory lumen.

When a total gastrectomy has been carried out macrocytic anaemia may eventually develop and it is wise to commence injections of Vitamin B12 while the patient is in hospital and advise that they be repeated monthly, otherwise they may be forgotten.

[*The illustrations for this Chapter on Operations for Carcinoma of the Thoracic Oesophagus and Cardia were drawn by Mrs. I. M. Prentice. Illustration 20 was drawn by Mr. R. N. Lane.*]

Index

Prince Charles Hospital Library

Prince Charles Hospital Library